Register Now for Online Access to Your Book!

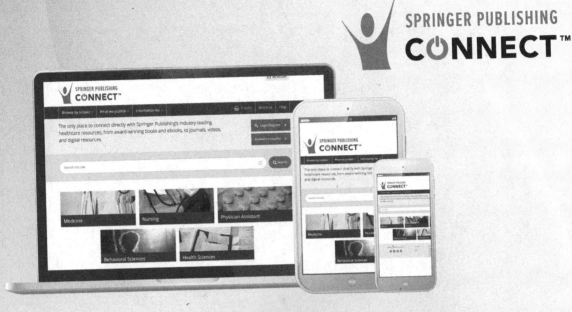

SPRINGER PUBLISHING
CONNECT™

Your print purchase of *Adult-Gerontology Clinical Nurse Specialist Certification Review* **includes online access to the contents of your book—** increasing accessibility, portability, and searchability!

Access today at:
http://connect.springerpub.com/content/book/978-0-8261-7417-8
or scan the QR code at the right with your smartphone
and enter the access code below.

2G3AWYLN

Scan here for quick access.

If you are experiencing problems accessing the digital component of this product, please contact our customer service department at cs@springerpub.com

The online access with your print purchase is available at the publisher's discretion and may be removed at any time without notice.

Publisher's Note: New and used products purchased from third-party sellers are not guaranteed for quality, authenticity, or access to any included digital components.

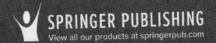

SPRINGER PUBLISHING
View all our products at springerpub.com

Adult-Gerontology Clinical Nurse Specialist Certification Review

Amy C. Shay, PhD, RN, APRN-CNS, FCNS, is a clinical assistant professor and clinical nurse specialist program coordinator at Indiana University. Amy is a pulmonary clinical nurse specialist and CCRN alumnus with over 20 years' experience in critical care. She has published and lectured nationally and internationally on clinical nursing topics. She is currently serving as a civilian research consultant/subject matter expert for military nursing research.

Jan Powers, PhD, RN, CCRN, CCNS, CNRN, NE-BC, FCCM, is currently the director of nursing research and professional practice at Parkview Health System in Fort Wayne, Indiana, and part-time faculty at the Indiana University School of Nursing. Jan has been a clinical nurse specialist for over 20 years and a nurse for 34 years, with experience in critical care, trauma, and neuroscience. She has published extensively on a variety of nursing and critical care topics. Jan is the current president elect of the National Association of Clinical Nurse Specialists (NACNS) Board of Directors.

Terry A. Doescher, MSN, RN, CNS-BC, CCRC, is a critical care clinical nurse specialist at Franciscan Health in Indianapolis, Indiana. Terry has over 30 years' nursing experience with specialty practice in critical care, pediatrics, nursing management, and research. She is a sitting board member of the Central Indiana Organization of Clinical Nurse Specialists and is currently completing her clinical doctor of nursing degree at Indiana University.

Adult-Gerontology Clinical Nurse Specialist Certification Review

Amy C. Shay, PhD, RN, APRN-CNS, FCNS
Jan Powers, PhD, RN, CCRN, CCNS, CNRN, NE-BC, FCCM
Terry A. Doescher, MSN, RN, CNS-BC, CCRC

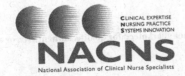

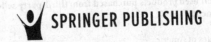

Springer Publishing Company, LLC
11 West 42nd Street, New York, NY 10036
www.springerpub.com
connect.springerpub.com/

Acquisitions Editor: Jaclyn Koshofer
Compositor: S4Carlisle Publishing Services

ISBN: 978-0-8261-7416-1
ebook ISBN: 978-0-8261-7417-8
DOI: 10.1891/9780826174178
21 22 23 24 25/ 5 4 3 2 1

The author and the publisher of this Work have made every effort to use sources believed to be reliable to provide information that is accurate and compatible with the standards generally accepted at the time of publication. Because medical science is continually advancing, our knowledge base continues to expand. Therefore, as new information becomes available, changes in procedures become necessary. We recommend that the reader always consult current research and specific institutional policies before performing any clinical procedure or delivering any medication. The author and publisher shall not be liable for any special, consequential, or exemplary damages resulting, in whole or in part, from the readers' use of, or reliance on, the information contained in this book. The publisher has no responsibility for the persistence or accuracy of URLs for external or third-party Internet websites referred to in this publication and does not guarantee that any content on such websites is, or will remain, accurate or appropriate.

Library of Congress Cataloging-in-Publication Data

Names: Shay, Amy C., editor. | Powers, Jan, RN, editor. | Doescher, Terry
  A., editor.
Title: Adult-gerontology clinical nurse specialist certification review /
  [edited by] Amy C. Shay, Jan Powers, Terry A. Doescher.
Description: New York, NY : Springer Publishing Company, [2022] | Includes
  bibliographical references and index.
Identifiers: LCCN 2021002646 (print) | LCCN 2021002647 (ebook) | ISBN
  9780826174161 (cloth) | ISBN 9780826174178 (ebook)
Subjects: MESH: Nurse Clinicians | Advanced Practice Nursing | Geriatric
  Nursing | Examination Questions | Outline
Classification: LCC RT55 (print) | LCC RT55 (ebook) | NLM WY 18.2 | DDC
  610.73076--dc23
LC record available at https://lccn.loc.gov/2021002646
LC ebook record available at https://lccn.loc.gov/2021002647

Amy Shay ORCID https://orcid.org/0000-0003-3064-2840

Publisher's Note: New and used products purchased from third-party sellers are not guaranteed for quality, authenticity, or access to any included digital components.

Printed in the United States of America.

Contents

Contributors

Natalie Baird, MSN, RNC-MNN, AGCNS-BC Clinical Nurse Specialist, Women and Children's Services, Indiana University Health, Bloomington, Indiana

Marianne Benjamin, DNP, RN, NE-BC Associate Chief Nursing Officer and Director of Professional Nursing Practice Franciscan Health, Indianapolis, Indiana

Eugena Bergvall, DNP, ACNP-BC, CNS-BC, ACCNS, CCRN, CNRN Clinical Nurse Specialist: Neuroscience Specialties, National Institute of Health Clinical Center, Bethesda, Maryland

Tamera Brown, MS, APRN, ACNS-BC, CWOCN Wound-Ostomy Clinical Nurse Specialist, Indiana University Health Ball Memorial Hospital, Muncie, Indiana

Julie Cahn, DNP, RN, CNOR, RN-BC, ACNS-BC, CNS-CP Perioperative Practice Specialist, Association of periOperative Registered Nurses (AORN), Denver, Colorado

Maria Carpenter, MSN, RN, AGCNS-BC, CCRN Clinical Nurse Specialist, Penn Presbyterian Medical Center, Philadelphia, Pennsylvania

Jose Chavez, MSN, RN, ACCNS-AG, CCRN, CVRN-BC, AACC Clinical Nurse Specialist, Critical Care Services, Cardiac Observation and Cardiac Intensive Care Unit, Cedars-Sinai Medical Center, Los Angeles, California

Monica D. Coles, DNP, RN-BC, ACNS-BC, CDP Gerontology Clinical Nurse Specialist, Carilion Roanoke Memorial Hospital, Roanoke, Virginia

Jennifer P. Colwill, DNP, APRN-CNS, CCNS, PCCN Clinical Nurse Specialist Cardiothoracic Surgery Stepdown, Heart and Vascular Institute, Cleveland Clinic, Cleveland, Ohio

Dianna Jo Copley, MSN, APRN-CNS, ACCNS-AG, CCRN Clinical Nurse Specialist, Advanced Practice Nursing, Nursing Institute, Cleveland Clinic, Cleveland, Ohio

Melissa Craft, PhD, APRN, CNS, AOCN Associate Professor, Interim Associate Dean of Academic Administration and Graduate Education, Director, PhD Program, University of Oklahoma Health Sciences Center, Oklahoma City, Oklahoma

Carmen R. Davis, MSN, RN, CCRN, CNS-BC Clinical Nurse Specialist, Indiana University Health, University Hospital, Indianapolis, Indiana

Lori Delaney, MS, RN, CNS, RN-BC, ACNS-BC Adult Health Medical Surgical Clinical Nurse Specialist, Indiana University Health Ball Memorial Hospital, Muncie, Indiana

Marissa Diefenderfer, MSN, AGCNS-BC, RN-BC Quality Initiative Nurse, Bon Secours DePaul Medical Center, Norfolk, Virginia

Caitlin Donis, MS, RN, AG-ACNP, ACCNS-AG Clinical Nurse Specialist, Critical Care, University of Maryland Upper Chesapeake Medical Center, Bel Air, Maryland

Diane M. Doty, MS, RN, CCNS, CCRN Critical Care Clinical Nurse Specialist, Community Health Network, Indianapolis, Indiana

Judy Dusek, DNP, MEd, APRN-CNS, CMSRN, ACNS-BC Clinical Nurse Specialist, Medical–Surgical and Orthopedic Nursing, Via Christi Hospitals, Wichita, Kansas

Elizabeth Duxbury, MS, RN, ACNS-BC, CCRN Clinical Nurse Specialist, Medical Intensive Care Unit, Rochester General Hospital, Rochester, New York

Jennifer Embree, DNP, RN, CCNS, NE-BC Clinical Associate Professor, Indiana University School of Nursing, Indianapolis, Indiana

Debra A. Ferguson, MSN, RN, CCRN-K, CNRN, SCRN Neuroscience Clinical Nurse Specialist, Community Health Network, Indianapolis, Indiana

Mary H. Fischer, MSN, ACNS-BC, ACHPN Palliative Care Clinical Nurse Specialist, St. Vincent Hospital, Indianapolis, Indiana

Nina M. Flanagan, PhD, GNP-BC, PMHCS-BC Clinical Nurse Specialist, Adult Psychiatric Mental Health, Clinical Professor, Binghamton University, Binghamton, New York

Jeanna Ford, DNP, APRN, ACNS-BC, ACHPN Palliative Care Clinical Nurse Specialist, Presbyterian Healthcare, Albuquerque, New Mexico

Patricia Gilman, PhD, RN, APRN, ACNS-BC Adult Clinical Nurse Specialist, Kaiser Permanente Foundation Hospitals, Modesto, California

Jessica Green, MSN, RN-BC, AGCNS-BC, CVRN Clinical Nurse Specialist, Indiana University Health, North Hospital, Carmel, Indiana

Earlie Hale, DNP, RN, GCNS-BC, CMSRN, VHA-CM Clinical Nurse Specialist, Richard L. Roudebush VA Medical Center, Indianapolis, Indiana

Jaime A. Hannans, PhD, RN, CNE Associate Professor, Nursing, California State University Channel Islands, Camarillo, California

Katrina Hawkins, MSN, RN, ACNS-BC, CNS-CP, CNOR Certified Perioperative Clinical Nurse Specialist, Richard L. Roudebush VA Medical Center, Indianapolis, Indiana

Benjamin Churchill Hickox, DNP, APRN, AGCNS-BC, CCRN-CMC Instructor of Nursing, Mayo Clinic College of Medicine and Science, Staff Registered Nurse, Medical Cardiology Intensive Care Unit, Mayo Clinic, Rochester, Minnesota

Elizabeth Hudson-Weires, MSN, APRN, ACCNS-AG Clinical Nurse Specialist, Dialysis and General Medicine, Emory University Hospital, Atlanta, Georgia

Nicole Huntley, MS, RN, APRN, ACCNS-AG Medical–Surgical Clinical Nurse Specialist and Sepsis Coordinator, University of Colorado, Denver, Colorado

Ramona S. Irabor, MSN, RN-BC, AGCNS-BC, CPAN Pain Management Clinical Nurse Specialist, Duke Health, Durham, North Carolina

Jackeline Iseler, DNP, RN, ACNS-BC CNS Program Director, Michigan State University College of Nursing, East Lansing, Michigan

Elsie A. Jolade, DNP, EdM, FNP-BC, ACNS, CDE, APRN, CCRN Clinical Professor, City University of New York, Hunter Bellevue School of Nursing, New York, New York

Alyson Keen, MSN, RN, ACNS-BC Clinical Nurse Specialist, Indiana University Health, Indianapolis, Indiana

K. Denise Kerley, MSN, RN, CNRN, AG-CNS Senior Partner, Medical Intensive Care Unit, Indiana University Health, University Hospital, Indianapolis, Indiana

Michelle J. Kidd, MS, APRN, ACNS-BC, CCRN-K Clinical Nurse Specialist, Critical Care, Indiana University Health Ball Memorial Hospital, Muncie, Indiana

Robina Kitzler, MSN, APRN, AOCNS, CCRN, CPAN Clinical Nurse Specialist, Memorial Sloan Kettering Cancer Center, New York, New York

Lynne Marie Kokoczka, MSN, APRN-CNS, ACCNS-AG, CCRN Clinical Nurse Specialist, Medical Intensive Care Units, Cleveland Clinic, Cleveland, Ohio

Francesca C. Levitt, DNP, RN-BC, ACNS-BC Perioperative Clinical Nurse Specialist, Hendricks Regional Health, Danville, Indiana

Tiffany Losekamp, MSN, RN, CNE, CHSE Assistant Professor of Practice and Coordinator of the Nursing Simulation Laboratory, Wittenberg University, Springfield, Ohio

Melissa Lowder, DNP, RN, ACNS-BC, CCRN Clinical Nurse Specialist, Franciscan Health, Indianapolis, Indiana

Angie Malone, DNP, APRN, ACNS-BC, OCN, AOCNS Director, Medical Oncology and Infusion, University of Louisville Hospital, James Graham Brown Cancer Center, Louisville, Kentucky

Karen S. March, PhD, RN, ACNS-BC Professor, The Stabler Department of Nursing, York College of Pennsylvania, York, Pennsylvania

Joan Miller, MSN, RN, CNS, PCCN Clinical Nurse Specialist, Indiana University Health, Methodist Hospital, Indianapolis, Indiana

Erica Newkirk, MSN, RN, AGCNS-BC, CMSRN Clinical Nurse Specialist, Indiana University Health Hospital, West, Indianapolis, Indiana

Adrianne Opp, MSN, RN, AGCNS Clinical Nurse Specialist, Franciscan Health, Indianapolis, Indiana

Sarah Pandullo, MSN, ARNP, CCRN, CCNS-BC Critical Care Clinical Nurse Specialist, UnityPoint Health, Des Moines, Iowa

Mechelle Peck, DNP, RN, ACNS-BC Cardiovascular Clinical Nurse Specialist, Franciscan Health, Indianapolis, Indiana

Valerie Pfander, DNP, RN, ACCNS-AG, CPAN, FASPAN Clinical Nurse Specialist, Munson Medical Center, Traverse City, Michigan

JoAnne Phillips, DNP, RN, CNS, CPPS, NEA-BC, FCNS Director of Clinical Practice, Virtua Health System, Marlton, New Jersey

Jan Powers, PhD, RN, CCNS, CCRN, NE-BC, FCCM Director, Nursing Research and Professional Practice, Parkview Health, Fort Wayne, Indiana

Cheryl L. Pullium, DNP, APRN, RN, ACNS-BC   Clinical Assistant Professor, Texas A & M University College of Nursing, Bryan, Texas

Suzanne Purvis, DNP, APRN, GCNS-BC   Clinical Nurse Specialist, NICHE, Beaumont Health, Royal Oak, Michigan

Tiffany L. Rader, MSN, RN, AGCNS-BC, CMSRN   Clinical Nurse Specialist, Indiana University Health, Methodist Hospital, Indianapolis, Indiana

Joan Rembacz, MS, APRN, CCNS, CCRN, CEN, TCRN   Clinical Nurse Specialist, Emergency Services, Northwestern Medicine McHenry Hospital, McHenry, Illinois

JoEllen Rust, MSN, RN, CNS, FCNS   Clinical Nurse Specialist, Rehabilitation Hospital of Indiana, Indianapolis, Indiana

Stacey Seggelke, DNP, APRN, ACNS-BC, BC-ADM, CDE   Assistant Professor of Medicine, University of Colorado School of Medicine, Aurora, Colorado

Amy C. Shay, PhD, RN, APRN-CNS, FCNS   Assistant Professor, CNS Program Coordinator, Indiana University, Indianapolis, Indiana

Megan Siebert, MSN, AGCNS, PCCN   Adult-Gerontology and Progressive Care Clinical Nurse Specialist, Community Health Network, Indianapolis, Indiana

Margaret Skoog, MSN, RN, AGCNS-BC   Clinical Nurse Specialist, Emergency Services, Swedish Medical Center, Seattle, Washington, DC

M. Jane Swartz, DNP, RN, ACNS-BC   Director, Center for Health Professions Lifelong Learning, University of Southern Indiana, Evansville, Indiana

Jo M. Tabler, MSN, RN, AGCNS-BC, CEN, CFRN   Clinical Nurse Specialist, Indiana University Health, Methodist Hospital, Indianapolis, Indiana

Misti Tuppeny, MSN, APRN, CNS, CCRN, CNRN, CCNS   Clinical Nurse Specialist for Neuroscience, Behavioral Health and Palliative Care, Florida Hospital, Orlando, Florida

Brittany Waggoner, MSN, RN, AGCNS-BC   Maternal/Child Clinical Nurse Specialist, Hendricks Regional Health, Danville, Indiana

Theodore J. Walker, Jr., APRN, A-CNS, CNS-CP, CNOR, CPPS, Paralegal   Perioperative Clinical Nurse Specialist, Providence Alaska Medical Center, Anchorage, Alaska

Donna Washburn, DNP, RN, CNS, ACNS-BC, AOCNS   Director, Professional Clinical Practice, Centra Health, Lynchburg, Virginia

Clarissa Welbaum, MSN, APRN, CCNS, CCTN   Clinical Nurse Specialist, Florida Hospital, Orlando, Florida

Anita White, MSN, APRN, ACNS-BC, CCRN   Acute Care Clinical Nurse Specialist, VA Northeast Ohio Healthcare System, Cleveland, Ohio

Melissa A. Wilson, PhD, APRN, CCNS-BC   Nurse Scientist, Air Force Research Laboratory, Wright-Patterson Air Force Base, Dayton, Ohio

Racheal L. Wood,* PhD(c), DNP, ACCNS-AG, CCRN-CMC, CEN   U.S. Army Nurse Corps, PhD student, Augusta University College of Nursing, Augusta, Georgia

Matthew J. Wren, MSN, APRN, AGCNS-BC, CEN   Clinical Nurse Specialist, Florida Hospital, Orlando, Florida

* The views and information presented are those of the author and do not represent the official position of the U.S. Army Medical Center of Excellence, the U.S. Army Training and Doctrine Command, or the Departments of Army/Navy/Air Force, Department of Defense, or U.S. government.

Foreword

Certification for clinical nurse specialists (CNS) has been available since 1973, when the American Nurses Association (ANA) started a certification program as a form of professional recognition. Being the first certification review resource to address the contemporary role and practice of the CNS, this book is a milestone in CNS certification. I am honored to provide these remarks. The editors, Dr. Shay, Dr. Powers, and Ms. Doescher, are stellar CNSs whose combined efforts culminated in a most excellent reference, *Adult-Gerontology Clinical Nurse Specialist Certification Review*. Designed in the framework of the three domains of CNS practice, known as the *spheres of impact*, the book provides a comprehensive overview of the knowledge a new CNS needs for entry into practice. More experienced CNSs needing a review will also find this reference most helpful.

Certification is a mechanism for validation of an individual's knowledge, skills, and abilities. Unlike the generalist registered nurse licensure examination, the National Council Licensure Examination NCLEX®, certification is offered by professional organizations and is recognition of knowledge in a specialty scope of practice. This review examines critical information for both the CNS role and the adult-gerontology population.

Certification for CNSs has changed since it was first introduced. Early certification was designed to validate excellence in practice. Eligibility for ANA's initial CNS certification included a graduate degree from a program that prepared graduates for the CNS role and a minimum of 2 years of experience in the CNS role. Internal motivation for recognition as excellent was the stimulus for achieving and maintaining the certification credential. Few states offered title protection for CNSs, making the certification credential a public validation of a qualified CNS.

In the 1990s, the purpose of certification began to shift. Since inception in the 1960s, the CNS role required a graduate degree in nursing. Other advanced practice roles were prepared primarily by postbaccalaureate/postdiploma certificate programs, where graduates relied on professional certification for validation of competency. With the shift to graduate education, the emphasis on certification was retained and reframed as validation of entry-level competency. CNS certification eventually shifted from a credential of excellence, becoming instead a credential for entry into practice.

Today, professional certification is an expectation for all advanced practice nurses, including CNSs. Validation of predetermined knowledge allows individuals to evaluate their competence in a specialty area and demonstrate to peers that they have met a national, professional standard. Although certification is important for the individual CNS, it has the additional advantage of serving to validate the unique, separate role of the CNS and the existence of a specialty body of knowledge, skills, and abilities that comprise the CNS role and practice. Certification achieves several additional objectives.

Certification provides evidence that a CNS remains current in practice. Certification must be renewed on a predetermined schedule, usually every 3 to 5 years, meaning certified CNSs must continue to update their knowledge and ascribe to lifelong learning. State boards of nursing rely heavily on certification credentials in granting authority to practice as an advanced practice nurse and to prescribe pharmaceutical therapies, diagnostic tests, selected medical interventions, and durable medical equipment.

Reimbursement also is linked to certification. The Centers for Medicare & Medicaid Services (CMS) mandates certification as a requirement for an advanced practice nurse to obtain reimbursement, whether a state requires certification or not. In addition, some insurance companies require certification for reimbursement.

This certification review text provides the support needed to prepare for a certification examination. Use it to assess areas of knowledge strengths and to identify areas needing more concentrated study. The Direct Patient Care section includes important topics such as diagnostic and clinical reasoning, pharmacology principles, nonpharmacologic interventions, and substance use and addiction in addition to advanced assessment and management of health problems. The Nurses and Nursing Practice section includes content on responses to illness, care of older adults, and advocating for patients and nurses. The Organizations and Systems section includes systems leadership, quality improvement, safety, evidence-based practice, and research.

Let this review guide the design of a study plan. Review of the content assists in identifying areas where greater knowledge or depth of content is needed. Supplement learning by reviewing articles and other materials related to selected topic areas. Use the practice questions to brush up on test-taking skills. With extreme pleasure, I offer these comments. I am confident this review book will be a treasured resource for students and practicing CNSs. On behalf of CNS colleagues everywhere, past, present, and future, I commend the editors for this outstanding landmark work. Congratulations!

Janet S. Fulton, PhD, RN, ACNS-BC, ANEF, FCNS, FAAN
Professor and Associate Dean for Graduate Programs
Indiana University School of Nursing
Editor, Clinical Nurse Specialist: The Journal for Advanced
Nursing Practice

Preface

Clinical nurse specialists (CNSs) play a critical role in ensuring the implementation of high-quality evidence-based care, improved patient outcomes, and reduced healthcare delivery costs. Professional certification is one way we distinguish our unique contributions and advanced practice nursing expertise from other advanced practice roles. This first edition of *Adult-Gerontology Clinical Nurse Specialist Certification Review* represents a compilation of CNS practice knowledge contributed by respected clinicians from across the nation for certification examination preparation. Successful certification examination performance is an important factor for employment opportunity as well an essential practice requirement in most states.

GOALS OF THIS BOOK

Adult-Gerontology Clinical Nurse Specialist Certification Review was designed to provide a current, comprehensive study guide for CNS program graduates preparing for the Adult-Gerontology Clinical Nurse Specialist (AGCNS) certification exam. This book provides one source for test review and practice based upon the most current National Association of Clinical Nurse Specialists (NACNS) Core Competencies (NACNS; 2019) and both the American Association of Critical-Care Nurses (AACN) and the American Nurses Credentialing Center (ANCC) Adult-Gerontology CNS certification examinations test plan content. Additionally, the book incorporates content from the American Association of Colleges of Nursing Adult-Gerontology Clinical Nurse Specialist Population Focused Competencies and the American Association of Critical Care Nurses Scope and Standards for Clinical Nurse Specialist Practice.

ORGANIZATION OF THE CONTENT

The book begins with an introduction to the current AGCNS examination options, test plans and processes, as well as test-taking strategies for success. The remainder of the book organizes test plan subject matter according to the three spheres of impact of CNS practice.

Section I: Patient Direct Care

The first section of the book includes 16 chapters presenting the overview, pathophysiology, etiology, assessment, diagnosis, treatment/management, and related pharmacology content according to each body system. This section also contains chapters on advanced health assessment, diagnostic and clinical reasoning, pharmacology principles, and substance use and addiction.

Section II: Nurses and Nursing Practice

The second section of the book addresses the nurse and nursing practice sphere of impact. Relevant content includes age-related response to illness and adult-gerontology-population-specific practice standards for care and advocacy of the older adult. Emphasis is placed upon culturally competent care and safe care transitions. Nursing practice content includes consultation, collaboration, education, mentoring, and communication skills. Nurse and nursing practice advocacy topics review public policy, professional practice issues, and ethical concerns.

Section III: Organizations and Systems

The third section of the book covers systems and systems leadership competencies of the CNS. Relevant content involves quality improvement principles, safety initiatives, financial stewardship, organizational level program development, and systems change. Clinical inquiry subject matter covers evidence-based practice, research methodology, and skills for dissemination of CNS work.

DISTINGUISHING FEATURES

Adult-Gerontology Clinical Nurse Specialist Certification Review is the first of its kind to be edited and authored entirely by qualified CNS practitioners and educators with demonstrated expertise in their respective content areas. The contributing authors hail from prestigious institutions and associations in 22 states across the United States. Content is thorough yet concise with formatting conducive to targeted, systematic review and retention of information. The book contains end-of-chapter practice questions with rationale as well as access to an online practice exam with appropriately weighted content areas.

Amy C. Shay and Jan Powers

*All content in this book is designed for certification examination review purposes only. This content is not intended for use in clinical practice.

REFERENCE

The complete reference list appears in the digital version of this chapter, at https://connect.springerpub.com/content/book/978-0-8261-7417-8/front-matter/fmatter3/

Acknowledgments

We extend our deepest and most sincere appreciation to the 70 clinical nurse specialist (CNS) contributors who volunteered to share their expertise with new generations of graduating CNS students. All of you sacrificed much time and energy to this important project. Some of you persevered through difficult times in this long journey and some of you came to the rescue later to see this journey to its conclusion. Your contributions are invaluable. We are personally very proud to see our names alongside such amazing, expert CNSs.

We also thank the staff at Springer Publishing Company, especially Margaret Zuccarini (retired), for helping us propose this book and Jaclyn Koshofer, acquisitions editor, for keeping the entire project organized.

Finally, we thank the National Association of Clinical Nurse Specialists (NACNS) for their copublication support of this book and their belief in its purpose.

Amy C. Shay, Jan Powers, and Terry A. Doescher

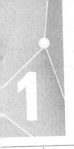

Introduction to AGCNS Examinations Process and Test Plans

M. Jane Swartz

Certification is the process by which a nongovernmental organization grants recognition to an individual who has met certain eligibility requirements. Certification can be voluntary or mandatory. Check your state board of nursing to see whether certification is mandatory for licensure or prescriptive authority. Many institutions may require certification as a condition for employment for your role as a clinical nurse specialist. Certification provides a validation of your competency and recognizes your accomplishments. There are currently two adult-gerontology CNS certification examination options. The two choices have similarities and differences (Box 1.1).

Consider the following before deciding which certification exam to take

- Your clinical experience
- Anticipated place of practice
- Eligibility requirements
- Renewal requirements
- Both examinations align with the National Association of Clinical Nurse Specialists and the American Association of Colleges of Nursing

ACUTE CARE CLINICAL NURSE SPECIALIST ADULT-GERONTOLOGY

- Board certification offered by American Association of Critical-Care Nurses (AACN)
- Webpage: www.aacn.org/certification/get-certified/accns-ag
- Credential is valid for 5 years
- Renewal by maintaining licensure and a combination of three options: 1,000 practice hours, continuing education, exam
- Testing at Applied Measurement Professionals, Inc.
- Exam allows 3.5 hours to answer 175 questions (25 questions are not scored; used to gather statistical data for future exams)
- Discount rate if a member of American Association of Critical-Care Nurses
- Organizing framework is AACN Synergy Model for Patient Care
- Content based on Advanced Practice Work Group. Bell, L. (Ed.). (2014). *Scope and standards for acute and critical care clinical nurse specialist practice*. American Association of Critical-Care Nurses.

ADULT-GERONTOLOGY CLINICAL NURSE SPECIALIST CERTIFICATION

- Board certification offered by American Nurses Credentialing Center (ANCC)
- Webpage: www.nursingworld.org/our-certifications/adult-gerontology-clinical-nurse-specialist/

Box 1.1 Comparison of Certification Test Plans

American Nurses Credentialing Center	American Association of Critical-Care Nurses
Wellness through acute care	Wellness through acute care
150 scored questions	150 scored questions
Assessment and diagnosis (28%)	Clinical judgment (65%)
Patient direct care	Cardiovascular (13%)
Nursing and organizational systems	Pulmonary (11%)
Planning and implementation (44%)	Endocrine (4%)
Patient direct care	Hematology/Immunology/Oncology (3%)
Nursing and organizational systems	Gastrointestinal (5%)
Evaluation (28%)	Renal/Genitourinary (4%)
Patient direct care	Integumentary (1%)
Nursing and organizational systems	Neurology (5%)
	Psychosocial/behavioral/cognitive health (4%)
	Factors influencing health status (4%)
	Multisystem (9%)
	Professional caring and ethical practice
	Advocacy/moral agency (4%)
	Caring practices (6%)
	Response to diversity (3%)
	Facilitation of learning (5%)
	Collaboration (5%)
	Systems thinking (6%)
	Clinical inquiry (6%)

Sources: From American Association of Critical-Care Nurses. (2019, May). *AGCNS-BC exam handbook*. https://www.aacn.org/~/media/aacn-website/certification/get-certified/handbooks/accnsage xamhandbook.pdf; American Nurses Credentialing Center. (2019, March). *AG-CNS board certification examination test content outline*. https://www.nursingworld.org/our-certifications/adult-gerontology-clinical-nurse-specialist

The complete reference list appears in the digital version of this chapter, at https://connect.springerpub.com/content/book/978-0-8261-7417-8/part/part01/chapter/ch01

- Credential is valid for 5 years
- Renewal by maintaining licensure and meeting renewal requirements.
- Test administered at Prometric Test Centers
- Exam allows 3.5 hours to answer 175 questions (150 are scored and 25 pretest questions that are not scored)
- Discount rate if a member of the American Nurses Association or a member of the American Association of Nurse Practitioners
- Content based on Adult-Gerontology Clinical Nurse Specialist Role Delineation Study Executive Summary (American Nurses Credentialing Center, 2019)

STUDYING TIPS

Reflect on previous positive outcomes with testing such as the NCLEX®. You have been preparing to take this certification exam for many years. Yet this exam raises anxiety due to its impact on your nursing career. So relax, WRITE a study plan and then WORK the study plan. The BEST studying strategy is to have a positive attitude towards the outcome based on your preparation to take the exam.

Choose the testing date and time carefully. Consider whether you are more alert in the morning or do better later in the day. Avoid testing on days when work or personal commitments can interfere with your focus. Before scheduling the exam, have at least two possible dates/times ready. Do not schedule an appointment after the exam. Your thoughts should be on the exam not on whether you will make your appointment.

1. After deciding which exam to take, review the registration process and submit the registration completely.
2. The best preparation is to review the test plan. Consider your strengths and weakness to develop a study plan at least three months prior to the anticipated testing day. Your study plan should be flexible and realistic. It is better to schedule shorter sessions rather than devoting an entire day to study.
3. Review content in your areas of weakness. Utilize available practice tests.
4. Consider a study partner or find someone who is already certified.
5. Use the exam resources from both AACN and ANCC. ANCC offers an online program on test taking strategies. Both organizations offer sample questions.
6. Seek a support person or group on social networking sites such as Facebook or LinkedIn.
7. To maximize your review of content, choose resources that match your learning style.
   a. Visual learners like reading, flashcards, videos.
   b. Auditory learners like videos, speaking aloud, or creating recordings.
   c. Kinesthetic learners like to read while taking notes or image teaching the content.
8. Practice, practice, practice taking exam questions using a timer.

9. Turn off distractions (phone, television, etc.) while studying.
10. Reward yourself when you follow your study plan.

The week prior to the test date
- Eat well-balanced meals.
- Practice driving to the testing site.
- Review the directions for taking the exam.

The day prior
- Get a good night's sleep.
- Avoid cramming the day before.
- Bring at least two current forms of ID (review the exam instructions booklet to know what is acceptable).
- Do something that you enjoy.

Day of the test
- Eat breakfast.
- Anxiety should be expected. This anxiety can be beneficial and enhance your focus.
- Arrive at the test site early.
- Dress in layers as room temperature can be variable.
- If provided scratch paper, write down information such as normal lab values or other lists. Use this as a reference rather than trying to remember numbers. This will allow you to focus on the question.
- Get comfortable in the seat. You earned the right to be in this seat so make the seat yours.
- Concentrate on the exam. Avoid distractions such as others moving in the room or noises.
- Employ relaxation techniques when feeling over-whelmed.
- Listen and read the directions on the day of the exam. Do you see only one question at a time? Can you go back to questions not answered? Where is the timer for the test?

TEST-TAKING STRATEGIES FOR MULTIPLE-CHOICE QUESTIONS

- Rely on your gut instinct. The first answer is usually the correct answer.
- Anticipate the answer, then look for the answer that matches.
- Consider all alternatives.
- Base your answer on the ideal or expected not on what you saw in a clinical rotation or in practice.
- Eliminate answers that are obviously incorrect or illogical. The more answers you eliminate the greater your ability to choose the correct answer.
- If two answers seem identical, then both are incorrect.
- If two answers are conflicting, you can at least eliminate one answer.
- Use critical thinking to determine the correct answer.
- Avoid spending too much time on one question. Better to make an educated guess and move on to the next question.

REFERENCES

The complete reference list appears in the digital version of this chapter at https://connect.springerpub.com/content/book/978-0-8261-7417-8/part/part01/chapter/ch01

Section I
Patient Direct Care

2

Advanced Health Assessment

Cheryl L. Pullium

OVERVIEW OF ADVANCED HEALTH ASSESSMENT

Advanced health assessment is required for the clinical nurse specialist (CNS) in any practice setting. Advanced health assessment is the systematic collection of subjective and objective patient data needed to evaluate a patient's current health status, predict a patient's future health risks, and identify appropriate health promotion measures.

Subjective patient data are collected in the health history interview and include:

■ Past medical history	■ Personal and social history
■ Family history	■ Review of systems

Objective patient data are findings collected by physical examination of body systems by using:

■ Inspection/observation	■ Palpation
■ Percussion	■ Auscultation

ASSESSMENT OF BODY SYSTEMS

The comprehensive health assessment collects subjective data in a general format and includes:

- Current patient history, including description of any specific symptoms and constitutional symptoms—fever/chills, malaise/fatigue, unintentional weight change

Mnemonic for Symptom Description—OLD CARTS

Onset	Characteristics
Location	Aggravating/alleviating factors
Duration	Radiation
	Timing
	Severity

- Past medical history, including:
  - Major adult illnesses, chronic or systemic problems
  - Hospitalizations and/or surgeries, serious injuries
  - Current medications, including all complementary/alternative therapies; note Beers criteria medications for older adults (The 2019 American Geriatrics Society Beers Criteria® Update Expert Panel, 2019)
  - Drug, food, environmental allergies; immunizations
  - Previous transfusions, recent labs and diagnostic or screening exams with results

- Family history—Three generations, including:
  - Major illnesses, genetic and/or familial disorders
- Personal/social history, including:
  - Cultural background, religious/cultural practices and/or preferences
  - Education/occupation, occupational exposure, and protective device use
  - Current stressors, support systems, hobbies and interests
  - Adequacy of economic resources, concerns about health-care costs
  - Usual diet, caffeine intake, exercise routine, sleep patterns
  - Tobacco, alcohol, recreational drug use
  - Relationship status, sexual history, prior sexually transmitted diseases
  - OLDER ADULTS—Functional assessment is an essential part of exam (see Chapter 19, "Care of the Older Adult")

Problem-Focused Assessments

A problem-focused assessment collects *focused* data based on the problem at hand. Problem-focused assessments are body-system specific, with data collected in the history determining which body systems are to be assessed. Below are important elements of the problem-focused assessment by body system:

Mental Status

- Patient history, including:
  - *OLD CARTS* for symptoms, associate with current events/stressors
  - Constitutional symptoms—Fever/chills, malaise/fatigue, unintentional weight change
  - Medications—Especially opioids, steroids, benzodiazepines, sedatives; complementary and/or alternative therapies; medications listed on Beers Criteria
  - Mania, panic attacks, depression, suicidal/homicidal thoughts
  - Hearing or vision concerns
- Past medical history, including:
  - Anxiety, depression, or confusion; psychiatric disorder or hospitalization(s)
  - Chronic illness, sexually transmitted disease(s)
  - Neurological issue, brain trauma/injury, vascular occlusion(s)
- Family history, including:
  - Psychiatric disorders/mental illness, intellectual disabilities, alcoholism
  - Alzheimer's disease
- Personal/social history, including:
  - Changes in sleep habits/patterns, appetite/usual diet, and/or sexual activity

The complete reference list appears in the digital version of this chapter, at https://connect.springerpub.com/content/ book/978-0-8261-7417-8/part/part01/chapter/ch02

- Changes in cognitive functioning or memory; changes in ability to perform activities of daily living (ADL)
- Alcohol and/or recreational drug use or withdrawal

Advanced Assessment Skills
- Inspect/observe:
  - Physical appearance and behavior; speech and mood; orientation; cognition

Skin, Hair, and Nails
- Patient history, including:
  - Constitutional and specific symptoms—*OLD CARTS*
  - Medications, including complementary and alternative; new medications—especially antibiotics
  - Changes in skin, hair, or nails; changes in tactile sensation and/or sensitivity
  - Recent bites/stings, exposure to infestation, changes in hygiene products
- Past medical history, including:
  - Previous skin issues, lesions, treatments; number of previous sunburns with severity
  - Susceptibility to skin infections, delayed healing response
  - Previous hair problems, previous nail trauma or infection
  - Cardiac, respiratory, liver, endocrine, hematologic issues; any other chronic/systemic problems
- Family history, including:
  - Dermatologic disorders, allergic hereditary disease(s)
  - Hair-loss patterns, hereditary/congenital conditions
- Personal/social history, including:
  - Current skin, hair, and nail habits; self-examination of skin
  - Recent/current stressors; recent travel; recent hazardous exposure—environmental, occupational, irritant—personal protection used
  - Alcohol, tobacco, recreational drug use
  - Sexual history, sexually transmitted diseases or infections

Advanced Assessment Skills
- Inspect (direct overhead lighting best):
  - Entire skin surface for:
    - Color, uniformity, hygiene, odor, lesions, breakdown
  - Lesions for:
    - Location, distribution, size, shape, color, elevation/depression, configuration, attachment at base
  - Overall condition of hair—color, distribution, hygiene, infestation
  - Overall condition of nails for:
    - Symmetry, ridging, pitting, peeling; clubbing
    - Redness, swelling, and/or exudate; cuticle integrity and hygiene
- Palpate:
  - Skin surface for moisture, temperature, texture, turgor, elasticity
  - Texture of hair; scalp lesions, nodules, masses
  - Smoothness and firmness of nails, attachment to nail bed

Head and Neck—General
- Patient history, including:
  - Constitutional and problem-focused symptoms—*OLD CARTS*
  - Medications, including complementary and alternative

- Dizziness, amnesia, general weakness and/or loss of balance, falls
- Headache with/without visual prodrome, nausea/vomiting
- Changes in level of consciousness (LOC), with independent observer account if available
- Any signs/symptoms of thyroid dysfunction, changes in bowel habits, changes in menses
- Past medical history, including:
  - Subdural hematoma, traumatic brain injury, radiation treatments head/neck, seizure disorder, headaches, head and/or neck surgeries
  - Recent lumbar puncture, prior meningitis
  - Cardiac, respiratory, neurologic, thyroid, or other chronic/systemic problems
- Family history, including:
  - Headaches with similar patterns/types as patient, thyroid issues
- Personal/social history, including:
  - Safety of environment—Work, home, personal; type of work—exposure to toxins/chemicals; use of protective equipment
  - Risks of injury—Use of assistive devices, sports participation—use of safety equipment
  - Usual dietary habits and nutritional status, current stressors/tension-provoking issues
  - Alcohol, tobacco, and/or recreational drug use

Advanced Assessment Skills
- Inspect:
  - Head shape and position, hair pattern
  - Facial features for symmetry, shape
  - Neck for position of trachea, symmetry, range of motion
- Palpate:
  - Head, scalp, and hair; temporal arteries
  - Trachea; thyroid for size, shape, consistency
- Auscultate:
  - Temporal arteries for bruit

Lymphatic System
- Patient history, including:
  - Constitutional and problem-focused symptoms—*OLD CARTS*
  - Medications, including complementary and alternative
  - Swelling of one or both extremities, swollen or painful nodes
  - Erythema, discoloration, or ulceration of extremity
  - Night sweats, abdominal pain/fullness
- Past medical history, including:
  - TB skin testing with result, recent chest x-ray with result
  - Trauma distal to nodes, surgical biopsy of lymph nodes
  - Cardiac, renal, HIV, known malignancies, recurrent infections
  - Autoimmune disease, organ transplant, blood transfusions
  - Allergies, immunization history
- Family history, including:
  - Malignancy, recent infectious diseases, blood disorders, immune disorder, tuberculosis
- Personal/social history, including:
  - Occupational exposure—Use of personal protective equipment
  - Recent foreign travel
  - Recreational IV drug use, sexual history, high-risk sexual practices

Advanced Assessment Skills

- Inspect:
  - Visible nodes and surrounding area
- Palpate:
  - Superficial nodes for consistency, tenderness, size, mobility, warmth

Eyes, Ears, Nose, and Throat

- *Eyes*—Patient history, including:
  - Constitutional and problem-focused symptoms—*OLD CARTS*
  - Medications, including complementary and alternative
  - Issues with vision, nocturnal eye pain, issues with depth perception
  - Dry eyes, excessive tearing, eye discharge, recent eye injury
- *Eyes*—Past medical history, including:
  - Eye surgery with cause and outcome, cataract removal, glaucoma
  - Diabetes, hypertension, hyperlipidemia, thyroid disorder, autoimmune disease, HIV, inflammatory bowel disease, seasonal allergies
- *Eyes*—Family history, including:
  - Glaucoma, macular degeneration, diabetes, hypertension, cataracts
  - Retinoblastoma, color blindness, retinitis pigmentosa
  - Strabismus, amblyopia, myopia, presbyopia
- *Eyes*—Personal/social history, including:
  - Corrective lens, contact lens with hygiene habits, last eye exam
  - Type of work—exposure to toxins/chemicals/machinery—use of protective equipment
  - Risk of injury—use of assistive devices, sports participation—use of safety equipment
  - Past or current tobacco use (shown to increase risk of age-related macular degeneration, cataracts, glaucoma, diabetic retinopathy, and dry-eye syndrome)

Eyes—Advanced Assessment Skills

- Inspect:
  - Visual acuity, pupils with accommodation, six cardinal fields of gaze, corneal light reflex
  - Eyebrows, orbital area, eyelids, lacrimal gland, conjunctiva, and sclera
  - Funduscopic: Red reflex, fundus, blood vessels, macula, optic disc
- Palpate:
  - Eyelids, eyes in sockets

- *Ears, nose, and throat*—Patient history, including:
  - Constitutional and problem-focused symptoms—*OLD CARTS*
  - Medications, including complementary and alternative
  - Ear pain and/or drainage, frequent ear infections, hearing loss, tinnitus, vertigo (older adult—falls)
  - Nasal discharge, snoring, sinus pressure or pain
  - Dental issues, dentures, lesions in mouth, hoarseness and/or voice change, pain in throat, swallowing issues
- *Ears, nose, and throat*—Past medical history, including:
  - Hypertension, cardiovascular disease, diabetes, renal disorder, bleeding disorder, gastrointestinal disorder, reflux esophagitis, asthma
  - Ear trauma, ear surgery, labyrinthitis

- Nose trauma, nose surgery, chronic epistaxis, chronic postnasal drip
  - Recurrent sinusitis, sinus surgery
  - Recurrent streptococcal infections
- *Ears, nose, and throat*—Family history, including:
  - Ménière's disease, hearing issues, hereditary renal disease
- *Ears, nose, and throat*—Personal/social history, including:
  - Type of work—exposure to toxins/chemicals/machinery/loud noises, use of protective equipment
  - Usual dietary habits, oral care habits, dental issues, xerostomia affecting ability to chew or swallow
  - Hearing loss, impact on ability to perform ADL
  - Tobacco use; alcohol use; recreational drug use, especially intranasal

Ears—Advanced Assessment Skills

- Inspect:
  - Size, shape, symmetry, position; lesions; external auditory canal
- Inspect with otoscope (largest speculum that fits comfortably):
  - Auditory canal; tympanic membrane for color, landmarks, mobility; cone of light
- Palpate:
  - Auricles and mastoid for tenderness
- Assess hearing:
  - Answers questions appropriately, whispered voice, tuning fork (Rinne and Weber tests)

Nose and Sinuses—Advanced Assessment Skills

- Inspect:
  - Shape/size/color external nose
  - Nares for symmetry, discharge; nasal mucosa and septum for color and condition
- Palpate:
  - Patency of nares, firmness of nasal bridge and tip, frontal and maxillary sinuses

Mouth—Advanced Assessment Skills

- Inspect:
  - Lips, teeth, buccal mucosa, gingiva, tongue, palate and uvula, oropharynx
- Palpate:
  - Gingiva, tongue, floor of mouth, gag reflex

Chest and Lungs

- Patient history, including:
  - Constitutional and problem-focused symptoms—*OLD CARTS*
  - Medications, including complementary and alternative
  - Cough, sputum, shortness of breath, pain in chest, dyspnea on exertion
  - Recent exposure to infectious agent/person, frequency of respiratory infections
  - Effects of weather on breathing, sedentary habits or immobility, coughing or choking when eating
- Past medical history, including:
  - Use of supplemental oxygen or other devices (e.g., continuous positive airway pressure [CPAP], bilevel positive airway pressure [BiPAP])
  - Trauma to thorax or trachea, hospitalizations or surgeries for pulmonary issue

- Chronic pulmonary diseases, tuberculosis, cardiac issues, clotting disorders, known cancer, dysphagia
- Recent pulmonary-related diagnostic testing, with results
- Immunizations—Influenza, pertussis, pneumococcal
  - Family history, including:
    - Tuberculosis, cystic fibrosis, chronic obstructive pulmonary disease(s) (COPD)
    - Malignancy, clotting disorders
  - Personal/social history, including:
    - Type of work and amount of effort required; exposure to toxins/chemicals, animals, vapors/fumes, known pulmonary irritants, allergens; use of protective equipment
    - Home environment—Ventilation, air-conditioner use, type of heating
    - Respiratory symptoms' impact on ADL
    - Amount of exercise—Tolerance or tolerance changes, travel exposures—valley fever (southwestern United States), tuberculosis, histoplasmosis (Ohio and Mississippi River valleys)
    - Hobbies—Birds, other animals, woodworking, painting
    - Tobacco usage—Number of pack years; exposure to secondhand smoke; alcohol use; recreational drug use, especially inhaled

Advanced Assessment Skills (Table 2.1)

- Inspect:
  - Size, shape, symmetry, landmarks of thorax; position of trachea
  - Compare anterior/posterior (a/p) versus transverse diameter, skin condition of posterior/anterior chest
  - Color of nails and lips, respiration rate and rhythm, symmetry of chest movement with breathing, effort of breathing (Table 2.2)
- Palpate:
  - Symmetry of thoracic expansion, tactile fremitus
- Percuss:
  - Thorax for resonance of tone, intensity, pitch—Compare bilaterally
- Auscultate:
  - Apex to base with side-to-side comparison; vocal resonance

Heart and Circulation

- Patient history, including:
  - Constitutional and problem-focused symptoms—OLD CARTS
  - Medications, including complementary and alternative
  - Chest pain and associated symptoms—Anxiety, dyspnea, diaphoresis, dizziness, nausea/vomiting, pallor, syncope, palpitations, excess fatigue
  - Leg cramps, pedal edema, leg pain, claudication, lower extremity skin changes
- Past medical history, including:
  - Cardiac surgery, hospitalization or workup for cardiac issue
  - Orthostatic hypotension, dysrhythmia, congenital heart disease, acute rheumatic fever
  - Hypertension, diabetes, thyroid issues, obesity, bleeding disorder, known coronary artery disease, stroke, transient ischemic attack (TIA), thrombosis, peripheral vascular disease

TABLE 2.1 PULMONARY ASSESSMENT TECHNIQUES

ASSESSMENT	TECHNIQUE	EXPECTED FINDING	ABNORMAL FINDING WITH POTENTIAL CAUSATION
Tactile Fremitus (*Spoken word is palpated*)	Palpation: Place palmar or ulnar surface of hands *posteriorly* on either side of spine between scapula (level of bifurcation of the bronchi), have patient say "99," compare sides for symmetry.	Vibration (fremitus) should be *symmetrical* and *palpable* with spoken word.	**Decreased or absent fremitus:** Pleural effusion, *bronchial* obstruction, emphysema **Increased fremitus (feels coarse):** Pneumonia (consolidation) **Asymmetrical fremitus:** See decreased, absent, or increased
Vocal Fremitus (Resonance; *spoken word is auscultated*)	Auscultation: Ask patient to recite their name while auscultating lung fields. Auscultate lung fields and ask patient to say "e"; auscultate lung fields and ask patient to whisper "1-2-3."	Spoken word is usually muffled in auscultation. "E" clearly is auscultated as "e"; whispered voice is faintly heard on auscultation.	**Bronchophony:** Increased loudness of spoken voice over area of consolidation **Egophony:** "E" sounds like "a" due to consolidation **Whispered pectoriloquy:** Whispered words auscultated clearly when consolidation present (same significance as increased tactile fremitus)
Resonance	Percussion: Ask patient to cross arms in front of chest, percuss over intercostal spaces posteriorly, moving downward and comparing sides (avoid the scapula).	Resonance	**Dullness:** Consolidation, pleural effusion **Hyperresonance:** Hyperinflation, pneumothorax, emphysema

TABLE 2.2 ADVENTITIOUS BREATH SOUNDS

DESCRIPTIONS/ IMPLICATIONS	FINE CRACKLES	COARSE CRACKLES	RHONCHI	WHEEZING	STRIDOR
Pitch	Soft and high	Loud and low	Low	High	High
Quality	Crackling	Gurgling	Rumbling	Musical	Whistling
Duration	Brief, discontinuous, does not clear with cough	Longer than fine crackles, discontinuous, does not clear with cough	Continuous, can clear with cough	Continuous	Continuous
Timing	Mid- to late inspiration	Inspiration or expiration	Expiration	Inspiration or expiration	Inspiration
Implications	Pneumonia, heart failure, aspiration, chronic bronchitis, pulmonary edema	Pneumonia, bronchitis, COPD, pulmonary fibrosis, bronchiectasis	Pneumonia, chronic bronchitis, bronchiectasis, COPD	Asthma, reactive airway disease, bronchitis,	Upper airway obstruction, laryngeal edema

COPD, chronic obstructive pulmonary disease.

- Family history, including:
  - Long QT syndrome; diabetes, hypertension, hyperlipidemia, obesity
  - Congenital heart disease; sudden death, thrombosis, peripheral vascular disease
- Personal/social history, including:
  - Type of work—Exposure to environmental hazards, stress of work, physical demands of work, hobbies, stress-reduction habits
  - Nutritional status; usual dietary habits; exercise—type, amount, and tolerance
  - Tobacco—type; pack-years, efforts to stop; alcohol—frequency, amount, duration
  - Recreational drugs—especially cocaine and intravenous drug use

Advanced Assessment Skills

- Inspect:
  - Apical impulse; skin or nail changes in extremities; varicosities performed while patient is standing, if possible
- Palpate:
  - Apical impulse; all arterial pulses for rate, rhythm, and amplitude (0–4)
  - Varicosities, pedal edema
- Auscultate:
  - Heart valves; heart sounds; murmurs, extra sounds; rhythm; rate
  - Five heart-valve areas for auscultation:
  - Aortic—Second right intercostal space (ICS) at right sternal border (RSB)
  - Pulmonic—Second left ICS at left sternal border (LSB)
  - Erb's (second pulmonic)—Third left ICS at lower LSB
  - Triscuspid—Fourth left ICS at lower LSB
  - Mitral—Fifth left ICS at MCL
- Suggested sequence and positioning for auscultation of heart valves:
  - Sitting up and leaning forward slightly: Auscultate all five areas, preferably in expiration.

- Supine: Auscultate all five areas.
- Left lateral recumbent: Auscultate all five areas.
- Additional assessments, including:
  - Carotid arteries, abdominal aorta, femoral arteries for bruit
  - Murmurs—Grade I through IV; jugular venous pressure (JVP) lower extremities for venous/arterial insufficiency
- *Technique for assessing JVP*: Begin with patient supine and gradually elevate head of bed/table until jugular pulsations become visible between the angle of the jaw and the clavicle. Illuminate across the right side of the patient's neck. Measure the distance vertically between the manubriosternal joint and the highest visible level of jugular vein pulsation.

Breasts and Axillae (Male and Female)

- Patient history, including:
  - Constitutional and problem-focused symptoms—*OLD CARTS*
  - Medications, including complementary and alternative—especially hormonal medications; anabolic steroids; males/hormonal therapy for prostate cancer
  - Use of diethylstilbestrol (DES; prescribed to women between 1940 and 1970 to prevent miscarriages and complications of pregnancy; increased risk of breast cancer for patients who received DES and patients with female breasts exposed to DES in utero)
  - Breast pain, nipple discharge; males—breast enlargement
- Past medical history, including:
  - Gender identity, sex assigned at birth
  - Previous breast disease—Cancer, fibroadenomas, fibrocystic changes, breast biopsy with results; surgeries—especially any breast-related surgeries
  - Known *BRCA1*, *BRCA2*, or other genetic issues; other related cancers (male and female)

- Female: Mammography and other breast imaging, menstrual history, pregnancies, lactation, menopause, endocrine issues
- Male: Undescended testicle, mumps as an adult, orchiectomy
- Male: Chest radiation (as for chest cancer treatment)
■ Family history, including:
  - Breast cancer, known *BRCA1* or *BRCA 2* in primary and secondary relatives (important to include questioning for both male and female, based on increased risk in both)
  - Other breast disease, related cancers
■ Personal/social history, including:
  - Breast awareness/use of self-breast exam—Timing to menses (female)
  - Caffeine usage; tobacco, alcohol, marijuana, or other recreational drug use

Advanced Assessment Skills
■ Inspect (male or female while seated):
  - Breast comparison for size, symmetry, contour, skin color and texture, venous patterns, lesions
  - Areolae and nipples bilaterally simultaneously for shape, color, surface, and appearance
■ Palpate (while seated or supine with arm overhead):
  - Chest wall sweep, digital bimanual exam, axillary lymph nodes
    ■ Nipple compression *no longer performed routinely* (nipple compression is indicated with report of *spontaneous* nipple discharge)

Abdomen
■ Patient history, including:
  - Constitutional and problem-focused symptoms—*OLD CARTS*
  - Medications, including complementary and alternative
  - Abdominal pain, nausea, vomiting, diarrhea, constipation, fecal incontinence, hematochezia, melena
  - Dysuria, urinary incontinence, hematuria; high-risk sexual encounters
  - Exposure to hepatitis, jaundice
■ Past medical history, including:
  - Gastrointestinal disease/disorder/infection/injury, prior pancreatitis, hyperlipidemia, hepatitis, liver cirrhosis
  - Urinary tract infections, abdominal or pelvic surgeries, sexually transmitted disease(s)
  - Major/chronic illness—Cardiac, kidney; cancer, especially colorectal, breast, ovarian, endometrial
  - Blood transfusions, hepatitis A and B immunization status
■ Family history, including:
  - Colorectal cancer, gallbladder disease, malabsorption syndrome, kidney disease
  - Adult-onset familial Mediterranean fever (characterized by acute onset of sporadic, recurrent fevers with chest pain, abdominal pain, and joint pain)
■ Personal/social history, including:
  - Nutritional status, usual dietary habits, changes in appetite, first day of last menstrual period
  - Occupational, environmental, and/or travel exposures (infectious)
  - Current major stressors, intimate partner violence (current or past), sexual abuse
  - Tobacco use; alcohol and recreational drug use

Advanced Assessment Skills
■ Inspect:
  - Color, contour, pulsations; abdominal musculature with raised head
■ Auscultate:
  - With diaphragm: Frequency and character of bowel sounds
  - With bell: Epigastric, aorta, renal, iliac, and femoral arteries
■ Percuss:
  - General tone in all four quadrants, liver span (6–12 cm adult), gastric bubble, spleen, costovertebral angle (CVA) bilaterally (direct or indirect percussion)
■ Palpate:
  - Light, moderate, deep for pain/tenderness; liver; spleen; kidney; aorta; bladder
■ Additional assessments (Table 2.3)

Female Genitalia
■ Patient history, including:
  - Constitutional and problem-focused symptoms—*OLD CARTS*
  - Medications, including complementary and alternative
  - Abnormal vaginal bleeding, menopause signs, abdominal pain
  - Dysuria, urinary incontinence, hematuria, dyspareunia, pelvic pain
  - Vaginal discharge, vaginal odor, vaginal itching, vaginal lesions
  - Change in libido (especially older adults)
■ Past medical history, including:
  - Gender identity, sex assigned at birth
  - Menstrual/menopause history, obstetric history, gynecologic history
  - Chronic diseases, related cancers, diabetes
■ Family history, including:
  - Diabetes, cancer, especially of reproductive organs
  - Multiple-birth pregnancies, congenital anomalies
■ Personal/social history, including:
  - Hygiene practices—Soap/powders/sprays/douching, self-exam practices, contraception history
  - Sexual history, history of sexually transmitted infection, sexual abuse or assault
  - Use of alcohol, recreational drugs; tobacco use

Advanced Assessment Skills
■ Externally inspect and palpate:
  - Mons pubis, labia majora and minora, clitoris, urethral orifice, vaginal introitus
  - Skene and Bartholin glands, muscle tone, perineum and anus
■ Internally inspect, palpate, and examine with speculum:
  - Cervix for color, position, size and shape, surface characteristics, discharge
  - Modify for sensory-impaired patients by raising head of exam table
  - Modify for comfort in older adults
■ Bimanually examine:
  - Uterus for size, shape, and contour; ovaries for shape and characteristics
■ Digitally examine:
  - Anal sphincter tone, walls of rectum

TABLE 2.3 ABDOMINAL ASSESSMENT

SIGN	DESCRIPTION	POSSIBLE ETIOLOGY
Aaron	Pain in heart or stomach when palpating McBurney's point	Appendicitis
Cullen	Ecchymosis around umbilicus	Hemoperitoneum, pancreatitis, ectopic pregnancy
Grey Turner	Ecchymosis in flank area(s)	Pancreatitis, hemoperitoneum
Kehr	RLQ bowel sounds absent	Renal calculi, splenic rupture, ectopic pregnancy
Markle	Heel jar causes abdominal pain	Appendicitis, peritoneal irritation
Murphy	Halts inspiration on palpation gall bladder	Cholecystitis
Rovsing	LLQ palpation causes RLQ pain	Appendicitis, peritoneal irritation

LLQ, left lower quadrant; RLQ, right lower quadrant.

Male Genitalia

- Patient history, including:
  - Constitutional and problem-focused symptoms—*OLD CARTS*
  - Medications, including complementary and alternative
  - Discharge or lesions on penis, curvature of penis with erection
  - Persistent erections, difficulty achieving or maintaining erection, ejaculation difficulty
  - Swelling in inguinal area, testicular pain or mass
- Past medical history, including:
  - Gender identity, sex assigned at birth
  - Congenital anomaly—Undescended testes, hypospadias, epispadias
  - Recent and/or past genitourinary (GU) surgery, hydrocele or varicocele, hernia, vasectomy
  - Sexually transmitted disease(s) history, hernia(s), priapism
  - Chronic illness, especially neurologic or vascular issues; testicular or prostate cancer; diabetes; cardiac disease
- Family history, including:
  - Prostate, testicular, penile, or breast cancer; hernias; Peyronie's disease
- Personal/social history, including:
  - Occupational risks, exposure to radiation and/or toxins, exercise/sports participation—use of protective equipment
  - Genital/testicular self-exam habits, number of children
  - Single or multiple sexual partners, sexual lifestyle; high-risk sexual behaviors, concerns about genitalia or sexual practices
  - Older adults—Change in frequency or desire of sexual activity; change in sexual response; fatigue, weakness, or pain from physical illness
  - Alcohol, tobacco, and/or recreational drug use

Advanced Assessment Skills

- Inspect:
  - Glans penis and pubic hair, external urethral meatus, scrotum and ventral surface
- Palpate:
  - Penis; inguinal canal for direct or indirect hernia, inguinal lymph nodes; testes, epididymides, vas deferens
  - Cremasteric reflex bilaterally (stroke inner thigh—scrotum and testicle rise on stroked side)

Anus, Rectum, and Prostate

- Patient history, including:
  - Constitutional and problem-focused symptoms—*OLD CARTS*
  - Medications, including complementary and alternative
  - Changes in bowel function/habits, anal/rectal discomfort, rectal bleeding
  - Changes in urinary function (patients with prostate)
- Past medical history, including:
  - Human papillomavirus (HPV) vaccination status, sexually transmitted disease(s), HIV
  - Gender identity, sex assigned at birth
    - Males and transgender women—Prostate cancer or hypertrophy
    - Females and transgender men—Laceration during pregnancy delivery
  - Hemorrhoids; spinal cord injury; colorectal cancer or related (ovarian, breast, endometrial); surgeries—anal, rectal, prostate
  - Known enlarged prostate (older adults)
- Family history, including:
  - Colon or prostate cancer; familial cancers
- Personal/social history, including:
  - Travel history, diet—High animal fat and low fiber content, travel history
  - High-risk sexual practices; tobacco, alcohol, or recreational drug use

Advanced Assessment Skills

- Inspect:
  - Perianal area—Infestation, inflammation, excoriation, scars, rashes
  - Anus—At rest and bearing down, skin characteristics
- Palpate:
  - Sphincter tone, anal ring, rectal walls
  - Prostate—2.5 cm size; medial sulcus contour; symmetrical, rubbery consistency; nontender

Musculoskeletal System

- Patient history, including:
  - Constitutional and problem-focused symptoms—*OLD CARTS*
  - Medications, including complementary and alternative

- Joint symptoms, injury and mechanism of injury
- Older adults: weakness, stumbling, falls, nocturnal muscle spasms, changes in exercise endurance
- Past medical history, including:
  - Bone infection, trauma, surgery on joint/bone, amputation, previous fractures
  - Chronic illness/disease: Sickle cell disease, hemophilia, cancer, arthritis, osteoporosis, neurologic issues, renal disease
  - Congenital anomalies, skeletal deformities
- Family history, including:
  - Congenital abnormalities; scoliosis; ankylosing spondylitis, gout, osteoarthritis, rheumatoid arthritis; genetic disorders—osteogenesis imperfecta; hypophosphatemia, hypercalcemia
- Personal/social history, including:
  - Occupation—Potential for unintentional injury, chronic stress on joints, safety precautions and/or protective devices
  - Exercise—Level of competition, overall conditioning, warm-up/cool-down habits
  - Functional abilities, nutrition, tobacco or alcohol use

Advanced Assessment Skills

- Inspect:
  - Overall body posture
  - Extremities: Size, alignment, contour, symmetry, skin over muscles, bones, joints
  - Muscles—Compare sides for size and symmetry
- Palpate:
  - Bones and joints, all muscles for tone and characteristics
  - Major joints for active and passive range of motion (compare sides)
  - Muscle strength comparison (by grading—0 to 5; Table 2.4)
  - Older adults—Functional assessment

Neurologic System

- Patient history, including:
  - Constitutional and problem-focused symptoms—*OLD CARTS*

- Medications, including complementary and alternative
- Seizures, pain, coordination of gait, parasthesia, weakness, tremor
- Older adults, pattern of falls, decreased agility, performance of ADL, social withdrawal, hearing loss, vision changes, anosmia, urinary or fecal incontinence, transient neurological deficits
- Past medical history, including:
  - Trauma—Concussion, spinal-cord injury, stroke; meningitis, encephalitis, lead poisoning, polio
  - Chronic disease/illness—Cardiac, hypertension, aneurysm, peripheral vascular disease, diabetes
  - Neurologic disorder(s), migraines, brain surgery, deformities, genetic syndromes, congenital anomalies
- Family history, including:
  - Hereditary disorders: Huntington's chorea, muscular dystrophy, pernicious anemia, alcoholism, diabetes; thyroid disease, diabetes, hypertension
  - Seizure disorder, migraine headaches
  - Learning disorders, intellectual disability
  - Gait disorder, cerebral palsy
  - Dementia—Alzheimer's, Parkinson's, vascular
- Personal/social history, including:
  - Environmental/occupational hazards; operation of large machinery or equipment; exposure to lead, insecticides, chemicals
  - Family patterns of dexterity and dominance; hand, eye, and foot dominance
  - Ability to fulfill work duties, ability for self-care, sleeping and eating patterns
  - Alcohol use, mood-altering recreational drug use

Advanced Assessment Skills

- Neurologic screening exam (Table 2.5)
  - CN I to CN XII
    - *Proprioception and cerebellar function*: Coordination, fine motor, balance, gait
    - *Sensory function*: Superficial touch and pain, point location
    - *Deep tendon reflexes*: Grade 0 through 4+
    - *Protective sensation* (monofilament)

GENERAL ASSESSMENT—OLDER ADULTS

Functional assessment elements, including:

- Detailed list of medications; use of assistive devices
- Degree of independence and/or need for caretaker assistance with basic ADL and instrumental ADL (IADL)
- Systems review, including:
  - Nutritional status, urinary incontinence, memory changes or signs of dementia
  - Depression, medication-induced delirium, falls or fear of falling
- Social/living situation—Caretaker, caretaker abilities; financial resources; advance directives and healthcare proxy
- Physical exam with focus on:
  - Mental status—Cognition, mood, memory
  - Respiratory—Dyspnea on exertion
  - Orthostatic hypotension
  - Musculoskeletal—Ability to rise from bed/chair and amount of assistance needed
  - Skin—Venous stasis or pressure areas

Older adult considerations:

- Additional assistance/time for position or position changes; may require alternate position

TABLE 2.4 MUSCLE STRENGTH AND RANGE-OF-MOTION ASSESSMENT

MUSCLE STRENGTH LEVEL OF FUNCTION	GRADE
No evidence of movement	0
Trace of movement	1
Full range of motion (only passive)	2
Full range of motion against gravity, but not against resistance	3
Full range of motion against gravity and some resistance, but weak	4
Full range of motion against gravity, full resistance	5

TABLE 2.5 CRANIAL NERVE ASSESSMENT

CRANIAL NERVE	CLASSIFICATION	ASSESSMENT
I Olfactory	Sensory (Some)	Identify familiar smell 1 nare at a time with eyes closed.
II Optic	Sensory (Say)	Visual acuity—Snellen chart; visual fields by confrontation test; fundoscopic exam
III Oculomotor*	Motor (Money)	Inspect eyelids for drooping, PERRLA, EOMs (Six Cardinal Fields of Gaze)
IV Trochlear*	Motor (Matters)	Inspect eyelids for drooping, PERRLA, EOMs (Six Cardinal Fields of Gaze)
V Trigeminal	Both (But)	Inspect face for fasciculation and/or tremors; palpate jaw muscles with teeth clenched for tone and strength; sharp/dull/light touch sensations on forehead, cheeks, jaw; corneal reflex
VI Abducens*	Motor (My)	Inspect eyelids for drooping, PERRLA, EOMs (Six Cardinal Fields of Gaze)
VII Facial	Both (Brother)	Inspect symmetry of face by smile, frown, puffed cheeks, raised eyebrows, bared teeth; and wrinkled forehead; taste—sweet and salty on each side of tongue
VIII Acoustic	Sensory (Says)	Test hearing with whisper test or audiometry, Weber and Rinne tests
IX Glossopharyngeal**	Both (Big)	Taste—Sour and bitter on each side of tongue, gag reflex, swallowing, voice quality
X Vagus**	Both (Brains)	Taste—Sour and bitter on each side of tongue, gag reflex, swallowing, voice quality
XI Spinal Accessory	Motor (Matter)	Shoulder shrug and head rotation against resistance
XII Hypoglossal	Motor (More)	Tongue movement and strength; speech quality of letters "l," "t," "d," "n"

*CN III, IV, and VI are the same assessment.
**CN IX and X are the same assessment
EOM, extraocular muscles; PERRLA, pupils equal, round, and reactive to light and accommodation.

- Perceptions of health and impact on life outlook
- Impact of life loss, family dynamics, changed living arrangements

REVIEW QUESTIONS

1. A neurologic past medical history should include data about:
   A. Family patterns of dexterity and dominance
   B. Circulatory issues
   C. Level of education
   D. Immunizations

2. A 55-year-old African American male is seeing the clinical nurse specialist (CNS) for a routine physical examination. He denies difficulty with urination or erectile dysfunction. He says he has "never had his prostate checked," but his medical record shows a negative prostate-specific antigen (PSA) test 10 months ago. The CNS performs a digital rectal examination and, upon palpation, expects the prostate gland to feel:
   A. Irregular
   B. Grainy
   C. Rubbery
   D. Hard

ANSWERS

1. **Correct answer: B. Rationale:** Circulatory problems may cause impairment of cerebral circulation, resulting in decreased blood flow to the brain. When cerebral circulation is impaired, neurological conditions, such as stroke, cerebral hemorrhage, cerebral hypoxia, and cerebral edema, may occur. Immunizations, familial patterns of dexterity/dominance, and education level are not pertinent information to the neurological history.

2. **Correct answer: C. Rationale:** This patient has minimal risk factors for prostate cancer and recent history of a normal PSA. A normal prostate exam finding is expected. A normal prostate in an older adult has a rubbery, soft, and smooth feel. Areas of the prostate that feel hard, grainy, or irregular in texture may indicate an abnormality that requires further diagnostic testing.

REFERENCES

The complete reference list appears in the digital version of this chapter, at https://connect.springerpub.com/content/book/978-0-8261-7417-8/part/part01/chapter/ch02

Diagnostic and Clinical Reasoning

Caitlin Donis

OVERVIEW OF DIAGNOSTIC AND CLINICAL REASONING

Clinical reasoning is a foundational part of clinical judgment and an essential component of clinical nurse specialist (CNS) practice competencies. Clinical reasoning requires a background of research-based knowledge and the ability to apply relevant evidence-based practices (Benner et al., 2008). It is also a process by which the CNS collects, processes, and interprets information to develop a plan of care and solve problems at the patient, family, healthcare surrogate, community, and population levels.

The epistemological basis of CNS practice regarding clinical reasoning is anchored in the domain of nursing—that is, phenomena that are concerned with nursing practice (Lyon, 2014). It is equally important for the CNS to develop a strong understanding of the pathophysiology, pharmacologic treatment, and medical management of common conditions that affect the adult-gerontology patient population.

The CNS should consider the following as foundational elements of CNS practice relating to clinical reasoning:

- The focus on wellness, a dynamic concept that is continuously redefined as the patient experiences exacerbations and remissions of comorbid conditions
- The critical differentiation between illness and disease:
  - Illness—A "subjective experience of discomfort greater than the person's normalized or expected level and a functional ability below perceived capability or expected level" (Lyon, 1990).
  - Disease—An "objective phenomenon with an identifiable group of signs and symptoms; a phenomenon that is observable and can be objectively measured" (Lyon, 2014).
- The goal of efficiency, accuracy, and fiscal responsibility in diagnostic decision-making
- The knowledge that poor diagnostic reasoning can lead to inappropriate, unnecessary, or missed treatment plans, which can all lead to patient harm

Clinical reasoning, as it pertains to CNS practice, encompasses an advanced scientific foundation that relies on synthesis of evidence to tailor nursing interventions from a holistic perspective. This holistic perspective bears in mind the most central concept within the domain of nursing: the patient. In general, the process of diagnostic reasoning can be intuitive, analytical, systematic, or a combination of these approaches. This chapter presents three different diagnostic reasoning models, each with a unique approach.

CLINICAL REASONING MODEL

The Clinical Reasoning Model published by Dr. Brenda Lyon (Figure 3.1; Lyon, 2014) is an inclusive model that promotes identification of etiologies with attention to nursing interventions, while acknowledging disease-specific etiologies as critical context. Nursing-required etiologies (NREs) are outlined in this model as etiologies that require and focus on nursing interventions (Lyon, 2014). In this model, the concept of clinical reasoning encompasses the differential diagnostic process, therapeutic/interventional reasoning, and evaluation of outcomes. For definitions of major concepts in this model, see Table 3.2.

Lyon's Clinical Reasoning Model

- Focuses on the CNS aspects of clinical inquiry and clinical judgment.
- Draws knowledge from all three spheres of CNS impact to identify etiologies and appropriate interventions.
- Includes diagnostic reasoning.
- Defines therapeutic/interventional reasoning.
  - Matches interventions with target etiologies.
  - Explores implementation of evidence-based interventions.
  - Validates the fidelity of the interventions.
  - Evaluates outcomes.
- Values the role and identification of target etiologies.
  - Depends on the clinical expertise of the CNS.
  - Once etiologies are hypothesized, data are systematically collected to rule in and rule out etiologies.

To further clarify Lyon's model of clinical reasoning from a nursing perspective, Figure 3.2 illustrates the unique contributions of both the medical and nursing domains while calling attention to the convergence of purpose: the goal of treating illness. This figure also explores the etiologies of illness as it relates to treatment categories, highlighting the vital interaction between domains. Exhibit 3.1 offers a further example of the Clinical Reasoning Model.

SYMPTOM ANALYSIS DIAGNOSTIC REASONING TOOL

Zunkel et al. (2004) conceptualized a symptom analysis teaching tool to aid in isolating symptoms, encourage critical thinking, and provide a structure for the process of differential diagnostic reasoning in advanced practice nursing. This teaching tool is designed to identify appropriate history questions, choose plausible leading hypotheses, explain expected physical examination findings, and guide diagnostic testing choices based on the known pathophysiology or etiologies associated with each hypothesis (Zunkel et al., 2004).

THE DIAGNOSTIC PROCESS MODEL

An alternative diagnostic reasoning model with application to advanced nursing practice is outlined by Stern et al. (2010). This step-wise method of diagnostic reasoning focuses on the development of a complete differential diagnosis in which hypotheses are

TABLE 3.1 DIAGNOSTIC AND CLINICAL REASONING COMPETENCIES, OUTCOMES, AND CURRICULAR RECOMMENDATIONS

CNS CORE COMPETENCIES	CNS OUTCOMES RELATED TO CORE COMPETENCIES	ESSENTIAL CORE CONTENT AREAS FOR DEVELOPING CNS COMPETENCIES
Synthesizes assessment findings by using advanced knowledge, expertise, critical thinking, and clinical judgment to formulate differential diagnoses	Phenomena of concern requiring nursing interventions are identified: ■ Diagnoses are accurately aligned with assessment data and etiologies. ■ Unintended consequences and errors are prevented.	■ Critical thinking, diagnostic reasoning, pattern identification, clinical decision-making, and problem-solving strategies

Source: From NACNS. (2019). *Statement on clinical nurse specialist practice and education* (3rd ed.). Author.

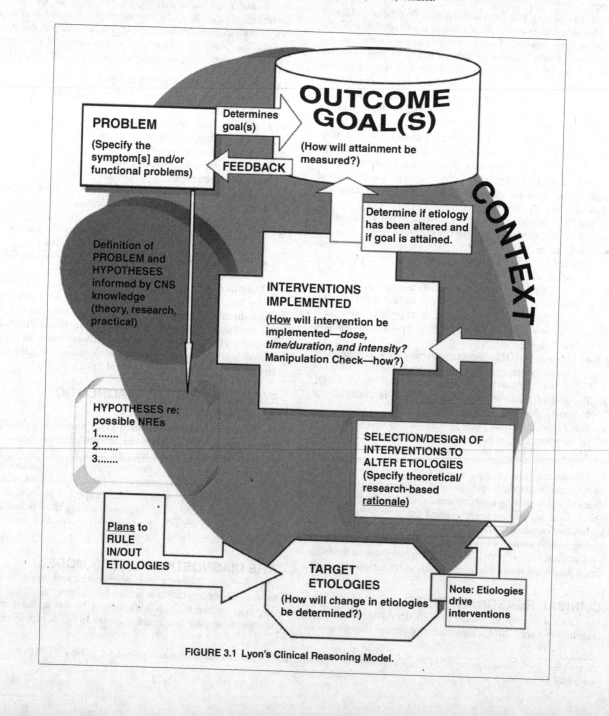

FIGURE 3.1 Lyon's Clinical Reasoning Model.

TABLE 3.2 DEFINITION OF MAJOR CONCEPTS IN LYON'S CLINICAL REASONING MODEL

Context	Background information (including but not limited to disease-specific traits, pathophysiology, historical or current signs and symptoms, age, gender, patient situation) that provides the foundation by which possible etiologies are selected.
Problem	The actual or potential problem that is identified in the initial assessment may be caused by one or more NREs.
Goals	"The predicted or desired outcomes of an intervention, which, if accomplished, represent a beneficial change in the problem" (Lyon, 2014).
Hypotheses	"Reasoned speculations about possible etiologies that could be contributing to the problem" (Lyon, 2014); includes etiologies in a holistic assessment, including NREs and medical diagnoses.
Interventions	Planned actions that are intended to cause beneficial changes with minimal risk of adverse outcomes.
Manipulation check	Confirm is whether the intervention acted as intended.

Source: From Lyon, B. (2014). Clinical reasoning model: A clinical inquiry guide for solving problems in the nursing domain. In J. Fulton, B. Lyon, & K. Goudreau (Eds.), *Foundations of clinical nurse specialist practice* (2nd ed., pp. 65–80). Springer Publishing Company.

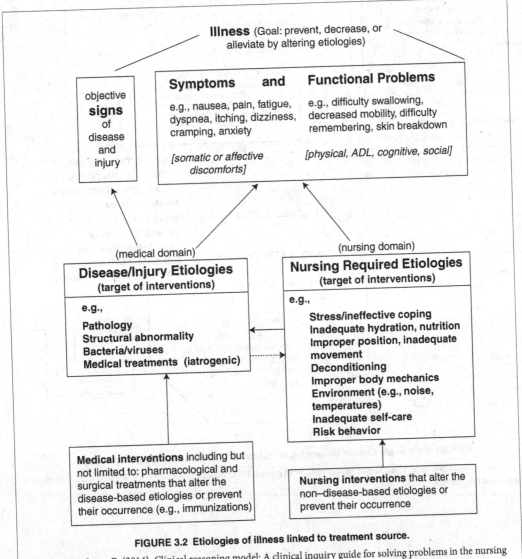

FIGURE 3.2 Etiologies of illness linked to treatment source.

Source: From Lyon, B. (2014). Clinical reasoning model: A clinical inquiry guide for solving problems in the nursing domain. In J. Fulton, B. Lyon, & K. Goudreau (Eds.), *Foundations of clinical nurse specialist practice* (2nd ed., pp. 65–80). Springer Publishing Company.

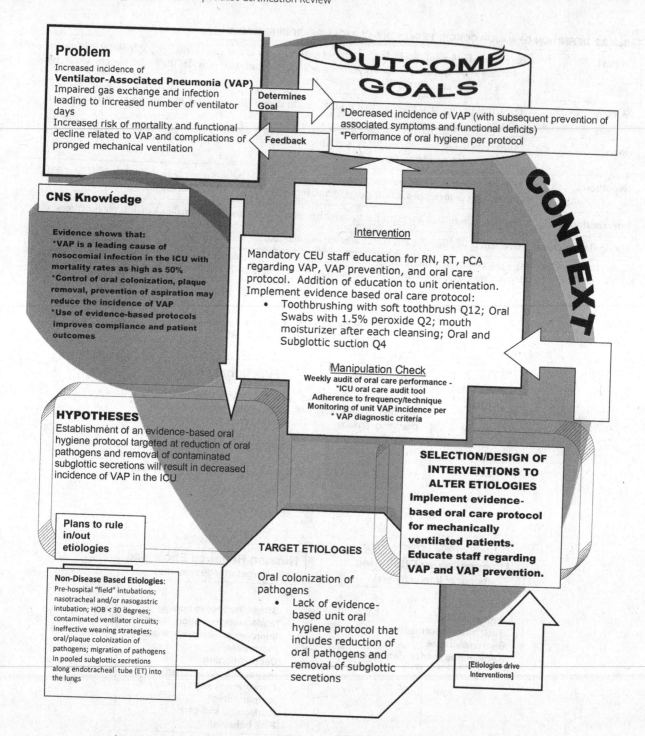

EXHIBIT 3.1 Sample Clinical Reasoning Model for ventilator-associated pneumonia.

CEU, continuing-education unit; CNS, clinical nurse specialist; HOB, head of bed; PCA, patient care technician; RT, respiratory therapist; VAP, ventilator-associated pneumonia.

prioritized, tested, reviewed, and confirmed. In this model, the focus is primarily on differential medical diagnosis and the process by which a provider confirms a suspected diagnosis (Stern et al., 2010). For definitions of major concepts in this model, see Table 3.3.

DIAGNOSTIC ERRORS

Diagnostic error can be defined as the "failure to establish an accurate and timely explanation of the patient's health problems or the failure to communicate that explanation to the patient" (Institute of Medicine [IOM], 2015). The pervasive nature of diagnostic error has gained more attention in the last two decades since the publication of the IOM's *To Err Is Human* report (2000). In this era of focus on patient safety, it is vital that CNSs strive to reduce diagnostic error in practice.

Each step of the diagnostic process has potential for error. Table 3.4 highlights the potential errors, adapted from Chase (2004) in an article by LaManna et al. (2018) This summary

TABLE 3.3 DEFINITIONS OF MAJOR CONCEPTS IN THE STERN CLINICAL REASONING MODEL

CLINICAL PROBLEMS	SYMPTOMS, PHYSICAL FINDINGS, TEST ABNORMALITIES, OR HEALTH CONDITIONS FOR WHICH DIAGNOSTIC EVALUATION CAN BE UNDERTAKEN
Pivotal points/context	Usually one of a pair of opposing descriptors used to compare and contrast conditions or clinical characteristics Ex: Chronic versus acute back pain, smoker versus nonsmoker, ongoing versus new gait disturbance
Accurate clinical problem representation	A concise, single sentence summary of the main clinical problem and its context
Fingerprints	Findings that are so specific that they are diagnostic Ex: Reed–Sternberg cells seen on biopsy results confirm diagnosis of Hodgkin's lymphoma
Frame/framework	An organizational method used to remember differentials Ex: Chest pain, anatomic framework: chest wall, pleura, esophageal, heart muscle Ex: Weight loss, system framework (good for symptoms with broad differential; each category or system has its own list of constructs): endocrine (hyperthyroidism, diabetes), pulmonary (cachexia, cancer), GI (short-gut, gastroparesis, cancers), cardiovascular (heart failure), etc. Others include pathophysiologic, mnemonic, or combinations thereof.
Leading hypothesis	The leading educated guess based on knowledge of fingerprints, typical presentations, and contextual knowledge
Must-not-miss hypotheses	Identify possible life-threatening conditions that cannot yet be ruled out according to context
Alternative hypotheses	Identify common conditions that cannot yet be ruled out according to context

GI, gastrointestinal.

Source: From Stern, S. D. C., Cifu, A., & Altkorn, D. (2010). *Symptom to diagnosis: An evidence-based guide* (2nd ed.). McGraw-Hill.

TABLE 3.4 POTENTIAL ERRORS IN THE STEPS OF THE DIAGNOSTIC REASONING PROCESS

STEP IN DIAGNOSTIC REASONING	POTENTIAL ERRORS
Data acquisition	■ Not listening to patient/family ■ Not using a systematic approach to data collection ■ Failing to develop situational awareness ■ Failing to note trends in data over time ■ Stopping data acquisition before process is complete
Hypothesis generation	■ Failing to generate multiple hypotheses ■ Ignoring the most obvious diagnosis ■ Ignoring the "not-to-be-missed" hypothesis ■ Allowing gender, age, or other bias to cloud hypothesis generation

(continued)

TABLE 3.4 POTENTIAL ERRORS IN THE STEPS OF THE DIAGNOSTIC REASONING PROCESS (continued)

STEP IN DIAGNOSTIC REASONING	POTENTIAL ERRORS
Hypothesis evaluation	■ Not using a systematic approach to evaluate hypotheses: body systems, anatomical, from the "skin in" ■ Not seeking further data to rule out a hypothesis ■ Not seeking further data to confirm a hypothesis ■ Not ordering tests to support data collection
Diagnostic choice	■ Premature closure on one hypothesis ■ Failure to consider "What else could this be?" ■ Delay in diagnostic consultation
Communication	■ Not providing team communication during hypothesis evaluation ■ Not providing patient/family communication regarding hypotheses
Goal setting	■ Not communicating with patient/family regarding preferences for goals of care ■ Not considering resources and demands on patient/family
Treatment choices	■ Not considering patient/family capacity for self-care ■ Not considering appropriate referral to specialists
Evaluation of effectiveness	■ Not checking back to assess the effect of care ■ Not involving patient's family in evaluating treatments, including medication side effects

Source: From Chase, S. K. (2004). *Clinical judgment and communication in nurse practitioner practice*. F. A. Davis; LaManna, J., Guido-Sanz, F., Anderson, M., Chase, S., Weiss, J., & Blackwell, C. (2019). Teaching diagnostic reasoning to advanced practice nurses: Positives and negatives. *Clinical Simulation in Nursing*, 26(C), 24–31.

table illustrates many of the potential biases and heuristic pitfalls that should be considered in the diagnostic reasoning process.

Tips for Reducing Diagnostic Error

■ Explicitly describe heuristics and how they affect clinical reasoning:
  ● A heuristic is a method of rapid problem solving. Heuristics can be mental shortcuts that allow for speed and flexibility in decision-making, but they are not necessarily guaranteed to be precise. There are many types of heuristics.
  ● *Availability heuristic* refers to when a diagnosis is made based on what is readily mentally accessible. Example: A patient presents with fever in the winter; the most readily accessible diagnosis is that of influenza.
  ● Heuristics in diagnostic decision-making can cause the CNS to choose one diagnosis while ignoring others, despite contrary evidence. This kind of mental process is called "cognitive bias," which contributes to diagnostic error.
■ Promote the use of "diagnostic time-outs":
  ● Taking a "diagnostic time-out" can promote reflection on the working diagnosis, review the current evidence supporting the working diagnosis, and potentially reframe the case with a new diagnosis that may be more appropriate.
  ● It can encourage skepticism in diagnostic decision-making, which leads to promotion of a more thorough workup.
  ● It can encourage students to slow down and avoid errors due to haste.

■ Promote the practice of "worst-case scenario medicine":
  ● The worse possible diagnosis should be considered and ruled out as part of the process.
  ● Embrace zebras. Considering rare diagnoses makes the learner more familiar with their presentation, even if the incidence of these diagnoses is limited.
■ Promote the use of a systematic approach to common problems:
  ● Using the same systematic approach to each problem will ensure that uncommon diagnoses don't get missed as a result of cognitive bias.
  ● Examples include anatomical approaches, use of mnemonics, and use of a step-by-step method when a specific symptom is present (Singh et al., 2014).
■ Ask why:
  ● This promotes examination of each case in detail to identify the root cause of patient conditions or symptoms.
■ Teach and emphasize the value of a clinical exam:
  ● It prioritizes the health history.
  ● It reduces dependence on diagnostic testing.
  ● It reduces dependence on previously documented information.
■ Teach Bayesian theory to direct the clinical evaluation and avoid premature closure:
  ● This allows providers to use mathematical reasoning to demonstrate the dangers of reaching a diagnostic decision too early.
  ● Many diagnostic tests have a likelihood ratio that is a measure of how well the test can confirm a targeted diagnosis. If a patient is low risk for a condition, and a diagnostic test with a high likelihood ratio shows that the

condition is present, the clinician may simply stop the workup. This can potentially result in a missed diagnosis due to premature closure. This is especially true if the posttest probability of the patient's having a certain diagnosis is not high (Trowbridge, 2008).

- Acknowledge how the patient makes the clinician feel:
  - Exploring the relationship between the clinician and patient focuses attention on potential emotional biases.

- Admit one's own mistakes:
  - Recalling cases in which diagnostic errors were made can encourage self-reflection and support learning for the next time a similar case is presented.

REFERENCES

The complete reference list appears in the digital version of this chapter, at https:// connect.springerpub.com/content/book/978-0-8261-7417-8/part/part01/ chapter/ch03

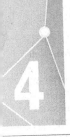

Pharmacology Principles and Nonpharmacologic Interventions

Benjamin Churchill Hickox and Tiffany L. Rader

PHARMACOKINETICS

OVERVIEW

Pharmacokinetics describes the time frame of drug action in the body through the stages of **absorption, distribution, metabolism, elimination,** and **excretion (ADMEE).**

ABSORPTION

Absorption describes the path by which a drug enters the body and is measured as bioavailability. Primary paths include the following:

- Enteral (i.e., through the gastrointestinal [GI] tract)
  - Oral, buccal, sublingual, or rectal
- Parenteral (i.e., other than the GI tract)
  - Intramuscular, subcutaneous, and intravenous (IV) injection; inhalation, or transdermal patch

DISTRIBUTION

Distribution refers to drug movement to the site of action and is a function of drug concentration, blood flow, protein binding, and other factors.

- Drug concentration
  - Because most drugs cross cell membranes by simple passive diffusion, the higher the concentration of the drug in the blood, the greater the movement of the drug into the capillary endothelial cells and subsequently into the sites of action.
- Protein binding
  - Protein binding is a mechanism by which a drug is eliminated from the blood, as drugs that are bound to protein are generally not active.
  - Many drugs are highly protein bound (e.g., warfarin, amiodarone). Thus, changes in the patient's protein levels (e.g., nutrition status) can dramatically affect the amount of free (active) drug in the blood. Likewise, administration of two drugs that are both highly protein bound can cause competition for binding and increase the level of free (active) amounts of the drug with less affinity.
  - There are two primary proteins in the blood that drugs bind to: albumin and α_1-acid glycoprotein. Acidic drugs typically bind to albumin, and basic drugs typically bind to α_1-acid glycoprotein.
- Volume of distribution (V_d)
  - The actual volume for drug distribution cannot be measured. However, the relationship of drug concentration in the blood and that in other body compartments can be measured, which is V_d, which is useful to estimate the amount of drug bound to plasma proteins or other tissue components.
  - V_d varies based on individual drug characteristics, such as binding to plasma or tissue components, lipophilic or hydrophilic properties of the drug, and the size of the drug molecule (Wecker et al., 2010).
- Measuring distribution: Peak and trough blood levels
  - Peak and trough blood levels describe drug concentration in the blood to ensure dosing is therapeutic and not toxic.
  - Peak drug levels are assessed immediately after IV drug administration and after expected absorption time (as per medication package insert guidelines) for oral medications.
  - Trough blood levels are obtained just prior to the scheduled dose.

METABOLISM

Metabolism refers to the conversion of a drug into other chemical species.

- Medications that must be converted into their active form by metabolism are called *prodrugs.*
- Primary locations of metabolism include the following:
  - **Liver (not all drugs experience all phases of hepatic metabolism)**
    - *Phase 1:* Chemical modification by oxidation, reduction, hydroxylation, primarily by the cytochrome P450 enzymes
      - The most important P450 isoenzymes are CYP3A4, CYP2D6, CYP2C9, CYP1A2, and CYP2C19 (Malhotra, 2016).
      - P450 enzyme pathways can be induced by, be inhibited by, or interact with genes; medications, food, and nutritional supplements can increase or decrease metabolic rate.
      - *Hepatic interactions:* Multiple medications that are metabolized by similar P450 pathways may experience competitive binding and subsequent variability in drug effect.
    - *Phase 2:* Conversion from lipid soluble to water soluble.
    - *Phase 3:* Binding with bile salts and secretion into bile.
  - GI tract
    - Brush border enzymes (enzymes located along the intestinal mucosa, contiguous with the luminal side of intestinal epithelial cells) play a significant role in drug metabolism in the GI tract (Li et al., 2016)
- **Bacteria within the GI tract also play an important role in drug metabolism; these bacteria can metabolize drugs and convert them into inactive or active metabolites prior to absorption by the intestinal epithelium.**
  - **Blood (plasma)**
    - Enzymes

ELIMINATION

Elimination refers to the removal of a drug from the body through metabolism and excretion.

Elimination Half-Life

- Elimination half-life ($t\frac{1}{2}$) is the time it takes for the concentration of a drug to decrease by one half. Conventionally, this is the concentration as measured in the blood.
- Half-life is dependent on clearance and volume of distribution. Anything that affects these parameters will affect half-life.
- It is generally accepted that a drug reaches *steady-state* concentration with regular dosing intervals after approximately five half-lives (Wecker et al., 2010a). Steady state is the point at which the rate of drug elimination = rate of drug absorption. Conversely, most of a drug will have been eliminated after five half-lives once the drug is discontinued.

EXCRETION

Excretion is the final removal of the drug and its metabolites from the body. Primary locations of excretion include the following:

- **Renal**
  - Renal clearance is the volume of plasma that is cleared of a substance in 1 minute.
  - *Creatinine clearance* is then used as a surrogate marker for how well a drug will be cleared by the kidneys because the same mechanisms are responsible for drug clearance.
  - **An individual's creatinine clearance, relative to how extensively a drug is excreted by the kidneys, is one of the most important pharmacokinetic parameters to consider when prescribing.**
- **Pulmonary**
  - Volatile agents (those that easily vaporize) are eliminated via exhalation, passing directly from the perialveolar capillaries into the alveoli for removal. Examples include alcohol and inhaled anesthetic agents.
- **GI tract**
  - Fecal drugs may be eliminated unchanged in the feces.
  - Drug metabolites may be eliminated after being secreted into the GI tract.
  - Some drugs are eliminated in the feces after being bound and secreted with bile salts during phase 3 hepatic metabolism.

ADDITIONAL FACTORS INFLUENCING DRUG ACTIONS

Transmembrane Transport

Transmembrane transport refers to the movement of drug molecules across cell membranes in body tissues. The most common mechanism of transmembrane transport is passive diffusion. Transmembrane transport is influenced by the charge, polarity, pH/pKa, molecular weight, and lipid solubility of the drug.

- Highly polar molecules (those with strong, separate charges, for example, sodium chloride) have difficulty crossing the lipid bilayer of the body's cells.
- The pKa of a drug and pH of the surrounding environment play a critical role in determining the ionization/dissociation, and subsequently the absorption, of a drug.
- Large molecules with a high molecular weight have difficulty crossing cell membranes and often require transmembrane proteins for active transport to site of action.
- Hydrophilic molecules (those that easily dissolve in water) also have difficulty crossing cell membranes.
- Lipophilic ("fat-loving") molecules, however, cross cell membranes easily.
- **The blood–brain barrier:** The capillaries that supply blood to the central nervous system are unique in that the endothelial cells that comprise them are joined by tight junctions, rather than by gap junctions that join peripheral capillary endothelial cells. The endothelial cells of the central nervous system also have far fewer specialized locations on the surface of the cells that can engage in pinocytosis (the transport of molecules from outside the cell to inside the cell via small vesicles).
- The net result of the blood–brain barrier is dramatically decreased absorption of drugs into the central nervous system from the blood.

Bioavailability

Bioavailability refers to the fraction of drug that reaches the systemic circulation after administration. Bioavailability is a function of

- Drug solubility,
- GI tract ability to absorb, and
- First-pass effect by the liver:
  - Orally administered drugs are subject to initial metabolism by the liver once absorbed by the GI tract (anywhere from esophagus to descending colon).
  - Sublingual, buccal, and rectal medications are not subject to the first-pass effect.

TIME–CONCENTRATION CURVE

The time–concentration curve (also called *plasma level profile*) is a function of all pharmacokinetic factors (Figure 4.1). Key components of the plasma concentration profile.

- Time is plotted on the x axis.
- Plasma drug concentration is plotted on the y axis.
- As concentration is plotted over time, a curve is formed.
  - The area under the curve (AUC) reflects the body's exposure to a drug during the full dosing interval.
  - The **median effective concentration (MEC)** is the plasma concentration that produces a specific intensity of effect in 50% of participants studied. This level is the benchmark for time of onset for a drug. That is, once the plasma drug concentration reaches this level, it is assumed that the drug is beginning to exert its therapeutic effect.
  - The time from when the plasma concentration crosses above the MEC to when it crosses below the MEC is considered the **duration of action**.
  - The **maximum therapeutic concentration (MTC)** is an important parameter as it marks the highest plasma drug concentration that is considered therapeutic. The range between the MEC and the MTC is considered the **therapeutic range**. An appropriate single dose should not cause the **maximum plasma concentration (C_{max})** to exceed the MTC. Likewise, a multidose schedule should not result in the plasma drug concentration exceeding the MTC.

PHARMACOKINETIC CHANGES WITH AGING

- General
  - Decrease in cardiac output = decreased blood flow through organs.
    - Aging affects all pharmacokinetic parameters.
- Absorption
  - Is largely unaffected by aging; however, increased gastric pH (more alkaline) may affect absorption of certain medications

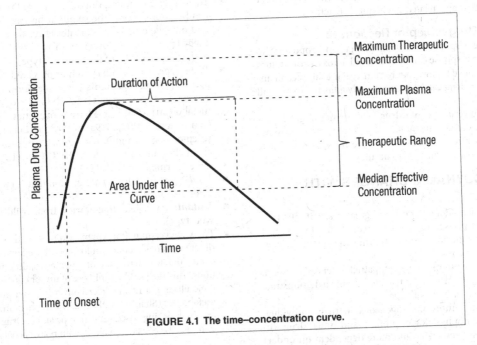

FIGURE 4.1 The time–concentration curve.

- Delayed gastric emptying (may allow for increased absorption)
- Distribution
  - There is a decrease in lean body mass and increase in adipose tissue.
    - This affects the V_d of many medications.
    - This increases the duration of the effect of lipophilic medications.
  - There is a decrease in plasma albumin and α1-acid glycoprotein concentrations.
    - This affects the V_d of many medications.
    - This increases the amount of free (active) drug.
  - There is a decrease in total body water.
    - This affects the V_d of many medications.
- Metabolism
  - Highly variable between individuals. Generally, there is a slight decrease in metabolic capacity, especially in the liver.
  - Greater sensitivity to hepatic inducers, inhibitors, and interactors.
- Excretion
  - Renal clearance is generally decreased. Renal function should be assessed prior to prescribing, and doses of drugs excreted by the kidneys should be decreased in the presence of impaired renal function. Creatinine clearance may overestimate renal function in older adults; consider using the Modification of Diet in Renal Disease (MDRD) study equation for glomerular filtration rate (GFR; Reuben et al., 2016).

PHARMACODYNAMICS

OVERVIEW

Pharmacodynamics refers to what a drug does to the body. Stated differently, pharmacodynamics are the biochemical and physiologic effects of drugs.

SITES OF DRUG ACTION

Drug site of action may be within a cell, at the cell membrane, or outside a cell.

Receptor Types

The most common receptor superfamilies are (Wecker et al., 2010) as follows:
- G-protein-coupled receptors (e.g., acetylcholine-muscarinic, adrenergic [α, β])
  - This is the most important superfamily of receptors. Many medications target this type of receptor.
- Ligand-gated ion channels (e.g., acetylcholine-nicotinic, Gamma-aminobutyric acid [GABA])
- Receptor tyrosine kinase (e.g., insulin)
- Nuclear hormone receptors (e.g., estrogen, androgens)

Drug Effect by Action on Receptor

Drugs that act on receptors are classified by the response that they elicit:
- An agonist activates a response.
  - A partial agonist activates a response but produces less than the maximum effect.
- An antagonist prevents or reverses a response.
  - A competitive antagonist causes blockade or reversal that can be overcome by an increased dose of agonist (uses same binding site). Most antagonists are of this type.
  - A noncompetitive antagonist causes blockade or reversal that can't be overcome by an increased dose of agonist (uses different binding site).
  - A physiologic antagonist produces an effect opposite that of the agonist but through a different receptor.
- An allosteric modulator increases or decreases a response to an agonist by binding to a different receptor.

Specificity and Affinity

Specificity is the ability of a drug to combine with a receptor to produce a particular effect. This effect is dependent on the three-dimensional chemical structure of that drug.

Affinity is the strength of attraction between the drug and the receptor. Affinity is also related to chemical structure.

Quantifying Drug-Receptor Responses

- *Graded:* The response to a drug changes in proportion to the dose. The response can be measured across a continuum from no response to maximal response. For example, an antihypertensive drug can be incrementally adjusted to a blood pressure goal.
- *Quantal:* The response to a drug is all or nothing. The response occurs either maximally or not at all. For example, if an antiepileptic is effective, there are no seizures. If it is ineffective, seizures continue to occur.

PHARMACODYNAMIC CHANGES WITH AGING

- Generally, older adults experience greater sensitivity (i.e., heightened response) to a given drug than do younger adults. This is especially true with drugs that affect the central nervous system.
  - A notable exception is the sympathetic nervous system, particularly β-adrenergic receptors, which demonstrate decreased sensitivity with age.
- Older adults are more heterogeneous in their individual physiologic/pathophysiologic profiles and thus drug responses are less predictable and more dependent on underlying morbidities and baseline health.
- Change in the number and function of receptors does occur (Wecker et al., 2010). Mechanisms include
  - Changes in receptor density or affinity,
  - Alterations in signaling pathways (refer to Receptor Types),
  - Alteration in biochemical responses such as glycogenolysis, and
  - Alteration in physiologic functions such as vascular tone.
- Aging is associated with impairment of homeostatic mechanisms, leading to increased vulnerability to drug toxicity and side effects (Wecker et al., 2010). Examples include:
  - Decreased activity of baroreceptors, leading to increased likelihood of orthostatic hypotension with administration of medications affecting blood pressure or fluid balance, and
  - Impaired thermoregulation, leading to hypothermia with administration of psychoactive agents, including alcohol.

PHARMACOGENOMICS

OVERVIEW

Pharmacogenomics is the study of the interaction between genetic variation and response to specific medications.

DEFINITIONS

- *Gene:* A sequence of DNA (i.e., cytosine, guanine, adenine, thymine) that corresponds to a sequence of amino acids (e.g., tyrosine, arginine) within a protein. Numerous genes are arranged on each chromosome. In humans, there are 23 pairs of chromosomes: 1 pair of sex chromosomes and 22 pairs of autosomal chromosomes.
- *Allele:* A gene that can have a variable sequence.
- *Polymorphism:* The ability of an allele to have more than one alternate sequence and thus the code for more than two phenotypes (e.g., blood type: A, B, or O).

- *Genotype:* The description of a pair of alleles. An allele pair can be homozygous (the same) or heterozygous (different), and one allele may have greater effect (dominant) over the other (recessive). In order for a recessive trait to be seen, both alleles must be of the recessive type.
- *Phenotype:* The manifestation or observed effect of an allele pair. In pharmacogenomics, examples include the activity of a certain enzyme (e.g., CYP2C19 and clopidogrel [Plavix] metabolism) (Clinical Pharmacogenetics Implementation Consortium [CPIC]2019a) or the function of an ion channel receptor (e.g., ryanodine receptor 1/ calcium voltage-gated channel subunit alpha 1 S [RYR1/CACNA1S] and malignant hyperthermia; CPIC, 2019b).
- *Wild-type:* The allele configuration that is most prevalent in a population.
- *Mutant:* An allele that varies from wild-type (i.e., not wild-type).
- *Phenoconversion:* Phenotypic expression that is opposite or different than what one would expect based on genotype. Often occurs due to external factors such as coadministered medications. The most studied subtype of this phenomenon is a genotypic ultrarapid metabolizer converting to a phenotypic poor metabolizer (Shah & Smith, 2015). This phenomenon can cause incorrect dosing based on genotype alone. Drug–drug interaction must be considered along with pharmacogenomics.

AREAS OF CONCERN

Hypersensitivity and Idiosyncratic Drug Reactions

- Hypersensitivity reactions to drugs are immune mediated. Some hypersensitivity reactions may be dependent on genotype and thus of interest in pharmacogenomics.
- Idiosyncratic drug reactions are those that do not have a known cause. It may be that some reactions historically considered idiosyncratic are actually related to variations in genotype.

Efficacy

- The ability of a drug to produce its intended effect can be highly influenced by genotype, particularly cytochrome P450 enzyme variations.
- Cytochrome P450 enzymes, concentrated in the liver but also found in various other locations throughout the body, such as the small intestine, are responsible for a large portion of drug metabolism. Certain isoenzymes, such as CYP2D6, are more prone to polymorphism than others and thus prone to variations in drug metabolism for drugs that use this enzyme.
- The variation in alleles for a given CYP isoenzyme determines an individual's ability to metabolize drugs that use that pathway. For example, individuals who have two mutant variants of the CYP2C19 allele may produce the CYP2C19 enzyme, which functions poorly, if at all. The result will be poor metabolism of any drug that uses the CYP2C19 isoenzyme. This can result in *treatment failure,* such as early in-stent thrombosis in patients with postpercutaneous coronary intervention who received a stent and were prescribed clopidogrel (Plavix), a prodrug that requires metabolism by CYP2C19 to be converted into its active form.
- Depending on genotype, an individual's ability to metabolize drugs using various CYP pathways can be graded as one of four phenotypes:
  - *Poor metabolizer*—Results in very slow or no metabolism.
  - *Intermediate metabolizer*—Results in slow metabolism.
  - *Extensive metabolizer*—Results in average metabolism.
  - *Ultrarapid metabolizer*—Results in very fast metabolism.

- P-glycoprotein (Pgp) is a transmembrane protein that is responsible for the transport of various molecules (including drugs) from within a cell to outside a cell. Pgp is coded for by the *ABCB1* and *ABCB4* genes. Variation in the alleles of these genes can change the degree to which a drug is effective. For example, if a person has extensive *ABCB1* activity due to allele variants, then there will be a large amount of Pgp expressed on the cell membrane, and a large amount of drug that was intended to remain inside the cell for activity will be removed and the drug will be ineffective. Examples of drugs that are affected by *ABCB1* and *ABCB4* genotypes include digoxin, several antiepileptic drugs, and certain antineoplastics (Malhotra, 2016).

Toxicity

- If a patient is a poor metabolizer for a specific CYP450 isoenzyme and is prescribed a drug that is metabolized via that specific pathway, there is a risk for toxicity, as the drug will not be metabolized or will be metabolized very poorly and the concentration of the drug will increase in the patient's tissues. Conversely, if a patient is an ultrarapid metabolizer for a specific CYP450 isoenzyme and the patient is prescribed a prodrug that utilizes that pathway, the concentration of drug in the patient's system will peak rapidly and possibly at a toxic level.
- Some drugs have specific metabolic pathways other than the cytochrome P450 system. These pathways may be dependent on enzymes that are coded for by a gene that is subject to polymorphism. If the allele variant codes for an enzyme that is less metabolically active than normal, there is a possibility that the drug may accumulate in the system and become toxic.

CLINICAL IMPLEMENTATION OF PHARMACOGENOMICS

- Potential indications for pharmacogenomic testing (Mayo Foundation for Medical Education and Research, 2019):
  - Symptoms suggestive of drug metabolism concerns:
    - Toxicity or adverse reactions
    - Problems with efficacy
  - Medication nonadherence due to side effects or lack of efficacy
  - Patient self-adjustment of medication dose or frequency
  - Contemplating prescription of a medication with a known adverse drug reaction (ADR)
  - Patient requests testing
- Guidelines
  - The CPIC, which is a service of the U.S. Department of Health and Human Services and is managed at Stanford University and St. Jude Children's Research Hospital, provides implementation guidelines for specific gene–drug interactions (CPIC, 2019c). See www.cpicpgx.org for more information.
    - These guidelines provide the rationale and suggested prescribing changes that are warranted based on allele variation. A number of the guidelines also include algorithms that can be incorporated into the electronic healthcare record for *clinical decision support*.
    - The CPIC website also includes an extensive list of gene–drug interactions and related information.
  - The *Pharmacogenomics Knowledgebase* (*PharmGKB*) is a database and working group related to the CPIC; it is funded by the U.S. Department of Health and Human Services and is managed at Stanford University (Whirl-Carrillo et al., 2012; see www.pharmgkb.org).

- PharmGKB provides a wealth of information, including data on drugs that have allele variants, pharmacokinetic or pharmacodynamic pathways affected by certain drugs, clinical guideline annotations, and drug label annotations.
- Other considerations
  - Pharmacogenomic testing can be expensive; with increased utilization, it is likely that the costs for these tests will come down. There are already many healthcare centers that offer pharmacogenomic testing and a number of centers that routinely utilize and incorporate test results in practice.
  - Pharmacogenomic testing should be considered in context. Be sure to take into account age, sex, race, or other individual characteristics that could account for variations in drug reaction.
  - Consider drug–drug and drug–food interactions when interpreting pharmacogenomic testing, since genotype may not reflect phenotype under conditions leading to phenoconversion.

GOOD PRESCRIBING PRINCIPLES AND MEDICATION MANAGEMENT

PROCESS OF RATIONAL PRESCRIBING

The World Health Organization's (WHO; de Vries et al., 1994) process of rational prescribing is the most commonly cited process for prescribing medications. The process includes six steps.

Step 1: Define the Patient's Problem

- Consider chief complaint/reason for visit, history of present illness, past medical history, social history, and review of systems/syndromes.
- Consider medication history and results of medication reconciliation.
- See Chapter 5 for special considerations when prescribing controlled substances.

Step 2: Specify the Therapeutic Objective

- Include the patient. Ask about cultural influences and personal beliefs about health and illness.
- Examples of objectives include curing illness, relieving symptoms, replacing deficiencies, and improving function.

Step 3: Verify That the Treatment Is Suitable for the Specific Patient

- Make an inventory of possible drug classes as well as nonpharmacologic treatments.
  - Reference reputable published guidelines, especially from professional societies (e.g., American College of Cardiology, American College of Rheumatology). Guideline-directed medical therapy (GDMT), when available, is considered best practice.
- Choose a drug class.
  - Consider formulary restrictions—This is often built into computerized provider order entry (CPOE).
  - Be aware of personal prescriber preferences:
    - Stay up to date with **prescribing recommendations**. Professional society websites are often helpful.
    - Familiarity with a drug can be good but not always. Be aware and curious about *personal prescribing patterns*.
    - Know that *pharmaceutical promotion* has an influence on practice, whether the prescriber is consciously

aware of it or not. Actively avoid **personal prescribing bias** due to pharmaceutical promotion.

- Choose a drug.
  - Consider using the I Can PresCribE A Drug (ICPCEAD) mnemonic (Iglar et al., 2007).
    - *Indication*—Consider things such as time-to-benefit versus life expectancy (e.g., statin drugs and very old/multi-morbid adults).
    - *Contraindications*—For example, always be aware that a woman of childbearing age may be pregnant and that a number of drugs are contraindicated in pregnancy.
    - *Precautions*—Consider drug disease/syndrome and drug–drug interactions (e.g., renal impairment, additive toxicity). See "Consider potential *interactions*" later in this section.
    - *Cost/compliance*—Things like once daily dosing, dual-drug pills, and depot injections improve adherence; consider current pill burden. Choose medications that can treat two conditions if possible. Consider affordable prescription programs (e.g., retail pharmacy $4 or $10 generic lists) and manufacturer assistance programs for specific drugs.
    - *Efficacy*—Consider pharmacokinetic, pharmacodynamic, and pharmacogenomic factors. Consider *pharmacoeconomics* (e.g., efficacy vs. cost) and evidence on absolute risk reduction.
    - *Adverse effects*—Consider pharmacokinetic and pharmacodynamic changes when prescribing for older adults. Consider drug-specific pharmacogenomics and family history of adverse effects. See section titled Adverse Drug Reactions in the following.
    - *Dose/duration/direction (plan)*—See Step 6 of the WHO process in the following text.
  - Consider potential *interactions*.
    - Drug–drug/drug–food:
      - Review potential metabolic modulation by hepatic induction, inhibition, or interaction (see Pharmacokinetics section).
      - Be aware of *additive toxicity*. Examples include
        - Increased risk for *bleeding* with coadministration of drugs such as aspirin, clopidogrel (Plavix), ginkgo biloba dietary supplement, nonsteroidal anti-inflammatory drugs (NSAIDs), and warfarin.
        - Increased risk for *hyperkalemia* with coadministration of drugs such as angiotensin-converting enzyme inhibitors, aldosterone antagonists, drospirenone/ethinyl estradiol (Yaz), and salt substitutes containing potassium chloride.
        - Increased risk for *central nervous system depression* with coadministration of drugs such as opioids, skeletal muscle relaxants, hypnotics (i.e., sleep aids), and alcohol.
        - Increased *QT segment prolongation* (of the EKG) with coadministration of a broad variety of drugs. A current and well-managed list is available (be found at http://crediblemeds.org).
        - Increased risk for *serotonergic toxicity* (e.g., serotonin syndrome) with coadministration of drugs such as selective serotonin reuptake inhibitors, linezolid (Zyvox), fentanyl (Sublimaze, Duragesic, Actiq), St. John's wort dietary supplement, buspirone (BuSpar), and many others.
        - Increased risk for *renal toxicity* with coadministration of drugs such as gentamicin (Garamycin), vancomycin (Firvanq, Vancocin), and amphotericin (Amphocin, Fungizone), NSAIDs, metformin (Glucophage), and many others.
        - Increased risk for *hepatic toxicity* with coadministration of drugs such as acetaminophen (Tylenol), azole antifungals (e.g., fluconazole [Diflucan]), carbamazepine (Tegretol), alcohol, and many others.
    - Drug condition:
      - Be aware of a patient's baseline renal function. Calculate creatinine clearance prior to prescribing medications that are excreted by the kidneys and adjust for any impairment.
      - Be aware of a patient's baseline hepatic function. Evaluate laboratory analyses that reflect the liver's metabolic function. Consider dose adjustments or alternative drugs if hepatic metabolic function is impaired.
      - Consider baseline cognitive status. Preexisting cognitive impairment (e.g., dementia) significantly influences prescribing decisions.
      - Conduct a full health history and be aware of any other conditions that may influence prescribing decisions. Consider the specific precautions and contraindications for the drug relative to the patient's health history.
    - Discuss a *backup treatment* in case the first-line therapy fails.

Step 4: Start the Treatment

Prescription writing/entry—Although CPOE has reduced the risk for many prescribing errors, there are still prescribers who write orders by hand. There are also important considerations for those who use CPOE, as it can decrease vigilance when writing prescriptions due to perceived "safety net" as well as *best practice alert* fatigue:

Critical Components of a Prescription

- *Prescriber information*: Name, title (be aware of what legal requirements there are for title in individual states), address, phone number
- *Patient information*: Name, date of birth, age, address, telephone number
- *Date*
- *Inscription* (drug name)
  - Generic name and trade name, if available
  - If a specific brand is required, include "*Dispense as Written*" or, for patients with Medicaid as payer, include "*Brand Medically Necessary*" and ensure trade name and brand are included in the inscription
- *Subscription* (details for fulfilling pharmacy)
  - *Dose/strength*—Avoid components on the do-not-use list (e.g., "U" or "u" as an abbreviation for units, trailing zeroes, etc.; The Joint Commission, 2018).
    - In most situations, use *metric units* (e.g., milliliters, milligrams).
    - Be familiar with *apothecary/avoirdupois units* (e.g., pound, ounce), but avoid using these. Know how to

convert from these units to metric (e.g., 1 fluid ounce ≈ 30 mL, 1 ounce ≈ 28 g).

- ■ For liquid medications, specify dose and volume (i.e., concentration): for example, 1,000 mg/250 mL or 20 mg/5 mL.
- *Quantity*—Spell out: "thirty," "sixty," and so forth. Do the math—the number of doses that a person receives should reflect the timing of a necessary follow-up visit or reevaluation of therapy. Pharmacies will also often only prescribe 1 month's worth of drug.
- *Form*—Indicate whether tablets, capsules, gel packs, suspension, and so forth.
- *Substitutions*—Specify whether pharmacy substitutions are allowed or not. A substitution may include using a generic rather than a trade formulation, using a different dose tablet and instructing the patient to cut the tablet, or filling with a different release form (e.g., immediate release vs. extended release). Therapeutically equivalent products are listed in the *Approved Drug Products with Therapeutic Equivalence Evaluations*, published by the U.S. Food and Drug Administration ([FDA], 2019).

■ *Transcription* (directions for use)
- Use plain language, not Latin (e.g., Take two tablets by mouth every 8 hours for anxiety).
- Include how many; what form; what route; how often— using time intervals is preferred (e.g., every 8 hours) over times daily (e.g., three times daily) because it helps assure appropriate dosing intervals and allows patients to tailor intervals to their lifestyle; and why (*indication*)—this is important, yet commonly omitted.
- Do not use "take as directed." This leads to confusion and can lead to therapeutic failure or overdose.
- Include important information such as "do not take with alcohol," "may cause drowsiness," or "take with food."

■ *Refills*
- Must be authorized by the prescriber.
- Most prescriptions are valid for one year; some are only valid for shorter durations.
- If no refills are desired, write "none" or "zero."
- If the refill quantity is left blank, it will default to none.
- Avoid using "PRN" for refills. If "as needed" is used for refill quantity, an indication must be included in the directions for use.

■ *Signature*
- A prescription can't be filled without a valid signature. With CPOE, the signature is electronic.
- Do not include your federal Drug Enforcement Administration (DEA) registration number on a prescription. If a pharmacy needs it, a representative can call by phone.
  - ■ As of 2010, controlled substances may be electronically prescribed if the provider's CPOE and the receiving pharmacy's software are compliant with the DEA rule (U.S. Department of Justice, 2010).

■ Avoid distractions when entering a prescription—this is a common source of prescribing error.

Step 5: Give Information, Instructions, and Warnings
- ■ Ensure that an appropriate support individual is present, if necessary.
- ■ Use plain language. Assess for health literacy. Use an interpreter if needed.

- ■ Ensure that the patient is able to read/hear and understand information given. Use a method, such as teach back, to ensure comprehension.

Step 6: Monitor the Treatment
- ■ *Safety*
  - *Food and Drug Administration (FDA) boxed warnings (i.e., black-box warnings)*: These must be included with drug packaging. These warnings draw attention to potential serious adverse reactions associated with the drug. Pay close attention to any black box warnings and consider applying the safety, tolerability, effectiveness, price, simplicity (STEPS; O'Connor, 2010) process to weigh the benefit versus risk of medications with a black box warning.
  - *Risk evaluation and mitigation strategy (REMS)*: The FDA requires this drug safety program for a very small number of medications that are associated with serious safety concerns. More information can be found on the FDA website (U.S. FDA, 2018a).
  - *FDA communications:* The U.S. FDA utilizes a broad range of strategies to communicate important drug-related information to providers and the public. These strategies include Drug Safety Communications, MedWatch Safety Alerts, and Adverse Event Reporting System. These are accessible on the FDA website (U.S. FDA, 2018b).
  - There are also a number of publications that offer timely updates on medication safety, such as *Pharmacist's Letter* and *Prescriber's Letter*; a prescriber's institution may have a subscription to such publications.

- ■ *ADR* is defined as harm to a patient that is the direct result of a drug (Nebeker et al., 2004).
  - Serious adverse drug reactions should be reported to the FDA through its Medwatch program, accessible online. Consumers and patients as well as providers can report events using this form.
  - ADRs can occur immediately or be delayed by days, weeks, or even up to years (Valdez et al., 2016).
    - ■ Rapid reactions occur immediately following administration.
    - ■ First-dose reactions occur, as the term implies, after the first dose. Dose reduction may need to be considered.
    - ■ Early reactions occur early in the treatment course and may resolve on their own as the patient develops a tolerance to the medication. They may require a reduction in dose but don't often require discontinuation.
    - ■ Intermediate reactions occur after a number of doses and are more difficult to predict. Drug discontinuation may or may not be required.
    - ■ Late reactions occur after prolonged exposure to a drug.
  - ADRs are broadly classified as pharmacologic or idiosyncratic (Valdez et al., 2016).
    - ■ *Pharmacologic* (comprise 85%–90% of reported events): Often a result of a greater-than-expected response to a medication or over-/under-dose.
    - ■ *Idiosyncratic* (comprise 10%–15% of reported events): May have an unknown cause, or may be related to things such as a unique immune response, genotype, or previously unknown biologic system.
    - ■ An ADR may result in a decrease in the dose of a drug or discontinuation of the drug. An alternative drug may need to be considered.

- *Adherence* (avoid using the paternalistic term *compliance*).
  - Active monitoring (de Vries et al., 1994)
    - Follow-up visit
      - Inquire about any adverse effects, especially "annoyances."
      - If concerns for nonadherence, bring "brown bag" with all pill bottles; perform pill count.
      - *Pharmacy refill inquiry* can inform the prescriber as to whether or not a patient has been getting refills on a schedule that would indicate adherence.
  - Passive monitoring (de Vries et al., 1994)
    - Patient self-report regarding adherence
  - Strategies to improve adherence may include
    - Simplifying the drug regimen,
    - Involving a pharmacist, and
    - Addressing sensory challenges
      - If needed, the prescriber must include the phrase "No child-safe packaging" in a prescription to eliminate these protective measures, which can be a barrier to accessing medications for certain patients (e.g., those with osteoarthritis). Ensure that such medication containers will be kept in a location inaccessible to children.
      - Inquire about medication setup, pill organizers, vision, fine-motor movement, and so forth.
- *Outcomes*
  - Active monitoring (de Vries et al., 1994)
    - Ask the patient about target symptom outcomes (refer to WHO step 2 earlier).
      - Consider using standardized rating scales for specific symptoms as well as overall functional ability (especially for older adults).
    - Order and review appropriate laboratory tests and other necessary monitoring.
    - Ask the patient about the stress of therapy, including the burden of number of pills, filling prescriptions, and medication setup.
  - Passive monitoring (de Vries et al., 1994)
    - Patient self-report regarding therapeutic effectiveness.
- *Follow-Up*
  - Considering the management phases of *initiation, stabilization, maintenance,* and *discontinuation,* create a plan for how frequently the patient will follow up, whom the patient will call with concerns or questions about therapy, and when the patient will be able discontinue treatment.

PRESCRIBING CONSIDERATIONS FOR OLDER ADULTS

Polypharmacy

Polypharmacy is generally defined as the concurrent administration of multiple medications; a number of sources cite five or more medications as indicative of polypharmacy (Masnoon et al., 2017). Polypharmacy may simply result from treatment of multiple chronic conditions or may be a consequence of the "prescribing cascade." Older adults are at risk of polypharmacy because they tend to have multiple chronic conditions and thus take more prescription drugs, over-the-counter (OTC) drugs, and dietary supplements.

The Prescribing Cascade

The *prescribing cascade* occurs when a medication is prescribed that results in an ADR; but instead of recognizing the ADR and having the drug dose reduced or stopped, the provider misdiagnoses it as a new condition and prescribes an additional drug counteract the adverse reaction. This cycle then repeats itself, resulting in polypharmacy (Rochon & Gurwitz, 1997). The prescribing cascade can also occur when a patient self-medicates with OTC drugs or dietary supplements.

Preventing Polypharmacy

Approaches to reduce or prevent polypharmacy include using tools, such as the *Medication Appropriateness Index* (Hanlon et al., 1992), the *Beers Criteria* (American Geriatrics Society 2015 Beers Criteria Update Expert Panel, 2015), the *Screening Tool to Alert Doctors to the Right Treatment* ([START], Barry et al., 2007), and the *Anticholinergic Risk Scale* (Rudolph et al., 2008), to identify the appropriateness of prescribing a drug in the first place and using additional tools such as the *Assess, Review, Minimize, Optimize, Reassess* tool ([ARMOR]; Haque, 2009) or the *Screening Tool of Older Persons' Potentially Inappropriate Prescriptions* ([STOPP]; Gallagher & O'Mahony, 2008) to evaluate patients' medication regimens for potentially inappropriate drugs after they've been prescribed.

Adverse Drug Reactions

Older adults are at increased risk for ADRs due to physical changes, pharmacokinetic and pharmacodynamic changes, and polypharmacy (Box 4.1). See sections "Pharmacokinetic Changes With Aging" and "Pharmacodynamic Changes With Aging."

Drug Selection

Older adults are much more heterogeneous with regard to pharmacokinetic and pharmacodynamic parameters and health profiles; thus, they require a more individualized approach to management. A guideline-directed approach may not be as applicable or beneficial for older adults; many randomized controlled trials of drugs exclude older and multi-morbid patients.

When prescribing for older adults, *start low* (dose) and *go slow* (adjustment interval; choose an older drug with more data on safety and efficacy; and monitor safety and efficacy closely.

NONPHARMACOLOGICAL INTERVENTIONS

OVERVIEW

Wellness is more than just the absence of disease; it encompasses an individual's perceived quality of life and functionality (Fulton & Baird, 2014). As an advanced practice nurse, the clinical nurse specialist, (CNS) uses clinical reasoning to address clinical problems within the nursing realm. Clinical reasoning

---

BOX 4.1 Adverse Drug Reactions: "Red Flags"

- Drowsiness
- Confusion/delirium
- Depressive symptoms
- Changes in speech or memory
- Changes in bowel or bladder function
- Insomnia
- Muscle weakness
- Falls or fractures
- Loss of appetite
- Parkinsonian symptoms (i.e., extrapyramidal effects)

Source: Guay, D. R. P. (n.d.). *Management of drug therapy* [classroom session]. University of Minnesota.

encompasses identifying etiologies appropriate for nursing interventions, choosing nursing interventions applicable for the identified problem, and evaluating the effectiveness of the intervention (Lyon, 2014). The CNS uses a holistic approach to identify problems, which are amenable to nursing interventions for optimal outcomes for the patient. The unique contribution of the CNS allows for a seamless integration of other healthcare disciplines while incorporating nursing interventions into the plan of care for patients to achieve wellness. This section reviews nonpharmacological interventions for several conditions.

Hypertension

- *Physical activity:* With or without weight loss has proven to reduce blood pressure
- *DASH (Dietary Approaches to Stop Hypertension) diet and reduction of salt intake:* There is a positive relationship between salt and blood pressure
- *Smoking cessation:* Leads to lower blood pressure and lower risk of cardiovascular disease
- *Alcohol can increase blood pressure:* Limiting alcohol consumption to 1 to 2 drinks a day is recommended (Helton, 2014)

Osteoporosis

- *Exercise:* Weight bearing and muscle strengthening increases bone density and decreases risk for falls by improving balance
- Calcium and vitamin D supplements
  - Without adequate calcium intake, the body will take calcium from bones.
  - Vitamin D helps the body absorb calcium and improves muscle function and balance.
- Fall prevention
  - Home safety evaluation
  - Evaluate gait and balance
  - Evaluate medication side effects
- Smoking cessation
- Limit alcohol consumption; 3 or more drinks per day can negatively impact bone (Nelson, 2014)

Pain

- *Acupuncture*—An ancient therapeutic technique involving insertion of needles into the body at specific locations to disrupt imbalances thought to influence symptoms and release opioid peptides.
- *Chiropractic*—This discipline focuses on supporting the body's own ability to heal itself without the use of drugs or surgery for pain (backache, neck ache, headache). Must be performed by a trained and licensed chiropractor provider.
- *Humor*—Humor is an important component of coping and has significant impact on an individual's spirituality, purpose, and meaning of life.
  - *Biologic effects:* Laughter boosts endorphins, which in turn may decrease the discomfort threshold in individuals.
- Massage therapy (Westman & Blaisdell, 2016)
  - Can be used for stress management, pain management, mobility, anxiety, and promote relaxation
  - *Types:* Compression, effleurage, friction, wringing, effleurage
  - *Contraindications:* Fractures, open wounds, burns, deep vein thrombosis
- Mindfulness (Day et al., 2014; Zeidan et al., 2012)
  - Associated with disruption of pain pathway and processing through cognitive reappraisal, emotional awareness, nonjudgmental consciousness, awareness of the transience of events, and acceptance.

- Heat and cold therapy (Zacharoff et al., 2010)
  - Can be used as an early treatment to acute injuries (first 24–48 hours)
    - *RICE:* Rest, ice, compression, elevation
    - May help with inflammation and edema
  - *Contraindications:* Impaired sensation, cognitive impairment, peripheral vascular disease, metastatic tumors, hypocoagulability
- Transcutaneous electrical stimulation—Uses low voltage electrical current for pain relief (Zacharoff et al., 2010)
  - Pain relief is effected through simulation of peripheral nerves to disrupt the nerve pathway.
  - Lack of rigorous randomized controlled trials to support efficacy and cost effectiveness (Rosenquist, 2019).
- Therapeutic exercise (Zacharoff et al., 2010)
  - Mobilizes and strengthens joints and muscles; increases balance and coordination.
  - Therapeutic exercise may be passive, active assisted, or active depending on the level of mobility.

Dementia: Behavior and Psychologic Symptoms

- *Occupational activities*—Geared toward patients' abilities, interests, roles. Increased self-efficacy and quality of life and reduced agitation and depression
- Music, aroma, and touch therapies—May reduce agitation and anxiety (Oliveira et al., 2015)

Delirium

- Assess, prevent, and manage pain
- Early mobilization
- Limit interruptions during sleep
- Family engagement (Marra et al., 2017; Rivosecchi et al., 2015)

Constipation

- *Bowel training*—Attempting to have a bowel movement 30 minutes after meals utilizes the gastrocolic reflex to facilitate evacuation; attempt to have a bowel movement first thing in the morning when the bowels are the most active.
- *Exercise*—A sedentary lifestyle or immobility increases risk for constipation.
- *Daily dietary fiber* <md>Ingest 25 to 30 g of bran, fruit, vegetables, nuts daily.
- *Hydration*—Keeping hydrated helps with GI motility (Hsieh, 2005; Toner & Claros, 2012).

Incontinence

- Fecal (Abrams et al., 2010)
  - *Diet*—High-fiber foods absorb fluid and add bulk. Determine trigger foods for allergies and/or intolerances and limit or eliminate from diet.
  - *Bowel training*—Use diet, scheduling, and enemas to assist with evacuation.
  - *Biofeedback*—This is a training mechanism to promote response to rectal distention.
- Urinary (Lukacz et al., 2011; MacLachlan & Rovner, 2015)
  - *Kegel exercises*—These strengthen the pelvic floor muscles; should be done a minimum of three times daily
  - *Bladder training*—This gradually lengthens the time between voiding while strengthening the pelvic floor and bladder muscles with Kegels
  - Diet
    - Avoiding caffeine, in any form, can increase the contractions of the detrusor muscle. This can cause increased pressure, leading to urgency and frequent urination.

■ Avoid bladder irritants.

■ Avoid artificial sweeteners, citrus drinks, and spicy foods because all can act as irritants to the bladder, resulting in overactive bladder and urge incontinence.

● Alcohol impacts the bladder as a diuretic

Insomnia

■ *Sleep diary*—Used to identify patterns and possible causes to sleep disturbances.

■ Promote sleep hygiene, sleep restriction, stimulus control, relaxation techniques.

■ *Diet*—Limit tobacco, caffeine, fluids, and heavy meals before bedtime (Touhy, 2016).

Anxiety

■ Nonpharmacologic interventions may be used alongside pharmacotherapy based on severity and response to treatment.

■ Encourage the use of

● Evidence-based thinking to combat catastrophizing events,

● Cognitive skills to increase problem solving,

● Time management and decision-making, and

● Progressive muscle relaxation to help combat tension.

■ *Mindfulness:* Focuses on learning how to be present in experiences and observe those experiences in a nonjudgmental manner (Craske, 2018).

Immobility, Gait Disturbance, and Falls

■ *Exercise*—Strengthening of the extensor groups has a positive impact on gait stability and endurance.

■ *Environmental assessment*—Well-lit areas and pathways clear of risks, such as wires or rugs, can improve the safety of patients with immobility or gait instability.

■ *Assistive devices*—Well-fitting shoes, walking cane, or walker can reduce pain on an affected limb or improve stability when ambulating (Alexander, 2014).

Depression

■ Nonpharmacologic interventions may be used alongside pharmacotherapy based on severity and response to treatment (Gaynes, 2019).

REVIEW QUESTIONS

1. Which of the following statements about nonpharmacologic care is accurate?

A. Symptoms will be relieved as much as possible.

B. Only physicians can order nonpharmacologic interventions.

C. All interventions will work the same for everyone.

D. There is no evidence to support nonpharmacologic interventions.

2. A 36-year-old patient with rheumatoid arthritis reports chronic pain despite the infliximab (Remicade) infusion therapy she receives. What is the clinical nurse specialist's (CNS's) most appropriate intervention?

A. Tell the patient to rest and avoid use of her joints.

B. Promote nonpharmacologic nursing interventions such as heat applications.

C. Start a ketogenic diet.

D. Recommend a nerve block.

ANSWERS

1. **Correct answer: A. Rationale:** Nonpharmacologic care provides symptom relief. However, not all interventions will provide the same amount of relief for everyone. Many nonpharmacologic interventions are well within the scope of nursing practice. There is an increasing body of evidence supporting the use of many types of nonpharmacologic interventions.

2. **Correct answer: B. Rationale:** The CNS is in the unique position to promote nonpharmacologic interventions such as heat, ice, exercise, and relaxation techniques. Avoiding use or immobility may decrease immediate pain but will contribute to worse long-term outcomes. Ketogenic diet and nerve blocks are not indicated for rheumatoid arthritis.

REFERENCES

The complete reference and additional reading lists appear in the digital version of this chapter, at https://connect.springerpub.com/content/book/978-0-8261-7417-8/part/part01/chapter/ch04

Substance Use and Addiction

Erica Newkirk

OVERVIEW

Substance abuse and addiction are becoming increasingly more prominent in the healthcare setting. The opioid epidemic has brought further attention to this patient population. It is important for adult-gerontology clinical nurse specialists to remain up to date on the many types of medications and treatments available for patients suffering from substance abuse or addiction.

Pathophysiology

Dopamine release creates a feeling of pleasure. Drug use stimulates the release of dopamine in higher doses than sex, food, and water. Repeated use of drugs causes the brain to decrease production of dopamine, resulting in the need to use more drug to stimulate the reward center (American Society of Addiction Medicine, 2011). Repeated drug use triggers neuroplastic changes in the midbrain dopamine neurons, enhancing the brain's response to drug cues, reducing sensitivity to nondrug rewards, weakening self-regulation, and increasing the sensitivity to stressful stimuli and depression (Volkow & Morales, 2015).

Definition

Addiction or substance use disorder is a chronic disease of the brain focusing on reward, motivation, and memory. It is characterized by inability to abstain, which results in impaired behavioral control and craving. The addict has diminished recognition of their own significant behavior problems and problems with interpersonal relationships. Like other chronic diseases, addiction often involves cycles of relapse and remission. Without treatment or engagement in recovery activities, addiction is progressive and may result in disability or premature death (American Society of Addiction Medicine, 2011).

Drug addiction is a chronic relapsing disease in which the use of drugs becomes the primary incentive that drives behavior regardless of consequence. As drug use becomes more compulsive, motivation for natural rewards that normally drive behavior decreases (Shippenberg et al., 2007). See Table 5.1 for information on commonly abused drugs.

ABCDE Characteristics of Addiction

a. Inability to consistently abstain
b. Impairment in behavioral control
c. Craving, or increased "hunger" for drugs or rewarding experiences
d. Diminished recognition of significant problems with one's behaviors and interpersonal relationships
e. A dysfunctional emotional response (American Society of Addict Medicine, 2011)

Terms

- *Tolerance* is the reduced response to a drug after repeated use. An increased dose of the drug is then required to achieve the same effect. Tolerance may not mean that one is addicted to the drug (National Institute of Drug Abuse, 2007).
- *Dependence* occurs when the brain adapts to repeated use of a drug. Physical dependence produces drug-specific withdrawal symptoms if the drug is stopped abruptly. Withdrawal may not mean one is addicted to the drug but may require further assessment. Tapering is recommended to decrease the experience of withdrawal symptoms (National Institute of Drug Abuse, 2007).
- *Withdrawal* is the experience of physical and mental symptoms that occur when long-term drug use is stopped (National Institute of Drug Abuse, 2007).

Assessment Tools

- *Withdrawal assessment*
  - The Clinical Opiate Withdrawal Scale (COWS) is an 11-item scale developed to rate the common signs and symptoms of opiate withdrawal (Wesson & Ling, 2003).
  - COWS assessment criteria:

Resting pulse rate	GI upset
Sweating	Tremor
Restlessness	Yawning
Pupil size	Anxiety or irritability
Bone or joint aches	Gooseflesh skin
Runny nose or tearing	

GI, gastrointestinal.

  - A copy of the COWS tool may be viewed online (www.drugabuse.gov/sites/default/files/files/ClinicalOpiateWithdrawalScale.pdf).
- *Substance and alcohol use disorder assessment*
  - The UNCOPE (**u**sed, **n**eglected, **c**ut down, **o**bjected, **p**reoccupied, **e**motional discomfort) tool is a six-item screen identifying alcohol and/or drug dependence (Hoffmann et al., 2003).
  - CAGE (**c**ut down, **a**nnoyed, **g**uilty, and **e**ye opener) is a set of four questions used to detect possible alcohol use disorder (Substance Abuse and Mental Health Services Administration, 2014).

Interventions for Substance and Alcohol Use Disorders

- *Screening, Brief Intervention, and Referral to Treatment (SBIRT)* is an evidence-based early intervention method

---

The complete reference list appears in the digital version of this chapter, at https://connect.springerpub.com/content/book/978-0-8261-7417-8/part/part01/chapter/ch05

TABLE 5.1 COMMONLY ABUSED DRUGS

DRUG	CLASS	DRUG ONSET/DURATION	SIDE EFFECTS	WITHDRAWAL SYMPTOMS
Marijuana (Cannabis, Mary Jane, weed, hash, pot)	Analgesics, herbal	Onset: Within seconds to minutes if smoked, 30–90 minutes if ingested. Duration: Smoke inhalation 2–3 hours; ingestion 4–12 hours depending on dose	Euphoria, relaxation, sleepiness, dry mouth, red eyes, impaired motor skills and/or perception, poor memory, increased appetite	Lasts 1–2 weeks; GI upset, night sweats, irritability, anxiety, restlessness, disturbed sleep, decreased appetite
Opioids (Hydrocodone/Norco; morphine; Suboxone; oxycodone-acetaminophen/Percocet; hydrocodone-acetaminophen/Vicodin; fentanyl, methadone; hydromorphne/Dilaudid; tramadol)	Opioids	Onset: PO 30–60 minutes; topical: 12–16 hours. Duration: PO: 3–4 hours; topical: 48–72 hours; IV: morphine solution = 3–4 hours, Dilaudid = 2–3 hours, fentanyl = 30 minutes–1 hour	Pain relief, drowsiness, nausea, constipation, euphoria, confusion, slowed breathing, death	Long acting: 12–48 hours after last dose; lasts 10–20 days. Short acting: 8–24 hours after last dose; lasts 4–10 days. Restlessness, muscle/bone pain, insomnia, diarrhea, vomiting, cold flashes/goose bumps, leg movements. Serotonin syndrome can occur with overdose
Cocaine (crack, coke)	Anesthetic	Onset: Seconds for IV or smoked;1–5 minutes if snorted. Peak: 5–10 minutes for IV/smoke; 1 hour if snorted. Duration: 1–1.5 hours	Increased HR, BP, and pupil dilation; decrease in skin temperature and heat perception along with impairment of sweating and skin blood flow; adverse cardiovascular events	Crash occurs a few hours after last dose; peaks after about 24 hours; fatigue, apathy, depression, anxiety, chills, body aches, pain, exhaustion, difficulty concentrating, inability to feel pleasure
Heroin (dope, smack)	Opioid	Onset: <1 minute. Peak: 10–30 minutes. Duration: 3–5 hours	Decreased breathing and HR, itching, nausea, vomiting, coma, death	Occurs 4–76 hours after last dose (average 21 hours); yawning, runny nose, panic, chills, lacrimation, restlessness, muscle and bone pain, insomnia, diarrhea, vomiting, cold flashes with goose bumps, leg movements
Amphetamine/methamphetamine (meth, speed, crystal)	Stimulants	Onset: Varies between routes, but usually within a few minutes. Peak: varies. Duration: 2–8 hours	Increased breathing, HR, BP, temperature; irregular heart beat	Occurs 24 hours after the last dose, lasts 7–10 days; subacute lasts about 3 weeks; depression, anxiety, tiredness
Nicotine	Stimulant	Onset: Within a few minutes	Increased HR, increased BP and weight loss; alertness, heartburn, peptic ulcer disease, dizziness, headache	Peaks in 3 days and lasts about 2 weeks; tingling in the hands and feet, sweating, headaches, irritability, difficultly concentrating

(continued)

TABLE 5.1 COMMONLY ABUSED DRUGS (*continued*)

DRUG	CLASS	DRUG ONSET/ DURATION	SIDE EFFECTS	WITHDRAWAL SYMPTOMS
Alcohol	Depressant	Varies depending on weight and amount consumed	Slurred speech, drowsiness, vomiting, diarrhea, upset stomach, headaches, breathing difficulties, distorted vision and hearing, impaired judgment, decreased perception and coordination, unconsciousness, coma, blackouts	Occurs 6–12 hours after last drink; withdrawal seizures occur between 24 and 48 hours after last drink; DTs usually begin between 48 and 72 hours after drinking has stopped; tremors, anxiety, nausea, vomiting, headache, increased HR, sweating, irritability, confusion, insomnia, nightmares, fever, hallucination
Synthetic cathinones ("bath salts")	Unregulated psychoactive substance	Onset: 15 minutes Duration: 4–6 hours	Increased HR, BP; euphoria; paranoia, agitation, hallucinations; psychotic/violent behavior; nosebleeds; sweating; nausea, vomiting; insomnia; irritability; dizziness; depression; suicidal thoughts; panic; reduced motor control	Depression, anxiety, tremors, paranoia, problems sleeping
Amphetamine (Adderall) **Methylphenidate** (Ritalin)	ADHA agents, stimulants	Immediate-release tablet: Onset: 30–60 minutes Peak: 1–2 hours Duration: 4–6 hours; for extended release capsule: onset: 30–60 minutes and 4 hours; later duration: 10–12 hours	Increased alertness, attention, energy; increased BP and HR; narrowed blood vessels; increased blood sugar; dilated breathing passages. High doses: dangerously high body temperature and irregular heartbeat, heart failure, seizures	Depression, tiredness, sleep problems
Alprazolam (Xanax) **Diazepam** (Valium) **Chlordiazepoxide** (Librium) **Clonazepam** (Klonopin) **Lorazepam** (Ativan)	Benzodiazepine, anxiolytic	Onset: 30 minutes Peak: 1–2 hours Duration: 2–6 hours	Drowsiness, slurred speech, poor concentration, confusion, dizziness, problems with movement and memory, lowered BP, slowed breathing	Insomnia, restlessness, disturbing dreams, feelings of tension, tachypnea, tachycardia, tremulousness, hyperreflexia, confusion, seizures
Zolpidem (Ambien) **Eszopiclone** (Lunesta) **Pentobarbital** (Nembutal) **Zaleplon** (Sonata)	Sedative, hypnotic	Onset: <30 minutes Duration: 4–8 hours	Drowsiness, slurred speech, poor concentration, confusion, dizziness, problems with movement and memory, lowered BP, slowed breathing	Insomnia, restlessness, disturbing dreams, feelings of tension, tachypnea, tachycardia, tremulousness, hyperreflexia, confusion, seizures

ADHA, attention deficit hyperactivity disorder; BP, blood pressure; DTs, delirium tremens; GI, gastrointestinal; HR, heart rate; IV, intravenous.
Sources: From National Institute of Drug Abuse. (2007, January). *National Institute on Drug Abuse.* www.drugabuse.gov; www.drugabuse.gov; National Institute of Drug Abuse. (2018, July). *National Institute of Drug Abuse.* www.drugabuse.gov; https://www.drugabuse.gov/drugs-abuse/commonly-abused-drugs-charts#Dextromethorphan

recommended by the U.S. Department of Health and Human Services, Substance Abuse and Mental Health Services Administration (SAMHSA). SBIRT is used to identify, reduce, and prevent problematic use, abuse, and dependence on alcohol and illicit drugs. SBIRT consists of three parts: screening, brief intervention, and referral to treatment (Substance Abuse and Mental Health Service Administration, n.d.). The

following assessment tools may be used for the screening phase of SBIRT:

● The Alcohol Use Disorders Identification Test (AUDIT-10) is a 10-item tool designed to assess alcohol intake, drinking behaviors, and alcohol-related problems (National Institute of Alcohol Abuse and Alcoholism, 2005).

- The Drug Abuse Screening Test (DAST) is a self-report tool with 10 or 20 items developed to identify individuals who are abusing drugs and to assess the degree of problems related to drug use (Substance Abuse and Mental Health Services Administration, 2014).
  - 12-step programs for addiction recovery are self-help groups that can complement and prolong the effects of professional treatment and medical management. The most well-known self-help groups are those affiliated with Alcoholics Anonymous (AA), Narcotics Anonymous (NA), and Cocaine Anonymous (CA), all of which are based on the 12-step model (National Institute of Drug Abuse, 2007).

Medication-Assisted Treatment

Medication-assisted treatment (MAT) is the use of Food and Drug Administration (FDA)-approved medications, in combination with counseling and behavioral therapies, for the treatment of substance use disorders (Table 5.2). MAT is frequently used for the treatment of addiction to heroin and prescription pain relievers that contain opiates. The purpose of MAT is to normalize brain chemistry, block the euphoric effects of alcohol and opioids, relieve physiologic cravings, and normalize body functions without the negative effects of the abused drug (U.S. Department of Health and Human Services, 2015).

TABLE 5.2 MEDICATION-ASSISTED TREATMENT

MEDICATION	CLASS	MECHANISM OF ACTION	INDICATIONS AND CONTRAINDICATIONS	DOSAGE	SIDE EFFECTS	SAFETY/PATIENT EDUCATION
Acamprosate (Campral)	Psychiatric agent	Not fully understood; may interact with glutamate and GABA neurotransmitter	Decreases the craving for alcohol/renal impairment	Oral: 666 mg PO TID	Diarrhea, anxiety, insomnia	Does not diminish withdrawal symptoms, assess for suicidal tendencies
Naltrexone (Vivitrol, Re-Via, Depade)	Opioid antagonists	Opioid competitive receptor	Prevent relapse after opioid detoxification/liver failure, acute hepatitis and precautions for other hepatic disease	Oral: 50–100 mg/d Intramuscular: 380 mg/mo	Dizziness, nausea, vomiting, injection site reaction, headache, decreased appetite	Assess for depression and suicide. Patients should be opioid free for at least 7–10 days before use
Disulfiram (Antabuse)	Alcohol deterrent	Produces a sensitivity to ETOH resulting in unpleasant reactions, including palpitations, chest pain, nausea, vertigo, and thirst	Expectation or experience of an adverse response to alcohol consumption; severe myocardial diseases, psychoses, liver failure, hypersensitivity to thiuram derivatives	Oral: 250–500 mg/d	Drowsiness, nausea, dizziness, metallic or garlic taste in mouth	Do not use any alcohol-containing products, never give to a patient who is intoxicated
Naloxone (Narcan)	Opioid reversal agent	Competitive opioid antagonist	Abrupt opioid reversal/known hypersensitivity	Injection: 0.4 mg/mL Inhalation: 2 mg	Abrupt opioid reversal, withdrawal reaction precipitated	Caution in patients with history of seizures, observe patients until there is no further risk of recurrent respiratory depression
Buprenorphine/naloxone (Suboxone)	Opioid antagonist	Binds to opioid receptors	Treatment of opioid dependence/use with caution with concurrent use of the central nervous system depressants	Sublingual: 2–12 mg	Headache, withdrawal syndrome, insomnia, pain, nausea, diarrhea	Respiratory depression

(continued)

TABLE 5.2 MEDICATION-ASSISTED TREATMENT *(continued)*

MEDICATION	CLASS	MECHANISM OF ACTION	INDICATIONS AND CONTRAIN-DICATIONS	DOSAGE	SIDE EFFECTS	SAFETY/ PATIENT EDUCATION
Methadone	Opioid analgesic	Narcotic agonist-analgesic receptors; inhibits ascending pathway, altering the response to pain	It is the only drug used in MAT approved for women who are pregnant or breastfeeding	Injection: 10 mg/mL Oral: 5–40 mg (many factors should be accounted for when dosing)	Agitation, anticholinergic, bradycardia	Risk of opioid addiction, abuse, and misuse, which can lead to overdose and death

ETOH, ethyl alcohol; GABA, gamma-aminobutyric acid; MAT, medication-assisted treatment.
Sources: From National Institute of Drug Abuse. (1994–2019). OUD treatments and practice guidelines 2015. *Medscape.* Medscape.com. https://reference.medscape.com/drugs; National Institute of Drug Abuse. (2007, January). *Drugs and diseases 2007.* National Institute on Drug Abuse. www.drugabuse.gov; www.drugabuse.gov; U.S. Department of Health and Human Services. (2015, September 28). *Providers clinical support system.* Substance Abuse and Mental Health Services Administration. www.samhsa.gov; https://www.samhsa.gov/medication-assisted-treatment/treatment

REVIEW QUESTIONS

1. The CNS (clinical nurse specialist) is seeing a 20-year-old female student at the university health clinic who is interested in oral contraception. The CNS conducts a health history, during which the patient admits to drinking at least 2 nights a week, consuming four to six beers per occasion. The most appropriate evidenced-based intervention approach at this time related to alcohol consumption would be which of the following?
   A. CAGE
   B. COWS
   C. SBIRT
   D. UNCOPE

2. The CNS (clinical nurse specialist) is seeing a heroin-addicted patient on medication-assisted treatment (MAT) for a follow-up visit. The patient is taking naltrexone. Which potential MAT-related problem should be addressed during this visit?
   A. Bradycardia
   B. Metallic taste in mouth
   C. Vitamin deficiency
   D. Suicidal thoughts and depression

ANSWERS

1. **Correct answer: C. Rationale:** High-risk drinking for females is defined as more than seven drinks per week or more than three drinks per occasion. Screening, Brief Intervention, and Referral to Treatment (SBIRT) is an evidence-based early-intervention method recommended by the U.S. Department of Health and Human Services, Substance Abuse and Mental Health Services Administration (SAMHSA). SBIRT is designed for use by any practitioner in any healthcare setting. SBIRT is used to identify, reduce, and prevent problematic use, abuse, and dependence on alcohol and illicit drugs. SBIRT consists of three parts: screening, brief intervention, and referral to treatment. CAGE, COWS, and UNCOPE are individual assessment tools rather than evidence-based early-intervention approach methods.

2. **Correct answer: D. Rationale:** Assess for depression and suicide risk. Naltrexone side effects include depression and thoughts of suicide. Bradycardia is a side effect of methadone. Metallic taste is a side effect of disulfiram. Vitamin deficiency is not associated with MAT.

REFERENCES

The complete reference list appears in the digital version of this chapter, at https://connect.springerpub.com/content/book/978-0-8261-7417-8/part/part01/chapter/ch05

6

Cardiovascular System

Diane M. Doty, Elsie A. Jolade, Jose Chavez, Jackeline Iseler, Sarah Pandullo, Mechelle Peck, Jessica Green, Racheal L. Wood, and Earlie Hale

CARDIOVASCULAR PATHOPHYSIOLOGY

OVERVIEW

The cardiovascular system is composed of the heart, blood vessels, lymphatic system, and blood. The main function of the cardiovascular or circulatory system is transport. The circulatory system transports and distributes oxygen and nutrients needed for metabolic processes to the tissues, carries waste products from cellular metabolism to the kidneys and other excretory organs for elimination, and circulates fluids, electrolytes, and hormones needed to regulate body function (McCance & Huether, 2014; Porth & Gaspard, 2015).

Heart

The heart (Figure 6.1) is a four-chambered muscular organ that pumps blood throughout the body.

- The right side of the heart (Porth & Gaspard, 2015):
  - Is composed of the right atrium and right ventricle (RV).
  - Pumps blood through the lungs (pulmonary circulation).
  - Delivers blood to the lungs for oxygenation.
  - Is a low-pressure system.
- The left side of the heart (Porth & Gaspard, 2015):
  - Is composed of the left atrium and left ventricle (LV).
  - Pumps oxygenated blood through the systemic circulation.
  - Delivers metabolic waste products to the lungs, kidneys, and liver.
  - Is a high-pressure system.

The heart wall has three layers (McCance & Huether, 2014; Porth & Gaspard, 2015; Story, 2018):

- *Epicardium:* Outer smooth layer
- *Myocardium:* Thickest layer of cardiac muscle, forming the walls of the atria and ventricles
- *Endocardium:* Innermost epithelial lining of the heart composed of connective tissue and a layer of squamous cells

Pericardium (McCance & Huether, 2014; Porth & Gaspard, 2015):

- A double-walled membranous sac that wraps around the heart
  - *Parietal:* Surface layer
  - *Visceral:* Inner layer
- Pericardial cavity (McCance & Huether, 2014; Porth & Gaspard, 2015):
  - Space between the parietal and visceral layers
  - Contains pericardial fluid (approximately 20 mL); the amount and character of the pericardial fluid are altered if the pericardium is inflamed

Fluids in the pericardial sac lubricate the outer wall of the heart so it can beat without causing friction, form a barrier against infections, and help keep the heart from overexpanding.

Valves of the Heart

One-way blood flow through the heart is ensured by the four heart valves (McCance & Huether, 2014; Porth & Gaspard, 2015; Story, 2018):

- Atrioventricular valves (AVs) are valves located between the atrium and the ventricles:
  - Blood flows one way from the atria to the ventricles.
  - Tricuspid valve on the right side of the heart has three leaflets or cusps.
  - Bicuspid (mitral) valve on the left side of the heart has two leaflets or cusps.
- Semilunar valves have three cuplike cusps that are attached to the valve rings. These are located between the great vessels and the ventricles:
  - One-way flow from the ventricles to either the pulmonary artery (PA) or the aorta

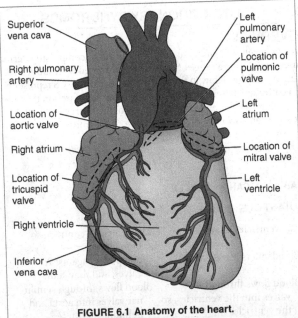

FIGURE 6.1 Anatomy of the heart.

Source: From Gawlik, K. S., Melnyk, B. M., & Teall, A. M. (2021). *Evidence-based physical examination: Best practices for health and well-being assessment.* Springer Publishing Company.

The complete reference and additional reading lists appear in the digital version of this chapter, at https://connect.springerpub.com/content/book/978-0-8261-7417-8/part/part01/chapter/ch06

- Pulmonic semilunar valve
- Aortic semilunar valve

The Great Vessels

Blood moves in and out of the heart through several large vessels (McCance & Huether, 2014; Porth & Gaspard, 2015; Story, 2018):

- Superior vena cava and inferior vena cava are two large veins that take blood from the rest of the body into the right atrium.
- The PA is a major blood vessel and connects to the RV.
- The RV pumps blood into the PA, which carries deoxygenated blood to the lungs.
- Pulmonary veins take oxygenated blood from the lungs to the left atrium.
- The aorta is the largest artery in the body and connects to the LV. The LV pumps blood into the aorta, which then carries it to the rest of the body.
- The aorta delivers oxygenated blood to systemic vessels that supply the body.
- Capillaries help exchange fluids between the blood and the interstitial space (McCance & Huether, 2014; Porth & Gaspard, 2015; Story, 2018).

The Coronary Vessels

- Coronary circulation supplies oxygen and other nutrients to the myocardium.
- The coronary arteries originate just beyond the aortic semilunar valve cusps and receive blood through the coronary ostia. The main branches are as follows:
  - Right coronary artery (RCA)
    - Conus artery—A small early branch off the RCA circulation
    - Right marginal branch
    - Posterior descending branch
  - Left coronary artery (LCA)
    - Left anterior descending (LAD) artery (or anterior interventricular artery)
    - Circumflex artery
- The coronary arteries are smaller in women because women's hearts weigh proportionately less than men's hearts.
- Coronary lymphatic vessels drain fluid to the paratracheal lymph nodes (Hanna, 2017; McCance & Huether, 2014; Story, 2018).

Collateral Circulation

When normal coronary circulation is impaired, new blood vessels develop under high pressure when normal coronary circulation is impaired to deliver adequate blood supply to the heart:

- Protects the heart from ischemia

Regulation of Blood Pressure

- *Vascular compliance* refers to the increase in volume a vessel is able to accommodate for a given increase in pressure; veins are more compliant than arteries (Hanna, 2017; McCance & Huether, 2014; Porth & Gaspard, 2015; Story, 2018)
- Arterial pressure (Hanna, 2017; McCance & Huether, 2014; Porth & Gaspard, 2015; Story, 2018; Table 6.1):
  - Mean arterial pressure (MAP) is the average pressure in the arteries throughout the cardiac cycle. It's calculated by using systolic blood pressure (SBP) and diastolic blood pressure (DBP) in the formula:

$$MAP = \frac{SBP + 2(DBP)}{3}$$

Example: BP = 120/80

$$MAP = \frac{120 + 160}{3} \quad MAP = 93$$

- Pulse pressure is the difference between systolic and diastolic pressures.
- Effects of total peripheral resistance (TPR) are primarily a function of the diameter of the arterioles (Table 6.1).
- Effects of cardiac output (CO):
  - CO can be changed by alterations in heart rate (HR), stroke volume (SV), or both.
- Neural control of resistance:
  - Baroreceptors:
    - Reduce blood pressure to normal by decreasing CO and peripheral resistance.
    - Can also increase blood pressure when needed.
  - Arterial receptors: chemoreceptors:
    - Are sensitive to oxygen, carbon dioxide, or pH.
    - Regulate blood pressure.
- Venous pressure (Hanna, 2017; McCance & Huether, 2014; Porth & Gaspard, 2015; Story, 2018):
  - Main determinants are the volume of fluid in the veins and compliance (distensibility) of the vessel walls.
- Coronary perfusion pressure is the difference between pressure in the aorta and pressure in the coronary vessels.
- Myoglobin in the heart muscle stores oxygen for use during the systolic phase.

ACUTE CORONARY SYNDROMES

OVERVIEW

Acute coronary syndrome (ACS) is an all-encompassing term used to describe a range of conditions associated with sudden reduction of blood flow to the heart (Hanna, 2017). ACS represents an entire spectrum of events from ischemia to infarction that occur at the cellular and muscular levels of the heart (Story, 2018):

- Sudden coronary obstruction due to thrombosis formation over a ruptured atherosclerotic plaque

TABLE 6.1 CARDIAC CYCLE

DIASTOLE	SYSTOLE
The ventricles relax.	The ventricles contract, so blood leaves.
Blood enters the atria.	Blood pushes against AV valves, and they shut.
Blood flows through AV valves into the ventricles, so the ventricles fill.	Blood flows through semilunar valves into aorta and pulmonary trunk.

AV, atrioventricular.

Sources: Hanna, E. B. (2017). *Practical cardiovascular medicine.* https://ebookcentral.proquest.com; McCance, K., & Huether, S. (2014). *Pathophysiology: The biologic basis for disease in adults and children* (7th ed.). Mosby; Story, L. (2018). *Pathophysiology: A practical approach* (3rd ed.). Jones & Bartlett.

- Unstable angina occurs due to partial occlusion of coronary artery.
  - *Myocardial infarction (MI)* refers to myocardial ischemia, injury, or necrosis from reduced coronary blood flow.
- Most common complications:
  - Dysrhythmias, congestive heart failure, and sudden death
Signs and symptoms of ACS are (Hanna, 2017; Porth & Gaspard, 2015; Story, 2018):
- Angina or chest discomfort, which is described as aching, pressure, tightness, or burning
- Pain radiating from the chest to shoulders, arms, upper abdomen, back, neck, or jaw
- Nausea or vomiting
- Indigestion
- Dyspnea
- Diaphoresis
- Lightheadedness, dizziness, or fainting
- Unusual or unexplained fatigue
- Restlessness or apprehension
Women are more likely to have vague signs and symptoms, such as back pain, fatigue, nausea, and vomiting, without chest pain or discomfort (Hanna, 2017; Story, 2018).

Angina
- Partial occlusion of coronary artery (Hanna, 2017; McCance & Huether, 2014; Story, 2018)
- Occurs when myocardial oxygen demand exceeds oxygen supply
- A reversible myocardial ischemia and an indication of impending infarction
- Transient episodes of thrombotic vessel occlusion and vasoconstriction occur at the site of plaque damage with a return of perfusion before significant myocardial necrosis occurs:
  - *Stable*—Occlusion with exertion or other precipitating event
  - *Unstable*—Occurs at rest
  - *Vasospastic*—Not related to activity; often at night
- Treatment (Hanna, 2017; McCance & Huether, 2014; Porth & Gaspard, 2015; Story, 2018):
  - Hospitalization with the administration of nitrates, antithrombotics, and anticoagulants if ACS, but not if stable angina or spasms like prinzmetal angina (Table 6.2)
  - Beta blockers and angiotensin-converting enzyme (ACE) inhibitors

Myocardial Infarction
- A complete occlusion of a coronary artery (Hanna, 2017; McCance & Huether, 2014; Story, 2018)
- Myocardial damage or necrosis due to ischemia from atherosclerotic disease of coronary arteries
- Prolonged ischemia causes irreversible damage to the heart muscle (myocyte necrosis):
  - Cellular injury, leading to cellular death

Types of MI
The two main types are subendocardial and transmural infarction (Hanna, 2017; McCance & Huether, 2014; Story, 2018):
- Individuals with ST segment elevations myocardial infarction (STEMI) on the EKG are at highest risk for complications and require immediate intervention.
- Smaller infarctions are not associated with non-ST segment elevations myocardial infarction (non-STEMI or NSTEMI):
  - Suggest that additional myocardium is still at risk for recurrent ischemia and infarction

- Clinical manifestations:
  - Infarcted myocardium is surrounded by a zone of hypoxic injury, which may progress to necrosis or return to normal; adjacent to this zone is a zone of reversible ischemia (Hanna, 2017; McCance & Huether, 2014; Porth & Gaspard, 2015; Story, 2018).
  - Sudden severe chest pain develops.
  - Some patients may present with hyperglycemia.

Diagnosis
- EKG changes with ST segment elevation as well as T wave abnormalities (Hanna, 2017; McCance & Huether, 2014; Porth & Gaspard, 2015; Story, 2018).
- Troponin I, troponin T: High specificity—troponin markers rise within 3 hours after onset of MI and can remain elevated for 7 to 10 days after injury.
- Creatine phosphokinase-myocardial band (CPK-MB):
  - Specific for myocardial injury; can exceed normal ranges within 4 to 8 hours and decline to normal within 2 to 3 days.
  - Is not specific to cardiac cell death.

Treatment
- Hospitalization
- Immediate administration of aspirin (160–325 mg; see also Table 6.3)
- Administer supplemental oxygen if arterial saturation is <90%, patient is in respiratory distress, history of heart failure (HF), or high risk for hypoxia
- Nitroglycerin
- Morphine sulfate if discomfort not relieved by nitroglycerin
- Bed rest
- Cardiac medications: thrombolytic, antithrombotic, vasodilators
- Percutaneous coronary intervention (PCI)
- Surgery
Cardiac cells do not regenerate and can survive a short time of ischemia before permanent cell death occurs. In the case of an MI, quick diagnosis and treatment can save heart muscle (Hanna, 2017; McCance & Huether, 2014; Porth & Gaspard, 2015; Story, 2018).

Complications
- Dysrhythmias
- HF
- Cardiogenic shock
- Pericarditis
- Ventricular aneurysm

Cardiac Conduction System
Heart muscle contains its own specialized cells that enable it to generate and transmit action potentials without input from the nervous system. The conduction system consists of (Figure 6.2; McCance & Huether, 2014):
- The sinoatrial (SA) node:
  - Pacemaker of the heart
  - Intranodal pathways
- AV node
- Bundle of His (AV bundle)
- Right and left bundle branches
- Purkinje fibers
- Ventricular myocardium

TABLE 6.2 ANTICOAGULANTS

MEDICATION: GENERIC NAME (BRAND NAME)	CLASSIFICATION: PHARMACOTHERAPEUTIC AND CLINICAL	MECHANISM OF ACTION: THERAPEUTIC	INDICATIONS AND CONTRAINDICATIONS	DOSAGE	ADVERSE EFFECTS	SAFETY AND PATIENT EDUCATION
A. COUMADIN						
Warfarin (Coumadin)	**Pharmacotherapeutic:** Vitamin K antagonist **Clinical:** Anticoagulant	Prevents further extension of existing clots, prevents new clot formation, secondary thromboembolic complications.	**Indications:** Prophylaxis, treatment of thromboembolic disorders and embolic complications arising from atrial fibrillation or valve replacement. Risk reduction of systemic embolism following MI. **Contraindications:** Hemorrhagic tendencies, recent or potential surgery of eye or central nervous system, neurosurgical procedures, open wounds, severe uncontrolled or malignant hypertension, spinal puncture procedures, uncontrolled bleeding, ulcers, unreliable or noncompliant patients, unsupervised patients, blood dyscrasias, pericarditis, or pericardial effusion, pregnancy; major regional lumbar block anesthesia or traumatic surgery, eclampsia/preeclampsia.	Dosing must be individualized with close monitoring of INR. Initially, 2–5 mg/d for 2 days OR 5–10 mg/d for 1–2 days, adjusting dose based on INR. Maintenance dose: 2–10 mg/d but may vary based on INR. Maximum: 10 mg/d. Dose should be verified by a second person prior to administration.	Bleeding complications, hepatotoxicity, blood dyscrasias, necrosis, vasculitis, local thrombosis occurs rarely. **ANTIDOTE:** Vitamin K. Amount based on INR, significance of bleeding. Range: 2.5–10 mg PO or slow IV infusion (refer to med reference for dose).	Obtain baseline and periodic CBC, PT/INR, monitor diligently. Screen and monitor for active bleeding, history of bleeding, recent bleeding, trauma, surgery or epidural anesthesia. Monitor for urine/stool occult blood, c/o of back or abdomen. Pain, severe h/a, confusion, aphasia, signs of bleeding. Patient should take precautions to avoid bleeding/bruising and immediately report any bleeding. Take medication at same time daily. Blood levels need to be monitored routinely. Do not take or d/c any other med except as prescribed by provider. Avoid alcohol, aspirin, drastic dietary changes. Consult with provider before surgery, dental work. Urine may become red-orange.

(continued)

B. HEPARIN, LOW-MOLECULAR WEIGHT HEPARINS

Drug	Pharmacotherapeutic/Clinical	Action	Indications/Contraindications	Dosage	Complications/Antidote	Nursing Implications
Enoxaparin (Lovenox)	**Pharmacotherapeutic:** Low-molecular weight heparin **Clinical:** Anticoagulant	Produces anticoagulation. Does not significantly influence PT, aPTT.	**Indications:** DVT prophylaxis hip or knee replacement surgery, abdominal surgery, or patients with severely restricted mobility during acute illness. Treatment of ACS, unstable angina, non-Q-wave MI, acute STEMI. Treatment of DVT with or without PE; without PE. **Contraindications:** Active major bleeding, concurrent heparin therapy, hypersensitivity to heparin, pork products, thrombocytopenia associated with positive in vitro test for antiplatelet antibodies.	**Prevention of long-term DVT in nonsurgical acute illness:** SQ: 40 mg once daily, continue until risk of DVT diminishes (usually 6–11 days). **Acute DVT (inpatient):** SQ: 1 mg/kg q12h or 1.5 mg/kg once daily (outpatient) 1 mg/kg q12h. **Refer to Kizior and Hodgson (2019) for surgically indicated or STEMI dosages.**	Bleeding complications HIT **ANTIDOTE:** IV injection of protamine sulfate (1% solution) equals dose of enoxaparin injected. One additional dose of 0.5 mg protamine sulfate per 1 mg enoxaparin may be given if aPTT tested 2–4 hours after first injection remains prolonged.	Receive full medical, surgical history for precautions. Ensure patient has not received spinal anesthesia or procedures. Assess for potential risk of or for active bleeding. Baseline and ongoing labs: CBC, platelet count, stool occult blood. Ensure active hemostasis of puncture sites following PCI. Assess for signs of bleeding. Educate patient on preparation and administration of medication. Do not discontinue current blood-thinning regimen or take any new prescribed medications unless approved by provider who started therapy. Suddenly stopping therapy may increase risk of blood clots or stroke. Report bleeding of any kind. If bleeding occurs, may take longer to stop. Immediately report signs of stroke. Minor blunt-force trauma may be life-threatening. Consult provider for any surgery/dental work.
Heparin	**Pharmacotherapeutic:** Blood modifier **Clinical:** Anticoagulant	Prevents further extension of existing thrombi or new clot formation. No effect on existing clots.	**Indications:** TE disorder and complication prophylaxis and treatment associated with atrial fibrillation. **Contraindications:** Severe thrombocytopenia, uncontrolled active bleeding (unless secondary to DIC), history of HIT, HITT, or patients who test positive for HIT antibody.	**ACS, IV infusion:** 60 units/kg bolus (maximum 4k units), then 12 units/kg/hr (maximum 1,000 units/hr). **DVT/PE IV infusion:** 80 units/kg bolus (maximum 5,000 units), then 18 units/kg/hr adjusted according to aPTT.	Bleeding complications occur more frequently in high-dose therapy, intermittent IV infusion, women 60 years and older. HIT may cause life-threatening TE.	Do not give by IM injection. Dose should be cross-checked before administration. Obtain baseline and ongoing CBC, PT/INR, aPTT per local protocol. Assess for bleeding risk. Ask about history of recent trauma, head injuries, GI/GU bleeding. Ensure patient has not received spinal anesthesia, spinal procedures.

(continued)

TABLE 6.2 ANTICOAGULANTS (continued)

MEDICATION: GENERIC NAME (BRAND NAME)	CLASSIFICATION: PHARMACOTHER- APEUTIC AND CLINICAL	MECHANISM OF ACTION: THERAPEUTIC	INDICATIONS AND CONTRAINDICATIONS	DOSAGE	ADVERSE EFFECTS	SAFETY AND PATIENT EDUCATION
				TE prophylaxis: SQ: 5,000 units q8–12h.	**ANTIDOTE:** Protamine sulfate 1–1.5 mg IV for every 100 units heparin SQ within 30 minutes of overdose, 0.5–0.75 mg for every 100 units heparin SQ if within 30–60 minutes of overdose, 0.25–0.375 mg for every 100 units heparin SQ if 2 hours have elapsed since overdose, 25–50 mg if heparin was given by IV infusion.	Diligently assess for bleeding. If platelet count decreases more than 50% from baseline, obtain stat HIT antibody test. If HIT antibody positive, discontinue heparin and consider treatment with direct thrombin inhibitor. Avoid IM injections due to potential for hematomas. When converting to warfarin therapy, monitor PT/INR results (will be 10%–20% higher while heparin is given concurrently). Educate patient on bleeding precautions (electric razor, soft toothbrush); patient should report signs of bleeding immediately. Do not use any OTC meds without provider approval. Wear or carry identification that notes anticoagulant therapy. Inform dentist, other providers of heparin therapy. Limit alcohol.
C. DIRECT THROMBIN INHIBITORS						
Bivalirudin (Angiomax)	**Pharmacotherapeutic:** Thrombin inhibitor **Clinical:** Anticoagulant	Decreases acute myocardial ischemic complications in patients with unstable angina pectoris.	**Indications:** Patients with unstable angina undergoing PTCA. Tx or px of HIT in patients undergoing PTCA. **Contraindications:** Hypersensitivity to bivalirudin. Active major bleeding.	**Unstable angina undergoing PTCA:** 0.75 mg/kg IV, then 1.75 mg/kg/hr during procedure. **HIT treatment or px in patients undergoing PTCA:** 0.75 mg/kg IV bolus, then 1.75 mg/kg/hr during procedure; may continue for up to 4 hours, then 0.2 mg/kg/hr for up to 20 hours if needed.	Fever, bleeding, h/a, hypotension, thrombocytopenia	Obtain baseline and periodic CBC, PT/INR, aPTT, renal function. Monitor for bleeding.

(continued)

Drug	Action	Indications	Dosage	Side Effects	Nursing Considerations
Dabigatran (Pradaxa)	Produces anticoagulation, preventing development of thrombus	of DVT, PE, stroke, systemic embolism in patients with atrial fibrillation. Px of DVT and PE post hip replacement surgery. **Contraindications:** Active major bleeding, patients with mechanical prosthetic heart valves.	**and prevention:** 150 mg PO BID (after 5–10 days treatment with parenteral anticoagulants) **Nonvalvular A-Fib:** 150 mg PO BID **Px following hip surgery:** 110 mg PO on day one (1–4 hours postoperative and established hemostasis), then 220 mg daily for up to 35 days.	fatal, hemorrhagic events may occur. Hypersensitivity reactions, including anaphylaxis, reported in less than 1% of patients.	CBC, platelet count, renal function test, PT, aPTT. Question hx of mechanical heart valve, recent surgery, hepatic, renal impairment, recent spinal, epidural procedures. Receive full medication and medical/surgical history. Monitor for bleeding. Patients should report signs of bleeding. Keep in original container. Once bottle is opened, must be used within 60 days. Report any difficulty speaking, h/a, paralysis, vision changes, seizures.
Argatroban	Produces anticoagulation.	**Indications:** Px or treatment of pts with HIT or at risk of HIT, at risk of HIT and undergoing PCI. **Contraindications:** Active major bleeding.	**HIT:** IV infusion: initially, 2 mcg/kg/min as a continuous infusion. After initial infusion, dose may be adjusted until steady-state aPTT is 1.5–3 times baseline value, not to exceed 100 seconds. Dosage should not exceed 10 mcg/kg/min. **PCI:** IV infusion: Initial bolus of 350 mcg/kg over 3–5 minutes, then infuse at 25 mcg/kg/min. Check ACT 5–10 minutes following bolus. If ACT is less than 300 seconds, give additional bolus of 150 mcg/kg; increase infusion to 30 mcg/kg/min. If ACT is greater than 450 seconds, decrease infusion to 15 mcg/kg/min. Once ACT of 300–450 seconds achieved, continue dose through duration of procedure.	Ventricular tachycardia, atrial fibrillation occurs occasionally. Major bleeding, sepsis occur rarely.	Obtain baseline and periodic CBC, PT, aPTT, ACT, platelet count. Determine initial BP. Minimize need for injection sites, blood draws, catheters. Monitor for signs of bleeding, vital signs, c/o abdomen/back pain, severe h/a. Monitor ACT, PT, aPTT, platelet count, Hgb, Hct. Question for increased signs of bleeding or hematuria. Patient should report signs of bleeding immediately.

(continued)

TABLE 6.2 ANTICOAGULANTS (*continued*)

MEDICATION: GENERIC NAME (BRAND NAME)	CLASSIFICATION: PHARMACOTHERAPEUTIC AND CLINICAL	MECHANISM OF ACTION: THERAPEUTIC	INDICATIONS AND CONTRAINDICATIONS	DOSAGE	ADVERSE EFFECTS	SAFETY AND PATIENT EDUCATION
D. FACTOR XA INHIBITORS						
Rivaroxaban (Xarelto)	**Pharmacotherapeutic:** Factor Xa inhibitor **Clinical:** Anticoagulant	Inhibits blood coagulation.	**Indications:** DVT px in hip or knee replacement surgery. Prevents stroke and systemic embolism in patients with NVAF. Treatment of acute DVT/PE. Reduces risk of recurrent DVT/PE following 6 months of treatment. **Contraindications:** Active major bleeding, severe renal impairment (CrCl less than 15 mL/min). Note: Avoid giving to patients with BMI greater than 40 kg/m² or weight greater than 120 kg due to lack of clinical data.	Administer doses of 15 mg or more with food. **DVT prophylaxis, knee/hip replacement:** PO: 10 mg daily for minimum 10–14 days up to 35 days. Initiate at least 6–10 hours after surgery once hemostasis established. **NVAF:** CrCl greater than 50 mL/min: 20 mg PO daily. CrCl 15–50 mL/min: 15 mg PO daily. **DVT/PE treatment:** PO: 15 mg BID for 3 weeks, then 20 mg once daily.	Increased risk for bleeding. Serious reactions, including jaundice, cholestasis, cytolytic hepatitis, Stevens-Johnson syndrome; hypersensitivity reaction, anaphylaxis reported.	Obtain baseline and periodic CBC, serum chemistries, PT/INR, vital signs, urine pregnancy if applicable. Obtain EKG for patients with hx of atrial fibrillation. Question for history of bleeding, recent surgery, bleeding disorders, spinal procedures, bleeding ulcers, anemia, open wounds, renal/hepatic impairment. Receive full medication history, including herbal supplements. Monitor for signs and symptoms of bleeding. Patient should immediately report suspected pregnancy; do not take or discontinue any medications except on advice of provider. Avoid alcohol, aspirin, NSAIDs, grapefruit products. Consult provider before surgery, dental work.

ACS, acute coronary syndrome; ACT, activated clotting time; aPTT, activated partial thromboplastin time; BMI, body mass index; BP, blood pressure; CBC, complete blood count; c/o, complaint of; d/c, discontinue; DIC, disseminated intravascular coagulation; DVT, deep vein thrombosis; GI, gastrointestinal; GU, genitourinary; h/a, headache; Hct, hematocrit; Hgb, hemoglobin; HIT, heparin-induced thrombocytopenia; HITT, heparin-induced thrombocytopenia thrombosis; h/x, history; IM, intramuscular; INR, international normalized ratio; IV, intravenous; MI, myocardial infarction; NSAIDs, nonsteroidal anti-inflammatory drugs; NVAF, nonvalvular atrial fibrillation; OTC, over-the-counter; PCI, percutaneous coronary intervention; PE, pulmonary embolism; PT, prothrombin time; PTCA, percutaneous transluminal coronary intervention; Px, prophylaxis; SQ, subcutaneous; STEMI, ST segment elevation myocardial infarction; TE, transthoracic echocardiogram; Tx, treatment.

TABLE 6.3 ANTIPLATELETS

MEDICATION: GENERIC BRAND NAME	CLASSIFICATION: PHARMACOTHER-APEUTIC AND CLINICAL	MECHANISM OF ACTION: THERAPEUTIC	INDICATIONS AND CONTRAINDICATIONS	DOSAGE	ADVERSE EFFECTS	SAFETY AND PATIENT EDUCATION
Aspirin (81 mg dose)	**Pharmacotherapeutic:** Nonsteroidal salicylate **Clinical:** Anticoagulant, antiinflammatory, antipyretic	Reduces inflammatory response, inhibits platelet aggregation, reduces intensity of pain, decreases fever.	**Indications:** Platelet aggregation inhibitor in the prevention of TIA, cerebral thromboembolism, MI or, reinfarction. **Contraindications:** Hypersensitivity to salicylates, NSAIDs. Aspirin triad (asthma, rhinitis, aspirin intolerance). Inherited or acquired bleeding disorders.	**Revascularization:** PO 80–325 mg/d **MI, stroke (risk reduction) PO:** Durlaza—162.5 mg once daily Avoid use in severe renal or hepatic impairment.	High doses of aspirin may cause GI bleeding or gastric mucosal lesions.	Do not use if vinegar-like odor noted, assess history of GI bleed, peptic ulcer disease, OTC product use with aspirin. Do not crush, chew, or split enteric-coated tablets. Avoid alcohol, OTC pain/cold products with aspirin. Report ringing of ears or persistent abdominal GI pain or bleeding.
Clopidogrel (Plavix)	**Pharmacotherapeutic:** Thienopyridine derivative **Clinical:** Antiplatelet	Inhibits platelet aggregation.	**Indications:** To decrease rate of MI and stroke in pts with NSTEMI ACS, acute STEMI, pts with hx of recent MI or stroke, established PAD. **Contraindications:** Hypersensitivity to clopidogrel. Active bleeding.	**Recent MI, stroke, PAD:** PO: 75 mg once daily **ACS, Unstable angina/STEMI:** PO: Loading dose of 300–600 mg, then 75 mg once daily (in combination with ASA for up to 12 months, then aspirin indefinitely). **ACS (STEMI):** PO: Continue for at least 14 days up to 12 months. Adults 75 years or younger: 300 mg loading dose, then 75 mg once daily. Older than 75: 75 mg once daily. **ACS (PCI):** PO: 600 mg loading dose, then 75 mg once daily (in combination with aspirin) for at least 12 months.	**Adverse effects:** Agranulocytosis, aplastic anemia/pancytopenia, TTP occurs rarely. Hepatitis, hypersensitivity reaction, anaphylactoid reactions have been reported.	Obtain baseline and periodic chemistries, CBC, LFT, renal function tests, platelet count. Perform platelet count before initiation, q2d during first week of treatment, and weekly thereafter until therapeutic maintenance achieved. Abrupt discontinuation of drug therapy produces elevated platelet count within 5 days. Patient should report any unusual bleeding but may take longer to stop bleeding during therapy. Inform provider, dentists if taking medication before any procedures.

ACS, acute coronary syndrome; ASA, acetylsalicylate acid; GI, gastrointestinal; hx, history; LFT, liver function test; MI, myocardial infarction; NSAIDs, nonsteroidal anti-inflammatory drugs; NSTEMI, NON-ST segment elevation myocardial infarction; OTC, over-the-counter; PAD, peripheral artery disease; PCI, percutaneous coronary intervention; pts, patients; STEMI, ST segment elevation myocardial infarction; TIA, transient ischemic attack; TTP, thrombotic thrombocytopenia purpura.

BOX 6.1 Risk Factors for Coronary Artery Disease

Nonmodifiable, Modifiable, and Nontraditional

Nonmodifiable
- Increasing age
- Male gender
- Genetic disorders of lipid metabolism
- Family history of premature coronary artery disease
- Postmenopausal

Modifiable
- Cigarette smoking
- Obesity
- Diabetes mellitus
- Hypertension
- Hyperlipidemia with elevated low-density lipoprotein and low high-density lipoprotein cholesterol; diet high in saturated fat; lack of exercise/sedentary lifestyle; cocaineamphetamine use

Nontraditional
- Inflammation marked by elevated C-reactive protein levels
- Hyperhomocysteinemia
- Increased lipoprotein (a) levels

Sources: Hanna, E. B. (2017). *Practical cardiovascular medicine.* https://ebookcentral.proquest.com; Porth, C., & Gaspard, K. J. (2015). *Essentials of pathophysiology* (4th ed.). Lippincott, Williams & Wilkins; Reeder, G. S., & Kennedy, H. L. (2019). Overview of the acute management of ST-elevation myocardial infarction. *UpToDate.* https://www-uptodate-com.proxy.wexler.hunter.cuny.edu/contents /overview-of-the-acute-management-of-st-elevation -myocardialinfarction?sectionName=Oxygen&search=Management %20of%20STEMI&topicRef=184&anchor=H167627380&source =see_link#H167627380

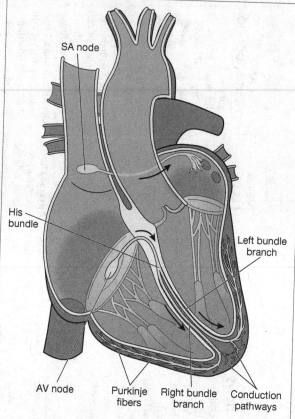

FIGURE 6.2 Electrophysiologic pathway of cardiac conduction.

AV, atrioventriculr; SA, sinoatrial.

Source: From Gawlik, K. S., Melnyk, B. M., & Teall, A. M. (2021). *Evidence-based physical examination: Best practices for health and well-being assessment.* Springer Publishing Company.

Normal EKG

The EKG is the sum of all cardiac action potentials (Figure 6.3; Hanna, 2017; McCance & Huether, 2014; Porth & Gaspard, 2015; Story, 2018):
- P wave represents atrial depolarization.
- The PR interval is the time from the onset of atrial activation to the onset of ventricular activation; it normally ranges from 0.12 to 0.20 second.
- The QRS complex represents the sum of all ventricular muscle cell depolarizations. The duration is normally between 0.06 and 0.10 second.
- The ST interval indicates when the entire ventricular myocardium is depolarized.
- The QT interval is sometimes called the *electrical systole of the ventricles* and varies inversely with the HR.
- U-waves.

Control of Heart Action

- The heart is composed of automatic cells that are capable of spontaneous depolarization.
- The SA node depolarizes spontaneously 60 to 100 times per minute (Hanna, 2017; McCance & Huether, 2014; Porth & Gaspard, 2015; Story, 2018).
- Autonomic nervous system influences the rate of impulse generation (firing), depolarization, and repolarization of the myocardium.

- Cardiac innervation:
  - **Adrenergic response—sympathetic nerves**—Increases electrical conductivity and the strength of the myocardial contraction:
    - Adrenergic receptors—Norepinephrine or epinephrine are the key neurotransmitters (Table 6.4).
  - **Vagal response—parasympathetic nerves**—Slows conduction of action potentials through the heart and reduces the strength of contraction.
    - Acetylcholine is the key neurotransmitter.

  Stimulation of both the beta-1 and beta-2 increases the HR (chronotropy) and force of the myocardial contraction (inotropy).
- If the HR is affected, then the effect is called *chronotropy*:
  - Negative chronotropy decreases HR.
  - Positive chronotropy increases HR.
- If the heart contraction is affected, then the effect is called *inotropy*:
  - Negative inotropy decreases force of contraction.
  - Positive inotropy increases force of contraction.
- Myocardial cells (Hanna, 2017; McCance & Huether, 2014; Porth & Gaspard, 2015):

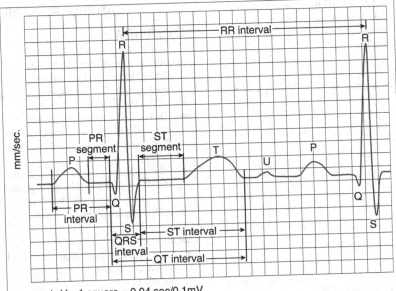

FIGURE 6.3 EKG waves.

Source: Reproduced with permission from R. Porter (Ed.). (2019). *Merck manual professional version* (known as the *Merck manual* in the United States and Canada and the *MSD Manual* in the rest of the world). Merck & Co. Copyright 2019 by Merck Sharp & Dohme Corp., a subsidiary of Merck & Co., Inc., https://www.merckmanuals.com/professional/cardiovascular-disorders/cardiovascular-tests-and-procedures/electrocardiography

TABLE 6.4 EFFECTS OF HORMONES

HORMONE	EFFECT
Epinephrine and norepinephrine	Vasoconstriction
Antidiuretic hormone	Increases blood volume by reabsorption of water from tubular fluid in the distal tubule and the collecting duct of the nephron
Renin–angiotensin–aldosterone system Aldosterone Angiotensin II	Stimulates reabsorption of sodium, chloride, and water to increase blood volume and stimulate thirst vasoconstrictor
Natriuretic peptides	Cause loss of sodium, chloride, and water through their effects on kidney function, decreasing blood volume
Adrenomedullin	Powerful vasodilatory activity
Nitric oxide Prostaglandins Endothelium-derived relaxing factor	Vasodilation

- Transmit action potentials faster through intercalated disks.
- Synthesize more adenosine triphosphate (ATP) because of a large number of mitochondria.

- Can access ions in the interstitium because of an abundance of transverse tubules.
- Enable the myocardium to work constantly, which skeletal muscles are not required to do.
- Contain (Hanna, 2017; McCance & Huether, 2014; Porth & Gaspard, 2015):
  - Actin, myosin, and the troponin–tropomyosin complex
    - Troponins T, I, and C
    - Titin (connectin), a protein that functions as a molecular spring responsible for the passive elasticity of muscle (Hanna, 2017; McCance & Huether, 2014; Porth & Gaspard, 2015; Story, 2018)

12-Lead EKG Interpretation

An EKG is used to assess for cardiovascular disease. The EKG can assist in the assessment of metabolic disorders, pharmacotherapy side effects, drug toxicities, implantable defibrillators, and pacemakers. It is the most important test for interpretation of the following:

- Cardiac rhythm
- Detection of myocardial ischemia or infarction
- Conduction abnormalities
- Preexcitation
- Prolonged QT interval
- Atrial abnormalities
- Ventricular hypertrophy
- Pericarditis

A 12-lead EKG is a representation of the heart's electrical activity. The EKG records electrical activity as it spreads through the heart from 12 different electrodes (leads). Each of the leads represents a different view of the heart.

It is important that the 12-lead EKG be recorded accurately to ensure proper diagnosis and management of the patient. Correct electrode placement and adequate skin preparation are key to ensure a true and reliable EKG.

Myocardial Damage

The following should be considered when reviewing a 12-lead EKG (Table 6.5):

- Rate
  - a. Normal
  - b. HR 60 to 100 bpm
  - c. Tachycardia
  - d. HR >100 bpm
  - e. Bradycardia
  - f. HR <60 bpm
- Rhythm
  - a. Normal sinus
  - b. Abnormal rhythm
- Intervals
  - a. PR
    - i. PR interval measured from the beginning of the P wave to the beginning of the QRS
    - ii. Normal PR interval is 0.12 to 0.20 sec
  - b. QRS
    - i. Measure ventricular depolarization
    - ii. Begins from the point where it first leaves the baseline to where the last wave ends
    - iii. Normal QRS width is 0.04 to 0.10 sec
  - c. QT
    - i. Measures the duration of ventricular depolarization and repolarization
    - ii. Begins from the beginning of the QRS complex to the end of the T wave
    - iii. Normal QT interval is 0.45 sec for men and 0.46 sec for women
- QRST duration
  - a. Q waves
  - b. R wave progression
  - c. ST segment depression/elevations
    - i. Measures early ventricular repolarization.
    - ii. Begins at the end of the QRS to the beginning of the T wave.
    - iii. Normal ST is an isoelectric line.
  - d. T wave changes

TABLE 6.5 CHARACTERISTIC LEAD CHANGES IN ACUTE MYOCARDIAL INFARCTION

WALL AFFECTED	LEADS	ARTERY INVOLVED
Anterior	V_1–V_4	Left coronary artery, LAD artery
Septal	V_1, V_2	LAD artery
Inferior	II, III, aV_F	RCA
Lateral	I, aV_L, V_5, V_6	Circumflex artery
Posterior	V_7, V_8, V_9	RCA and circumflex artery
Right ventricular infarct	V_4R, V_5R, V_6R	Marginal branch of RCA

LAD, left anterior descending; RCA, right coronary artery.
Source: From Clutter, P. (2015). *ECG for nursing demystified.* McGraw-Hill.

CARDIAC REHABILITATION

OVERVIEW

Cardiac rehabilitation (CR) is a comprehensive program used to restore or improve the physiologic and psychologic well-being of patients after an acute occlusive cardiovascular event, such as heart attack, HF, angioplasty, or heart surgery (Al Quait & Doherty, 2017; Foster et al., 2017):

- CR requires a multidisciplinary team of physicians, nurses, physical therapists, nutritionists, respiratory therapists, psychologists, and vocational counselors (Al Quait & Doherty, 2017).
- All disciplines work collaboratively to restore the physiologic and psychologic well-being of patients, including assisting in their prompt and safe return to appropriate work (Al Quait & Doherty, 2017; Foster et al., 2017).

Goal

- Help patient return to as normal a life as possible by maintaining an adequate level of cardiovascular fitness (Goel et al., 2011).
- Ensure the psychologic well-being of the patient by addressing social and emotional needs.

Phases

- Begin concurrently with the inpatient treatment of the acute illness and then extends through a physician-supervised recovery (Al Quait & Doherty, 2017)
- Independent exercise program that embodies many core components, including ongoing functional and cardiovascular risk assessments and aggressive modification of risk factors, including hypertension and hyperlipidemia through therapeutic lifestyle changes (Goel et al., 2011)
- Adjunctive drug therapies of proven benefit as well as nutritional and psychologic counseling (Foster et al., 2017)

Indications

Generally accepted indications for CR include the following (Al Quait & Doherty, 2017; Foster et al., 2017; Goel et al., 2011):

- MI
- Coronary artery bypass graft (CABG)
- PCI
- Valve repair or replacement
- Angina
- Patients with HF and heart transplants

Clinical Benefits

- CR is associated with a 40% decrease in all-cause mortality for patients after MI or revascularization (Foster et al., 2017).
- CR participation after PCI is associated with a significant reduction in mortality rates (Al Quait & Doherty, 2017).

Risks and Contraindications

- These surround the exercise component of the program, especially during the first phase of rehabilitation, and occur during the acute treatment period (Al Quait & Doherty, 2017).
- CR is contraindicated in unstable patients, including those with decompensated HF, ventricular arrhythmia, unstable angina, and severe pulmonary hypertension due to the risk for decreased myocardial perfusion when engaging in moderate exercise with these conditions (Al Quait & Doherty, 2017; Foster et al., 2017).

DYSLIPIDEMIA

OVERVIEW

Dyslipidemia is abnormally elevated cholesterol or fats (lipids) in the blood. It is one of the leading contributors to the development of coronary heart disease (CHD) and one of the most modifiable risk factors (Box 6.2 and Table 6.6):

- Hypertriglyceridemia is a highly prevalent lipid disorder in the adult population.
- Adults over the age of 20 have shown an increased prevalence of triglycerides (TGs) >150 mg/dL.
- The risk of CHD increases significantly as the low-density lipoprotein cholesterol (LDL-C) increases. LDL-C has been the predominate target of dyslipidemia treatment efforts.
- Elevated TGs and low levels of high-density lipoprotein cholesterol (HDL-C) are also independent predictors of CHD.

Types of Lipoprotein

- **LDLs** (also called *bad cholesterol*) are the main carrier of cholesterol. LDL particles are rich in cholesterol and cholesterol esters.
- **High-density lipoproteins (HDLs;** often referred to as *good cholesterol*) are synthesized by several pathways, including direct secretion by the intestine and liver and transfer of lipids.
- **Diagnosis of dyslipidemia** is based on complete lipid profile (fasting).

Treatment

- Primary target is a reduction in LDL cholesterol (Table 6.7; Hanna, 2017; Porth & Gaspard, 2015; Reeder & Kennedy, 2019).
- When dietary and therapeutic lifestyle changes are unsuccessful, pharmacologic treatment is considered (Hanna, 2017; Porth & Gaspard, 2015; Reeder & Kennedy, 2019):
  - The five lipid-lowering drugs are stains, bile acid–binding resins, cholesterol-absorption inhibitor agents, niacin and its congeners, and the fibrates.
- Pharmacologic treatment with statins is also an option (Table 6.7).

BOX 6.2 Major Risk Factors for Atherosclerotic Cardiovascular Disease

Age	Male ≥45 y/o
	Female ≥55 y/o
Family history	<55 y/o in a male first-degree relative
	<65 y/o in a female first-degree relative
Elevated blood pressure	≥140/≥90 mmHg or currently on blood pressure medication
Low HDL-C	Male <40 mg/dL
	Female <50 mg/dL
Current smoker	

HDL-C, high-density lipoprotein cholesterol.

Lipid-Lowering Agents: Prescription and Management

- These agents are among the most commonly prescribed drugs in the United States. Because elevated cholesterol and TG are risk factors for heart disease, lipid-lowering agents are recommended by the American Heart Association (AHA) when total cholesterol is >200 mg/dL and for TG >150 mg/dL.
- A healthy lifestyle that includes a nutrient-dense diet and regular physical activity remains a focal point of the 2018 American Heart Association/American College of Cardiology (AHA/ACC) cholesterol guidelines, with lipid-lowering agents used as an adjunct to a healthy lifestyle (Box 6.3).
- Clinicians are recommended to assess for medication adherence and efficacy at 4 to 12 weeks with a fasting lipid test and then at every 3 to 12 months.
- Proprotein convertase subtilisin/kexin type 9 (PCSK9) inhibitors are indicated as an effective nonstatin agent, particularly as add-on therapy to a statin, but few long-term data are available on safety in patients with hypercholesterolemia.

TABLE 6.6 CRITERIA FOR ATHEROSCLEROTIC-CARDIOVASCULAR DISEASE: RISK ASSESSMENT, TREATMENT GOALS, AND LEVELS

RISK	CRITERIA	TREATMENT GOAL Non-HDL-C, LDL-C (mg/dL)	CONSIDER DRUG THERAPY Non-HDL-C, LDL-C (mg/dL)
Low	0–1 major ASCVD risk factors	<130, <100	≥190, ≥160
Moderate	2 major ASCVD risk factors	<130, <100	≥160, ≥130
High	≥3 major ASCVD risk factors	<130, <100	≥130, ≥100
	Diabetes		
	CKD stage 3B or 4		
	LDL-C >190 mg/dL		
Very high	ASCVD	<100, <70	≥100, ≥70
	Diabetes		
	≥2 major risk factors		
	Evidence of end-organ damage		

ASCVD, atherosclerotic-cardiovascular disease; CKD, chronic kidney disease; HDL-C, high-density lipoprotein cholesterol; LDL-C, low-density lipoprotein cholesterol.

TABLE 6.7 LIPID-LOWERING AGENTS

MEDICATION: GENERIC BRAND NAME	CLASSIFICATION: PHARMACOTHER-APEUTIC AND CLINICAL	MECHANISM OF ACTION: THERAPEUTIC	INDICATIONS AND CONTRAINDICATIONS	DOSAGE	COMMON ADVERSE EFFECTS	SAFETY AND PATIENT EDUCATION
BILE ACID SEQUESTRANTS						
Cholestyramine (Prevalite, Questran)	**Pharmacotherapeutic:** Bile acid sequestrants **Clinical:** Antihyperlipidemic	Decreases LDL-C, increases HDL-C, TG	**Indications:** Primary hypercholesterolemia **Contraindications:** Pregnancy, breastfeeding	4 g 1–2 times/d With constipation may start with 4 g once a day. May increase over 1-month interval. Usual dose: 8–16 g/d in 2 divided doses Maximum: 24 g/d	Constipation to fecal impaction, increased bleeding tendencies	Do not take with other medications. Do not give in dry form; mix with water, milk, or juice. Take with meals.
COLESTIPOL (COLESTID), COLESEVELAM (WELCHOL)						
CHOLESTEROL ABSORPTION INHIBITOR						
Ezetimibe (Zetia)	**Pharmacotherapeutic:** Antihyperlipidemic **Clinical:** Anticholesterol agent	Reduces total serum cholesterol, LDL-C, and TG; increases HDL-C	**Indications:** Primary hypercholesterolemia (in combination with diet therapy and/or statins) Homozygous familial hypercholesterolemia (combined with atorvastatin or simvastatin) Mixed hyperlipidemia (in combination with fenofibrate) **Contraindications:** Hypersensitivity to ezetimibe; concurrent use of a statin in patients with active hepatic disease or unexplained persistent elevations in serum transaminase; pregnancy and breastfeeding (when used with a statin)	10 mg PO once daily May give at same time as statins. Give at least 2 hours before or 4 hours after bile acid sequestrants. Give with or without food.	Hepatitis, hypersensitivity reaction, myopathy, rhabdomyolysis occur rarely.	Receive full diet and medication history, medical history. Obtain serum cholesterol, serum TG, hepatic function test, blood counts. Question history of hepatic/renal impairment. Treatment should be discontinued if hepatic enzyme levels persist at more than 3 times normal limit. Monitor daily bowel activity, stool consistency. Assess and teach patient to report back pain, abdominal disturbances, muscle, or bone pain. Monitor serum cholesterol, TG for therapeutic response. Periodic lab tests and compliance are essential. Speak to provider before stopping medication.

(continued)

FIBRIC ACID						
Fenofibrate (Antara, Lofibra, Tricor, Triglide) Fenofibric acid (Fibricor, Trilipix)	Pharmacotherapeutic: Fibric acid derivative Clinical: Antihyperlipidemic	Decreases TG and LDL-C; increases HDL-C	Indications: Adjunct to diet for reduction of LDL-C, total cholesterol, TG, apo-lipoprotein B, and to increase HDL-C in patients with primary hypercholesterolemia, mixed dyslipidemia Contraindications: Hypersensitivity to fenofibrate; active hepatic disease, preexisting gallbladder disease, severe renal/hepatic dysfunction (including primary biliary cirrhosis, unexplained persistent hepatic function abnormality), breastfeeding	Dosages (mg/d): Antara: 43–130 *Lofibra 67–200 Tricor: 48–145 Triglide: 50–160 *Fenoglide: 40–120 *Lipofen: 50–150 Trilipix: 45–135 Fibricor: 35–105 *Give with meals.	Decreased libido, ED, flu-like symptoms, hepatic impairment, myalgia, pancreatitis, nausea, rash	May increase levels of ezetimibe. Concomitant use of statins may increase rhabdomyolysis, elevate CPK levels, and cause myoglobinuria.
Gemfibrozil (Lopid)	Pharmacotherapeutic: Fibric acid derivative Clinical: Antihyperlipidemic	Lowers serum cholesterol, TG (decreases VLDL, LDL-C; increases HDL-C)	Indications: Hypertriglyceridemia (adjunct to diet/exercise) Reduction of CAD in patients unresponsive to traditional therapies Contraindications: Hypersensitivity to gemfibrozil; hepatic impairment, preexisting gallbladder disease, severe renal impairment, concurrent use with dasabuvir, repaglinide, or simvastatin; pregnancy, breastfeeding	600 mg 2 times a day 30 minutes before morning and evening meals Adjust dose with renal or hepatic impairment.	Abdominal pain, blurred vision, cataract development, dizziness, dyspepsia, eczema, epigastric pain, eosinophilia, fatigue, gallstone development, headache, hepatotoxicity, leukopenia, n/v/d, rhabdomyolysis	Use only if strongly indicated and lipid studies show definite response. Give 30 minutes before breakfast and dinner. Concomitant use of statins may increase rhabdomyolysis, elevate CPK levels, and cause myoglobinuria. Patient should report muscle pain with fever, urine/stool changes, upper abdominal pain.

(continued)

TABLE 6.7 LIPID-LOWERING AGENTS (continued)

MEDICATION: GENERIC NAME (BRAND NAME)	CLASSIFICATION: PHARMACOTHER-APEUTIC AND CLINICAL	MECHANISM OF ACTION: THERAPEUTIC	INDICATIONS AND CONTRAINDICATIONS	DOSAGE	COMMON ADVERSE EFFECTS	SAFETY AND PATIENT EDUCATION
D. NIACIN						
Niacin, nicotinic acid (Niacor, Niaspan)	**Clinical:** Antihyperlipidemic, vitamin	Decreases LDL-C, TG; increases HDL-C	**Indications:** Dyslipidemia CAD, post-MI **Contraindications:** Hypersensitivity to niacin, nicotinic acid; active peptic ulcer disease, arterial hemorrhage, significant or unexplained persistent elevations in hepatic transaminases, active hepatic disease	Dyslipidemia: Immediate release: 100 mg PO TID, increased to 1 g PO TID ER: 500 mg/d PO at bedtime for 4 weeks, then 1 g/d PO HS for another 4 weeks Maximum: 2 g/d. CAD, post MI: 500 mg/d HS, titrated at 4-week intervals to maximum 1–2 g/d	Flushing, GI upset, glucose intolerance, hyperuricemia, n/v/d, rash	Diabetics may experience a dose-related elevation in glucose. Do not substitute ER form for immediate-release form at equivalent doses; severe hepatotoxicity possible. ASA 325 mg 30 mg prior to dose may help with flushing. Do not combine with a statin. Take at bedtime; avoid hot foods/drinks, alcohol around dose time to decrease flushing. Patient should report rash, unusual bleeding, or bruising.
e. Omega Fatty Acids						
Icosapent (Vascepa) Lovaza Epanova	Omega-3 fatty acid Antihypertriglyceridemic	Decreases TG	**Indications:** Adjunct to diet to reduce triglyceride levels in adults with severe (500 mg/dL or higher) hypertriglyceridemia **Contraindications:** Hypersensitivity to omega-3 fatty acids; use cautiously with known sensitivity or allergy to fish/shellfish.	4 g/d, given as a single dose (4 capsules), or 2 capsules BID	Arthralgia, bleeding, hepatic impairment, hypersensitivity reaction	Patient should continue to adhere to lipid-lowering diet. Periodic lab tests are essential. Discontinue therapy if no response after 2 months. Monitor baseline and ongoing TG levels, LFTs.

(continued)

F. PCSK9 INHIBITORS

Alirocumab (Praluent) Evolcumab (Repatha)	**Pharmacotherapeutic:** PCSK9 inhibitor **Clinical:** Antihyperlipidemic	Decreases serum cholesterol levels	**Indications:** Alirocumab and Evolcumab: Heterozygous familial hypercholesterolemia with maximal tolerance to statin therapy or clinical atherosclerotic CV disease Evolcumab: MI and stroke risk reduction, revascularization in patients with established CV disease	Alirocumab: 75 mg SQ once q2wk Maximum: 150 mg SQ once q2wk Evolcumab: 140 mg SQ once q2wk; or 420 mg SQ (three 140-mg injections given in 30 minutes) once a month	Flu-like symptoms, hypersensitivity reactions, injection-site reactions, nasopharyngitis	Monitor LDL at baseline and periodically. Monitor for severe hypersensitivity reaction. Use caution in pregnancy/breastfeeding. Patient should rotate injection sites, report difficulty breathing, rash, injection site pain/inflammation.
g. HMG-CoA Reductase Inhibitors (Statins)					
Atorvastatin (Lipitor)	**Pharmacotherapeutic:** HMG-CoA reductase inhibitor **Clinical classification:** Antihyperlipidemic	Decreases LDL-C, VLDL, and TG; increases HDL-C	**Indications:** Adjunct to diet therapy in management of hyperlipidemia Primary prevention of cardiovascular disease in high-risk patients Reduces risk for stroke and heart attack in patients with type 2 diabetes mellitus with or without evidence of heart disease **Contraindications:** Active hepatic disease, breastfeeding, pregnancy, unexplained elevated liver-function tests	Initially, 10–20 mg /d (40 mg with patients requiring greater than 45% reduction in LDL-C; range: 10–80 mg/d Maximum dose with strong CYP3A4 inhibitors: 20 mg/d Administer in evening	Cataracts, photosensitivity, myalgia, rhabdomyolysis, hepatotoxicity	Obtain baseline and periodic serum cholesterol, TG, LFT, CPK. Receive full medical, diet, and medication history. Monitor for h/a, rash, pruritus, rash, malaise. Patient should follow prescribed diet; periodic lab tests are essential. Do not take other medications without speaking to provider. Patient should report dark urine, unexplained muscle pain, bone pain. Avoid excessive alcohol intake, large intake of grapefruit products.

(continued)

TABLE 6.7 LIPID-LOWERING AGENTS (continued)

MEDICATION: GENERIC NAME (BRAND NAME)	CLASSIFICATION: PHARMACOTHER- APEUTIC AND CLINICAL	MECHANISM OF ACTION: THERAPEUTIC	INDICATIONS AND CONTRAINDICATIONS	DOSAGE	COMMON ADVERSE EFFECTS	SAFETY AND PATIENT EDUCATION
Pravastatin (Pravachol)			**Uses:** Diet adjunct in treatment of primary hyperlipidemias and mixed dyslipidemias. Risk reduction of MI, revascularization, and mortality in hypercholesterolemia without clinically evident CHD.	Give without regard to meals. Prior to therapy initiation, patient should be on standard cholesterol-lowering diet for 3–6 months. Adults/older adults: Initially, 40 mg/d. Titrate to desired response. Renal impairment: Give 10 mg/d initially. Titrate to desired response.	Potential for malignancy, cataracts, myopathy, rhabdomyolysis	Question possibility of pregnancy. Be alert for malaise, muscle cramping/ weakness; if accompanied with fever, may need to discontinue medication. Report immediately any muscle pain/weakness. Use nonhormonal contraception. Avoid direct exposure to sunlight.
Simvastatin (Zocor)			**Indications:** Hyperlipidemias FH, secondary prevention of cardiovascular events in patients with hypercholesterolemia and CHD or at high risk for CHD **Contraindications:** Concurrent use of clarithromycin, cyclosporine, gemfibrozil	**Prevention of cardiovascular events:** 10–20 mg once daily, range 5–40 mg/d. **Hyperlipidemias:** Initially 10–20 mg once daily. Patients with CHD or CHD-risk equivalents: initially, 40 mg/d, range 5–40 mg/d. Note: Limit 80 mg dose to patients taking simvastatin longer than 12 months without evidence of myopathy. Dosage adjustment needed for renal impairment.	Potential for ocular lens opacities, hepatitis, myopathy	Question for possibility of pregnancy before initiating therapy. Monitor daily pattern of bowel activity, stool consistency; assess for h/a, myopathy; educate on appropriate contraceptive measures; avoid grapefruit products; report unexplained muscle pain, weakness.

ASA, acetylsalicylate acid; CAD, coronary artery disease; CHD, coronary heart disease; CPK, creatine phosphokinase; CV, cardiovascular; ER, extended release; FH, familial hypercholesterolemia; GI, gastrointestinal; h/a, headache; HDL-C, high-density lipoprotein cholesterol; HMG-CoA; LDL-C, low-density lipoprotein cholesterol; LFT, liver function test; MI, myocardial infarction; n/v/d, nausea, vomiting, diarrhea; TG, triglyceride; VLDL, very-low-density lipoprotein.

BOX 6.3 Lifestyle Changes for Low-Density Lipoprotein Goal

Diet
- Saturated fat <7% of calories
- Cholesterol <200 mg/d
- Fiber 10–25 g/day

Weight management
Increased physical activity
Smoking cessation

- The 2018 guidelines recommend the following statin regimen based upon intensity level to lower LDL-C:
  - *High-intensity therapy:* 80 mg atorvastatin (40 mg: down titration if intolerable to 80 mg) and 20 mg rosuvastatin (40 mg)
  - *Moderate-intensity therapy:* 10 mg atorvastatin (20 mg) and 10 mg rosuvastatin (5 mg) and 20 to 40 mg simvastatin or 40 mg pravastatin (80 mg) and 40 mg lovastatin (80 mg) and 80 mg Fluvastatin XL and 40 mg Fluvastatin BID and pitavastatin
  - *Low-intensity therapy:* 10 mg simvastatin or 10 to 20 mg pravastatin and 20 mg lovastatin and 20 to 40 mg Fluvastatin

ATHEROSCLEROSIS

This is thickening and hardening caused by the accumulation of lipid-laden macrophages in the arterial wall. It is a leading cause of coronary artery and cerebrovascular disease (Hanna, 2017; Porth & Gaspard, 2015; Reeder & Kennedy, 2019):

- Plaque development is a process that occurs throughout the body:
  - Monocytes attach to the endothelium → macrophages.
  - Macrophages release free radicals → oxidized LDL.
  - Macrophages ingest oxidized LDL → foam cells.
  - White blood cells (WBCs), platelets, and vascular endothelium release chemicals that promote plaque formation.
  - Plaques can rupture → clot forms (thrombus):
    - May completely block the artery.
    - May break free and become an embolus.

Refer to Box 6.1 for risk factors of atherosclerosis.

Clinical Manifestations

- Atherosclerosis usually doesn't cause signs and symptoms until it severely narrows or totally blocks an artery. Usually 70% to 80% stenosis is reached before patients have symptoms.
- Several patients are asymptomatic until they have a medical emergency, such as a heart attack or stroke.
- Symptoms and signs are the result of inadequate perfusion of tissues.

  Signs and symptoms depend on the vessels involved and the extent of vessel obstruction (Hanna, 2017; Porth & Gaspard, 2015; Reeder & Kennedy, 2019).

Treatment

- Focuses on reducing risk factors, removing the initial causes of vessel damage, and preventing lesion progression
- Exercising, smoking cessation, and controlling hypertension and diabetes when appropriate while reducing LDL cholesterol levels by diet or medications or both (Hanna, 2017; Porth & Gaspard, 2015; Reeder & Kennedy, 2019)

ACUTE INFLAMMATORY DISEASE

OVERVIEW

Inflammation is the first line of defense against injury or infection (Table 6.8). It is a normal response of the body to protect tissues from infection, injury, or disease. The inflammatory response begins with the production and release of chemical agents by cells in the infected, injured, or diseased tissue. This inflamed tissue generates additional signals that recruit leukocytes to the site of inflammation. Leukocytes destroy any infected agent and remove cellular debris from damaged tissue. The inflammatory response usually promotes healing; however, if uncontrolled, it may become harmful. Acute inflammation typically lasts only a few days.

CARDIAC TAMPONADE

Cardiac tamponade is a compression of the heart resulting from fluid accumulation in the pericardial sac. This fluid in the pericardial sac can cause enough pressure to prevent the atria and ventricles from filling completely during diastole. This results in decreased CO, SV, and hypotension. The body compensates with tachycardia. Eventually, the compensatory mechanisms fail, and hemodynamic instability ensues (Carlson, 2009).

Signs and Symptoms

Many signs and symptoms of cardiac tamponade are often subtle (Dries & Brobst, 2012). As a result, the diagnosis of cardiac tamponade is often overlooked:

- Anxiety
- Progressive shortness of breath, chest pain, and cough
- Hypotension
- Tachycardia
- Distant heart sounds
- Jugular vein distention (JVD)
- Pulsus paradoxus: Exaggerated fall in blood pressure during inspiration by >10 mmHg
- Beck's triad:
  - Three classic symptoms of cardiac tamponade:
    - Hypotension/distended neck veins/distant heart sounds
    - Lightheadiness/dizziness
    - Weakness/fatigue

Diagnostic Testing

- Echocardiogram:
  - Quickest and most accurate method used to diagnosis cardiac tamponade.
  - Shows fluid in pericardial sac and compression of the heart chambers.
- EKG:
  - Tachycardia
  - Waveform changes: P-wave shorter, diffuse ST elevation
- Radiology (Hoit, 2019):
  - *Chest x-ray:* Shows cardiac enlargement and mediastinal widening
  - *CT:* Reveals pericardial effusion
  - *MRI:* Exposes pericardial effusion and provides an estimate of the extent of the effusion
- PA catheterization:
  - Evaluates PA pressure
  - Decreases CO
  - Increases systemic vascular resistance (SVR)

TABLE 6.8 INFLAMMATORY CONDITIONS

DEFINITION	SIGNS AND SYMPTOMS	DIAGNOSTIC TESTING	TREATMENT
Myocarditis Inflammatory disease of the heart's myocardium (Kindermann et al., 2012). Caused by a broad source of triggers, including infectious agents, viruses, bacteria, parasites, and fungi, as well as non-infectious triggers, such as toxins and hypersensitivity agents. Viral infections are the most prevalent cause of myocarditis (Sinagra et al., 2016). Acute myocarditis develops over 3 months or less. Chronic myocarditis develops after 3 months.	Heterogeneous, ranging from asymptomatic state with vague signs and symptoms to severe cardiogenic shock and arrhythmias (Fung et al., 2016). In mild cases of myocarditis, pts may have no symptoms. In serious cases, the signs and symptoms vary, depending on the cause of the disease. Common signs and symptoms of myocarditis are as follows: Heart failure Chest pain Arrhythmias Shortness of breath, at rest or during physical activity Fluid retention, edema of lower extremities Fatigue Other signs and symptoms of a viral infection, such as a headache, body aches, joint pain, fever, sore throat, or diarrhea	Noninvasive testing (Fung et al., 2016; Kindermann et al., 2012) EKG assists in distinguishing between MI and myocarditis. Myocarditis presents on EKG with nonspecific T waves and ST segment changes. Echocardiography is a useful measurement tool in the diagnostic assessment of myocarditis and to rule out heart failure. Cardiac magnetic resonance imaging EMB is the only way to definitively diagnose myocarditis. Chest x-ray, cardiac biomarkers, and BNP if symptoms of heart failure are evident. Troponin is usually elevated.	Treatment of myocarditis should be focused on the causal pathophysiology (Fung et al., 2016) Antiviral agents Immunosuppression Corticosteroids
Endocarditis Inflammation of the heart's endocardium (inner lining), usually involving the heart valves. Bacteria enter the bloodstream. The bacteria commonly enter the bloodstream via the mouth, GI or urinary tract, or skin. They can also enter via venous catheters or after an invasive medical or surgical procedure (Cahill et al., 2017).	Endocarditis can present as either acute or subacute disease. Acute endocarditis: Sudden onset High fever, rigors, sepsis Subacute endocarditis: Can be difficult to diagnose. Patients present with non-specific symptoms that last for several weeks to months: Fatigue Dyspnea Weight loss	Blood cultures are drawn from three separate venipuncture sites. Determination of the causative pathogen is extremely important. Echocardiography is the ideal imaging modality for the diagnosis of endocarditis. Echocardiographic features vegetations, abscess, fistula, leaflet perforation, valve regurgitation, and prosthetic valve dehiscence. TE has a 70% sensitivity for diagnosis of new valve endocarditis. TEE offers higher sensitivity and better visualization than TE. Cardiac CT is for visualization of abscess or aneurysms.	Pathogen-specific antibiotics given for a prolonged period, usually 4–6 weeks. Good oral hygiene needed. Gum disease increases the risk of bacteria entering the bloodstream and the development of endocarditis. Indications for surgical inventions are acute complications, such as valve dysfunction. This could result in heart failure and increase the risk of mortality.

(continued)

TABLE 6.8 INFLAMMATORY CONDITIONS (continued)

DEFINITION	SIGNS AND SYMPTOMS	DIAGNOSTIC TESTING	TREATMENT
Pericarditis Inflammation of the pericardium caused by a broad source of triggers, which include infectious agents, viruses, bacteria, parasites, and fungi. Pericarditis develops suddenly and may last up to several months. It is categorized according to symptom duration (Cremer et al., 2016). Incessant pericarditis symptoms last more than 4–6 weeks. Chronic pericarditis symptoms persist for 3 months or longer.	Chest pain Sharp and stabbing; worsens with inspiration, cough, or when supine Decreased pain when patient is sitting up and leaning forward	Acute pericarditis: At least two of the following clinical criteria are required: Chest pain (typically sharp and pleuritic) that improves with sitting up and leaning forward Pericardial friction rub Changes in EKG with diffuse ST elevation or PR depression New or worsening pericardial effusion Narrowing pulse pressures	Anti-inflammatory drugs Aspirin: 750–1,000 mg TID for 1–2 weeks NSAIDs Ibuprofen 600 mg TID for 1–2 weeks Colchicine 0.5 mg BID for 3–6 months Corticosteroids—prednisone for 2–4 weeks, then start to taper (for recurrent pericarditis)

BNP, B-type natriuretic peptide; EMB, endomyocardial biopsy; GI, gastrointestinal; MI, myocardial infarction; NSAIDs, nonsteroidal anti-inflammatory drugs; pts, patients; TE, transthoracic echocardiogram; TEE, transesophageal echocardiography.

Treatment

- Overall management of cardiac tamponade focuses on relieving pressure on the heart and improving CO (Hoit, 2019).
- Stabilize the patient:
  - Perform volume resuscitation to increase preload.
  - *Avoid* medication that decreases SVR or preload (vasodilators).
  - Severe hemodynamic compromise requires decompression with pericardiocentesis.
- Pericardiocentesis:
  - Insert a catheter into the pericardial space to drain fluid.
  - Catheter can be left in place up to 24 hours. When less than 50 mL/d drains, the catheter can be removed:
    - Complications with pericardiocentesis:
      - Dysrhythmias
      - Pneumothorax
      - Laceration of coronary arteries
      - Laceration of lung
      - Puncture of right atrium or ventricle
      - Infection
      - Introduction of air into heart
      - Hypotension
  - Echocardiogram-guided pericardiocentesis:
    - Procedure of choice to remove pericardial fluid
  - Pericardial window:
    - Performed on patients who do not respond to other treatments
    - Entails removing a section of pericardium, creating an opening in pericardium to drain fluid from the pericardial sac:
      - Complications:
        - Infection
        - Atelectasis
        - Pleural effusion
        - Pneumothorax
        - Pain
        - Dysrhythmia

CARDIOMYOPATHY

Cardiomyopathy is a disease involving destruction of the cardiac muscle fibers, resulting in myocardial function impairment and decreased CO. It may affect the myocardial heart layer:

- The cause of cardiomyopathy is often idiopathic with no identified cause. Cardiomyopathies are classified into three types: dilated, hypertrophic, and restrictive (Table 6.9; Braunwald, 2017; Burns, 2014).

CARDIAC SURGERY

OVERVIEW

CABG has been recognized as an effective way of revascularization in treating patients with extensive coronary artery disease. It has been shown to statistically increase survival in high-risk patients:

- The surgical procedure entails the harvesting of the patient's own arteries or veins.
- These arteries or veins are used as grafts to bypass coronary arteries that are partially or completely obstructed by atherosclerotic plaque.
- Atherosclerotic lesions that narrow the lumen by 50% are considered significant.
- The decision to perform CABG is based on data obtained during a cardiac catheterization.
- The CABG is performed using a midline sternotomy.
- There are two basic ways the CABG procedure is performed: on-pump CABG and off-pump CABG:
  - On-pump CABG:
    - Utilizes the cardiopulmonary bypass machine:
      - Blood is diverted outside the body to a pump that mechanically provides perfusion and oxygenation to the blood and then returns it to arterial circulation.
    - Is performed while the heart is stopped (heart is arrested):

- This is accomplished by occluding the ascending aorta and perfusing the heart with cold, high-potassium cardioplegia solution.
  - Risk factors:
    - Stroke
    - Kidney failure
    - Liver failure
    - Decreased mental function
    - Bleeding
    - Infection
    - Irregular heart rhythms
- Off-pump CABG:
  - Is performed without using a cardiopulmonary bypass machine
  - Is performed on beating heart

- The pericardium is opened, and a stabilizing device is used to minimize wall motion at the site of anastomosis.

Risk Factors

- Infection
- Bleeding
- Irregular heart rhythms
- Blood clots
- Kidney failure

The most commonly used conduits in bypass surgery are the left internal thoracic artery and the saphenous vein. Sections of a vessel are attached between an arterial blood source and the targeted coronary vessel. Arterial conduits are preferred because of their patency rates.

TABLE 6.9 TYPES OF CARDIOMYOPATHIES

CARDIOMYOPATHIES	DEFINITIONS	SIGNS AND SYMPTOMS	DIAGNOSTIC TESTING	TREATMENT
Dilated	Dilated cardiomyopathy is the most common type of cardiomyopathy. Commonly caused by coronary artery disease, it impairs myocardial contractility and increased ventricular filling pressure. Coronary artery disease contributes to ventricular remodeling, which causes a reduction in ejection fraction. Dilated cardiomyopathy begins with the gradual destruction of myocardial fibers.	Fatigue Tachycardia Narrowed pulse pressure Decreased CO Dyspnea Arrhythmias Abnormal hemodynamics JVD	Chest x-ray 12-lead EKG Echocardiography	Oxygen Inotropic agents Diuretics Beta blockers ACE/ARB inhibitors
Hypertrophic	Hypertrophic cardiomyopathy is categorized as obstructive or nonobstructive. Both cause ventricular hypertrophy. Obstructive hypertrophic cardiomyopathy diagnosis is made if hypertrophy of the intraventricular septum is present. The hypertrophied septum obstructs the left ventricular outflow just below the aortic valve, resulting in limited ejection. The ventricle becomes rigid, resulting in reduced ventricular compliance and distensibility.	Angina Syncope Tachycardia Ventricular Fibrillation CO is initially normal and then decreases Dyspnea Orthopnea Palpitations Abnormal hemodynamics	Chest x-ray 12-lead EKG Echocardiography	Beta blockers Reduced physical and psychological stress Cardiac surgery Ethanol ablation
Restrictive	Restrictive cardiomyopathy involves ventricular fibrosis. The ventricular fibrosis is often caused by infiltration of the cardiac myocytes with abnormal tissue, such as sarcoid or amyloid disease. The fibrotic muscle tissue becomes rigid, with decreased compliance inhibiting distention during diastole.	Weakness Arrhythmias Dyspnea Decreased CO Abnormal hemodynamics JVD Peripheral edema Jaundice	Chest x-ray 12-lead EKG Echocardiography	Diuretics Sodium restriction Fluid restriction Vasodilator

ACE, angiotensin-converting enzyme; ARB, angiotensin receptor blocker; CO, cardiac output; JVD, jugular vein distention.

Indications
- Three-vessel coronary artery disease
- Left ventricular ejection fraction <35%
- Significant disease in left main coronary artery

Contraindications
- Older adults
- Debilitated patients
- Patients with severely diseased distal coronary vasculature
- Left ventricular ejection fraction <5% to 15%
- Contraindications to anesthesia:
  - Pulmonary edema
  - Severe chronic pulmonary disease
  - Pulmonary hypertension

Postoperative Management
- Maintain hemodynamic stability:
  - *MAP:* 70 to 80 mmHg
  - *Cardiac index (CI):* 2.0 to 3.5 L/min/m^2
  - *PA obstructive pressure:* 10 to 12 mmHg
  - *Central venous pressure:* 5 to 10 mmHg:
    - HR: 80 to 100 bpm
- Maintain ventilation and oxygenation.
- Prevent postoperative complications:
  - Bleeding from vascular graft sites
  - Cardiac tamponade:
    - Frequently assess for signs and symptoms of tamponade.

- Infection
- Cardiac arrhythmia:
  - Monitor EKG continuously.
  - Treat unstable arrhythmias.
  - Maintain potassium and magnesium within normal limits.
- Control of pain and anxiety

VALVULAR HEART DISEASE
Heart valve disease causes either stenosis or insufficiency of the valve:
- Stenosis occurs when the valve narrows, preventing it from opening fully. Pure stenosis blocks the flow of blood from one heart chamber to another or prevents adequate ejection of blood from a ventricle into circulation (Table 6.10).
- Insufficiency is the result of the valve's inability to close tightly, resulting in leaking. The leaking of blood back is referred to as *regurgitation.*
- The three common causes of valvular disorders:
  - Degenerative disease:
    - Valve is damaged over time due to mechanical stress, such as age or hypertension.
  - Rheumatic disease:
    - Causes gradual fibrotic changes of the valve
    - Causes valve cusps to become calcified
    - Commonly affects mitral valve
  - Infective endocarditis:

TABLE 6.10 TYPE OF VALVE INSUFFICIENCY AND STENOSIS

	DESCRIPTION	SIGNS AND SYMPTOMS
Mitral valve stenosis	Valve leaflet edges gradually become fused and fibrotic. Valve leaflets may also have an infusion of calcium deposits. Mitral valve becomes increasingly stenotic. Left atrium pressure increases. Dilation of the left atrium occurs as the stenosis worsens. Right ventricular failure develops because of increased left atrium pressure.	Diastolic murmur; Atrial arrhythmia (premature atrium contraction); Dyspnea; Hemoptysis; JVD; Orthopnea; Cough; Fatigue
Mitral valve insufficiency	Closure of mitral valve is needed for blood to be ejected into left atrium during ventricular systole. Insufficient mitral valve closure results in blood flowing backward into the left atrium. It is often associated with cardiomyopathy. As the left ventricle dilates, papillary muscles stretch, resulting in the failure to close the mitral valve. Left atrium pressure increases. Dilation of the atrium may occur. Right ventricular failure develops because of increased left atrium pressure.	Nocturnal dyspnea; Orthopnea; S3 and/or S4; Crackles; Systolic murmur; Atrial arrhythmias
Aortic valve stenosis	Valve leaflet edges gradually become fused and fibrotic. Valve leaflets may also have an infusion of calcium deposits. Aortic valve becomes increasingly stenotic. Worsening effects of aortic stenosis can lead to heart failure. Left ventricular pressure increases. Dilation and hypertrophy of the left ventricle occur as the stenosis worsens. Cardiac output decreases. Left atrium pressure increases, as the left atrium must generate more pressure to eject blood into the left ventricle.	Angina; Syncope; Decreased systemic vascular resistance; S3 and/or S4; Systolic murmur; Narrowed pulse pressures

(continued)

TABLE 6.10 TYPE OF VALVE INSUFFICIENCY AND STENOSIS (continued)

	DESCRIPTION	SIGNS AND SYMPTOMS
Aortic valve insufficiency	Closure of aortic valve is needed for blood to be ejected into left ventricle during ventricular systole. Insufficient aortic valve closure results in blood flowing backward into the left ventricle. Left ventricular pressure increases. Dilation and hypertrophy of the left ventricle occur as the result of increased left ventricle pressure. Cardiac output decreases.	Angina S3 Diastolic murmur Widening pulse pressures De Musset's sign (nodding of head)
Tricuspid valve stenosis	Valve leaflet edges gradually become fused and fibrotic. Valve leaflets may also have an infusion of calcium deposits. Tricuspid valve becomes increasingly stenotic. Right arterial pressure increases as result of right atrium attempting to propel blood into the right ventricle. Right atrium pressure increases. Right atrium dilatation increases.	Dyspnea Fatigue Increased RA pressure Peripheral edema Hepatomegaly JVD Atrial arrhythmia Diastolic murmur Decreased cardiac output
Tricuspid valve insufficiency	Damage to tricuspid valve prevents it from completely closing during ventricular systole. Insufficient tricuspid valve closure results in blood flowing backward into the right atrium. It is often associated with cardiomyopathy. As the right ventricle dilates, papillary muscles stretch, resulting in the failure to close the tricuspid valve. Right atrium pressure increases. Right atrium dilates. Right side cardiac output decreases.	Dyspnea Fatigue Increased RA pressure Peripheral edema Hepatomegaly JVD Conduction delays Supraventricular tachycardia Systolic murmur
Pulmonic valve stenosis	Valve leaflet edges gradually become fused and fibrotic. Valve leaflets may also have an infusion of calcium deposits. Pulmonic valve becomes increasingly stenotic. Right ventricular pressure increases. Right ventricle dilates. Right side cardiac output decreases. Pressure and volume in the venous system increase.	Dyspnea Fatigue Increased RA pressure Peripheral edema Hepatomegaly JVD Cyanosis Systolic murmur
Pulmonic valve insufficiency	Damage to pulmonic valve prevents it from completely closing during ventricular systole. Insufficient pulmonic valve closure results in blood flowing backward into the right ventricle. Right ventricular volume and pressure increase. Right side cardiac output decreases. Right ventricle dilates. Volume and pressure in venous system increase.	Dyspnea Fatigue Increased RA pressure Peripheral edema Hepatomegaly JVD Diastolic murmur

JVD, jugular vein distention; RA, right arterial.

- Results from a secondary infection
- Destroys valve tissue

Diagnostic Testing
- Chest x-ray:
  - Useful in identifying specific cardiac chamber enlargement, pulmonary congestion, and valve calcification.
- 12-Lead EKG:
  - Useful in the diagnosis of right ventricular, left ventricular, and left atrial hypertrophy.
- Echocardiogram:
  - Shows the size of the four cardiac chambers.
  - Useful in identifying the presence of hypertrophy and amount of regurgitant flow.
- Radionuclide studies:
  - Useful in identifying abnormal ejection fraction during inactivity and activity.
- Cardiac catheterization:
  - Identifies cardiac chamber pressures, ejection fraction, regurgitation, and pressure gradients.

Treatment
- Maximize cardiac function:
  - Medical management (Table 6.11)
  - Improve oxygen delivery:
    - Ventricular dilatation causes increased ventricular wall tension, myocardial workload, and oxygen consumption.

TABLE 6.11 BETA BLOCKERS

MEDICATION: GENERIC NAME (BRAND NAME)	CLASSIFICATION: PHARMACOTHER- APEUTIC AND CLINICAL	MECHANISM OF ACTION: THERAPEUTIC	INDICATIONS AND CONTRAINDICATIONS	DOSAGE	ADVERSE EFFECTS	SAFETY AND PATIENT EDUCATION
Propranolol (Inderal)	Beta blocker, antihypertensive, antianginal, antiarrhythmic, antimigraine	Slows heart rate, decreases BP, myocardial contractility, myocardial oxygen demand	**Indications:** Tx of angina, supraventricular arrhythmias, HTN, V tach, symptomatic obstructive hypertrophic cardiomyopathy, prevention of MI **Contraindications:** Hypersensitivity to propranolol, bronchial asthma, severe sinus bradycardia, cardiogenic shock, sick sinus syndrome, heart block greater than first degree, uncompensated HF	**HTN:** Immediate release: initially, 40 mg BID. May increase dose q3–7d. Usual dose: 120–240 mg/d in 2–3 doses. Maximum: 640 mg/d **Angina:** Immediate release: PO 80–320 mg/d in 2–4 divided doses **Arrhythmia:** PO: Immediate release: 10–30 mg q6–8h or 10–40 mg TID–QID times/d **Obstructive cardiomyopathy:** PO: Immediate release: 20–40 mg TID–QID times a day or 80–160 mg once daily as extended release capsule	Overdose may produce profound bradycardia, hypotension. Abrupt withdrawal may cause diaphoresis, palpitations, h/a. May precipitate HF, MI in patients with cardiac disease. Thyroid storm may occur in patients with thyrotoxicosis. Hypoglycemia may occur in patients with diabetes. **Antidote:** Glucagon	Obtain baseline and ongoing renal function, LFT, ECG as indicated, vital signs. Monitor for signs of HF; edema, monitor I/O. Patient should not stop abruptly. Compliance with regimen is essential. Restrict salt, alcohol intake. Do not use nasal decongestants, OTC cold preparations without approval from provider.
Atenolol (Tenormin)	Beta blocker, antihypertensive, antianginal, antiarrhythmic	Slows sinus node heart rate, decreasing cardiac output, BP; decreases myocardial oxygen demand	**Indications:** HTN, management of angina, management of definite/suspected MI to reduce CV mortality **Contraindications:** Hypersensitivity to atenolol; cardiogenic shock, uncompensated HF, second- or third-degree heart block, sinus bradycardia, sinus node dysfunction, pulmonary edema, pregnancy	**HTN:** PO: initially, 25–50 mg once daily. After 1–2 weeks, may increase up to 100 mg/d. Older adults: initial dose 25 mg once daily. **Angina:** PO: Initially 50 mg once daily. May increase dose up to 200 mg once daily. Older adults, initial dose 25 mg daily. **Post-MI:** PO: 100 mg once daily or 50 mg BID for 6–9 days post MI.	Overdose may produce profound bradycardia, hypotension. **Antidote:** Glucagon	Obtain baseline and ongoing EKG as indicated, vital signs, renal and hepatic function tests. Monitor for difficulty breathing, bowel activity, stool consistency; assess for HF; dyspnea, nocturnal cough, edema. Monitor I/O. Diabetics should monitor blood glucose. Do not abruptly discontinue medication. Compliance is essential. Report bleeding/bruising, dizziness, rash. Restrict salt, alcohol. Outpatients should monitor BP prior to taking medication.

(continued)

TABLE 6.11 BETA-BLOCKERS (continued)

MEDICATION: GENERIC NAME (BRAND NAME)	CLASSIFICATION: PHARMACOTHERAPEUTIC AND CLINICAL	MECHANISM OF ACTION: THERAPEUTIC	INDICATIONS AND CONTRAINDICATIONS	DOSAGE	ADVERSE EFFECTS	SAFETY AND PATIENT EDUCATION
Metoprolol (Lopressor)	Beta blocker, antihypertensive, antianginal, antiarrhythmic	Slows heart rate, decreases cardiac output, reduces BP; decreases myocardial ischemia severity	**Indications:** Tx of AMI to reduce CV mortality, HTN, angina **Contraindications:** Hypersensitivity to metoprolol; MI, severe sinus bradycardia, MI with heart rate <45 bpm, SBP <100 mmHg, moderate to severe, significant first-degree heart block, second- or third-degree block	**HTN:** Initially, 50 mg PO BID. Increase at weekly intervals. Maintenance 100–450 mg/d in 2–3 doses. **Angina:** PO: Initially, 50 mg PO BID. Usual range: 50–200 mg BID. Maximum 400 mg/d.	Overdose may produce profound bradycardia, hypotension. Abrupt withdrawal may cause diaphoresis, palpitations, h/a. May precipitate HF; MI in patients with cardiac disease. Thyroid storm may occur in patients with thyrotoxicosis. Hypoglycemia may occur in patients with diabetes. **Antidote:** Glucagon	Obtain baseline and ongoing EKG as indicated, vital signs, renal and hepatic function tests. Monitor for difficulty breathing, bowel activity, stool consistency; assess for HF, dyspnea, nocturnal cough, edema. Monitor I/O. Diabetics should monitor blood glucose. Do not abruptly discontinue medication. Compliance is essential. Report bleeding/bruising, dizziness, rash. Restrict salt, alcohol. Outpatients should monitor BP prior to taking medication.
Carvedilol (Coreg)	Antihypertensive	Reduces cardiac output, reduces peripheral vascular resistance	**Indications:** treatment of mild to severe HF, left ventricular dysfunction following MI, HTN **Contraindications:** Hypersensitivity to carvedilol. Cardiogenic shock marked sinus bradycardia, overt HF, second- or third-degree AV block. Sick sinus syndrome, severe hepatic impairment	**HTN:** Initially 6.25 mg PO BID, may double at intervals of 1–2 weeks to 12.5 mg BID, then to 25 mg BID. Maximum 25 mg BID. **HF:** PO: Initially, 3.125 mg BID. May double at 2 weeks intervals to highest tolerated dosage. Maximum for greater than 85 kg: 50 mg BID. Less than 85 kg: 25 mg BID. **Left ventricular dysfunction following MI:** PO: Initially 3.125–6.25 mg BID. Increase at intervals 3–10 days up to 25 mg BID.	Overdose may produce profound bradycardia, hypotension. Abrupt withdrawal may cause diaphoresis, palpitations, h/a. May precipitate HF; MI in patients with cardiac disease. Thyroid storm in patients with thyrotoxicosis. Hypoglycemia may occur in patients with diabetes.	Obtain baseline vital signs, EKG, renal and hepatic function tests. Monitor vital signs, dyspnea, EKG, daily bowel activity, stool consistency, assess for HF, dyspnea, nocturnal cough, edema. Monitor I/O. Diabetics should monitor blood glucose. Do not abruptly discontinue; compliance is essential. Report bleeding/bruising, dizziness, rash. Restrict salt, alcohol. Outpatients should monitor BP prior to taking medication.

AMI, acute myocardial infarction; AV, atrioventricular; BP, blood pressure; CV, cardiovascular; h/a, headache; HF, heart failure; HTN, hypertension; I/O, intake/output; LFT, liver function test; MI, myocardial infarction; OTC, over-the-counter; SBP, systolic blood pressure; Tx, treatment.

- Measure oxygenation consumption:
  - Pulse oximetry
  - SVO_2 mixed venous oxygenation
  - Arterial blood gases
- Decrease preload:
  - Decrease excess fluid and ventricular end-diastolic volumes (VEDVs).
  - Restrict fluids and sodium.
  - Patients with aortic insufficiency are exceptions to this.
- Decrease afterload:
  - Diuretics
  - Vasodilators
  - Inotropic agents:
    - Milrinone
    - Dobutamine
- Improve contractility:
  - Increase myocardial contractility and improve CO.
  - Inotropic agents:
    - Milrinone
    - Dobutamine
- Modify activity:
  - Limiting activity helps reduce myocardial oxygen consumption.
- Perform balloon valvuloplasty:
  - Option is for stenotic mitral and aortic valve.
  - Balloon is inflated at the stenotic lesions to force open the fused commissures and improve valve leaflet mobility.
- Surgical management:
  - Cardiac surgery is indicated when medical management is ineffective:
    - Valve repair:
      - Repair instead of replacing dysfunctional valve.
      - Hemodynamic function is better with a repaired valve as opposed to a prosthetic valve.
    - Valve leaflet reconstruction
    - Chordae tendineae reconstruction
    - Annuloplasty ring—Corrects dilatation of the valve annulus
    - Prosthetic valve replacement
    - Transcatheter aortic valve replacement (TAVR):
      - Minimally invasive aortic valve replacement
      - Avoids the use of cardiopulmonary bypass

Postoperative Management

- Maintain hemodynamic stability:
  - *MAP:* 70 to 80 mmHg
  - *CI:* 2.0 to 3.5 L/min/m^2
  - *PA obstructive pressure:* 10 to 12 mmHg
  - *Central venous pressure:* 5 to 10 mmHg
  - *HR:* 80 to 100 bpm
- Maintain ventilation and oxygenation.
- Maintain adequate preload.
- Monitor for conduction disturbances:
  - Conductive disturbances may be treated with temporary or permanent cardiac pacing.
- Offer anticoagulation therapy.

Prevention of Postoperative Complications

- Prosthetic valve dysfunction:
  - Biologic valve dysfunction develops slowly with gradual signs and symptoms: new murmur, dyspnea, and syncope.
  - Mechanical valve dysfunction may occur slowly or suddenly.
  - Rapid valve dysfunction requires emergency intervention:
    - Patient presents with acute cardiac failure:
      - Hypotension
      - Tachycardia
      - Low CO
      - HF
      - Cardiac arrest
- Cardiac tamponade:
  - Frequently assess for signs and symptoms of tamponade.
- Infection prevention:
  - Administer antibiotic prophylaxis.
- Cardiac arrhythmia:
  - Monitor EKG continuously.
  - Treat unstable arrhythmias.
  - Maintain potassium and magnesium within normal limits.
- Control pain and anxiety

HEART FAILURE

OVERVIEW

HF is a complex progressive clinical syndrome that results from any structural or functional cardiac disorder that affects the ability of the cardiac ventricles to fill or eject blood, resulting in volume overload and inadequate tissue perfusion (Eisen, 2017; Box 6.4):

- HF is classified as left-sided HF or right-sided HF and HF with reduced ejection fraction (HFrEF), also known as *HF with systolic dysfunction*, or *HF with preserved ejection fraction* (HFpEF), also known as *HF with diastolic dysfunction* (see Figure 6.1).
- The ACC and the AHA have created clinical staging guidelines that are correlated with the patient's symptoms and progression of HF (Feng et al., 2015; Table 6.12).

Pathophysiology

Multiple underlying etiologies and disease abnormalities may cause HF; the majority of HF cases are caused by one or more factors (Givens & Schulze, 2017; Table 6.13):

- Damage to the heart causes a compensatory response due to the decreased perfusion, causing vasoconstriction and sodium and water retention.
- HF begins with myocardial injury or stress, which initiates the series of compensatory mechanisms.

BOX 6.4 Causes of Heart Failure

- Coronary heart disease
- Valvular heart disease
- Cardiomyopathies
- Hypertension
- Diabetes mellitus
- Toxins
- Hypo/hyperthyroidism
- Infection/inflammation
- Congenital heart disease
- Substance abuse

TABLE 6.12 AMERICAN COLLEGE OF CARDIOLOGY/AMERICAN HEART ASSOCIATION GUIDELINES AND NEW YORK HEART ASSOCIATION HEART FAILURE CLASSIFICATION

CLINICAL STAGES AND FUNCTIONAL CLASSES OF HEART FAILURE			
ACC/AHA STAGE	**OBJECTIVE ASSESSMENT**	**NYHA CLASSIFICATION**	**PATIENT SYMPTOMS**
A	Risk factors for HF but no structural heart disease or symptoms	I	No limitation in any activities; no symptoms from ordinary activities
B	Structural evidence of heart disease but no symptoms	I	No limitation in any activities; no symptoms from ordinary activities
C	Structural evidence of heart disease and signs or symptoms of HF	I, II, III	Slight or marked limitation of physical activity; comfortable at rest; less than ordinary activity causes fatigue, palpitation, or dyspnea
D	Structural evidence of advanced heart disease and marked symptoms and signs of HF	II, III, IV	Unable to carry on any physical activity without discomfort; symptoms of heart failure at rest; if any physical activity is undertaken, discomfort increases

ACC, American College of Cardiology; AHA, American Heart Association; HF, heart failure; NYHA, New York Heart Association.
Source: Adapted from the American College of Cardiology Foundation/American Heart Association Task Force on Practice Guidelines. (2013). ACCF/AHA guideline for the management of heart failure: Executive summary. *Journal of the American College of Cardiology, 62*(16), 1495–1535. http://dx.doi.org/10.1016/j.jacc.2013.05.020

TABLE 6.13 LEFT-SIDED HEART FAILURE AND RIGHT-SIDED HEART FAILURE

	LEFT-SIDED HF	**RIGHT-SIDED HF**
Pathophysiology	The left ventricle is enlarged due to increased workload and end-diastolic volume. Usually associated with coronary artery disease, decreased oxygen supply causes the ventricle to expand, stretching the myocytes and decreasing the functionality of the ventricle. The abnormal contraction leads to abnormal electrical conduction and may result in ventricular and atrial dysrhythmias.	The right ventricle becomes enlarged or stretched, causing ventricular hypertrophy. The stretched right ventricle impairs the contractility, also reducing the electrical conduction and functionality of the ventricle. The increased pressure of the right ventricle increases the pressure and congestion into the superior and inferior vena cava, causing distension into the GI tract, liver, and peripheral tissues.
Etiology	■ Hypertension ■ Cardiomyopathy ■ Valve disease ■ Substance abuse ■ Coronary artery disease	■ Tricuspid regurgitation ■ Left ventricular failure ■ Pulmonary hypertension ■ Pulmonary valve stenosis ■ Pulmonary emboli
Signs/symptoms	■ Changes in mental status ■ Rales ■ Atrial dysrhythmias ■ Dyspnea ■ Hyperventilation ■ Fatigue and activity intolerance ■ Cool and pale skin ■ Tachycardia ■ Pulmonary edema ■ Cough with frothy sputum ■ Hypoxia ■ S3 and S4	■ Pitting edema ■ Venous congestion ■ Ascites ■ Decreased appetite, nausea, vomiting ■ Positive hepatojugular reflex (abdominal distension) ■ Jugular vein distention ■ Weight gain ■ S3 (early) ■ S4 (possible)

GI, gastrointestinal; HF, heart failure.
Source: Givens, R., & Schulze, P. (2017). Molecular changes in heart failure. In H. Eisen (Ed.), *Heart failure: A comprehensive guide to pathophysiology and clinical care* (pp. 1–18). Springer-Verlag London.

- Myocardial dysfunction and dilation cause the compensatory neurohormonal response to activate the renin–angiotensin–aldosterone system (RAAS) and the sympathetic nervous system (SNS).
- Remodeling occurs with a reduction of urinary excretion, resulting in excess total body fluid.
- Epinephrine levels begin to elevate, as do as norepinephrine, vasopressin, angiotensin II, aldosterone, and endothelin, leading to increased blood pressure, increased HR, increased afterload, increased preload, and increased cardiac workload, which produces a toxic injury on cardiac cells.
- Compensatory mechanisms promote cardiac function initially; eventually, the hypertrophied myocytes lose the ability to contract efficiently, causing the ventricular wall to increase in stiffness.
- Chronic volume overload causes dilation of the ventricular chamber, stretching the myocardial fibers and causing myocyte hypertrophy (myocyte cell proliferation), which initiates a remodeling process to the myocardium.
- Function of the heart deteriorates and performance is reduced.

- Calcium levels begin to increase in the myocardium, which causes the myocytes to augment contractability, impairing myocardial relaxation; this increases myocardial energy and further decreases CO.

Heart Failure Preserved Ejection Fraction Diastolic Heart Failure

HF*p*EF, or normal ventricular systolic function without valve lesions, is also referred to as *HF with diastolic dysfunction* (Figure 6.4).

Primary diastolic dysfunction is often observed in patients with hypertension or restrictive cardiomyopathy. It is characterized by a low CO from a thickened ventricle wall (increased left ventricular mass) with a small cavity. The LV becomes stiff and produces a slow relaxation in early diastole and increased resistance to late diastole filling, causing elevated diastolic pressures (Aziz et al., 2015; Michalska-Kasiczak et al., 2018).

Heart Failure Reduced Ejection Fraction

HF*r*EF is also known as *HF with systolic dysfunction* (see Figure 6.4). It is observed when there is an inadequate or

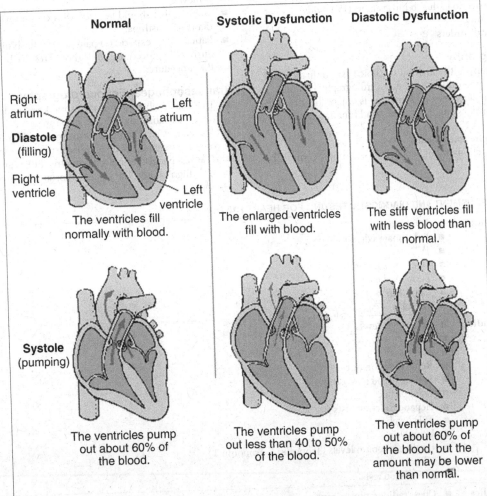

FIGURE 6.4 Systolic and diastolic dysfunction.

Source: From the *Merck Manual Consumer Version* (known as the *Merck Manual* in the United States and Canada and the *MSD Manual* in the rest of the world). (2019). In R. Porter (Ed.), Copyright 2019 by Merck Sharp & Dohme Corp., a subsidiary of Merck & Co., Inc., https://www .merckmanuals.com/home/heart-and-blood-vessel-disorders/heart-failure/heart-failure

diminished contraction of the ventricles, decreasing the CO. The left ventricular ejection fraction is less than 40%. HFrEF can be precipitated by coronary artery disease, hypertension, or dilated cardiomyopathy (Michalska-Kasiczak et al., 2018; Tables 6.14 and 6.15).

Clinical Practice Guidelines

For detailed guidelines, refer to 2017 ACC/AHA/HFSA *Guideline for the Management of Heart Failure* (ACC/AHA/HFSA, 2017; https://doi.org/10.1016/j.jacc.2017.04.025).

Pulmonary Edema

Pulmonary edema is an acute response to left ventricular HF (Table 6.16):

- When the filling pressure of the LV increases, the increased pressure in the pulmonary capillaries then causes extravasation of fluid into the interstitial spaces and alveoli, causing pulmonary edema.
- The precipitating causes of pulmonary edema originate from:
  - Acute coronary ischemia
  - Lack of adherence to dietary or medication therapy
  - HF decompensation
  - Volume overload due to intravenous (IV) fluids
  - Arrhythmia
  - Valvular disorders

Echocardiography

Echocardiography is the method of choice for confirming HF. The two- and three-dimensional echocardiography (2D and 3D echo) with Doppler ultrasound imaging is one of the most reliable tools when assessing the anatomy and function of the heart (Volpe & Lima, 2017).
Echocardiography assessment:

- Assesses functionality of ventricles, wall motion, and valve abnormalities.
- Assesses cardiac size, position, and wall thickness.
- Measures ejection fraction (normal ventricular ejection fraction: 55%–70%).
- Assesses structural remodeling.
- Assesses cardiac function, blood-flow speed, and direction.

Exercise Stress Echocardiography

- Evaluates the cardiac function under physical, exercise-induced stress.
- Helps identify the origin of the chest pain, cardiac function post MI, cardiac dysrhythmias, and cardiac perfusion post intervention.

Dobutamine Stress Echocardiography

- This is used for patients who are unable to tolerate the exercise stress echocardiography.
- Patients receive dobutamine to induce stress similar to the stress of exercise.
- Echocardiography is conducted at different intervals: once before medication administration, after medication administration, and a final test is done once the goal HR is achieved.
- Dobutamine should be used with caution when testing patients with asthma.
- Patients may experience palpitations, flushing, or chest pain during the procedure, but it should resolve by completion of the procedure.

Transesophageal Echocardiography

- This is a combination of ultrasound and endoscopy to produce a visualization of heart structures.
- Transducer attached to a gastroscope and inserted into the esophagus generates images of the posterior heart.
- Transesophageal echocardiography (TEE) can also visualize with high quality the thoracic aorta, PA, coronary arteries,

TABLE 6.14 ASSESSMENT AND DIAGNOSTIC TESTING FOR HEART FAILURE

Assessment findings	■ Dyspnea ■ Pulmonary edema ■ JVD ■ Chest discomfort ■ Peripheral edema ■ Cool skin ■ Oliguria
Laboratory studies	■ Electrolyte levels ■ CBC ■ BNP assay ■ Renal function test ■ Fasting blood glucose level ■ Lipid profile ■ Hepatic function tests ■ TSH level ■ Urinalysis ■ Cardiac troponin levels (Troponin I, Troponin T) ■ HIV ■ Serum iron tests
Diagnostic studies	■ Chest radiography (x-ray) ■ EKG ■ 2D echocardiography with Doppler ultrasound imaging ■ Exercise stress test ■ Cardiac MRI

BNP, B-type natriuretic peptide; CBC, complete blood count; JVD, jugular vein distention; TSH, thyroid-stimulating hormone.

TABLE 6.15 ACUTE, CHRONIC, AND ADVANCED HEART FAILURE

ACUTE HEART FAILURE	CHRONIC HEART FAILURE	ADVANCED HEART FAILURE
Acute HF is an initial response to ischemia, infarction, or myocardial insult: ■ The reaction leads to a loss of myocytes, decreasing the EF and resulting in pump failure. ■ As the pump fails, there is an increase of pressure in the venous system, which causes congestion when returning to the heart, increasing right and left atrial pressure. ■ Decreased cardiac output with an inability to produce systemic perfusion causes an increase in sympathetic nervous tone.	Chronic HF occurs after the ischemic injury (initial insult), which alters loading conditions. The compensatory mechanisms maintain an adequate cardiac output. This adaption sustains the heart rate, blood pressure, and cardiac output. Compensation begins as a response to the changes in the cardiac pump; fluid retention starts to occur due to the changes in renal perfusion.	Advanced HF occurs when the adaptive mechanisms in chronic HF no longer sustain adequate output. The presence of progressive and persistent severe signs and symptoms of HF begin to occur with no response to therapies or symptom management.

Pharmacology management
First line
- Inotropic (poor tissue perfusion and hypotension)
- Vasodilator (pulmonary congestion)
- Loop diuretic (fluid overload)
- ACE inhibitors
- Beta blockers
- ARBs

Second line
- ARNI
- Iron replacement
- Omega 3 fatty acids
- Digoxin
- Anticoagulation

Treatments for patients with advanced HF include cardiac transplantation, LVAD, CRT, ICD, and IABP. Cardiac transplantation is the primary treatment for advanced HF, but organ shortage and increased wait times lead to candidates not receiving donor hearts. LVAD placement can be used as a bridge to transplantation or destination therapy for patients who are not surgical candidates (Taghavi & Mangi, 2017).

Monitoring
Invasive hemodynamics:
- PAP monitoring differentiates patients with HF from patients with pulmonary disorders and measures function of the left ventricle with pulmonary wedge pressure.

ACE, angiotensin-converting enzyme; ARBs, angiotensin receptor blockers; ARNI, angiotensin receptor neprilysin inhibitor; CRT, cardiac resynchronization therapy; EF, ejection fraction; HF, heart failure; IABP, intra-aortic balloon pump; ICD, implantable cardioverter defibrillator; LVAD, left ventricular assist device; PAP, pulmonary artery pressure.

TABLE 6.16 PULMONARY EDEMA: ASSESSMENT, SYMPTOMS, AND TREATMENT

ASSESSMENT FINDINGS/ DIAGNOSTIC	SYMPTOMS	TREATMENT
Pulmonary crackles Chest x-ray Dyspnea	Dyspnea Diaphoresis Wheezing Blood-tinged frothy sputum	Oxygen Nitrates (intravenous) Diuretics Inotropes (HFrEF) Mechanical ventilation or BiPAP ventilation

BiPAP, bilevel positive airway pressure; HFrEF, heart failure with reduced ejection fraction.

cardiac valves, left and right atria, atrial septum, and left atrial appendage.
- It requires IV sedation and continuous monitoring during and after the procedure.
- Esophageal varices or obstructions are contraindicated for this test.

HYPERTENSION

OVERVIEW

Hypertension is a chronic disease of elevated blood pressure associated with considerable morbidity and mortality and is often masked in the early years of onset.

- Hypertension is the result of an array of abnormalities that include ventricular hypertrophy, systolic and diastolic dysfunction, arrhythmias, and symptomatic HF.
- A compensatory mechanism of hypertensive heart disease is that the left ventricular wall thickens in response to elevated blood pressure to minimize wall stress (Table 6.17).
- As the heart transitions to failure, the LV dilates, and the ventricular ejection fraction declines. All hypertensive patients' morbidity and mortality can be directly related to their hypertension.

Signs and Symptoms

High blood pressure is mostly symptomless. It has been referred to as the "silent killer."

Diagnostic Testing

Blood pressure monitoring

Treatment

- Lifestyle changes:
  - Smoking cessation
  - Exercise at least 30 min/d
  - Heart-healthy diet
    - Low sodium: Ingest less than 2.4 g/d
    - Less than 30% fat
    - Avoid trans fats
  - Maintain healthy weight
- Medications
  - ACE inhibitors (Table 6.18)
  - ARBs (Table 6.19)
  - Diuretics (thiazide diuretics)
  - Beta blockers (see Table 6.10)
  - Calcium channel blockers (Table 6.20)

Hypertensive Crisis

Hypertensive crisis an acute episode or exacerbation that infrequently occurs in a small number of hypertensive patients. It may be a primary or secondary condition in seriously ill patients.

- Patients in hypertensive crisis frequently have an underlying diagnosis of chronic hypertension.
- Blood pressure is often >180/120 mmHg, and there is no specific blood pressure value. The rate at which the blood pressure increases is more important than the value.
- Organs most significantly impacted by elevated blood pressure are the brain, heart, and kidneys; injury can manifest as encephalopathy, stroke, intracranial hemorrhage, unstable angina, MI, left ventricular dysfunction, or aortic dissection.

There are two types of hypertension crisis.

- **Hypertensive urgency**
  - Severely elevated blood pressure without evidence of organ failure.
  - The goal is to reduce the pressure over hours to days to a safer level. It is managed with oral or IV agents and gradual blood pressure control over 24 to 48 hours.
- **Hypertensive emergency**
  - Refers to new or progressive end-organ injury secondary to elevated blood pressure.
  - The goal is to reduce mean arterial blood pressure by no more than 20% to 25% in the first few hours.
  - Treatment requires continuous monitoring of blood pressure, neurologic status, urine output, and other parameters.
  - Parenteral and titratable agents are utilized to lower the blood pressure within minutes to hours.
  - If blood pressure is lowered too rapidly, it may result in hypoperfusion of major arterial beds and can result in cerebral infarction or MI.

TABLE 6.17 AMERICAN HEART ASSOCIATION CLASSIFICATION OF BLOOD PRESSURE

CLASSIFICATION OF BP			
BP CATEGORY	SYSTOLIC BP	DIASTOLIC BP	TREATMENT OR FOLLOW-UP
Normal	<120 mmHg	<80 mmHg	Evaluate yearly; encourage healthy lifestyle changes to maintain BP
Elevated	120–129 mmHg	<80 mmHg	Encourage healthy lifestyle changes and reassess 3–6 months
Hypertension stage 1	130–139 mmHg or	80–89 mmHg	Assess the 10-year risk for heart disease and stroke with the atherosclerotic cardiovascular disease risk calculator: ■ If risk is less than 10%, start with healthy lifestyle recommendations and reassess in 3–6 months. ■ If risk is greater than 10% or the patient has known clinical cardiovascular disease, diabetes mellitus, or chronic kidney disease, recommend lifestyle changes and one BP-lowering medication; reassess in 1 month for effectiveness of medication: • If goal is met after 1 month, reassess in 3–6 months. • If goal is not met after 1 month, consider a different medication or titration. • Continue monthly follow-up until control is achieved.
Hypertension stage 2	>140 mmHg or	>90 mmHg	■ Encourage healthy lifestyle changes and two BP-lowering medications of different classes; reassess in 1 month for effectiveness: • If goal is met after 1 month, reassess in 3–6 months. • If goal is not met after 1 month, consider a different medication or titration. • Continue monthly follow-up until control is achieved.

BP, blood pressure.

TABLE 6.18 CARDIAC MEDICATIONS

MEDICATION	CLASS	MECHANISM OF ACTION	MAJOR INDICATIONS/CONTRAINDICATIONS	DOSAGE	SIDE EFFECTS	SAFETY/PATIENT EDUCATION
Captopril (Capoten), Benazepril (Lotensin), Enalapril (Vasotec), Enalaprilat, Lisinopril (Prinivil, Zestril), Ramipril (Altace)	ACE inhibitors	Inhibits ACE Prevents conversion of angiotensin I to angiotensin II Leads to decreased levels of angiotensin II, which results in increased plasma renin activity and decreased in aldosterone release	**Indications:** Hypertension Heart failure Left ventricular dysfunction after myocardial infarctions **Contraindications:** Hypersensitivity ACE inhibitor Angioedema related to previous treatment with ACE Pregnancy (cause renal abnormalities in fetus)	**For hypertension:** Capotril: 25 mg PO BID or TID Benazapril, Lisinopril, and Fosinopril: 10 mg PO daily Enalapril: 5 mg PO daily Ramipril 2.5 mg PO daily **For heart failure:** Captopril: 6.25 mg PO TID Enalapril: 2.5 mg PO daily Lisinopril: 2.5–5 mg PO daily Ramipril: 1.25–2.5 mg PO BID	Chest pain, palpitations, increased serum creatinine, hyperkalemia, dysgeusia (loss of taste), bronchospasm, cough, rash, fetal toxicity	Encourage taking medication 1 hour prior to meals. Instruct to report urinary retention, hematuria, change in urine output or weight gain. Report signs of hyperkalemia (confusion, dizziness), severe cough, and chest pain. Interacts with loop diuretics, NSAIDs, and potassium-sparing diuretics, allopurinol, ciprofloxacin, and eplerenone. Increased rate of angioedema in African Americans.
Losartan, Candesartan (Atacand), Irbesartan (Avapro), Valsartan (Diovan)	Angiotensin II receptor blockers	Block the vasoconstrictor and aldosterone-secreting effects of angiotensin II Interacts reversibly at the AT_1 and AT_2 receptors of many tissues	**Indications:** Hypertension management Diabetic nephropathy Hypertension with left ventricular hypertrophy **Contraindications:** Hypersensitivity Pregnancy (cause renal abnormalities in fetus)	Initial dose of 50 mg daily Dose range 25–100 mg once or BID with maximum dose 100 mg/d in 1 or 2 divided doses 25 mg/d in patients receiving diuretics or intravascular volume depletion	Hypotension, chest pain, orthostatic hypotension, myasthenia, dizziness fatigue, hyperkalemia, diarrhea, cough back pain, intraoperative hypotension in surgical patients	Can take without food. Instruct to report urinary retention, hematuria, change in urine output or weight gain. Report signs of hyperkalemia (confusion, dizziness), severe cough, and chest pain.

(continued)

TABLE 6.18 CARDIAC MEDICATIONS *(continued)*

MEDICATION	CLASS	MECHANISM OF ACTION	MAJOR INDICATIONS/CONTRAINDICATIONS	DOSAGE	SIDE EFFECTS	SAFETY/PATIENT EDUCATION
Diazoxide (Hyperstat) Hydralazine (Apresoline) Minoxidil (Loniten) Sodium nitroprusside (Nitropress) Tolazoline (Priscoline)	Peripheral vasodilators	**Hydralazine (Apresoline)** Vasodilation of arterioles **Sodium nitroprusside (Nitropress)** - Direct action of vasodilation on arteriolar and venous smooth muscle, leading to reduced peripheral resistance	**Indications:** Management of moderate to severe hypertension **Contraindications:** Mitral valve disease, renal impairment, coronary artery disease, postural hypertension, lupus-like syndrome, peripheral neuritis	Hydralazine dosing Hypertension: PO—Initial 10 mg QID/increase to 25 mg QID; then 50 mg QID Hypertensive emergency: IM, IV dosing—initial 5–10 mg; can repeat in 20–30 minutes if BP remains elevated above threshold; maximum dose 20 mg Sodium nitroprusside dosing: 0.3–0.5 mcg/kg/min IV, can increase by 0.5 mcg/kg/min q5min	Hydralazine: Headache, anorexia, nausea, vomiting, diarrhea, palpitations, tachycardia, angina pectoris Sodium nitroprusside: Chest pain or discomfort, rapid, irregular heartbeat or pulse, lightheadedness, dizziness, bradycardia, difficulty breathing, unusual tiredness	Hydralazine: Instruct patient to report lupus symptoms, urinary hesitancy, severe dizziness, fainting, angina, tachycardia. Nitroprusside: Instruct patient to report dyspnea, tachycardia, severe dizziness, agitation, diaphoresis, muscle rigidity, or nausea.
Thiazide diuretics: (Hydrochlorothiazide, Chlorthalidone) Loop diuretics: (Furosemide, Bumetanide, Torsemide) Potassium-sparing diuretics: (Amiloride, Spironolactone)	Diuretics	Thiazide Diuretic: inhibits reabsorption of Na+ and Cl⁻ in the distal convoluted tubule, resulting in retention of water in the tubule. Loop diuretic: inhibits the Na+/K+/2Cl⁻ cotransport in the ascending loop of Henle, resulting in retention of Na+, Cl⁻, and water in the tubule. Potassium-Sparing diuretic: Spironolactone inhibits the aldosterone-mediated reabsorption of Na+ and secretion of K+. Amiloride and triamterene block Na+ channels.	**Indications:** Edema due to heart failure, hepatic cirrhosis, or renal function Management of mild to moderate hypertension **Contraindications:** Known drug hypersensitivity; electrolyte imbalance; anuria	Hydrochlorothiazide: 12.5–50 mg PO once daily; for edema, 25–100 mg PO once daily or BID Chlorthalidone: 12.5–25 mg/d PO for hypertension; 50–100 mg/d PO or 100 mg PO QOD for edema not to exceed 200 mg/d Furosemide: Initial: 20–40 mg/d PO. Maintenance: 40–220 mg/d PO Torsemide: Initial: 5–10 mg/d PO Maintenance: 10–50 mg/d PO Bumetanide: Initial: 0.5–1 mg/d PO Maintenance: 1–5 mg/d PO Amiloride: Hypertension 5–10 mg/d PO daily or divided q12h Spironolactone: 25–100 mg PO daily or divided q12h initially for hypertension and edema	Necrotizing angiitis, orthostatic hypotension, dizziness, vertigo, restlessness, headache, paresthesia interstitial nephritis, renal failure, glycosuria, hypercalcemia, hypokalemia, nausea, vomiting, diarrhea, constipation, pancreatitis, pulmonary edema, Stevens-Johnson syndrome, erythema multiform	Instruct patient to report signs of hyperglycemia, fluid and electrolyte imbalance, urinary retention, hematuria, severe abdominal pain, nausea, back pain, vomiting, shortness of breath.

(continued)

					Side effects	
Organic nitrates: Nitroglycerin, isosorbide dinitrate (Isordil), isosorbide mononitrate **Beta blockers** **Calcium channel blockers** **Nondihydropyridines: Diltiazem (Cardizem), verapamil (Calan, Verelan)** **Dihydropyridines: amlodipine (Norvasc, Lotrel), felodipine (Plendil), nifedipine (Adalat, Procardia),**	Antianginals	Organic nitrates: Enter smooth muscle cells and relax all types of vessels, with the venules and veins being particularly sensitive. Beta blockers: Block beta receptors in the heart and juxtaglomerular apparatus of the kidneys. Calcium channel blockers: Block inward flow of Ca^{2+} through voltage-gated L-type calcium channels by binding to the channel alpha1 subunit.	**Indications:** Nitrates: Angina pectoris, intractable congestive cardiac failure, left ventricular failure Beta blockers: Tachycardia, hypertension, myocardial infarction, congestive heart failure, cardiac arrhythmias, hyperthyroidism, glaucoma Calcium channel blockers: Hypertension, chronic stable angina or angina from coronary spasm Nondihydropyridines: Hypertension, angina pectoris, arrhythmias, headache Dihydropyridines: Hypertension, angina pectoris, migraine **Contraindications:** Acute myocardial infarction, severe anemia Beta blockers: Asthma, cocaine-induced coronary spasm, acute or chronic bradycardia, hypotension	Nitroglycerin dosing: 0.3–0.6 mg SL q5min up to 3 times for angina pectoris; 1 tablet SL 5–10 minutes before activities likely to provoke angina attacks for angina pectoris (Prophylaxis) Isosorbide dinitrate dosing for angina pectoris: SL (prophylaxis): 2.5–5 mg 15 minutes before performing activities likely to cause angina SL (treatment): 2.5–5 mg; may be repeated q5–10min; not to exceed 3 doses in 15–30 minutes Isosorbide mononitrate: immediate release: 5–10 mg PO BID initially (5 mg in small patients) given each dose 7 hours apart; increased to 10 mg PO q12h by day 2 or 3; maintenance: 20 mg PO q12h Beta blockers: Dosage dependent on renal function Calcium channel blockers: Cardizem (most commonly prescribed) dosing: extended-release capsule, 120 mg daily, range 120–320 mg daily	Nitrates: Hypotension, dizziness, paresthesia, hyperkalemia, abdominal pain, dyspnea, diaphoresis Beta blockers: Bradycardia, fatigue, depression, worsening of chronic lung disease and peripheral artery disease, coronary artery spasm Calcium channel blockers: Headache, flushing, dizziness, dyspepsia, constipation, impaired cardiac conduction, reflex tachycardia, decreased contractility, shortness of breath, peripheral edema	Report bradycardia, tachycardia, fainting, severe headache; report chest tightness, wheezing, seizures, shortness of breath, and excessive weight gain, or facial, lip, or tongue swelling. Monitor for signs of hypotension, dizziness, and tolerance and need for dose adjustment.

(continued)

TABLE 6.18 CARDIAC MEDICATIONS (continued)

MEDICATION	CLASS	MECHANISM OF ACTION	MAJOR INDICATIONS/CONTRAINDICATIONS	DOSAGE	SIDE EFFECTS	SAFETY/PATIENT EDUCATION
			Calcium channel blockers: Atrial fibrillation, atrial flutter with RVR Nondihydropyridines: Hypersensitivity, bradycardia acute MI, post MI Dihydropyridines: Hypersensitivity, aortic stenosis			
Digoxin	Antiarrhythmics	Digoxin: Shortens atrial and ventricular refractory periods, causing prolonged AV nodal conduction and AV nodal refractory periods	Digoxin: Atrial fibrillation, heart failure **Contraindications:** Ventricular fibrillation	Digoxin: 0.4–0.6 mg IV over >5 min; may repeat 0.1–0.3 mg IV over >5 min	Digoxin: Arrhythmias, nausea, and vomiting	Monitor for digoxin toxicity (nausea, vomiting, visual changes, cardiac arrhythmias).
Adenosine	Antiarrhythmics	Adenosine: Slows or blocks AV nodal conduction to prevent tachyarrhythmias	Paroxysmal supraventricular tachycardia **Contraindications:** Asthma, second- or third-degree AV block, sinus node disease	Adenosine: 6 mg IV rapid bolus over 103 sec followed by a 20-mL bolus of NS; repeat with 12 mg in 1–2 min	Adenosine: AV block, flushing, chest discomfort due to bronchospasm	

ACE, angiotensin-converting enzyme; AV, atrioventricular; BP, blood pressure; IM, intramuscular; IV, intravenous; NSAIDs, nonsteroidal anti-inflammatory drugs; RVR, rapid ventricular rate.

TABLE 6.19 ALPHA ADRENERGIC BLOCKERS

MEDICATION: GENERIC NAME (BRAND NAME)	CLASSIFICATION: PHARMACO-THERAPEUTIC AND CLINICAL	MECHANISM OF ACTION: THERAPEUTIC	INDICATIONS AND CONTRAINDICATIONS	DOSAGE	ADVERSE EFFECTS	SAFETY AND PATIENT EDUCATION
Doxazosin (Cardura) Prazosin (Minipress) Terazosin (Hytrin)	Pharmacotherapeutic: Alpha-adrenergic blocker **Clinical:** aAntihypertensive	Causes peripheral vasodilation, lowering BP.	**Indications:** Treatment of mild to moderate HTN; used alone or in combination with other antihypertensives **Contraindications:** Hypersensitivity to doxazosin or other quinazolines	**Doxazosin:** PO (immediate-release): initially, 1 mg once daily. May be increased to 2 mg once daily. Can increase over several weeks to maximum of 16 mg/d. **Prazosin:** PO: 6–20 mg/d **Terazosin:** PO: 1–20 mg/d	First-dose syncope may occur 30–90 minutes following initial dose of 2 mg or more, to rapid an increase in dosage, addition of another antihypertensive agent. First-dose syncope may be preceded by tachycardia. Dizziness, light-headedness, palpitations.	Give first dose at bedtime. If given during daytime, patient must remain recumbent 3–4 hours. Assess vital signs immediately prior to and q15–30min until BP stabilizes. Assess for edema, h/a. Full therapeutic effect may not occur for 3–4 weeks. Avoid tasks that require alertness until response to drug is established. If not taken for several days, restart at initial dose.

BP, blood pressure; h/a, headache; HTN, hypertension.

Signs and Symptoms
- Symptoms often reflect the organ affected:
  - Headache
  - Blurred vision
  - Nose bleed
  - Dizziness
  - Diminished peripheral pulses
  - GI bleed
  - Pulmonary edema
  - Short of breath
  - Fatigue
  - Malaise
  - Nausea and vomiting
  - Hematuria or dysuria

Diagnostic Testing
- EKG to assess for cardiac ischemia
- Chest x-ray to evaluate pulmonary edema or widening mediastinum
- CT of brain if altered mental status or focal neurologic deficits
- Specific tests to target organ damage:
  - Renal angiography
  - Coronary angiography
  - Carotid/cerebral angiography

Treatment
- Rapid-acting antihypertensives are preferred:
  - Labetalol
  - Esmolol
  - Nitroprusside
  - Nicardipine
  - Nitroglycerin
  - Fenoldopam
- Oral antihypertensives can be initiated within 6 to 12 hours of presentation and parenteral agents weaned.

CARDIOVASCULAR PROCEDURES AND SKILLS

OVERVIEW
It is imperative that CNSs be knowledgeable of the most current recommendations for effective cardiopulmonary resuscitation:
- CPR is defined as a first-aid technique used for ineffective breathing or the absence of a heartbeat (Healthdirect, 2017).
- The CPR sequence is as follows: Chest compression, assess airway, provide rescue breaths (acronym: CAB).
- The 2017 AHA Updates for outside hospital cardiac arrest include providing chest compression–only CPR (Kleinman et al., 2017).

Effective chest compressions are essential to improving survival from cardiac arrest. High-quality CPR must be maintained to ensure adequate blood flow throughout the body supplying oxygen to the heart and brain (Kleinman et al., 2015).

PERFORM SYNCHRONIZED CARDIOVERSION
- Synchronized cardioversion is an intervention that delivers a low energy shock to the heart, which is accurately timed to the QRS complex. Synchronization ensures no inappropriate

TABLE 6.20 CALCIUM CHANNEL BLOCKERS

MEDICATION: GENERIC NAME (BRAND NAME)	CLASSIFICATION: PHARMACOTHERAPEUTIC AND CLINICAL	MECHANISM OF ACTION: THERAPEUTIC	INDICATIONS AND CONTRAINDICATIONS	DOSAGE	ADVERSE EFFECTS	SAFETY AND PATIENT EDUCATION
Verapamil (Calan Isoptin)	Calcium channel blocker Antihypertensive, class III antiarrhythmic	Decreases heart rate, myocardial contractility, slows SA, AV conduction. Decreases total peripheral vascular resistance by vasodilation.	**Indications:** **Parenteral:** Management of SVT, temporary control of rapid ventricular rate in atrial flutter/fibrillation. **PO:** Tx of HTN, angina pectoris, SVT, rate control for atrial flutter/fibrillation. **Contraindications:** Hypersensitivity to verapamil. Atrial flutter/fibrillation in presence of accessory bypass tract (e.g., WPW), severe LV dysfunction, cardiogenic shock, second or third AV block, hypotension, sick sinus syndrome, current use of IV beta-blocking agents, v tach.	**Angina:** PO: Initially, 80–120 mg TID. For older adults or patients with hepatic dysfunction, initially 40 mg TID. Titrate to optimal dose. Maintenance: 240–480 mg/d in 3–4 divided doses. Usual range: 80–160 mg TID. **HTN:** PO: Initially, 40–80 mg TID. Range: 240–480 mg/d in divided doses. **Chronic atrial fibrillation (rate control)/SVT:** PO: 240–480 mg/d in 3–4 divided doses. Usual range: 120–360 mg/d.	Rapid ventricular rate in atrial flutter/fibrillation. Marked hypotension, extreme bradycardia, HF, asystole, second or third AV block.	Obtain baseline EKG, vital signs. Assess and monitor vital signs, EKG changes; monitor daily pattern of bowel activity, stool consistency. Therapeutic serum level: 0.08–0.3 mcg/mL. Compliance with therapy is essential; do not abruptly discontinue medication. Limit caffeine and avoid or limit alcohol. Report cardiac symptoms, dyspnea, swelling, dizziness, constipation. Avoid grapefruit products.
Diltiazem (Cardizem) (PO)	Calcium channel blocker, class IV antiarrhythmic, antihypertensive	Relaxes coronary vascular smooth muscle, decreases heart rate, increases myocardial oxygen delivery	**Indications:** Tx of angina due to coronary artery spasm, chronic stable angina, HTN	**Angina:** PO: Initially, 30 mg QID. Range 120–320 mg/d. **HTN:** Extended-release PO capsules used, dosage range varies based upon formulation.	Abrupt withdrawal may increase frequency or duration of angina, HF; second- or third-degree HB occurs rarely. **Antidote:** Glucagon, insulin drip with continuous calcium infusion.	Obtain baseline and periodic vital signs, EKG, renal/hepatic function tests. Monitor vital signs, patient report of pain (angina description), edema, bradycardia. Do not abruptly discontinue. Compliance is essential with regimen. Report palpitations, dyspnea, dizziness, nausea, constipation, avoid alcohol.

(continued)

Drug	Classification	Action	Indications/Contraindications	Dose	Adverse Effects/Antidote	Nursing Considerations
Nifedipine XL (Procardia XL, Adalat CC)	Calcium channel blocker, antianginal, antihypertensive	Increases heart rate, myocardial oxygen delivery, cardiac output. Decreases systemic vascular resistance, BP.	**Indications:** Tx of angina due to coronary artery spasm. **Extended release:** HTN. **Contraindications:** Hypersensitivity to nifedipine. STEMI.	**Angina:** PO (immediate-release): Initially, 10 mg TID. Increase at 7- to 14-day intervals. Maintenance 10 mg TID up to 30 mg QID. Maximum: 180 mg/d. Extended release: PO: Initially 30–60 mg/d. Maximum 120 mg/d. **HTN:** PO: Extended release: initially 30–60 mg/d. Max 90–120 mg/d.	HF, MI in patients with cardiac disease, peripheral ischemia. Overdose produces nausea, drowsiness, confusion, slurred speech. **Antidote:** Glucagon.	Obtain baseline anginal pain description, BP. Assess for peripheral edema. Assess skin for flushing. Monitor LFT, observe for HF. Patient should report dyspnea, dizziness, palpitations, exacerbations of angina. Avoid alcohol, grapefruit juice.
Amlodipine (Norvasc)	Calcium channel blocker, antihypertensive, antianginal	Dilates coronary arteries, peripheral arteries/arterioles. Decreases total peripheral vascular resistance and BP by vasodilation.	**Indications:** Management of HTN, CAD **Contraindications:** Hypersensitivity to amlodipine	**HTN** PO: Initially, 5 mg/d as a single dose (older adults: 2.5 mg/d). May titrate q7–14d. Maximum: 10 mg/d. **CAD:** PO: 5–10 mg/d as single dose. Older adults with hepatic impairment: 5 mg/d single dose.	Overdose may produce excessive peripheral vasodilation, marked hypotension with reflex tachycardia, syncope.	Obtain baseline and periodic renal/hepatic function tests, vital signs. If SBP < 90 mmHg, hold medication, contact provider. Assess for flushing or edema. Question for h/a, asthenia. Compliance with therapy is essential. Do not abruptly discontinue regimen. Do not ingest grapefruit products.

AV, atrioventricular; BP, blood pressure; CAD, coronary artery disease; h/a headache; HB, heart block; HF, heart failure; HTN, hypertension; IV, intravenous; LFT, liver function test; LV, left ventricle; MI, myocardial infarction; SA, sinoatrial; SBP, systolic blood pressure; STEMI, ST segment elevation myocardial infarction; SVT, supraventricular tachycardia; Tx, treatment; v tach, ventricular tachycardia; WPW, Wolff–Parkinson–White.

shocks are delivered that could result in ventricular fibrillation (ACLS, 2018; Zoll, 2018).
- Cardioversion is used in the treatment of certain arrhythmias and may be used in conjunction with medical management.
- Common arrhythmias for which cardioversion may be indicated include atrial flutter, atrial fibrillation, and supraventricular tachycardia (Zoll, 2018).
- Sedation should be administered prior to cardioversion to reduce patient discomfort.

MANAGE PATIENT WITH LIFE VEST

The CNS should understand proper management of patients with life vests and ensure patients and their families understand the importance of adherence to the AHA, ACC, and the Heart Rhythm Society recommendations.
- Currently, the life vest is recommended for patients at risk for sudden cardiac arrest/death, including postMI, post-PCI (cardiac artery stenting), and nonischemic cardiomyopathy (Zoll, 2017).
- The life vest can usually deliver its shock in under a minute once an arrhythmia is detected. It has a 98% success rate with first shock delivery and a 92% shock survival rate (Zoll, 2017). Patients should wear their life vest at all times; it should be removed only when showering/bathing (Zoll, 2017).

HEMODYNAMIC INTERPRETATION

OVERVIEW

Hemodynamic is a term referring to the interrelationship of blood pressure, blood flow, vascular volumes, HR, ventricular function, and the physical properties of the blood. The parameters obtained from hemodynamic monitoring provide specific, accurate, and timely physiologic data.
- The aim of hemodynamic management is to optimize perfusion pressure and oxygen delivery to maintain and/or restore adequate cellular metabolism.
- Hemodynamic management guides the administration of fluids and vasoactive agents to optimize cardiopulmonary function.

Parameters

- Heart rate
  - Normal value: 60 to 100 bpm
- Stroke volume
  - The amount of blood ejected from the ventricles with each heartbeat:

$$SV = CO/HR \times 1000$$

  - It is the difference between end diastolic volume (EDV) and end systolic volume (ESV).
  - Normal value is 50 to 100 mL/heartbeat.
- Stroke volume index (SVI)
  - It is SV adjusted to body size:

$$SVI = CI/HR$$

  - Normal value: 35 to 60 mL/heartbeat/m^2.
- Cardiac output
  - It is the amount of blood pumped by the ventricles each minute.
  - It is the result of HR and SV:

$$CO = HR \times SV$$

  - Normal value: 4.0 to 8.0 L/min.
- Cardiac index
  - The cardiac index is the CO adjusted to patient body size.
  - It is calculated by dividing the CO by body surface area (BSA):

$$CI = CO/BSA$$

  - Normal value: 2.5 to 4.3 L/min/m^2.
  - CO is the volume of blood flowing through either the systemic or the pulmonary circuit.
  - It is calculated by multiplying the HR in beats per minute by the SV and is expressed in liters per minute. Normal adult CO at rest is about 5 L/min (Amsterdam et al., 2014; Cannon et al., 2013).

Factors Affecting Cardiac Output

- *Ejection fraction* refers to the amount of blood ejected per heart beat; it is an indicator of ventricular function.
  - Calculated by dividing the SV by the end-diastolic volume; normal value is 66% for women and 58% for men (Cannon et al., 2013).

Preload

- Also called *VEDV* and *ventricular end-diastolic pressure (VEDP)*.
- It is the volume of blood filling the ventricles during diastole.
- Preload is determined by the amount of venous return to the heart.
- The volume causes the myocardial fibers of the ventricles to stretch.
- As the myocardial fibers stretch, the heart's contractility force increases.
- Increase in preload is an increase in the volume of blood delivered to the ventricles, which causes an increase in myocardial fiber stretch, which in turn results in a more forceful ventricular contraction.
- A forceful ventricular contraction produces an increased SV and CO.
- Afterload
  - SVR or TPR is the resistance to ejection during systole.
  - It is the resistance the ventricles must overcome to open the aortic and pulmonic values to pump blood into the systemic and pulmonary vasculature.
  - An increase in afterload means the harder the heart must work to eject the volume.

Systemic Vascular Resistance

  - It reflects changes in arterioles that affect emptying of the LV.
  - It is key to knowing why the SVR is elevated.
  - Normal value: 800 to 1,200 dynes/sec/cm^{-5}.

Pulmonary Vascular Resistance

- It reflects changes in arterioles that affect emptying of the RV.
- Normal value: 100 to 250 dynes/sec/cm^{-5}.
- **Frank-Starling law** of the heart (Amsterdam et al., 2014; Cannon et al., 2013):
  - This refers to the volume of blood at the end of diastole.
  - Myocardial stretch determines the force of myocardial contraction.
  - More stretch = Increased force of contraction.

- It is the major way that the RV and LV maintain equal minute outputs, despite stroke (beat) output variation.
- **Laplace's law** (Amsterdam et al., 2014; Cannon et al., 2013):
  - The contractile force within a chamber depends on the radius of the chamber and the thickness of its wall.
    - Smaller chambers and thicker chamber walls result in increased contraction force.
    - In ventricular dilation, the force needed to maintain ventricular pressure lessens available contractile force.
- **Myocardial contractility** (Amsterdam et al., 2014; Cannon et al., 2013):
  - Refers to SV:
    - Volume of blood ejected during systole
  - Determinants of the force of contraction:
    - Changes in the stretching of the ventricular myocardium, caused by changes in ventricular volume (preload)
    - Alterations in nervous system input to the ventricles
    - Adequacy of myocardial oxygen supply
  - Neural reflexes:
    - *Baroreceptor reflex:* When blood pressure falls, HR increases and arterioles constrict.
    - *Bainbridge reflex:* This refers to changes in HR from IV infusions.

Hemodynamic Effects of Cardiovascular Agents

- Inotropic agents:
  - Positive inotropic agents increase the force of contraction:
    - Norepinephrine
    - Epinephrine
  - Negative inotropic agents decrease the force of contraction:
    - Acetylcholine released from the vagus nerve
  - Hypoxia decreases contractility

BASIC HEMODYNAMICS

Hemodynamic values provide information on how the body is responding to maintain adequate perfusion due to injury, disease, or treatment. It is important to remember that the patient's hemodynamic values are only a portion of the information needed to provide quality care (Tables 6.21–6.23).

Noninvasive Monitoring

- Korotkoff sounds (turbulent flow) correspond directly to systolic and diastolic blood pressure.
- Palpation only measures systolic blood pressure.

Hemodynamic Monitoring Devices
Invasive Monitoring
- Arterial catheter:
  - Used to measure arterial pressures
  - Single lumen
  - Arteries most commonly used are radial and femoral
- PA catheter:
  - Used to measure right-sided and left-sided intracardiac pressures and CO.
  - Multi-lumen catheter inserted into the PA.
  - Veins used for PA catheter include internal jugular, subclavian, femoral, and brachial.
  - PA catheter is located within the heart.

Minhimally Invasive
- Esophageal Doppler
  - It utilizes sound to measure aortic blood flow velocity.
  - A waveform is used to capture a blood flow velocity.
  - Doppler CO provides an immediate measurement of blood flow velocity as opposed to delayed measurements when using a PA catheter.
  - A transducer probe is inserted into the esophagus.
  - Contradictions for use of transesophageal doppler monitoring are as follows:
    - Coarctation of the aorta
    - Esophageal pathology
    - Coagulopathies
    - Intra-aortic balloon pumps
  - Sedation may be required for monitoring.
- Thoracic bio impedance
  - The resistance of current flow (impedance) across the chest is inversely related to the thoracic fluid.
  - It measures current from outer electrode to inner sensor.
  - Changes in impedance occur when there is a change in blood flow and velocity through the ascending aorta.
    - This bio impedance change reflects aortic flow, which is directly related to the contractility function of the ventricles.
  - Thoracic bio impedance is not accurate enough for diagnostic interpretation.

PERIPHERAL VASCULAR SYSTEM

OVERVIEW

The peripheral vascular (PV) system transports oxygenated blood from the left side of the heart to other body systems and

TABLE 6.21 NONINVASIVE HEMODYNAMIC VALUES

PARAMETER	DEFINITION	FORMULA	NORMAL RANGE
Heart rate			60–100 pm
Blood pressure			Less than 120/80 mmHg
Cardiac index	The amount of blood in liters per minute per square meter	$\dfrac{\text{Cardiac output}}{\text{Body surface area}}$	2.5–4.3 L/min/m^2
Cardiac output	The amount of blood pumped in liters per minute	Stroke volume × heart rate	4–8 L/min
Mean arterial pressure	Amount of pressure perfusing the organ	$\dfrac{2\,(DBP) + SBP}{3}$	65–110 mmHg
Stroke volume	Amount of blood pumped per beat	CO/HR × 1000	50–100 mL/beat
Stroke index	Amount of blood pumped per beat relative to the body surface area	CI/HR × 1000	35–60 mL/beat/m

CI, cardiac index; CO, cardiac output; DBP, diastolic blood pressure; HR, heart rate; SBP, systolic blood pressure.

TABLE 6.22 MANAGE PATIENT HEMODYNAMICS WITH PHARMACOLOGIC INTERVENTION

DRUG CLASS	COMMON MEDICATIONS	PURPOSE
ACEI	Captopril Enalapril Lisinopril	Reduces afterload Lowers blood pressure by acting on the renin–angiotensin–aldosterone system
ARBs	Losartan Candesartan Irbesartan	Reduces preload Lowers blood pressure by acting on the renin–angiotensin–aldosterone system
Calcium channel blockers	Nondihydropyridine calcium channel blockers: Diltiazem Verapamil Dihydropyridine calcium channel blockers: Amlodipine Nicardipine	Reduces afterload Myocardial relaxation ■ Angina ■ Hypertension ■ Select tachycardia In Black adults with hypertension but without heart failure or chronic kidney disease, including those with diabetes mellitus, initial antihypertensive treatment should include a thiazide-type diuretic or CCB. Do not use with nondihydropyridine calcium channel blockers with patients with heart failure.
Inotropes	Dobutamine Dopamine Milrinone Digoxin	Improves ventricular contractility in acute care.
Diuretics	Furosemide Bumetanide Ethacrynic acid Chlorothiazide Metolazone Mannitol Hydrochlorothiazide	Reduces preload. Reduces blood volume. In Black adults with hypertension but without heart failure or chronic kidney disease, including those with diabetes mellitus, initial antihypertensive treatment should include a thiazide-type diuretic. Thiazide diuretics are contraindicated for use in patients with anuria and sulfonamide allergies.
Vasodilator	Dopamine Nitroglycerin	Reduces preload
Smooth muscle relaxants and alpha inhibitors	Nitroprusside Nitroglycerin Diazoxide Hydralazine Methyldopa Trimethaphan Phentolamine	Reduces afterload in acute care

ACEI, angiotensin-converting enzyme inhibitor; ARBs, angiotensin II receptor blockers; CCB, calcium channel blockers.

tissues through the arteries. The deoxygenated blood is then transported back to the heart via the veins to the right heart for reoxygenation by the lungs. The vascular system also transports lymph fluid. If peripheral blood flow is impeded, then vascular lymph flow is also impeded (ACC, 2016):

- Peripheral artery disease (PAD; only disease of a peripheral artery)
- Peripheral vascular disease (PVD; both peripheral arterial and venous disease)

HUMAN AGING AND THE VASCULAR SYSTEM

The vascular system ages with human aging. The main layers of the vascular system, with connective tissue, are the intima (inner lining), media or medial muscular layers, and adventitia or outer rough layer. The layers of the vessel work with the valves in the vessels to continue the movement of blood through the body to perfuse tissues (American Heart Association [AHA], 2019; John Hopkins Medicine, n.d.).

PERIPHERAL VASCULAR DISEASE

PVD refers to diseases/disorders of the blood vessels outside of the heart, including blood vessels supplying the brain, gut, kidneys, or limbs.

- It is caused by blockage (i.e., blood clot, fatty buildup, cholesterol, atherosclerosis, plaque, calcification) or damage to blood vessels.

TABLE 6.23 EFFECTS OF CARDIOVASCULAR AGENTS ON HEMODYNAMICS

DRUG	HR	MAP	CO	PAOP	SVR	CVP	PVR
Norepinephrine (Levophed)	↑ ↔	↑	↑ slightly	↑	↑	↑	↑
Phenylephrine (Neosynephrine	↔↓	↑	↔↓	↑	↑	↑	↑
Epinephrine (Asthmahaler)	↑	↑	↑	↑	↑	↑	↑
Dobutamine (Dobutrex)	↔↓	↑	↑	↓	↓	↓	↓
Dopamine (intropin)		↑	↑	↑		↑↑	↔
< 5 mcg/kg/min	↑	↑ slightly	↑	↑↑	↑ slightly	↑↑	↑
>5 mcg/kg/min		↑↑			↑↑		
Digoxin (Lanoxin)	↓	↔	↑	↔	↔	↔	↔
Isoproterenol (Isuprel)	↑	↓	↑	↓	↓	↓	↓
Levosimendan (Simdax)	↔↓	↑	↔↓	↑	↑	↑	↑
Vasopressin	↔↓	↑	↔↓ related to SVR	↑	↑	↑	↑
Milrinone (Primacor)	↔ (↑in preload-sensitive patients)	↔ (↓ in preload-sensitive patients)	↑	↓	↓	↓	↓
Nitroglycerin (Tridil)	↔	↔	↔	↓	↔	↓	↔
20–40 mcg/min	↑	↓		↓	↓	↓	↓
50–250 mcg/min							
Nitroprusside (Nipride)	↑	↓	↑	↓	↓	↓	↓

CO, cardiac output; CVP, central venous pressure; MAP, mean arterial pressure; PAOP, pulmonary artery occlusion pressure; PVR, pulmonary vascular resistance; SVR, systemic vascular resistance.

■ Vasculitis is inflammation in the vascular system and can lead to decreased perfusion or occlusion of a vessel (ACC, 2016; John Hopkins Medicine, n.d.).

Risk Factors for PVD
Risk factors include both modifiable and nonmodifiable factors. Controlling modifiable risk factors is the best way to prevent PVD. Modifiable risk factors can be affected by lifestyle change and change in behavior and may also be treated with a pharmacologic agents or medical therapy to affect risk factors (i.e., antihypertensive agents, lipid lowering agents). Nonmodifiable risk factors are genetic and/or the process of aging (Aronow, 2018).

Signs/Symptoms of Venous Insufficiency/Deep Vein Thrombosis
■ *Claudication*—Pain in the legs with walking; resolves with rest
■ *Dependent edema*—Fluid in a limb (often feet and hands) that is peripheral to the bodice or heart
■ Change in color, temperature, or sensation in an extremity (Henke, n.d.; John Hopkins Medicine, n.d.)
Venous insufficiency often is evidenced by peripheral edema, due to the inability of the veins to efficiently transport fluid back to the heart.

DEEP VEIN THROMBOSIS
A *deep vein thrombosis (DVT)* specifically refers to a blood clot in a deep vein located in a muscle. Decreased movement of blood and lymph fluid may result in venous stasis or DVT or vessel occlusion (John Hopkins Medicine, n.d.).

CAROTID ARTERY DISEASE
The carotid arteries are the main arteries that carry oxygenated blood to the brain. Coronary artery disease, a blockage or narrowing of the carotid arteries, reduces or interrupts oxygenated blood delivery to the brain.

Acute arterial occlusion refers to an artery with no direct blood flow past the occlusion. This is an acute emergency. Types of occlusion include the following:
■ Anatomical occlusion of a vessel:
  ● Injury to the vessel, resulting in loss of blood flow
  ● Tissue growth inside the vascular system (i.e., mass)
  ● Calcium, fatty, or atherosclerotic occlusion related to vascular disease
  ● Blood clot obstruction of blood flow
  ● Dissection (separation of the layers of the vessel) of the intima of the vessel resulting in occlusion (this can happen with vascular intervention—see Interventions later)

Changes in Extremities Distal to the Arterial Occlusion
Intermittent changes may be a sign of interruption of blood flow and PVD without occlusion.

Change in appearance, color, and/or sensitivity of an extremity distal to the occlusion due to lack of perfusion may include:
■ Swelling,
■ Skin redness,
■ Skin paleness,
■ Slow capillary refill,

- Skin coolness,
- Skin mottling,
- Skin chaffing,
- Lack of hair growth on legs,
- Loss of strength or use of an extremity,
- Blue skin (i.e, tissue ischemia/lack of blood flow/perfusion), and
- Serum lab findings that include muscle injury resulting in increased troponin (creatine kinase [CK]).

The **classic signs** and **symptoms** of arterial occlusion or limb ischemia include the **six P's** (Abu-Fadel, 2017; MacKensie et al., 1991; Smith & Lilie, 2019):

- Pain
- Pallor—Change in color, paleness
- Paresthesia—Change in feeling/sensation
- Paralysis—Inability to move
- Pulselessness
- Poikilothermia—Inability to maintain core temperature

Testing

Ankle/Brachial Index

The ankle/brachial index (ABI) measurement is a test to help identify PVD:

- ABI—Systolic blood pressure in the ankle divided by the brachial systolic blood pressure.
- ABI less than 0.9 is indicative of PAD (MediCalc, 2018; The Society of Cardiovascular Angiography and Intervention [SCAI], 2018).

Doppler and Ultrasound Flow Studies

- Doppler flow studies use the doppler sound to listen to the flow or interruption of flow from vessels to detect PVD.
- Ultrasound uses ultrasound waves to create a picture of the blood flow to detect interruption of blood flow.

Peripheral Vascular Disease Treatment

- Risk factor modification/behavior modification
- Pharmacologic/medical therapy
- Catheter-based therapy (interventional) in a catheterization or interventional radiology laboratory
- Surgical therapy (Cardiovascular Coalition, 2019)

Interventions

- **Catheter-directed anticoagulation/thrombolysis**—Dependent upon the ability to get a catheter to the area of significant PVD. Medications to dissolve a clot may be given directly via a catheter inserted into the vessel to deliver the medication directly to the clot (catheter-directed therapy).
- **Systemic anticoagulation**—Provides quick access for thrombolysis/anticoagulation and may be preferable if the patient requires quick therapy to avoid immediate stroke or organ or limb loss or if the PVD is not amenable to catheter-based therapy.
- **Catheter-based therapy—Percutaneous interventions** (catheterization lab or interventional radiology)—Percutaneous access is dependent upon access to the artery related to the size, shape (tortuosity), and extent of disease in the artery.
- **Angioplasty**—Use of a catheter in a vessel; a balloon is inflated to compress the blockage in the artery against the vessel wall.
- **Stent**—The stent is inflated with a balloon and provides a structure to hold open the artery wall. The stent is imbedded against the artery wall for security.
  - Drug-eluting stent—A stent with a medication imbedded/coated on the stent to release drug to prevent restenosis.
- **Atherectomy catheters/systems**—Often used to debulk very hard/irregular lesions (i.e., calcified) to prepare the artery for better adherence of the balloon and/or stent placement. The devices can cut, shave, sand, or vaporize atherosclerotic or calcified lesions (Charitakis & Feldman, 2015).

Possible Catheter-Based Therapy (Interventional) Complications

- Bleeding related to access of the vessel and/or injury to the vessel.
- *Dissection*—A separation of the intima in the vessel that creates a tunnel between the layers of the vessel and may impede circulation.
- *Aneurysm*—A ballooning out of the artery wall creating risk for clotting, bleeding, and disturbance in circulation.
- *Perforation*—A breakthrough of all layers of the artery wall, creating bleeding and disturbance in circulation (Abu-Fadel, 2017).

Surgical Interventions Performed by a Vascular Surgeon

- *Endarterectomy*—The surgical opening of an artery and scraping of the artery wall to remove blockage.
- *Bypass surgery*—Use of a vessel to bypass the partial or total occlusion and provide circulation distal to the occlusion.
- *Vascular repair*—Surgical repair of the artery or vein with suture, grafting material, and so on to restore the anatomy and function of the artery for transportation of blood and nutrients (Feldman et al., 2018).
- *Amputation*—Last resort; performed if the dead/infected limb/anatomical area creates a risk for infection and/or for further interruption of blood flow/perfusion (The Society for Vascular Surgery [SVS], n.d.-b. Vascular Treatments).

Patient Care After Peripheral Vascular Disease Treatment

Many order sets and protocols provide guidance for patient care when thrombolytics or anticoagulation is administered and after catheter-based therapies.

- Schedule neurologic and vascular assessment frequently.
- Scheduled blood work per the order set and directed for the location of the clot may include the following:
  - *Troponin*—Inflammatory marker for muscle to detect inflammation possibly related to decreased perfusion
  - *Hemoglobin/hematocrit*—H/H—red blood cell count
  - Clotting studies (i.e., prothrombin time [PT], partial thromboplastin time [PTT], D-dimer)
  - Complete blood count (CBC; includes H/H)
- Scheduled testing for bleeding:
  - Hematest for stools and urine

AORTIC ANEURYSM

- The aortic artery is referred to in multiple anatomical parts: the aortic root (which may include the aortic valve), the transverse aorta or aortic arch, and the descending or abdominal aorta in the thoracic aorta.
- Layers—The internal smooth intima; medial, thicker muscular layers; and an outer rough layer. When the aorta balloons out due to high pressure, the wall of the aorta becomes weak and is more prone to rupture. The aortic aneurysm is

described in relation to the section of the aorta (i.e., ascending, transverse, abdominal/descending, or thoracic).

- When the aorta is involved in a cardiac or vascular interventional procedure, there is a risk for aortic dissection (separation of the layers interrupting blood flow to the remainder of the body), with guidewire and catheter disturbance of the vessel layers (SCAI, 2017; Wiesenfarth, 2018).

Aortic Aneurysm Signs and Symptoms

- A pulsating feeling near the navel
- Constant deep pain in or on the side of the abdomen
- Back pain

AORTIC DISSECTION

Aortic dissection is an emergency, can mimic a heart attack, and is always a reason for emergent care (i.e., call 911).

The symptoms of an aortic dissection include sudden onset:

- Chest pain, often described as tearing pain in the upper back
- Dizziness or fainting
- Nausea or vomiting
- Severe anxiety, feeling of impending doom
- Shortness of breath
- Difficulty speaking, sudden vision loss or weakness, loss of functioning on one side. Can also be sign of a stroke (Powers et al., 2018; SCAI, 2017; Seligson & Marx, 2018).

Types of Aortic Dissection

The dissection may be a partial or a complete dissection, placing the aorta at risk for rupture with the high pressure of blood pumped from the heart into the aorta.

Ruptured Aorta

- A ruptured aorta is a complete break in the artery wall, which results in blood leaking out of the artery. A ruptured aorta may result from a ruptured dissection, a ruptured aortic aneurysm, or traumatic injury/aortic transection. A ruptured aorta is always a medical emergency to prevent massive blood loss and death. Emergent surgical intervention is a priority for aortic repair with graft placement as needed (Seligson & Marx, 2018).
- Signs and symptoms of a ruptured aorta are similar to those of an aortic dissection and may result in immediate loss of consciousness, blood pressure, and respirations (code blue) with mortality. Approximately 20% of patients with aortic ruptures survive to the hospital for emergent repair (Seligson & Marx, 2018).

Testing for Aortic Aneurysm, Dissection, Ruptured Aorta

- Computed tomography angiography (CTA) or magnetic resonance angiography of the chest and abdomen is highly sensitive.
- CT of chest and abdomen.
- Echocardiography.
- Chest x-ray, if patient is too unstable to receive CT (The Society for Vascular Surgery [SVS], n.d.-a).

Arterial or Venous Sheath

Catheter-based therapy (intervention) for PAD treatment requires a sheath to be inserted in the peripheral artery to provide access for guidewire and catheter exchanges (Ginapp, 2009).

- Often, a protocol exists for sheath removal with scheduled serum PTT or activated clotting time (ACT) levels until the PTT or ACT approaches a level consistent with the blood clotting process to decrease the risk for bleeding with sheath removal from the vessel (i.e., ACT less than 180) (Cohen & Merschon, 2010; Ginapp, 2019; Shaffer, 2017a, 2017b).

Education and Competency

Education and competency for sheath removal are essential to help prevent complications related to sheath removal.

Common risk factors for increased complications, mortality, and morbidity with sheath removal:

- Advanced age (aging of vessels)
- Female (generally smaller vessels with PVD at higher age with more comorbidities)
- Tortuosity of the vessel
- Change in mental status
- Baseline abnormal bleeding/clotting labs/disorders—notify physician/allied health provider of abnormal labs prior to sheath removal
- Comorbidities (i.e., extensive PVD, coronary artery disease, history of stroke, hypertension, chronic lung disease, etc.)
- Not using a hemostasis pad or closure device (Ortiz et al., 2014)

A baseline neurovascular assessment, history, and physical of the patient are essential prior to sheath removal to compare with postsheath removal assessment. Peripheral vascular assessment includes color, temperature, sensation, swelling, and ability to move/control the extremities.

- **Vital signs** are assessed prior to sheath removal. If the systolic blood pressure is greater than or equal to 160 mmHg, then notify the physician/allied health provider prior to sheath removal.
- Blood pressure management assists with hemostasis.

Patient Preparation for Sheath Removal

- Patient education for sheath removal is essential (Shaffer, 2017a, 2017b).
- Pain relief during sheath removal is important, as blood pressure tends to rise with pain, and blood pressure management assists hemostasis.
- A vaso-vagal response is possible with manual pressure at the femoral site. The vaso-vagal response may include light-headedness, feeling dizzy, bradycardia, hypotension, nausea, and/or loss of consciousness (fainting).
- If resistance is met with sheath removal, **do not remove** the sheath and notify the physician/allied health professional.

Sheath Removal and Vessel Closure

- Multiple methods exist to close the peripheral vascular access site after intervention.
- Manual pressure is to be held at least 20 minutes for an arterial access site and at least 10 minutes for a venous access site without other closure assistance.
- It is generally recommended to discontinue the arterial sheath first, obtain hemostasis at the arterial site, and then remove the venous sheath.
- Refer to organizational and assistance devices (i.e., compression devices) for specific instruction to help prevent A-V fistula (Cohen & Merschon, 2010; Ortiz et al., 2014).

PERIPHERAL ARTERY DISEASE AND FEMORAL POPLITEAL SURGICAL BYPASS

If PVD is not amenable to percutaneous intervention or catheter-based therapy, then surgical bypass may be indicated and is generally the last intervention offered before amputation.

■ ***Femoral popliteal bypass or fem-pop***—If blood flow is obstructed between the femoral artery and the popliteal artery, then a bypass graft may be sewn from the femoral artery to the popliteal arter. This is the most common peripheral bypass surgery (Starr, n.d.).

Any peripheral bypass surgery requires the same neurovascular assessment as an intervention or catheter-based therapy. The goal is to supply blood past the severe area of PVD or occlusion to maintain blood flow and healthy tissue (Starr, n.d.).

Risks

■ Failure of the bypass, lack of perfusion
■ MI
■ Wound/Incision Infection and/or nonhealing:
  ● Antibiotics are given routinely before and after surgery.
  ● Wound healing is dependent upon healthy tissue, postoperative care of the incision, blood glucose (glycemic control), and adequate nutrition.
  ● Risk factor modification:
    ▪ Nutrition
    ▪ Smoking/tobacco use
■ Injury to nearby nerves (Starr, n.d.; U.S. National Library of Medicine [USNLM], 2019a)

Prescribing and Management

■ Lower blood pressure slowly in geriatric patients and monitor for signs and symptoms of worsening HF and myocardial ischemia (Ayan et al., 2016).
■ For all cardiac medications, monitor EKG, HR, blood pressure, and renal function; assess fluid status.
■ For diuretics, monitor weight, intake and output, serum electrolytes, blood urea nitrogen (BUN), and creatinine.
■ Check for black-box warnings prior to prescribing medication.
■ Slowly taper doses.

REVIEW QUESTIONS

1. When developing a teaching plan for a 61-year-old patient with multiple risk factors for coronary artery disease (CAD), the nurse should focus primarily on the
   A. elevated low-density lipoprotein (LDL) level
   B. increased risk associated with the patient's gender
   C. increased risk of cardiovascular disease as people age
   D. increased risk due to family history of CAD

2. A patient with newly diagnosed heart failure is admitted to the cardiac unit. A nurse consults the clinical nurse specialist because the patient has orders for exercise stress echocardiography, but the patient is unable to walk. Which statement best reflects the options of completing the echocardiography?
   A. Cancel the order until the patient can walk.
   B. Place order for physical therapy to see patient and reschedule the exercise stress test.
   C. Assess patient for dobutamine stress echocardiography.
   D. Assist the nurse in ambulating the patient during the exercise stress test.

3. A patient comes into the ED with complaints of substernal, sharp, pleuritic chest pain that worsens on inspiration. The pain radiates to both shoulders. The patient states that the pain lessens when sitting up and leaning forward. It has been present for the past 2 days and has progressively worsened.

The patient complains of dyspnea. Vital signs show patient tachycardia at 120 beats per minute with a blood pressure of 110/70 mmHg. EKG shows diffuse ST elevation. Follow-up vital signs show tachycardia at 125 beats per minute and blood pressure of 100/80 mmHg, and a pericardial rub is auscultated at the apex. What type of diagnosis would the clinical nurse specialist anticipate?
   A. Endocarditis
   B. Pericarditis
   C. Myocarditis
   D. Cardiomyopathy

ANSWERS

1. **Correct answer: A. Rationale**: Because family history, gender, and age are nonmodifiable risk factors, the nurse should focus on the patient's LDL level. Decreases in LDL will help reduce the patient's risk for developing CAD. The CNS cannot change the nonmodifiable risk factors (family history, gender, and age); however, it is important that the patient be aware of their increased risk based on these factors.

2. **Correct answer: C. Rationale**: Echocardiography is the most useful tool for the diagnosis and management of heart failure. It is used to assess the cardiac anatomy and physiology. Two-dimensional echocardiography allows for the assessment of left ventricular volume and valvular disease. Three-dimensional echocardiography has enhanced the accuracy and reliability to assess chamber volume and function as well as the mechanistic evaluation—regurgitation. Patients who are unable to walk for an exercise stress echocardiography may be candidates for the dobutamine stress echocardiography

3. **Correct answer: B. Rationale**: Pericarditis is an inflammation of the pericardium. The signs and symptoms include the following: chest pain that is sharp and stabbing and worsens with inspiration, cough, or supine; pain decreases when sitting up and leaning forward; EKG shows ST elevation and/or PR depression; ta narrowing of pulse pressures; a new or worsening pericardial effusion and pericardial friction rub. Endocarditis is an inflammation of the heart's endocardium (inner lining), usually involving the heart's valves. Its clinical manifestations includessudden onset, high fever, rigors, and/or sepsis. The clinical manifestation of myocarditis is heterogeneous, ranging from asymptomatic state with vague signs and symptoms to sever cardiogenic shock and arrhythmias. Common signs and symptoms of myocarditis are chest pain; rapid or abnormal heart rhythms (arrhythmias); shortness of breath, at rest or during physical activity; fluid retention with swelling of legs, ankles, and feet; and fatigue. Cardiomyopathy is a disease involving destruction of the cardiac muscle fibers, resulting in myocardial function impairment and decreased cardiac output. It is commonly caused by coronary artery disease, which impairs myocardial contractility and increased ventricular filling pressure.

REFERENCES

The complete reference and additional reading lists appear in the digital version of this chapter, at https://connect.springerpub.com/content/book/978-0-8261-7417-8/part/part01/chapter/ch06

Respiratory System

Jo M. Tabler, Mechelle Peck, Amy C. Shay, Megan Siebert, Maria Carpenter, and Elizabeth Duxbury

PULMONARY AIR-LEAK SYNDROMES

PNEUMOTHORAX OVERVIEW

Definition

Pneumothorax occurs when air accumulates in the pleural space and leads to partial or complete collapse of the lung.
Pneumothorax types are as follows:

- *Primary spontaneous pneumothorax*—No obvious cause
- *Secondary spontaneous pneumothorax*—Underlying lung disease is present
- *Iatrogenic pneumothorax*—Is a consequence of a therapeutic intervention
- *Traumatic pneumothorax*—Penetrating or nonpenetrating injury
- *Tension pneumothorax*—Medical emergency

Pathophysiology

Pressure in the pleural space is negative to both alveolar pressure and atmospheric pressure throughout the respiratory cycle. The negative pressure gradient is a result of the natural elastic recoil of the lung. Pneumothorax develops when there is communication between the pleural space and another intrapulmonary air space, resulting in equal pressure between the air spaces. A pneumothorax can also occur if there is a communication between the atmosphere, through the chest wall, to the pleural space.

Etiology

Primary spontaneous pneumothorax is believed to result from a rupture of a subpleural bleb in the apex of the lung. Patients tend to be young, tall, thin, and cigarette smokers. Observation and follow-up x-ray may be appropriate treatment for asymptomatic primary spontaneous pneumothorax. Symptomatic primary spontaneous pneumothorax may be successfully treated with needle aspiration.

Secondary spontaneous pneumothorax occurs in patients who have underlying lung disease, such as chronic obstructive pulmonary disease (COPD), and tumors. Patients who have COPD should be evaluated for pneumothorax if they demonstrate sudden onset of chest pain or sudden worsening of shortness of breath. Chest tube placement is the appropriate treatment.

Iatrogenic pneumothorax occurs after procedures such as needle aspiration, central line placement, or mechanical ventilation. Other procedures associated with iatrogenic pneumothorax risk include thoracentesis, lung biopsy, cardiopulmonary resuscitation, tracheostomy, and insertion of nasogastric tubes.

Traumatic pneumothorax is caused by blunt or penetrating injury and is often accompanied by hemothorax. Appropriate treatment is chest tube placement (Light & Lee, 2015).

Tension pneumothorax occurs when the intrapleural pressure is greater than the atmospheric pressure throughout most of the respiratory cycle. This is typically seen in patients who are receiving positive pressure mechanical ventilation or during resuscitation. In tension pneumothorax, air continues to enter the pleural space but is unable to exit. Pressure continues to build with each respiration cycle and eventually collapses the lung, causes mediastinal shift to the opposite side, and impairs venous return to the heart. If not resolved quickly, tension pneumothorax can lead to systemic hypotension and cardiopulmonary arrest. Diagnosis should be based upon clinical findings. *Treatment should not be delayed by chest x-ray confirmation of the diagnosis.* Treatment is considered a medical emergency calling for needle decompression (Burns & Delgado, 2019).

Assessment

Signs and symptoms of pneumothorax include sharp and sudden chest pain, asymmetrical chest wall movement, shortness of breath, hypotension, absent breath sounds on the affected side, hyperresonance to percussion, absent tactile fremitus, decreased cardiac output, tracheal deviation to the opposite side, or distended jugular veins.

Diagnosis

Chest x-ray confirms diagnosis. Radiograph findings include air in the pleural space and possible mediastinal shift; the visceral pleural line runs paralleling the chest wall from lung apex to base (Light & Lee, 2015).

Interventions
- Monitoring
- Supplemental oxygen
- Chest tube placement
- Needle aspiration
  - Treatment option for *symptomatic primary spontaneous pneumothorax*
  - Needle aspiration uses a small-bore (16 G or 18 G) over-the-needle catheter, tubing, three-way stopcock, and a 50- or 60-mL syringe. The catheter is inserted at the *midclavicular line, second intercostal space*, on the affected side. Air is withdrawn from the pleural space through the stopcock and syringe and expelled into the atmosphere. This process is repeated until the lung reexpands.
- Needle decompression
  - This is an emergency procedure.

The complete reference and additional reading lists appear in the digital version of this chapter, at https://connect.springerpub.com/content/book/978-0-8261-7417-8/part/part01/chapter/ch07

- It is a treatment option for *tension pneumothorax*.
- Insertion of a 14-G to 16-G angiocatheter at the *midclavicular line, second intercostal space*, on the affected side (Light & Lee, 2015).
  - Thoracostomy with pleurodesis
  - Thoracoscopy (video-assisted thoracic surgery [VATS])
  - Open thoracotomy

Complications of pneumothorax treatment include

- Air leaks,
- Failure to reexpand, and
- Reexpansion pulmonary edema.

Small-bore chest tube (less than 20 Fr) placement is the treatment of choice for pleural drainage. Small-bore chest tubes are typically placed to a water seal without suction for the first 24 hours to help avoid incidence of pulmonary edema upon reexpansion. Once the lung has reexpanded and air leak has resolved, the chest tube can be removed and the patient monitored for tolerance.

For patients who have failed aspiration or with recurrent pneumothorax, VATS is the preferred treatment. The VATS procedure attempts to eliminate the blebs that contribute to pneumothorax. VATS offers shorter hospitalization and fewer complications than an open thoracotomy. Open thoracotomy can be used if VATS is not available. Open thoracotomy has a lower incidence of recurrent pneumothorax than VATS (Light & Lee, 2015).

PNEUMOMEDIASTINUM

Pneumomediastinum is the presence of air in the mediastinum that may travel to the subcutaneous tissues of the neck and scalp. Many patients present with a spontaneous pneumothorax; chest pain that may radiate to the back and neck and subcutaneous emphysema. Most cases only require symptom management. In severe cases, air can dissect into the pericardial sac and may cause pneumopericardium. If this air is not reabsorbed by the body, a tension pneumothorax, cardiac tamponade, and eventual cardiopulmonary arrest may occur. For those severe cases, VATS or thoracotomy may be required (Kouritas et al., 2015).

PULMONARY EMBOLISM

OVERVIEW

Pulmonary embolism (PE) occurs when venous thromboemboli obstruct a portion of the pulmonary arterial bed. This obstruction leads to ventilation/perfusion (V/Q) mismatch with subsequent arterial hypoxemia. The size and location of the clot determines the degree of blood flow obstruction. Pulmonary capillary bed obstruction can cause increased right ventricular afterload, dilation of the right ventricle (RV), and cor pulmonale.

Submassive PE: The RV is stressed, but the patient is hemodynamically stable. Patients with submassive PE have a better in-hospital survival rate, but mortality risk persists after hospitalization. Continued follow-up after hospital discharge facilitates early identification of morbidity and signs/symptoms of repeat PE.

Massive PE: The patient is hemodynamically unstable, showing signs/symptoms of cardiogenic shock, or has a period of pulselessness. Patients with massive PE have a higher in-hospital mortality rate. Both submassive and massive PE require follow-up after discharge from the hospital for monitoring and prevention of a subsequent event.

Nonthrombotic Sources of Pulmonary Embolism

- *Air embolus*—A large amount of air seen in the veins or right side of heart via venous catheters, surgery, or blunt trauma. Place patient in left lateral decubitus Trendelenburg position.
- *Fat embolus*—Fat or bone marrow; risk associated with long-bone fracture and orthopedic procedures.
- *Infected material*—Septic embolism resulting from infective endocarditis or thrombophlebitis.
- *Amniotic fluid*—Amniotic fluid embolism that occurs during labor.
- *Foreign bodies*—Particulate matter by intravenous (IV) injection (e.g., talc).
- *Tumors*—Tumor cells enter venous circulation.

Symptoms of Pulmonary Embolism

PE symptoms can range in severity from no symptoms to an emergency that results in permanent damage or death. Symptoms of PE often occur suddenly and may include the following:

- Sudden onset shortness of breath, tachycardia and tachypnea
- Sharp chest or back pain; may be aggravated by cough or movement
- Cough with or without sputum production; sputum may be heme positive
- Feeling of doom expressed by the patient
- Patient anxiety with shortness of breath
- Light-headedness and/or dizziness
- Cyanotic lips or nail beds and/or mottling/discoloration from the chest nipple line up to the top of head

Risk Factors

- Trauma, particularly large bone fracture (i.e., femur, hip, knee)
- Repair of large bone fracture
- Abdominal surgery repair
- Cancer/cancer treatment (i.e., chemotherapy)
- Long periods of inactivity (bed rest, extended travel, travel with long periods of sitting, such as in an automobile or airplane)
- Cardiovascular (CV) disease (clot and/or blockage breakaway)
- Irregular heart rate (atrial or ventricular arrhythmias that may alter systole and/or diastole, contributing to incomplete filling and emptying of the heart; possible stasis of blood)
- Pregnancy and first 6 weeks after delivery (changes in blood volume/contents)
- Oral contraceptives
- Hormones taken for menopausal symptoms
- Autoimmune diseases (e.g., lupus)
- Inherited blood disorders (e.g., thrombophilia)
- Inflammatory bowel disease
- Smoking
- Obesity
- Vascular intervention/procedures (see Chapter 6)
- Pacemaker or implantable defibrillator

Diagnosis

Patient and family history helps identify risk factors. Physical exam and diagnostic testing confirm PE.

Diagnostic Testing

- Computerized tomography angiogram (CTA)
- Chest x-ray (basilar atelectasis, pleural effusion, diaphragm elevation)

- Echocardiogram (for risk stratification)
- V/Q lung scan
- Doppler testing for deep vein thrombosis (DVT)—possible etiology of PE
- EKG (signs of RV strain: R axis deviation, R bundle branch block)
- Serum blood testing may include the following:
  - Arterial blood gas (ABG)—respiratory alkalosis, hypoxemia
  - D-dimer
  - Troponin
  - Beta natriuretic peptide (BNP; Secemsky et al., 2018)

Pulmonary Embolism Response Team

Interdisciplinary teams have been developed to assist with early, rapid identification, testing, analysis, and treatment of PE. One example of a detailed pulmonary embolism response team (PERT) guideline has been made available online by The University of Texas M.D. Anderson Cancer Center at www.mdanderson.org/content/dam/mdanderson/documents/for-physicians/algorithms/clinical-management/clin-management-pert-web-algorithm.pdf (Barnes et al., 2017).

Treatment
Anticoagulation/Thrombolysis

Similar to peripheral vascular disease (Chapter 6), a PE may be treated with either systemic or catheter-directed anticoagulation/thrombolysis/fibrinolysis. Systemic anticoagulation/lysis therapy is often used when the patient cannot tolerate the diagnostic workup and procedural time for catheter-based therapies. Heparin is commonly used to treat PE in combination with thrombolysis.

Catheter-Based Interventions

- Catheter-directed thrombolytic delivery
- Catheter-based/endovascular aspiration device (clot retrieval) to remove the clot
- Inferior vena cava (IVC) filter placement for prevention of PE (percutaneous—catheter-based filter placed in the IVC)

Surgical Interventions

Surgical therapy is an option with careful consideration of risks and benefits or if other options are not possible (i.e., unable to tolerate catheter-based therapy or vascular system not amenable to catheter-based therapy).

- Extracorporeal membrane oxygenation (ECMO) may be used to oxygenate the patient until the PE can be dissolved with thrombolytic therapy or other therapy can be initiated (requires cardiothoracic surgery consult).
- Surgical removal of the clot is also an option (embolectomy; Barnes et al., 2017).

ASTHMA

OVERVIEW

Asthma is a chronic illness characterized by airway hyperreactivity, inflammation, and reversible bronchospasm. The airway reacts to triggering stimuli, leading to tightening of respiratory smooth muscle, narrowing airways, reduction in airflow, and mucus hypersecretion. Wheezing is commonly associated with asthma; however, not all asthmatics wheeze. It is important to note that adults with a history of wheezing and asthma who present with decreased air movement or decreased breath sounds may be in severe distress requiring rapid bronchodilator interventions. Wheezing that dissipates in the presence of severe bronchospasms due to impaired air movement is an ominous sign and marks the need for intubation. Differential diagnoses associated with wheezing include COPD, pneumonia, bronchitis, croup, PE, allergic reactions, and heart failure. Understanding the asthma patient's history of hospital admissions and/or history of intubation should guide the medical interventions.

Asthma Triggers

Adults with a history of asthma since childhood usually know their triggers. Triggers can change, however. Assessment of triggers should include both the home and the work environments. Common triggers include the following:

- Food allergies (e.g., sulfites in food and drink)
- Inhalant allergies (e.g., pollen, latex, mold, animal dander, dust)
- Irritants (e.g., cigarette smoke, smog, air pollution, aerosolized chemicals, perfumes)
- Exposure to cold weather
- Exercise
- Viral upper respiratory illness
- Sinusitis, rhinitis
- Gastroesophageal reflux disease (GERD)
- Nonsteroidal anti-inflammatory drugs (NSAIDs) or aspirin

Signs and Symptoms

Assessment should include daytime and nighttime frequency of symptoms, symptoms over the previous 2 to 4 weeks, and activity limitations. A simple tool, such as the Asthma Control Test, can be used to define and describe how asthma affects the patient: www.allergyasthmanetwork.org/cms/wp-content/uploads/2014/06/Asthma-Control-Test.pdf.

Common signs and symptoms include the following (Brashers, 2014)

- Expiratory wheezing is most common; inspiratory wheezing may also be present
- Dyspnea
- Tachypnea
- Coughing
- Orthopnea
- Low oxygen saturations
- Chest tightness
- Peak expiratory flow rate (PEFR) less than 50% of predicted value
- Use of accessory muscles
- Anxiety
- Halting speech
- Diaphoresis

Interventions

The 2007 National Asthma Education and Prevention Program (NAEPP) supports a stepwise approach based upon asthma severity. The stepwise approach should be used to augment clinical decision-making. Four categories of severity are based on reported symptoms, current lung function, and number of exacerbations that required oral steroids (see Table 7.1).

Prevention

Management interventions to prevent exacerbation include the following:

- Annual flu vaccination is recommended to prevent complications related to influenza.

TABLE 7.1 THERAPEUTIC INTERVENTIONS BY SEVERITY AND SYMPTOMS

ASTHMA SEVERITY CATEGORY	SYMPTOMS	THERAPEUTIC INTERVENTIONS
Intermittent	<ul><li>Daytime symptoms less than two times per week</li><li>Waking two times or less during sleep</li><li>Waking two or less times during sleep</li><li>No activity limitations</li><li>FEV_1 within normal</li><li>FEV_1/ FVC ratio normal</li><li>≤ 1 exacerbations needing oral steroids</li></ul>	<ul><li>Position of comfort</li><li>Monitor oxygen saturation</li><li>Provide oxygen if saturation less than 92%</li><li>Measure PEFR before and after medication interventions</li><li>Ensure proper use of MDI and spacer</li><li>Teach adherence to trigger control/question trigger exposure</li><li>Quick-acting inhaled beta-2-selective adrenergic agonist</li><li>If symptoms are exacerbated by exercise or cold air, teach use of inhaled beta agonist ~10 min prior to event</li></ul>
Mild persistent	<ul><li>Symptoms less than daily but more than 2 days per week</li><li>Three to four times per week waking during sleep</li><li>Use of SABAs less than daily but more than 2 days per week</li><li>Minor activity limitations</li><li>FEV_1 within normal range</li><li>FEV_1/FVC normal range</li><li>Two or more exacerbations requiring oral steroids</li></ul>	<ul><li>Mild persistent includes interventions from Intermittent and adds the following:</li><li>Low-dose inhaled GC.</li><li>Additional interventions could include the following:</li><li>Leukotriene receptor agonist</li><li>Theophylline</li><li>Cromoglycates</li></ul>
Moderate persistent	<ul><li>Daily individual asthma symptoms</li><li>more than 1 time per week awakening from sleep</li><li>Daily SABA use</li><li>Some activity limitations</li><li>FEV_1 within normal range</li><li>FEV_1/FVC below normal</li></ul>	<ul><li>Moderate persistent interventions include intermittent care plus the following:</li><li>Low dose of inhaled GC plus a LABA *or* medium dose of inhaled GC</li><li>Alternative methods include leukotriene modifier or theophylline</li><li>Theophylline is rarely introduced with moderate symptomology</li></ul>
Severe persistent	<ul><li>Daily asthma symptoms</li><li>Nightly awakening</li><li>Use of SABAs several times per day for symptom relief</li><li>Severe activity limitation</li><li>FEV_1 less than 60% predicted</li><li>FEV_1/FVC below normal</li></ul>	<ul><li>Severe persistent interventions include intermittent care plus the following:</li><li>Medium to high dose of inhaled GC PLUS</li><li>LABA</li><li>Triple threat therapy is considered to be GC + leukotriene modifier + LABA</li><li>*Severe* asthma PO GC daily or QOD</li><li>Occasionally, anti-IgE therapy is considered if evidence of sensitivity to a perennial allergen</li><li>With eosinophilic severe asthma, monoclonal antibodies against interleukin-5 may be considered</li></ul>

Note: Interventions deemed to be *of little use* in asthma include sputum cultures, antibiotics, complete blood count, chest x-ray, arterial blood gas, and intravenous aminophylline.

FEV_1, forced expiratory volume in one second; FVC, forced vital capacity; GC, glucocorticoid; IgE, immunoglobulin E; LABA, long-acting beta$_2$ agonist; MDI, metered-dose inhaler; PEFR, peak expiratory flow rate; SABA, short-acting beta$_2$ agonist.

- Pneumococcal vaccination is recommended to prevent complications related to pneumococcal infection for adults whose asthma is severe enough to require controller medication.
- For immunization prescribing guidelines, see the U.S. Advisory Committee on Immunization Practices (ACIP) website (www.cdc.gov/vaccines/acip/recommendations.html).
- Optimization of pharmacotherapy reduces exacerbations and need for ED or hospital admissions.
- *Asthma action plan:* Maximizing the use of an ongoing asthma action plan based on the patient's long-acting medication, short-acting medication, peak flow meter daily levels, knowledge of triggers, and symptom knowledge assists the patient in adjusting medication management prior to alerting the physician or practitioner (Table 7.2). The asthma action plan should be easily accessible to the patient, family, and healthcare provider. Encourage regular practitioner visits, use of the asthma action plan, and maintaining a log of symptoms.

Management

- *Stepwise management approach (NAEPP):* Evidence-based interventions to reduce symptoms and improve quality of life.
- Referral to a higher level of care is necessary if the patient experiences a life-threatening asthma exacerbation or has been intubated *once.*

- *Pulmonology or immunology consult:* For patients not responding to the stepwise treatment plan within 3 to 6 months of appropriate therapy (Edwards, 2005; Kosinski et al., 2006; U.S. Department of Health and Human Services, 2012).

CHRONIC OBSTRUCTIVE PULMONARY DISEASE

OVERVIEW

Definition

COPD is a chronic, irreversible condition with symptoms of chronic cough, expectoration of phlegm, and dyspnea. COPD should be suspected in persons presenting with cough, dyspnea, increased sputum production, and a history of smoking or other inhalation exposure. Spirometry, rather than physical assessment findings, confirms the diagnosis of COPD. COPD is divided into two categories: chronic bronchitis and emphysema. Chronic bronchitis is a clinical diagnosis in the presence of chronic cough with sputum production on a daily basis for 3 months per year for 2 successive years. Emphysema is the focus of the following chronic lung disease discussion.

Pathophysiology

Pathophysiologic changes of emphysema include increased size of tracheobronchial mucous glands, goblet cell hyperplasia, metaplasia of the epithelial mucous cells, increased bronchial wall thickness, increased V/Q abnormalities, hypoxemia, and acidemia. Smoking (or other environmental exposures) causes oxidative stress, increased macrophages, CD-8 T lymphocytes, and loss of antiproteinase protection. This results in a sustained, chronic inflammatory response leading to parenchymal tissue destruction, small airway fibrosis, and mucus hypersecretion. Emphysema is characterized by airflow limitation, gas trapping, decreased ventilation, and CO_2 retention. Over time, hypoxic vasoconstriction can lead to pulmonary hypertension (PH) and RV dysfunction (cor pulmonale).

Etiology

- Cigarette smoking
- Inhalation of noxious particles due to environmental or occupational pollution
- Alpha1-antitrypsin deficiency (Brashers, 2014)

Assessment

- Subjective findings include chronic cough and sputum production, DOE with possible progression to dyspnea at rest, inability to complete activities of daily living (ADL), history of smoking, or environmental exposure and family history of emphysema.
- Physical examination findings include the following:
  - *Observation*
    - Barrel chest, nail clubbing, use of accessory muscles
  - *Palpation*
    - Decreased vocal fremitus (air trapping)
  - *Percussion*
    - Hyperresonance (air trapping)
  - *Auscultation*
    - Coarse crackles, expiratory wheezes, distant lung sounds
  - *Signs and symptoms of RV dysfunction*
    - Jugular vein distension (JVD), peripheral edema, gallop, hepatomegaly, cyanosis, dusky skin color

Diagnostic Testing

- *Pulmonary function testing:* Diagnoses airflow limitation and confirms presence of COPD. Establishing disease severity is essential in determining the appropriate therapy.
  - Reduced FEV_1
  - Postbronchodilator FEV_1/FVC ratio <0.7 in combination with an FEV_1 of less than 80% of predicted value
- *Chest x-ray:* Flattened diaphragm and hyperlucent vasculature.
- *ABG:* Hypercarbia and hypoxemia; compensated respiratory acidosis is common with the patient with long-term COPD.
- *CBC:* Polycythemia is typically present (Brashers, 2014; Global Initiative for Chronic Obstructive Lung Disease, 2019).

Nursing Interventions

- The patient may use the tripod position to reduce work of breathing.
- Pursed-lip breathing technique improves oxygenation by delaying alveolar collapse during exhalation.
- Oxyge is worn continuously for patients with severe resting hypoxemia (oxygen saturation ≤ 88%).
- Use the lowest FiO_2 to keep oxygen saturations at the patient's baseline level. Titration to keep saturation level greater than or equal to 92% may be recommended. If saturations are less than 92%, an ABG may be recommended.
- Trend and observe for CO_2 retention. Assess alertness and level of consciousness (LOC).
- Anxiety and altered LOC should be assumed to be CO_2 retention until ruled out.
- Smoking-cessation teaching needed for patient, family, and significant others (e-cigarettes as a cessation aide is uncertain).
- Pulmonary rehabilitation: encourage participation.
- Teach the patient about inhaled bronchodilator and glucocorticoid (GC) medications.
- Teach proper technique for use of medication delivery device: metered-dose inhaler (MDI), spacer, nebulizer.
- Advise patient of the importance of pneumococcal and influenza vaccinations.
- Support energy conservation measures such as bundling care to decrease symptoms of breathlessness.
- *Palliative care and hospice:* assist patient and family to understand options as disease progresses.
- *Closely monitor intake and output:* Trend patient's weight (Brashers, 2014).

PULMONARY REHABILITATION

OVERVIEW

Patients with COPD often experience worsening shortness of breath with physical exertion. Exertional dyspnea leads to increased anxiety, with a subsequent reduction in physical activity. Over time, this decreased activity and fear of exertion leads to a vicious cycle of progressive deconditioning and diminished quality of life. Pulmonary rehabilitation (PR) interventions can break this cycle of inactivity while improving dyspnea and exercise tolerance. PR has little or no effect on the abnormal lung function of COPD but rather addresses extrapulmonary factors contributing to dyspnea and fatigue. Endurance exercise training is the cornerstone intervention, supplemented by health-promoting behavior education and psychologic support. Other conditions for which PR is appropriate include asthma, cystic fibrosis, and interstitial lung disease (Bartelome & Celli, 2016: Spruit et al, 2013).

TABLE 7.2 ASTHMA PHARMACOLOGY

CLASS	SABA					
MECHANISM OF ACTION	**RELAXES BRONCHIAL SMOOTH MUSCLE AT THE BETA₂ SITE**					
MEDICATION	**INDICATIONS**	**CONTRAINDICATIONS**	**DOSAGE**	**COMMON ADVERSE EFFECTS**	**SAFETY/PATIENT EDUCATION**	
Albuterol (Proventil, Ventolin, ProAir, ProAir RespiClick*, ProAir Digihaler*) Levalbuterol (Xopenex)	Bronchospasm in asthma; exercise-induced asthma	Precaution: CV disorders; hyperthyroidism *Inhalation powder is contraindicated in patients with severe milk protein hypersensitivity	1–2 puffs q4–6h as needed; maximum 8 puffs a day *2 inhalations q4–6h as needed 2 puffs q4–6h as needed	Nervousness, tremor, tachycardia, throat irritation	Store at room temperature. May feel excitable with elevated heart rate. *Dry powder inhalers: Never wash or put any part of the inhaler in water.	

CLASS	INHALED GC				
MECHANISM OF ACTION	**SUPPRESSES AIRWAY INFLAMMATION**				
MEDICATION	**INDICATIONS**	**CONTRAINDICATIONS**	**DOSAGE**	**COMMON ADVERSE EFFECTS**	**SAFETY/PATIENT EDUCATION**
Flunisolide (*Aerobid) Budesonide (*Pulmicort Flexhaler) Fluticasone (*Flovent Diskus: Flovent HFA)	Mild to severe asthma maintenance	Contraindicated in acute asthma episodes *Inhalation powder is contraindicated in patients with severe milk protein hypersensitivity	Use lowest effective dose once asthma is stable Dose is dependent upon specific drug, inhaled aerosol or inhaled powder form, and disease severity	Fatigue, malaise, oral candidiasis, sinus infection, throat irritation, nasal congestion	Powder inhalation does not need spacer. Rinse mouth after use. Be aware of any white or red patches in the mouth. Avoid being near anyone with chicken pox or measles if the patient has not been exposed. Check blood sugar if the patient is diabetic. Osteoporosis can occur with long-term use.

CLASS	LABA				
MECHANISM OF ACTION	**RELAXES BRONCHIAL SMOOTH MUSCLE AT THE BETA₂-RECEPTOR SITE/ SALMETEROL ACTS LOCALLY IN THE LUNG**				
MEDICATION	**INDICATIONS**	**CONTRAINDICATIONS**	**DOSAGE**	**COMMON ADVERSE EFFECTS**	**SAFETY/PATIENT EDUCATION**
Salmeterol (Serevent) Budesonide (Symbicort) Fluticasone and Salmeterol (Advair) Formoterol (Foradil)	Asthma maintenance Asthma and COPD maintenance Asthma and COPD maintenance COPD maintenance	LABA should not be used as the only asthma medication. LABAs increase the risk for asthma-related death as a monotherapy; black box warning in the United States	1 puff (50 mcg) q12h 1 puff q12h 2 puffs q12h 20 mcg/20 mL via nebulizer q12h	Headache, dizziness, dyspepsia, increased liver enzymes, throat irritation	Do not take if milk allergy. Check blood sugar if diabetic. Rinse mouth after use. Do not double dose. Store at room temperature.

(continued)

CLASS				
LEUKOTRIENE RECEPTOR AGONISTS				
MECHANISM OF ACTION				
INHIBITS THE CYSTEINYL LEUKOTRIENE RECEPTOR REDUCING AIRWAY EDEMA, SMOOTH MUSCLE CONTRACTION; DECREASES INFLAMMATION				
MEDICATION	INDICATIONS	CONTRAINDICATIONS	DOSAGE	COMMON ADVERSE EFFECTS	SAFETY/PATIENT EDUCATION
Montelukast (Singulair) Zafirlukast (Accolate)	Allergic rhinitis, asthma, exercise-induced bronchoconstriction	Caution in: hepatic disease, avoid use with aspirin or NSAIDs in patients with aspirin sensitivity	10 mg qPM 20 mg BID	Headache, dizziness, pyuria, increased AST and ALT, viral infection, cough	Do not use to treat an asthma attack. Use rescue inhalers. Signs of liver problem: dark urine, feeling tired, stomach pain, light-colored stool, or yellow eyes or skin. Do not take two doses at a time if you miss a dose.

CLASS				
THEOPHYLLINE				
MECHANISM OF ACTION				
BRONCHODILATOR				
MEDICATION	INDICATIONS	CONTRAINDICATIONS	DOSAGE	COMMON ADVERSE EFFECTS	SAFETY/PATIENT EDUCATION
Theo-Dur Theo-24	Poorly controlled asthma on adequate dose of inhaled glucocorticoids, LABA creating no benefit, failed beta₂ selective agents and IV magnesium fail to control symptoms	Hypersensitivity, allergy to corn-related products (IV only)	Loading dose of 5–7.5 mg/kg to provide a peak serum level of 10–15 mcg/mL	Tachycardia, tremors, abdominal pain Toxicity can be severe and fatal. Clearance may be decreased in patients with fever, CHF, pulmonary edema, liver disease, shock, and sepsis.	Do not take with St. John's wort. Notify physician if hives, itching, shortness of breath, or other signs of allergic reaction. Do not take with alcohol. Do not smoke tobacco or marijuana while taking theophylline.

CLASS				
CROMOGLYCATE				
MECHANISM OF ACTION				
STABILIZES AIRWAY MAST CELLS AND DECREASES THE INFLAMMATORY EFFECT				
MEDICATION	INDICATIONS	CONTRAINDICATIONS	DOSAGE	COMMON ADVERSE EFFECTS	SAFETY/PATIENT EDUCATION
Cromolyn	Adjunct in mild asthma maintenance	Hypersensitivity to cromoglycate	2–4 puffs TID–QID 20 mg per nebulized dose TID–QID	Drowsiness, irritation of nose, nausea, cough, and wheezing	This medication is used to treat asthma but not an asthma flare. Take rescue inhaler if you experience a flare. Stop taking if you experience allergic reaction such as swelling the lips or tongue. Full effect of the medication can take up to 1 month if the patient is taking for exercise induced asthma.

(continued)

TABLE 7.2 ASTHMA PHARMACOLOGY (continued)

CLASS					
LEUKOTRIENE MODIFIER					
MECHANISM OF ACTION	**SELECTIVE LEUKOTRIENE RECEPTOR AGONIST THAT INHIBITS CYSTEINYL LEUKOTRIENE RECEPTOR DECREASING AIRWAY EDEMA, SMOOTH MUSCLE CONTRACTION; DECREASING INFLAMMATORY PROCESS**				
MEDICATION	**INDICATIONS**	**CONTRAINDICATIONS**	**DOSAGE**	**COMMON ADVERSE EFFECTS**	**SAFETY/PATIENT EDUCATION**
Montelukast (Singulair) Zafirlukast (Accolate) Zileuton (Zyflo CR)	Allergic rhinitis, asthma, exercise-induced bronchoconstriction (prevention)	Precautions; follow for eosinophilia and vasculitis	Singulair 4 mg daily Accolate 10–20 mg daily Zileuton 600 mg QID	Headache, dizziness, fatigue	Take in the evening. May take with food. This is a prevention medication. A rescue inhaler must be used for an asthma attack.
CLASS					
GLUCOCORTICOID (ORAL)					
MECHANISM OF ACTION	**SUPPRESSES MIGRATION OF POLYMORPHONUCLEAR LEUCOCYTES AND REVERSES INCREASED CAPILLARY PERMEABILITY**				
MEDICATION	**INDICATIONS**	**CONTRAINDICATIONS**	**DOSAGE**	**COMMON ADVERSE EFFECTS**	**SAFETY/PATIENT EDUCATION**
Prednisone Dexamethasone Cortisone acetate	Asthma when symptoms are not controlled by inhaled agents first	Hypersensitivity to prednisone or components of the formulation, administration of live or live-attenuated vaccines with immunosuppressive doses of prednisone and systemic fungal infections.	Dose will vary depending on route of administration Anticipate dose taper	Hypertension, euphoria, insomnia, mood swings, edema, GI distress, impaired wound healing and increases in blood glucose	Do not abruptly stop dose. Take as directed. Monitor blood sugar in diabetic patients.
CLASS					
SMOOTH MUSCLE RELAXER					
MECHANISM OF ACTION	**RELAXATION OF BRONCHIAL SMOOTH MUSCLE**				
MEDICATION	**INDICATIONS**	**CONTRAINDICATIONS**	**DOSAGE**	**COMMON ADVERSE EFFECTS**	**SAFETY/PATIENT EDUCATION**
Magnesium sulfate	Per guidelines in *acute severe exacerbations*	Heart block, myocardial damage, or sensitivity to any of the component of the formulation	IV: 2 g as a single dose over 20 minutes for severe symptoms that remain after 1 hour of intensive conventional therapy	Flushed skin Decreased respirations Hypotension Vasodilation	Alert patient to the potential flushing feeling. Advise the patient about the feeling of sluggishness, slow movement, or shortness of breath. Monitoring of vital signs q15–30min may be necessary.

ALT, alanine aminotransferase; AST, aspartate aminotransferase; CHF, congestive heart failure; COPD, chronic obstructive pulmonary disease; CV, cardiovascular; GC, glucocorticoid; GI, gastrointestinal; HFA, hydrofluoroalkane; IV, intravenous; LABA, long-acting beta₂ agonist; NSAIDs, nonsteroidal anti-inflammatory drugs; SABA, short-acting beta₂ agonist.

Source: From Lexicomp Online Clinical Drug Information. (2019). Wolters Kluwer. https://www.wolterskluwercdi.com/lexicomp-online

Definition
PR is part of the recommended treatment program for patients with symptomatic airflow obstruction. It is a comprehensive intervention strategy designed to improve physical function, quality of life, and adherence to health-enhancing behaviors.

Components of Pulmonary Rehabilitation
- *Exercise endurance training:* Improves skeletal muscle oxidative capacity and weakness
  - *Upper extremity strength:* Improves task performance
  - *Lower extremity strength and endurance:* Improves function, exercise endurance, and perception of dyspnea
- Respiratory muscle training: Pursed-lip breathing and airway clearance techniques
- Education
- Self-management of disease
- Pacing of activity: Energy conservation
- Smoking cessation: Nicotine replacement and counseling
- Adherence to medication regimens
- Healthy nutrition
- Advanced care planning
- Psychologic support: Self-efficacy, coping strategies, and anxiety and depression screening

Patients are assessed prior to PR to establish an individually tailored exercise prescription and to assess for conditions that might place the patient at risk during exercise (e.g., uncontrolled cardiac disease, severe arthritis, neurologic impairment). Patients are carefully supervised and monitored during exercise. Exercise is halted if the patient develops severe dyspnea, chest pain, dizziness, tachycardia, hypotension, or refractory hypoxemia.

Patient-centered outcomes: Improved quality of life, improved dyspnea and fatigue symptoms, improved functional performance, improved adherence to treatment, and decreased healthcare utilization (Bartelome & Celli, 2016; Spruit et al, 2013).

PLEURAL EFFUSION

OVERVIEW

Definition
Pleural effusion refers to an abnormal fluid collection in the pleural space. Fluid occupies the space in the thoracic cavity and decreases lung capacity. There are two types of effusions: transudative and exudative.

Etiology
- *Transudative pleural effusions*—Causes: Congestive heart failure (CHF), pericardial disease, PE, peritoneal dialysis, cirrhosis
- *Exudative pleural effusions*— Causes: Lupus, rheumatoid arthritis, infectious diseases, neoplastic disease, trauma (chyle, blood)

Assessment
- *Signs and symptoms*—Dyspnea, cough, decreased breath sounds on affected side, decreased chest wall movement, egophony, friction rub, dull and aching pleuritic chest pain. Dullness with percussion.

Diagnostic Testing
- Chest x-ray: Blunting of the costophrenic angle; dense homogeneous opaque area; approximately 200 mL fluid is needed to detect an effusion on x-ray.
- Fluid shifts occur with change in body position.
- CBC: May reveal elevated white blood cell (WBC).
- Chemistry: Test results depend upon underlying cause of effusion (e.g., elevated ALT and AST in cirrhosis).

Interventions
- Thoracentesis may be necessary to drain the fluid. Fluid is sent for pathology, cultures, and Gram stain.
- Chest tube placement is done for rapid accumulation of pleural fluid.
- Chemical pleurodesis may be indicated for recurrent malignant pleural effusion.

Nursing Interventions
- Head of bed (HOB) >45° to facilitate lung expansion.
- Splinting of the thoracic cavity during deep inspiration may assist with minimized pain during deep breathing exercises.
- Keep oxygen saturation >92%.
- Incorporate multimodal pain interventions with NSAIDs and acetaminophen as indicated. Refer to the Centers for Disease Control and Prevention (CDC) guidelines for prescribing opioids.
- Monitor thoracentesis site for signs of infection.
- *Chest tubes*: Maintain suction at prescribed levels. Assess FOCA—fluctuation, output amount, color of output, and monitoring for air leak. Follow individual manufacturer instructions.
- Home pleural drainage systems are available and indicated for intermittent drainage of recurrent and symptomatic pleural effusions. This system is also appropriate for inpatient use (C. R. Bard, Aspira Drainage System, 2012).

THORACIC SURGERY

OVERVIEW
Definition
Thoracic surgery is the surgical repair of organs in the thoracic cavity, including lungs, trachea, mediastinum, chest wall, and diaphragm. The most common indications for noncardiac thoracic surgery include treatment for lung cancer, chest trauma, esophageal cancer, and emphysema.

Indications for Thoracic Surgery
- Lung cancer
- Pulmonary bleb affecting oxygenation, repeated pneumothorax
- Empyema
- Other dysfunctions of the lung (e.g., injury, chronic emphysema, scar tissue, fibrotic or connective tissue disease [CTD]; AACN, 2019)

Types of Thoracic Surgery
- Thoracotomy
  - Approaches:
    - Anterolateral chest
    - Lateral chest
    - Posterolateral/inferolateral chest
- *Mini thoracotomy*—Smaller incision for access with the goal to decrease risks for large incision, decrease pain, avoid spreading of the ribs, and improve progressive mobility.
- *VATS*—Small incisions provide access for video-assisted equipment. Avoids full thoracotomy incision in order to decrease risks for larger incision, decrease pain, avoid rib spreading, and improve progressive mobility.
  - *Robotic-assisted VATS*—Uses small incisions to manipulate robotic tools.

Thoracotomy Procedures

- **Wedge resection**—Resection of a small wedge-shaped portion of lung for treatment of benign or malignant lesions.
- **Segmentectomy**—Removal of bronchovascular segment of a lobe; this procedure offers better pulmonary function preservation than lobectomy.
- **Lobectomy**—Resection of the entire lobe of the lung.
- **Pneumonectomy**—Resection of an entire lung; mesothelioma is the most common indication.
- **Pleurectomy**—Removal of the pleura to reduce the risk of symptomatic pleural effusions and recurrence of spontaneous pneumothorax.
- **Decortication**—Scraping/removal of the restrictive fibrous membrane covering the pleura to allow the lung to reexpand.
- **Thoracoscopy**—Direct endoscopic visualization of the pleura. Most often used for pleural fluid drainage, parietal pleural biopsy, and pleurodesis. Conversion to thoracotomy is possible for access to tissues as needed.

Thoracic Procedures

- **Pleurodesis**—Artificial obliteration of the pleural space to prevent recurrent pleural effusion, persistent pneumothorax, or chylothorax. Pleurodesis may be a mechanical procedure (i.e., abrasion or partial pleurectomy) or instillation of a chemical irritant into the pleural space. The chemical irritant causes inflammation and fibrosis to facilitate adherence of the visceral and parietal pleural layers.
- **Pleural biopsy**—Diagnostic pleural tissue sample.
- **Chest tube or pleural drainage catheter**—Percutaneous placement of a flexible tube to drain air or fluid from the pleural space or mediastinum (see "Management of the Patient With Chest Tubes" in this chapter; American Lung Association, 2019).

Management Principles for Thoracic Surgery

- Thoracotomy incision is one of the most painful of all surgical incisions; pain control is paramount to facilitating patient mobility, lung expansion, and prevention of atelectasis.
- **Pain control**—Epidural, intercostal block, intrapleural anesthetic, and patient-controlled analgesia (PCA) narcotic methods may be used.
- **Positioning**—Frequent side-to-side repositioning and progressive out-of-bed mobility needed.
- **Pneumonectomy positioning**—Use high Fowler's position (60–90°). Avoid lateral position on nonoperative side (side of remaining lung; AACN, 2019).

RESTRICTIVE LUNG DISEASE

OVERVIEW

Definition

Restrictive lung diseases are a category of extrapulmonary or parenchymal diseases that restrict lung expansion, resulting in decreased lung volume, increased work of breathing, with inadequate ventilation and/or oxygenation. Pulmonary function tests show decreased total lung capacity. Restrictive lung disease may be classified as intrinsic or extrinsic.

Intrinsic (diseases of lung parenchyma):

- Interstitial lung disease
- Idiopathic pulmonary fibrosis

- Pulmonary fibrosis
- Sarcoidosis
- Pneumoconiosis
Extrinsic (extrapulmonary—Chest wall, pleura, respiratory muscles):
- Obesity
- Pleural effusion
- Myasthenia gravis
- Kyphoscoliosis
- Neuromuscular disease (e.g., muscular dystrophy, amyotrophic lateral sclerosis [ALS])

Intrinsic Presentation

- Velcro crackles
- Clubbing

Extrinsic Presentation

- Dull percussion, decreased tactile fremitus—Pleural effusion
- Accessory muscle use, paradoxical breathing—Neuromuscular diseases
- Deformities of spinal column
- Obese body habitus

Interventions

- Pleural drain or chest tube for drainage of pleural effusion, retained blood, or purulent fluid is used
- Pleurectomy for restriction related to pleura
- Thoracotomy, VATS, and robotic-assisted VATS are interventions used to treat lung mass or tissue dysfunction
- Oxygen therapy
- PR
- Noninvasive ventilation for gas exchange abnormalities during sleep (extrinsic; Lung Institute, 2019)

PULMONARY INFECTIONS

PNEUMONIA

Pneumonia is an inflammatory process of the lung parenchyma and alveolar spaces. Pneumonia is typically acute; however, chronic pneumonia can be the result of chronic micro-aspiration in older adults or patients with reduced cough or gag reflex.

Pathophysiology

Inflammation leads to phagocytosis and fluid transfer from pulmonary capillaries into the alveoli. Alveoli become filled with fluid and leukocytes, leading to alveolar consolidation.

Etiology

Pneumonia is classified as community acquired or hospital acquired. Hospital-acquired pneumonia is further differentiated into ventilator-associated events (VAEs), ventilator-associated pneumonia (VAP), or nonventilator-associated hospital-acquired pneumonia (nv-HAP). Both VAP and nv-HAP employ bundled care interventions to reduce incidence. Translocation of bacteria in the oral cavity can lead to both VAP and NVHAP.

- **Streptococcus pneumoniae:** Most common cause of pneumonia in older adults and chronically ill
- **Mycoplasma pneumoniae:** Spread by droplet and may produce epidemics
- **Haemophilus influenza:** Associated with bacteremia in older adults

- *Viral pneumonia:* Most often caused by influenza A; older adults and patients in residential facilities are at greater risk for outbreaks
- *Fungal pneumonia:* Aspergillosis is typically associated with construction and renovation sites; it is more common in immunocompromised patients and patients with preexisting lung disease. Histoplasmosis is linked to soil contaminated with bird or bat droppings; it is found in central and eastern states, particularly the Ohio and Mississippi River valleys Giuliano et al., 2014).

Assessment
- *Assess for risk factors:* Smoking, upper respiratory infection, influenza, alcohol use, advanced age, underlying pulmonary or cardiac disorders, altered LOC, malnutrition, compromised immune system, immobility, and exposure to inhalants.
- *Sign and symptoms:* Intercostal retractions, cyanosis, hypoxemia, tachycardia, tachypnea, fever, chest pain, myalgia, cough, dyspnea, and anxiety.
- Asymmetric chest expansion and/or tactile fremitus may be noted during palpation.
- Percussion may reveal dullness in the area of consolidation.
- *Auscultation:* Crackles, wheezes, bronchophony, whispered pectoriloquy, and egophony.
- Older patients may present with change in mental status, dehydration, and with or without fever.

Diagnostic Testing
- ABG, chest x-ray, CBC, blood cultures, respiratory cultures.
- *Chest x-ray:* Infiltrates and possible consolidation.
- Sepsis screening should be completed utilizing the evidence-based suggestions in the Surviving Sepsis Campaign. Refer to the Society of Critical Care Medicine Surviving Sepsis for the current bundle requirement: www.survivingsepsis.org.

Interventions
- **HOB greater than 30°** unless contraindicated.
- Perform bedside dysphagia exam prior to oral medication or fluids. If the patient fails the initial exam, consider a referral for modified swallow evaluation by speech therapy.
  Blood and respiratory cultures prior to antibiotic therapy if patient condition indicates (ICU admission or outpatient antibiotic [ATB] failure) or if sepsis is a differential diagnosis.
- Initiate empiric broad-spectrum antimicrobial therapy that will cover all suspected pathogens.
- Antibiotic therapy should be started within the first hour of sepsis identification. Do not delay administration of the first dose of antibiotics if cultures cannot be obtained.
- *Procalcitonin levels:* Biomarker rises in response to bacterial infections and may be considered with the community-acquired pneumonia to help guide duration of therapy. Serial levels may be useful.
- *C-reactive protein (CRP):* Less sensitive than procalcitonin for the detection of bacterial pneumonia. CRP clinical correlation in conjunction with testing should be utilized to improve outcomes.
- *De-escalation of antibiotics:* As soon as the pathogen is identified and sensitivities established.
- *Antibiotic stewardship:* Collaboration with pharmacy to assist with the antibiogram for the specific facility and region.
- *Hydration:* IV fluids may be necessary as a response to sepsis guidelines.

- *Pain control:* Encourage pharmacologic and nonpharmacologic pain interventions.
- *Airway clearance:* Consider use of expectorants and nebulized bronchodilators.
- NVHAP bundled care includes the following:
  - Oral care is tiered interventions based on patient condition include tooth brushing, denture care, or oral suction/swab brushing therapy
  - Incentive spirometry
  - Turn, cough, and breathe deeply
  - Early mobilization
- VAP/VAE bundled care includes the following:
  - HOB elevated >30°.
  - *Early mobilization*—Chair position, turning every 2 hours, or early ambulation.
  - Closed suction system.
  - *Oral care*—Brush teeth, gums, and tongue at least twice a day using a soft, compact head (pediatric or adult) toothbrush; provide oral mucosa moisturizing every 2 to 4 hours; use oral chlorhexidine gluconate (0.12%) rinse twice a day in intubated patients to reduce risk of VAP; subglottic suction.
  - Subglottic suction prior to repositioning the endotracheal tube (ETT).
  - DVT and peptic ulcer prophylaxis may be included in the care bundle (Storzer, 2017).

TUBERCULOSIS
Mycobacterium tuberculosis causes the respiratory disease tuberculosis (TB). TB is transmitted via infected respiratory droplets. Airborne droplet nuclei may remain suspended in room air currents for several hours. Disseminated tuberculosis is a mycobacterial infection that has spread from the lungs to multiple parts of the body via the bloodstream or lymph system.

TB may occur in three stages. Mycobacterium tuberculosis bacilli initially causes a *primary infection*, which is usually asymptomatic, followed by a *latent or dormant phase* of infection. *Active TB* refers to active signs and symptoms of disease. Infection is usually not transmissible in the primary phase and is not contagious in the latent phase.

TB resistance has become a public health concern. TB can be endemic in areas of overcrowding, in poor living conditions, and in immigrant populations. Older adults and immunosuppressed people are at high risk for latent TB. TB is the leading killer of patients infected with HIV.

Pathophysiology
TB may occur in three stages. *Mycobacterium tuberculosis* bacilli initially causes a primary infection, which is usually asymptomatic, followed by a latent or dormant phase of infection. *Active TB* refers to active signs and symptoms of disease. Infection is usually not transmissible in the primary phase and is not contagious in the latent phase (CDC, 2019).

Assessment
- *Signs and symptoms include:* Cough for greater than 2 weeks, hemoptysis, fever, chills, night sweats, fatigue, and unexplained weight loss

Diagnostic Testing
- CBC, chemistry panel, and sputum for acid-fast organisms; blood cultures, respiratory culture, and sensitivity

- Chest x-ray has high sensitivity but poor specificity in diagnosis of active TB
  - Chest x-ray findings suggestive of TB: Linear opacities, calcified hilar nodes, Ghon's complex.
- Mantoux tuberculin skin test (TST)
- Interferon-gamma release assay (IGRA) blood test detects TB bacterial infection

Interventions

- **RIPE** therapy (rifampin, isoniazid, pyrazinamide, and isoniazid) is the first-line treatment. Alterative medications are needed for drug-resistant TB, children, pregnant women, and those with HIV infection.
- Side effects of RIPE therapy include gastrointestinal (GI) upset and aversion to foods, thus resulting in weight loss, poor compliance, and decreased absorption.
- Infectious disease specialist collaboration is key to optimizing therapy. Compliance is often difficult as treatment is needed for up to 10 months.
- Collaborate with state departments of health.
- Airborne precautions, proper mask, or powered airpurifying respirator (PAPR) use is essential for healthcare professionals.
- Teach the patient to contain cough and respiratory secretions. Proper hand hygiene should be taught to the patient and family.
- Consistent follow-up with a primary care practitioner is needed following discharge.

PULMONARY ASPIRATION

OVERVIEW

Pulmonary aspiration is usually caused by regurgitation and vomiting. **Aspiration pneumonitis** is acute lung injury resulting from inhalation of gastric contents. The risk for gastric content aspiration increases as LOC decreases. Aspiration of large particles can obstruct the major airway and can cause immediate asphyxia and death. Immediate interventions to clear the airway such as the Heimlich maneuver or deep tracheal suctioning is required. Most pulmonary aspirations are of clear acidic liquid with a pH <2.5. The greater the volume of aspirate, the more severe the pulmonary insult.

Aspiration pneumonia develops after the inhalation of colonized oropharyngeal bacteria, leading to the development of a radiographic infiltrate in patients at increased risk for oropharyngeal aspiration.

Pathophysiology
Aspiration Pneumonitis

Aspiration of gastric contents results in a chemical burn of the tracheobronchial tree and pulmonary parenchyma, triggering a highly inflammatory cellular reaction. The pathophysiology of acidic aspiration includes the destruction of type II alveolar cells, leading to a decrease in surfactant production. There is caustic injury to the alveolar–capillary interface, leading to acute lung injury. Acidic gastric contents are sterile under normal circumstances; however, bacterial infection may occur at later stages of the acute lung injury. Grossly contaminated materials, such as those that occur with bowel obstruction, may be rapidly fatal. Patients with aspiration pneumonitis who require mechanical ventilation are at high risk for developing adult respiratory distress syndrome (Brashers, 2014).

Aspiration Pneumonia
Assessment

- **Signs and symptoms:** Cough, dyspnea, hypoxemia, tachypnea, increased secretions, and fever. Observe for increased work of breathing. Assess for stridor and cyanosis. Tactile fremitus may be present with obstruction of large bronchial airways. Dullness may be percussed over the infiltrated region. Auscultation of wheezing or crackles may be heard in the affected airway. Absent breath sounds are common in occluded bronchus.
- **Aspiration pneumonitis risk factors:** Altered LOC, history of dysphagia, history of stroke, ingestion of narcotics, benzodiazepines, or alcohol.
- **Aspiration pneumonia risk factors:** Older adults, history of GERD, alcoholism, anesthesia, history of dysphagia, history of stroke

Diagnostic Testing

- **Chest x-ray:** Infiltrates—Right lower lobe is most common.
- Fiberoptic bronchoscopy if necessary to obtain a specimen for culture and sensitivity.

Interventions

- If acute, position the patient with head of bed elevated or turn patient to the side. Suction oropharynx without further irritation of the gag reflex and induction of vomiting.
- Fiberoptic bronchoscopy is used for retrieval of large volume aspirate or food particles.
- Emergent intubation is warranted for patients unable to protect the airway.
- Consider naso or orogastric tube placement postintubation.
- When the patient is extubated, strongly consider a formal dysphagia evaluation.
- **Antibiotic therapy**—Aspiration pneumonitis: For symptoms persisting >48 hours—consider bacterial infection and treat as per aspiration pneumonia guide as noted in Table 7.3.
- **Antibiotic therapy**—Aspiration pneumonia: Indicated immediately; treat as community-acquired aspiration pneumonia if onset within 72 hours of admission or as hospital-acquired aspiration pneumonia if indicated >72 hours after admission.
- Deescalate antibiotics as soon as sensitivity is received.
- Switch to oral antibiotic therapy when the patient passes the dysphagia screen, the patient is hemodynamically stable, and the GI tract is stable.
- Consider ongoing sepsis screening (Bartlett, 2019a).

OBSTRUCTIVE SLEEP APNEA

OVERVIEW

Obstructive sleep apnea (OSA) is one of the most common chronic upper airway obstructions. Apnea is the loss of airflow for more than 10 seconds. Sleep apnea is hypopnea with repeated episodes during sleep accompanied by daytime drowsiness. Upper airway dysfunction in association with narrowing or closure of the posterior pharynx and trachea is influenced by neuromuscular tone, muscle synchrony, and the stage of sleep. OSA is most common during rapid eye movement (REM) sleep. Patients are at risk for hypertension, PH, dysrhythmias, heart failure, heart attack, and stroke. Late signs of OSA are hypoxemia, hypercapnia, polycythemia, and cor pulmonale (Storzer, 2017).

TABLE 7.3 MEDICATIONS FOR TREATMENT OF PULMONARY ASPIRATION

CLASS	GLUCOCORTICOID			
MEDICATION	SOLUMEDROL			
MECHANISM OF ACTION	DECREASED INFLAMMATION			
INDICATIONS	**CONTRAINDICATIONS**	**DOSAGE**	**COMMON ADVERSE EFFECTS**	**SAFETY/PATIENT EDUCATION**
Controversial therapy; off-label use as short-term treatment of COPD exacerbation	Patients with systemic fungal infections	1–2 mg/kg Typically 125 mg IV, decreasing subsequent doses	Hyperglycemia Irritability Adrenal insufficiency	Inform patient and family about hyperexcitability Alert about delayed wound healing
CLASS	ANTIBIOTIC, PENICILLIN			
MEDICATION	AMPICILLIN-SULBACTAM (UNASYN)			
MECHANISM OF ACTION	INHIBITS BACTERIAL CELL WALL SYNTHESIS BY BINDING TO THE PBPX-INHIBITING CELL WALL BIOSYNTHESIS			
INDICATIONS	**CONTRAINDICATIONS**	**DOSAGE**	**COMMON ADVERSE EFFECTS**	**SAFETY/PATIENT EDUCATION**
Anaerobic pathogens probable	Allergy to components of medication or previous hypersensitivity to penicillin	1.5–3 g IV q6h for normal renal function	Watch for allergic reaction or Stevens-Johnson syndrome Diarrhea Thrombophlebitis Rash Superinfection such as *Clostridium difficile*	Should be adjusted for creatinine clearance in patients with a history of renal insufficiency and should alert provider Teach patient about signs of allergic reaction Include patient in antibiotic stewardship discussion
CLASS	ANTIBIOTIC, BETA-LACTAM			
MEDICATION	AMOXICILLIN-CLAVULANATE (AUGMENTIN)			
MECHANISM OF ACTION	BINDING PROPERTIES TO THE CELL WALL INHIBIT CELL WALL BIOSYNTHESIS			
INDICATIONS	**CONTRAINDICATIONS**	**DOSAGE**	**COMMON ADVERSE EFFECTS**	**SAFETY/PATIENT EDUCATION**
Anaerobic pathogen probable and oral therapy is indicated	Patients with history of hypersensitivity/extended release; should not be used in patients with renal failure or dialysis	875 mg PO BID	GI upset Nausea Vaginitis Rash	Do not take with probenecid. Alert provider if coadministration with blood thinners. Watch for superinfections. Some formulations contain phenylalanine alert; provide if PKU history. Take with food.
CLASS	ANTIBIOTIC, CARBAPENEM			
MEDICATION	MEROPENEM (MERREM)			
MECHANISM OF ACTION	BINDS TO CELL WALL INHIBITING WALL BIOSYNTHESIS, ENDING IN CELL WALL DESTRUCTION			
INDICATIONS	**CONTRAINDICATIONS**	**DOSAGE**	**COMMON ADVERSE EFFECTS**	**SAFETY/PATIENT EDUCATION**
Hospital-acquired pneumonia aerobic bacteria especially Gram-negative bacilli and *Staphylococcus aureus*. Patients with poor dentation	Hypersensitivity to beta lactams	1.5–6 g daily divided q8h	Headache Rash Elevated liver enzymes Increased BUN and creatinine	Tell provider is patient is taking probenecid or valproic acid. Watch for diarrhea. Check for signs of allergic reaction. Include patient in antibiotic stewardship discussion

(continued)

TABLE 7.3 MEDICATIONS FOR TREATMENT OF PULMONARY ASPIRATION (continued)

CLASS	ANTIBIOTIC, GLYCOPEPTIDE			
MEDICATION	VANCOMYCIN			
MECHANISM OF ACTION	HINDERS BACTERIAL CELL WALL SYNTHESIS; INTERFERES WITH RNA SYNTHESIS			
INDICATIONS	CONTRAINDICA-TIONS	DOSAGE	COMMON ADVERSE EFFECTS	SAFETY/PATIENT EDUCATION
MRSA is considered. Dose must be adjusted in patients with poor renal function.	Hypersensitivity to drug or drug compounds	Initial dose is dependent on patient severity of illness but is usually 10–20 mg/kg/dose with maximum 2 g dose initially; given q8–12h. Ensure optimal therapeutic dosing: serum vancomycin trough level can be drawn 30 min before the fourth dose in patients receiving q8h or 12h dosing. Earlier vancomycin trough levels are indicated in patients receiving once-daily dosing	Renal toxicity—eGFR dosing regimens required Maculopapular rash of face and trunk—Red man syndrome requires a slower rate for next infusion Hypotension and shock have been reported to rapid administration	Notify staff if pain or redness at infusion site. Intradermal hyaluronidase may be considered for refractory extravasated areas. Notify provider if experiencing chills or itching with infusion. Alert care providers of any history renal insufficiency. Tell prescriber if experiencing decreased hearing.

BUN, blood urea nitrogen; COPD, chronic obstructive pulmonary disease; eGFR, estimated glomerular filtration rate; GI, gastrointestinal; IV, intravenous; MRSA, methicillin-resistant *Staphylococcus aureus*; PBPX, penicillin-binding protein 2X gene; PKU, phenylketonuria.

Source: From Lexicomp Online Clinical Drug Information. (2019). Wolters Kluwer. https://www.wolterskluwercdi.com/lexicomp-online

Etiology and Risk Factors

- Obesity
- Advancing age
- Male gender
- History of smoking
- Menopause
- Nasal obstruction
- Tonsillar hypertrophy
- Macroglossia
- Vocal cord paralysis
- Central nervous system abnormalities

Assessment

- *Subjective symptoms*—Excessive daytime sleepiness, personality changes, fatigue-related work injuries, loud snoring, headaches, decreased libido
- *Objective signs*—Presence of one or more of the subjective symptoms, family history, social confirmation of loud snoring, gasping, or choking episodes during sleep
- Physical assessment
  - Inspect for obesity, work of breathing, duskiness or cyanosis, patient's ability to concentrate; inspect the nose and throat for blockage.
  - Palpate for sinus tenderness.
  - Auscultate upper airway for stridor, wheezing, coarse rhonchi, or decreased breath sounds for occluded bronchus.
- *Diagnostic tests:* Sleep study, ABG, and pulmonary function tests. Formal diagnosis of OSA is based upon a combination of increased frequency of obstructive apnea events during sleep and daytime sleepiness and a positive sleep study.

Interventions and Patient Management

- Multidisciplinary approach to improve quality of life
  - Continuous positive airway pressure (CPAP) use
  - Patient and family teaching on CPAP compliance
  - Improved blood pressure control
  - Reducing risk related to automobile accidents or workplace injury
  - Weight loss strategies
  - Controlling insulin resistance and type 2 diabetes
  - Ensuring perioperative assessment to reduce postoperative cardiac or respiratory events
  - Stress reducing techniques such as mindfulness or meditation prior to sleep
  - Avoiding stimulants in the afternoon to promote sleep

OSA treatment should include an assessment of adherence to CPAP use and review of barriers to nighttime compliance. Face mask alternatives should be considered to reduce pressure injuries associated with nasal masks (Storzer, 2017).

AIRWAY OBSTRUCTIVE ATELECTASIS

OVERVIEW

Definition

Atelectasis is the collapse of lung tissue with loss of volume. Atelectasis is categorized as obstructive or nonobstructive according to the underlying pathophysiologic process.

Pathophysiology

Obstructive atelectasis is a potential consequence of airway blockage. Trapped air distal to the occlusion is resorbed from nonventilated alveoli. Affected lung regions become totally gasless and then collapse. A shunt occurs as blood perfuses unventilated lung units, resulting in hypoxemia. Postobstruction alveoli fill with secretions and cells. The heart and mediastinum shift toward the atelectatic area.

Complications

- Acute pneumonia
- Bronchiectasis
- Hypoxemia and respiratory failure
- Postobstructive fluid accumulation
- Sepsis
- Pleural effusion and empyema

Etiology

Causes and risk factors of obstructive atelectasis include the following:

- **Mucus plugs**
  - Upper-abdominal or thoracic surgery
  - Advanced age
  - Obesity
  - Smoking history
  - Reduced mobility
  - Sedation
  - Neuromuscular disorders
  - Chronic lung disease
  - Pain with deep breathing
- **Risk factors**
  - Smoking
  - Asbestos worker
  - Age >35
  - First-degree relatives with lung cancer

Presentation

Symptom presentation is determined in part by the factors listed in Table 7.4.

Diagnostic Testing

See Table 7.5 for diagnostic testing details.

Assessment

Physical Examination

- Dullness to percussion over affected area
- Diminished or absent breath sounds
- Reduced chest excursion of the involved lung
- Tracheal deviation toward the affected side (large area of collapse)

TABLE 7.4 AIRWAY OBSTRUCTIVE ATELECTASIS SYMPTOMS

FACTORS	SYMPTOMS
Speed of onset of the bronchial occlusion	**Slow** onset: Atelectasis may be asymptomatic or cause only minor symptoms initially **Rapid** bronchial occlusion: Sudden onset of dyspnea, and cyanosis; possible hypotension, tachycardia
Size of the lung area affected	**Large** area of lung collapse causes pain on the affected side, sudden onset of dyspnea, and cyanosis **Major bronchus** obstruction: May cause severe hacking or coughing
Infection: Complication	**Presence of Infection:** Fever, leukocytosis

TABLE 7.5 DIAGNOSTIC TESTING

TEST	RESULTS
ABG	Hypoxia—Resulting from V/Q mismatch and areas of right to left shunt
CXR	Increased opacity (with signs of volume loss), air bronchograms (distal lung fields obstructed by secretions)
CT scan	Evidence of lobar collapse
Bronchoscopy	Etiology identification: Mucus plugging, tumor Histology: Brushing, washing, biopsy specimens

ABG, arterial blood gas; CXR, chest x-ray; V/Q, ventilation/perfusion.

Source: Madappa, T. (2018). Atelectasis workup. https://emedicine.medscape.com/article/296468-workup#c6

In the beginning stages of atelectasis development, prior to obstruction, breath sounds will show late inspiratory crackles (caused by sudden opening of distal airways). The initial onset of atelectasis can be slow with subtle changes in symptoms (respiratory rate, heart rate, oxygenation).

Treatment for obstructive atelectasis depends upon the etiology.

Treatment for Mucus Plug Obstruction

- *Chest physiotherapy*—Postural drainage, chest wall percussion, and vibration
- *Huff cough*—Forced expiration technique
- *Bronchodilators and humidification*—May improve ventilation and sputum expectoration
- *Nasotracheal suctioning*—Necessary if ineffective cough and secretion clearance
- *Continuous positive airway pressure*—May be effective in improving oxygenation and reexpanding the collapsed lung.
- *Fiberoptic bronchoscopy*—For mucus plug removal if standard techniques (chest physiotherapy, cough and deep breathing, suctioning) are not effective.
- *Intubation and mechanical ventilation* may be needed for severe hypoxemia with respiratory distress. Intubation provides oxygenation, ventilation, and access for airway suctioning. Positive pressure ventilation and delivery of larger tidal volumes (TVs) helps to reexpand collapsed lung units (Thanavaro & Foner, 2013).
- *Broad-spectrum antibiotics*—Indicated for postobstruction infection and pneumonia
- *N*-acetylcysteine aerosol *is not* routinely recommended due to risk for bronchoconstriction and the lack of documented evidence of efficacy.

Prevention

Atelectasis, retained secretions, and mucus plugging can be prevented by enhancing lung expansion and airway clearance. Postoperative pain control, early ambulation, cough and deep-breathing exercises, or incentive spirometry improve lung expansion. A proper technique is essential for effective use of incentive spirometry (IS), which should always be within the patient's easy reach. Airway clearance techniques such as positive expiratory pressure (PEP) may be used to help move secretions into the larger airways and prevent alveoli collapse on expiration. Systemic hydration and adequate airway humidification help prevent thickened mucus that impedes secretion clearance.

Prevention in high-risk surgical patients begins with preoperative patient education. Information should include expectations of pain control, mobility, and cough and deep-breathing exercises. Postoperatively, nurses should maintain heightened clinical suspicion when caring for at-risk patients.

Treatment for Tumor Obstruction

Treatment may involve surgical reduction or removal of the tumor and/or shrinkage of the tumor with chemotherapy or radiation.

Surgical options are further described under Thoracic Surgery section in this chapter (Cassidy et al., 2013).

PULMONARY ARTERIAL HYPERTENSION

OVERVIEW

Pulmonary arterial hypertension (PAH) is a life-threatening disease without a cure. Early diagnosis and specialty care are essential for treatment optimization. PAH is generally underdiagnosed with specialty treatment delayed for up to 2 years. Patients with unexplained dyspnea on exertion (DOE), exercise limitation, syncope or pre-syncopal episodes, and/or signs of RV dysfunction should be considered for evaluation of PAH (Hoeper et al., 2013).

Definition

PAH is a chronic, progressive, debilitating disease affecting the pulmonary vasculature. PAH is characterized by severe remodeling of the distal pulmonary arteries in the absence of other cardiopulmonary disease, increased pulmonary vascular resistance (PVR), and RV dysfunction that promotes heart failure. PAH is definitively diagnosed by right-heart catheterization (RHC) mean pulmonary artery pressure (mPAP) values greater than 25 mmHg, PVR greater than 3 Wood Units (WU), and a pulmonary artery wedge pressure (PAWP) less than 15 mmHg.

Diagnosis

Noninvasive screening for PAH should begin with transthoracic echocardiogram (TTE) evaluating the condition of the right side of the heart. Subsequent testing includes definitive diagnosis by RHC and diagnosis of cause. Complete pulmonary function testing, thoracic computed tomography, and nocturnal plethysmography to evaluate sleep-disordered breathing are to be evaluated (Maron & Galie, 2016; Stewart et al., 2017).

The WHO functional classification is used to grade the severity of functional limitations of PH (see Box 7.1):

- *Class I:* Patient with PH without limitation of physical activity. Ordinary physical activity does not cause undue dyspnea or fatigue, chest pain, or near syncope.
- *Class II:* Patient with PH with slight limitation of physical activity; patients are comfortable at rest. Ordinary physical activity causes undue dyspnea or fatigue, chest pain, or near syncope.
- *Class III:* Patient with PH with marked limitation of physical activity, although patients are comfortable at rest; less than ordinary activity causes undue dyspnea or fatigue, chest pain, or near syncope.
- *Class IV:* Patient with PH with the inability to carry out any physical activity without symptoms. Patients have signs of right-heart failure, dyspnea, and/or fatigue at rest. Discomfort is increased by any physical activity.

Treatment

Advanced therapies should be prescribed by experienced clinicians at centers of excellence in PH care. The evaluation of a patient's disease should be done using a systematic and consistent approach using the WHO functional capacity (FC), exercise capacity, and echocardiographic, laboratory, and hemodynamic variables to inform therapeutic decisions. Supportive therapies, such as diuretics, supplemental oxygen, digoxin, anticoagulation, and physical therapy, are important to continue in the management of PAH. Newly diagnosed patients are risk stratified low, medium, or high according to the expected 1-year mortality. Monotherapy, double, or triple combination therapy algorithms exist to guide treatment plans. According to the risk status of the patient, multiple drugs approved for PAH, interfering with the endothelin, nitric oxide, and prostacyclin pathways, can be utilized in varying and individualized strategies. Lung transplantation may be required in the most advances cases on maximal medical therapy (Galie et al., 2016; Galie et al., 2018).

Goals of Treatment

- Improvement of FC to class I or II, 6-minute walk distance (6MWD) of greater than 380 to 440 m
- Cardiopulmonary exercise test measured peak oxygen consumption greater than 15 mL/min/kg
- Ventilatory equivalent for carbon dioxide (VE/VCO$_2$) less than 45

Box 7.1 Classification of Pulmonary Hypertension

> *World Health Organization*
> **WHO group I:** PAH causes include the following: IPAH; HPAH; DPAH; PAH related to CTD, such as SLE-PAH and SSc-PAH; Po-PH; HIV-PAH; CHD-PAH; PVOD or PCH, and schistosomiasis.
> **WHO group II:** PH due to left-heart disease.
> **WHO group III:** PH due to lung disease or chronic hypoxia.
> **WHO group IV:** CTEPH.
> **WHO group V:** PH due to multifactorial issues: hematologic disorders such as chronic hemolytic anemia, myeloproliferative disease, and splenectomy; systemic disorders such as sarcoidosis, histiocytosis, vasculitis, neurofibromatosis, and lymphangioleiomyomatosis; metabolic disorders such as glycogen storage disease, Gaucher's disease, and thyroid disorder; and other diseases such as chronic kidney disease, tumor obstruction, fibrosing mediastinitis.

CHD-PAH, congenital heart disease-PAH; CTD, connective tissue disease; CTEPH, chronic thromboembolic pulmonary hypertension; DPAH, drug-induced PAH; HIV-PAH, HIV-pulmonary arterial hypertension; HPAH, genetic/heritable PAH; IPAH, idiopathic PAH; PAH, pulmonary arterial hypertension; PCH, pulmonary capillary hemangiomatosis; PH, pulmonary hypertension; Po-PH, portopulmonary hypertension; PVOD, pulmonary veno-occlusive disease; SLE-PAH, systemic lupus erythematosus-PAH; SSc-PAH, scleroderma-PAH; WHO, World Health Organization.

Source: From Klinger, J., Elliott, G., Levine, D. J., Bossone, E., Duvall, L., Fagan, K., Frantsve-Hawley, J., Kawut, S. M., Ryan, J. J., Rosenzweig, E. B., Sederstrom, N., Steen, V. D., & Badesch, D. B. (2019). Therapy for pulmonary arterial hypertension in adults. *Chest, 155*(3), 565–586.

- BNP level toward normal
- TTE and/or cardiac MRI demonstrating normal/near normal RV size and function
- Hemodynamics showing normalization of RV function with right-atrial (RA) pressure less than 8 mmHg and cardiac index greater than 2.5 to 3 $L/min/m^2$ (McLaughlin et al., 2013)

Pharmacologic Treatment
Patient Education
In order for a treatment plan to be successful, patients with PAH must be engaged, committed, and have support. Consider patient preference in route of drug administration, lifestyle, social support, financial resources, and insurance when beginning a treatment plan See Table 7.6 for PAH pharmacotherapies.

Prescribing and Management
Experienced PH teams and evidence-based guidelines are available for the diagnosis and treatment of PAH in PH centers of excellence.
- *Maximize the benefit of prostacyclin pathway therapies*: Identify, accurately assess, and appropriately manage prostacyclin side effects, which otherwise would lead to discontinuation of therapy. Educate patients and care givers of adjunctive therapies to ease side effects.
- Routinely monitor drug therapy.
- Monitor patients for signs of right-heart failure, which could indicate medication failure.
- Begin therapy at a low dose. Titrate up to tolerance of side effects until maintenance dose is achieved.
- Monotherapy and/or combination therapy for PAH are approved treatments by the Food and Drug Administration (FDA).
- Avoid pregnancy.
- Educate on low-sodium diet.
- Incorporate palliative care services (Galie, 2013; Kingman et al., 2017; Klinger, 2019).

ACUTE RESPIRATORY FAILURE

OVERVIEW
Definition
Acute respiratory failure (ARF) occurs when the pulmonary system is not able to meet the body's metabolic demands by providing adequate oxygenation to the blood and/or elimination of carbon dioxide.
Respiratory failure is categorized as hypoxemic or hypercapnic failure:
- Hypoxemic
  - $PaO_2 < 50$
  - Inadequate oxygen exchange
- Hypercapnic
  - $PaCO_2 > 50$ with pH < 7.35
  - Decreased elimination of CO_2
  - Airflow obstruction, central respiratory failure, or neuromuscular failure

Pathophysiology
Hypoxemic Respiratory Failure
- *V/Q mismatch:* Normal ventilation (V) to perfusion (Q) ratio is 1:1.
  - Low V/Q (<1)

Examples: Pneumonia, atelectasis, bronchospasm, mucus plug
  - High V/Q (>1)
Example: PE
- *Intrapulmonary shunt:* Blood flows through the pulmonary capillaries without participating in gas exchange.
  - Examples: Acute lung injury, acute respiratory distress syndrome (ARDS), pulmonary edema, atelectasis

Hypercapnic Respiratory Failure
- Alveolar hypoventilation
  - Reduced minute ventilation (MV)
  - Example: COPD, drug overdose

Etiology
Extrapulmonary

- TBI	- ALS
- Central nervous system lesion	- Myasthenia gravis
- Spinal cord lesion	- Morbid obesity
- Pleura (pneumothorax, pleural effusion)	- Chest trauma

ALS, amyotrophic lateral sclerosis; TBI, traumatic brain injury.

Intrapulmonary

- COPD	- Cystic fibrosis
- Pulmonary embolism	- ARDS
- Pneumonia	- Asthma

ARDS, acute respiratory distress syndrome; COPD, congestive obstructive pulmonary disease.

Sources: Burns, S. M., & Delgado, S. A. (2018). *AACN essentials of critical care nursing* (4th ed.). McGraw-Hill; Morton, P. G., & Fontaine, D. K. (2018). Critical care nursing: A *holistic approach* (11th ed.). Lippincott Williams & Wilkins.

Assessment
History needed for medical conditions and precipitating events.

Signs and Symptoms

- Hypoxemia ($PaO_2 < 50$)	- $SpO_2 < 90$
- Dyspnea	- Hypercarbia ($PaCO_2 > 50$)
- Use of accessory muscles	- Tachypnea
- Restlessness	- Somnolence (late sign)
- Cyanosis (late sign)	- Loss of consciousness (late sign)

Diagnostic Findings
Arterial blood gas: ABG analysis confirms the diagnosis of respiratory failure (see Chapter 11, "Renal System," Acid–Base Imbalances, Arterial Blood Gas Analysis sections).
- $PaO_2 < 50$
- $PaCO_2 > 50$
- pH ≤ 7.30
Diagnostic Tests to Determine Etiology:
- Chest x-ray (CXR), CT scan, bronchoscopy, echocardiogram, thoracentesis, sputum culture, pulmonary angiography

Treatment
Immediate intervention is needed to address gas exchange problems and resolve the underlying condition. Assessment to

TABLE 7.6 VASCULAR-TARGETED PHARMACOTHERAPIES FOR PULMONARY ARTERIAL HYPERTENSION

MEDICATION, CLASS, MECHANISM OF ACTION	INDICATIONS	DOSAGE	COMMON SIDE EFFECTS	KEY SAFETY/ PATIENT EDUCATION INFORMATION
Epoprostenol (Flolan) IV (Veletri) IV Cardiovascular agent, Prostacyclin Potent vasodilator, inhibitor of platelet aggregation	WHO group I PAH Indication: to improve exercise capacity	Continuous IV infusion with a 6-minute half-life Initial: 2 ng/kg/min, titrate upward in increments of 2 ng/kg/min every 15 minutes or longer until dose-limiting effects or intolerance develops: avoid abrupt withdrawal	Flushing, jaw pain, diarrhea, headache, nausea, GI upset, vomiting, supraventricular tachycardia, hypotension, anxiety, thrombocytopenia	Seek immediate medical attention for interruption in therapy, keep a second pump and medication cassette ready as a backup, half-life of IV Veletri and Flolan approximately 6 minutes; manage side effects; rebound PH will occur if abruptly discontinued.
IV **Treprostinil** (Remodulin) Cardiovascular agent, Prostacyclin Potent vasodilator, inhibitor of platelet aggregation, inhibition of smooth muscle proliferation **Subcutaneous** (Remodulin) Cardiovascular agent, Prostacyclin Potent vasodilator, inhibitor of platelet aggregation, inhibition of smooth muscle proliferation **Inhaled** (Tyvaso) Cardiovascular agent, Prostacyclin Potent vasodilator, inhibitor of platelet aggregation, inhibition of smooth muscle proliferation	WHO group I PAH WHO group I PAH WHO group I PAH WHO group I PAH WHO group I PAH	**IV** 4-hours half life Initial: 1.25 ng/kg/min continuous via central line IV infusion; decrease to 0.625 ng/kg/min if initial dose cannot be tolerated; increase dose in increments of 1.25 ng/kg/min per week continuous via central line IV infusion for the first 4 weeks and then by 2.5 ng/kg/min per week continuous via central line IV infusion for remaining duration; may increase dose more often if tolerated. **Subcutaneous** 4-hour half-life Initial: 1.25 ng/kg/min continuous subcutaneous infusion; decrease to 0.625 ng/kg/min if initial dose cannot be tolerated; increase dose in increments of 1.25 ng/kg/min per week continuous subcutaneous infusion for the first 4 weeks and then by 2.5 ng/kg/min per week continuous subcutaneous infusion for remaining duration; may increase dose more often if tolerated. Initial: 3 breaths (18 mcg) via oral inhalation per treatment session, four times daily during waking hours (approximately 4 hours apart with each treatment session taking 2 to 3 minutes); reduce to 1 or 2 breaths if 3 breaths not tolerated and subsequently increase to three breaths. Maintenance: titrate by additional 3 breaths via PO inhalation at approximately 1–2-week intervals as tolerated, to a target dose of 9 breaths (54 mcg) per treatment session, QID during waking hours (approximately 4 hours apart).	**IV** Extremity pain, headache, nausea, vomiting, diarrhea, jaw pain, fatigue, dizziness, dyspnea, flushing, palpitations, peripheral edema **Subcutaneous** Infusion site pain, reaction, abscess, headache, flushing, nausea, vomiting, diarrhea, jaw pain, rash, dizziness **Inhaled** Hypotension, cough, throat irritation, headache, nausea, diarrhea, flushing, dizziness, increased risk of bleeding **Oral** Headache, flushing, nausea, vomiting, diarrhea, jaw pain, extremity pain	**IV** This medicine may cause dizziness. Caution patient to stand up slowly when getting out of bed or rising from a sitting position, manage side effects. **Subcutaneous** Site pain management: use ice or warmth as needed, topical anesthetic agents, vasoconstrictive agents, corticosteroid creams or sprays, oral H1 and H2 blockers, nonopioid analgesics, GABA analogs, antidepressants, opioids for severe pain. Subcutaneous site pain typically occurs during the first 2–5 days after starting a new infusion site. Pain will subside and should be monitored for up to 6 or more weeks. A site change is indicated when the site begins to become irritated or infected. Seek consultation from specialty pharmacy or provider for site pain management. **Inhaled** Maintain normal breathing pattern with treatment; do not hold breath once medication is inhaled; use the pause button between breaths if needed; swish and spit after treatment; use cough medication, warm or cold drinks to sooth throat; improves exercise ability; use only with Tyvaso inhalation system.

(continued)

TABLE 7.6 VASCULAR-TARGETED PHARMACOTHERAPIES FOR PULMONARY ARTERIAL HYPERTENSION (continued)

MEDICATION, CLASS, MECHANISM OF ACTION	INDICATIONS	DOSAGE	COMMON SIDE EFFECTS	KEY SAFETY/ PATIENT EDUCATION INFORMATION
Oral Treprostinil (Orenitram) Cardiovascular agent, Prostacyclin Potent vasodilator, inhibitor of platelet aggregation, inhibition of smooth muscle proliferation		Reduce to 1 or 2 breaths if 3 breaths not tolerated and subsequently increase to 3 breath. Maintenance: titrate by additional 3 breaths via PO inhalation at approximately 1–2-week intervals as tolerated, to a target dose of 9 breaths (54 mcg) per treatment session, QID during waking hours (approximately 4 hours apart). **Oral** Initial: 0.25 mg PO BID *or* 0.125 mg TID with food. Maintenance: titrate by 0.25 mg or 0.5 mg BID OR 0.125 mg TID q3–4d to achieve optimal response; maximum dose determined by tolerability; if not tolerated, consider slower titration or decrease dose in increments of 0.25 mg		If adverse effects preclude titration to target dose, continue treatment at the highest tolerated dose; maximum dose of 9 breaths per treatment session, QID (FDA dosage). **Oral** Should be taken with food; should be swallowed whole; must not be crushed, chewed, or split. Contact your provider if you miss two or more doses. Do not abruptly discontinue.
Ventavis Inhalation solution (Ioprost) Cardiovascular agent, Prostacyclin Synthetic analog of prostacyclin PGI(2) that dilates systemic and pulmonary arteries	WHO group I PAH	Initial: 2.5 mcg inhaled using a specially designed adaptive aerosol delivery device: if tolerated, increase dose to 5 mcg inhaled 6–9 times per day (no more than q2h) during waking hours; maximum daily dose 45 mcg (5 mcg, 9 times per day)	Cough, throat irritation, flushing, jaw pain, headache, hypotension, body aches, nausea, diarrhea, dizziness, pulmonary edema	Maintain normal breathing pattern with treatment; do not hold breath once medication is inhaled; use the pause button between breaths if needed; swish and spit after treatment; use cough medication, warm or cold drinks to sooth the throat. Patient should watch for and report signs/ symptoms of hypotension with initial dosing and dose changes. Stand up slowly when getting out of bed or rising from a sitting position.
Selexipag (Uptravi) Cardiovascular agent, Prostacyclin IP receptor agonist Selexipag is an oral prostacyclin receptor (IP) agonist, structurally distinct from prostacyclin.	WHO group I PAH WHO group IV CTEPH	Initial: 200 mcg PO BID; increase to the highest tolerated dose in 200-mcg BID increments at weekly intervals, up to 16,000 mcg BID. If dose is not tolerated, reduce to the previously tolerated dose	Headache, nausea, vomiting, diarrhea, jaw pain, myalgia, flushing, pain in extremities	Advise patient to report symptoms of pulmonary edema. Instruct patient to take a missed dose as soon as possible, but if next dose is in less than 6 hours, skip the missed dose. Instruct patient to contact healthcare professional for instructions if treatment for 3 days or more is missed.

(continued)

TABLE 7.6 VASCULAR-TARGETED PHARMACOTHERAPIES FOR PULMONARY ARTERIAL HYPERTENSION (continued)

MEDICATION, CLASS, MECHANISM OF ACTION	INDICATIONS	DOSAGE	COMMON SIDE EFFECTS	KEY SAFETY/ PATIENT EDUCATION INFORMATION
Revatio (Sildenafil, Tadalafil) Cardiovascular agent, nitric oxide pathway, PDE-5-inhibitor Vasodilation of the pulmonary vascular bed	WHO group I PAH	Sildenafil 20 mg q8h Tadalafil 20 mg BID or 40 mg daily	Hypotension, epistaxis, seizures, headache, dyspepsia, flushing, dyspnea, vision, and hearing loss	Do not use with nitrates or Viagra.
Riociguat (Adempas) Guanylate cyclase stimulator Nitric oxide pathway	WHO group I WHO group IV CTEPH	**Oral** Initial: 1 mg TID; may initiate dose at 0.5 mg TID in patients who may not tolerate the hypotensive effects. If systolic blood pressure remains >95 mmHg and the patient has no signs or symptoms of hypotension, increase the dose by 0.5 mg TID at intervals of ≥2 weeks to the highest tolerated dosage. Maximum dose: 2.5 mg TID	Teratogenicity, hypotension, palpitations, peripheral edema, headache, dizziness, dyspepsia, nausea, diarrhea, anemia, epistaxis	Monitor blood pressure for signs and symptoms of hypotension, significant peripheral edema. Females of childbearing potential must have a negative pregnancy test prior to the initiation of therapy, monthly during treatment, and 1 month after discontinuation of therapy. Monitor for signs/symptoms of hypotension, bleeding, and pulmonary edema. Screen for smoking. Dose adjustment may be required with smoking or smoking cessation. Advise patient that if a dose is missed, take the next regularly scheduled dose. If treatment is interrupted for ≥3 days, retitration is required.
Bosentan (Tracleer), **ambrisentan** (Letairis), **macitentan** (Opsumit) Endothelin receptor antagonist, endothelin pathway Potent vasoconstrictor	WHO group 1 PAH idiopathic, associated with connective tissue disease, and Eisenmenger's syndrome	Bosentan 62.5 mg BID, increase to 125 mg BID. Ambrisentan 5 or 10 mg once daily Macitentan 10 mg once daily	Teratogenicity, headache, flushing, severe fluid retention, liver toxicity, anemia	Patient may experience headache, flushing, cough, or rhinorrhea. Have patient report immediately to prescriber signs of liver problems (dark urine, fatigue, lack of appetite, nausea, abdominal pain, light-colored stools, vomiting, or jaundice), difficulty breathing, edema, weight gain, or severe loss of strength and energy.
Amlodipine, nifedipine, diltiazem Calcium channel blockers Use only in documented AVR Potent vasodilator	Idiopathic PAH WHO group I with AVR; (Medarov & Judson, 2015)	Titrate up to high doses as tolerated	Hypotension, headache, nausea, edema, negative inotropy	Has vasodilatory effects on blood vessels of the heart, lungs, fingers—Raynaud's phenomenon.

AVR, acute vasoreactive response; CTEPH, chronic thromboembolic pulmonary hypertension; FDA, Food and Drug Administration; GABA, gamma-aminobutyric acid; GI, gastrointestinal; IP, I-prostanoid; IV, intravenous; PAH, pulmonary arterial hypertension; PDE-5 inhibitor, phosphodiesterase-5 inhibitor; PGI$_2$, prostacyclin; PH, pulmonary hypertension; WHO, World Health Organization.

Source: From Klinger, J., Elliott, G., Levine, D. J., Bossone, E., Duvall, L., Fagan, K., Frantsve-Hawley, J., Kawut, S. M., Ryan, J. J., Rosenzweig, E. B., Sederstrom, N., Steen, V. D., & Badesch, D. B. (2019). Therapy for pulmonary arterial hypertension in adults. *Chest, 155*(3), 565–586.

determine the need for endotracheal intubation and mechanical ventilation must be performed rapidly (Table 7.7; Burns & Delgado, 2018; Hess et al., 2016; Morton & Fontaine, 2018).

MECHANICAL VENTILATION

Indications
- Apnea
- Severe oxygenation deficit
- Acute or impending ventilatory failure

Goals of Mechanical Ventilation
- Reverse of hypoxemia (oxygenation).
- Reverse of respiratory acidosis (ventilation).
- Decrease work of breathing (resting the muscles of respiration).

Mechanical ventilation is needed when respiratory failure cannot be corrected by noninvasive treatment options.

Positive Pressure Ventilation
Positive pressure ventilation is categorized as either volume mode or pressure mode (Table 7.8):
- **Volume:** TV and MV are guaranteed with each breath:
  - TV delivered is set for each breath regardless of airway resistance or lung compliance.
  - Peak pressure is variable with each breath.
  - **Respiratory muscle rest:** Must increase respiratory rate (RR) until spontaneous respirations cease.
  - Consistent pattern of gas flow delivery.
- **Pressure:** Pressure level is guaranteed with each breath.
  - Pressure level delivered for each breath is set.
  - Amount of TV delivered is variable dependent upon the set pressure level, lung compliance, and airway resistance. TV delivered must be monitored.
  - **Respiratory muscle rest:** Pressure support is increased until RR rate is ≤20/min and TV of 6 to 10 mL/kg of predicted body weight (PBW) is achieved (Burns & Delgado, 2018; Hess et al., 2016).
  - Decelerating pattern of gas flow delivery (better gas distribution).

Modes of Ventilation
Positive pressure modes of ventilation are described in Table 7.9.

Additional Mechanical Ventilation Terms
Tube compensation: Ventilator support to compensate for airway resistance due to endotracheal tube (ET) diameter.

TABLE 7.7 ACUTE RESPIRATORY FAILURE MANAGEMENT

MANAGEMENT GOAL	INTERVENTION
Airway: Establish and maintain	Endotracheal intubation - Patent airway - Remove secretions - Prevent aspiration
Oxygenation	Delivery of increased FiO_2 via mechanical ventilation to correct hypoxemia
Correct acid–base imbalance	Improve alveolar ventilation in hypercapneic acidosis

Source: From Morton, P. G., & Fontaine, D. K. (2018). *Critical care nursing: A holistic approach* (11th ed.). Lippincott Williams & Wilkins.

Trigger Sensitivity
- Determines the amount of effort required for the patient to trigger the ventilator to deliver a breath; sensitivity must be high enough for minimal patient effort to trigger breaths while avoiding patient–ventilator dyssynchrony.
- Triggering may be flow triggered or pressure triggered. Flow triggering is generally more sensitive.

Auto-PEEP: happens when exhalation of a ventilator breath is not complete before the next delivered breath. This results in air trapping and a buildup of pressure. Risk for auto-PEEP is associated with higher respiratory rates and prolonged expiratory times associated with COPD and asthma. This buildup of pressure may cause hemodynamic instability, barotrauma, and volutrauma. Auto-PEEP cannot be observed on the ventilator airway pressure display at end expiration and thus may be difficult to diagnose.

Management of the Patient on Mechanical Ventilation

To Improve Oxygenation
- Increase FIO_2.
- Increase mean alveolar pressure.
  - Increase PEEP.
  - Increase I:E ratio.
- Reopen alveoli.
  - Increase PEEP.

To Improve CO_2 Elimination
- Increase respiratory rate.
- Increase TV.

Complications Related to Mechanical Ventilation
- **Decreased cardiac output:** Increased mean airway pressure impedes venous return to the heart.
- **Barotrauma:** Alveolar rupture due to excessive airway pressure or overdistention of alveoli; may cause subcutaneous emphysema and pneumothorax.
- **Volutrauma:** Damage to alveoli from large volume ventilation causing alveolar fracture and flooding.
- Auto-PEEP and air trapping.
- **Oxygen toxicity**—Attempt to reach an FIO_2 of ≤ 60% within the first 24 hours of mechanical ventilation.
- **Atelectasis, mucus plugging**—See Airway Obstructive Atelectasis.
- **Tracheal edema, lesions**—ETT maintenance includes monitor cuff pressure (20–30 cm H_2O) and oral and endotracheal suctioning as indicated; verify position and document the centimeter mark at teeth; rotate regularly; secure in place.
- **VAP**—See Pulmonary Infections.
- **Upper GI bleed**—Provide prophylaxis for increased risk of stress ulcer (Burns & Delgado, 2018; Morton & Fontaine, 2018).

Weaning Fom Short-Term Mechanical Ventilation
- **Short-term ventilation:** Equals <72 hours on the ventilator.
- Underlying cause of respiratory failure is resolved.
- Decreasing level of ventilatory support is needed.
- Pressure support 5 cm/H_2O above PEEP indicates reduced patient dependence.

Assessment of Readiness to Wean
Weaning Parameters
- FiO_2 ≤0.50, MV ≤ 10 L/min, PEEP ≤ 5 cm H_2O
- Negative inspiratory pressure (NIP) at least 20 cm H_2O

TABLE 7.8 VENTILATORY PARAMETERS

PARAMETER	DEFINITION	DETAILS
TV	Volume of air delivered to the patient with each breath	Calculated based on predicted body weight
Rate	Number of breaths per minute	Set rate: minimum ventilator breaths per minute Total rate: set rate plus patient breaths
Minute ventilation	Tidal volume times respiratory rate (TV × RR)	Minute ventilation has an inverse relationship to $PaCO_2$
FiO_2	Concentration of inhaled oxygen	Use the lowest FiO_2 to achieve targeted oxygenation Prolonged FiO_2 >0.60 may cause oxygen toxicity
PIP	Pressure required to deliver prescribed tidal volume. Highest level of pressure during inhalation.	Target PIP is <35 cm H_2O High PIP may cause lung injury
Plateau pressure	Measure of end-inspiratory distending pressure Plateau pressure is estimated using an end-inspiratory hold maneuver	Plateau pressure is predictive of lung injury (overdistention of alveoli) Plateau pressure should be <28 cm H_2O
PEEP	Pressure remaining in the lungs after resting exhalation The residual volume to splint open the alveoli	Maintains alveolar recruitment Higher levels of PEEP may decrease venous return to the heart thereby decreasing cardiac output
Inspiratory time	Time to deliver TV	There is an inspiratory time point at which the expiratory time becomes too short resulting in air trapping and Auto-PEEP
I:E ratio	Inspiratory time to expiratory time ratio (normal ratio is 1:2)	Inverse ratio: Longer inspiratory time improves oxygenation by increasing the mean airway pressure over the entire respiratory cycle; more even gas distribution Risk of gas trapping, intrinsic PEEP and barotrauma as a result of shorter expiratory time Less well tolerated by the patient; requires deeper sedation

FiO_2, fraction of inspired oxygen; PEEP, positive end-expiratory pressure; PIP, peak inspiratory pressure; RR, respiratory rate; TV, tidal volume.

- Spontaneous TV ≥5 mL/kg
- VC ≥10 mL/kg
- RR <30 breaths/min
- Rapid-shallow breathing index (RSBI) <105 breaths/min/L
Recommended bundled approach to weaning: ABCDEF bundle (Table 7.10)

Weaning Methods for Short-Term Mechanical Ventilation

- T-piece
- CPAP
- Pressure support (Burns & Delgado, 2018; Hess et al., 2016)

CHRONIC RESPIRATORY FAILURE

Chronic respiratory failure is characterized by a combination of chronic hypoxemia, hypercapnea, and compensatory metabolic alkalosis (elevated bicarbonate levels with normalized pH). Patients with chronic respiratory failure can experience worsening symptoms, resulting in acute or chronic respiratory failure requiring mechanical ventilation.

Weaning From Long-Term Mechanical Ventilation

Long-term mechanical ventilation: >3 days on the ventilator. Patients on long-term mechanical ventilation suffer from many conditions that interfere with weaning in addition to the condition that originally led to respiratory failure. They are also often in a malnourished and deconditioned state. This physiologic complexity requires a comprehensive approach to evaluation of weaning readiness. The Burns' Wean Assessment Program (BWAP; Burns & Delgado, 2018) is an excellent example of a tool used to identify and resolve impediments to weaning using a systematic approach: www.academia.edu/25771748/The_Relationship_of_26_Clinical_Factors_to_Weaning_Outcome.

General Guidelines for Weaning Long-Term Mechanically Ventilated Patients

- *Endurance conditioning principles:* Gradual increases in respiratory muscle work
- *Pressure support ventilation:* Allows the gradual decrease of pressure support (PS) over time
- Ensure adequate respiratory muscle rest between breathing trials

Extubation Procedure

- Identify the postextubation oxygen delivery plan: High-flow nasal cannula, mask, noninvasive ventilation, oral suction, and other supports as needed.
- Perform baseline cardiac and pulmonary assessment to evaluate patient response post extubation.

TABLE 7.9 COMMONLY USED MODES OF VENTILATION

VENTILATION MODE	PARAMETERS OF THE MODE	CLINICAL USE
VOLUME-CONTROL MODES		
CMV	Set volume, rate, PEEP.	Maximum support; for heavily sedated or paralyzedpatients unable to initiate spontaneous breaths
A/C	Set volume, rate, PEEP. Sensitivity is set: when patient initiates a breath, a full volume breath is delivered.	Maximum support; initial mode used for many patient situations
SIMV (with pressure support)	Set volume, rate, PEEP, and pressure support. Patients can breathe spontaneously at their own rate and depth; mandatory breaths are delivered at the prescribed rate and volume and are synchronized with patient breaths. Spontaneous breaths are pressure supported above the PEEP (not volume supported).	SIMV requires more patient WOB and carries the potential for respiratory muscle fatigue. Not normally used as an initial ventilator mode. Least efficient mode for ventilator weaning May be used for patients who breathe too rapidly on A/C.
Mandatory minute ventilation (automode) Switches between control mode and spontaneous mode based on the patient's breathing efforts	Set PEEP, tidal volume, rate, pressure support. Set minimum minute ventilation. Patient breathes spontaneously. Spontaneous breaths will be pressure supported above the PEEP (not volume supported). If minute ventilation requirement is not met, the machine will cycle a breath to provide the minute ventilation deficit. Patient spontaneous rate is irrelevant as long as minute ventilation is met.	Potential option for Cheyne-Stokes respiration, operating room setting, or postanesthesia patients
PRESSURE-CONTROL MODES		
CPAP	Set FiO$_2$, PEEP, pressure support. (No set rate or tidal volume.) Patient breathes spontaneously with continuous monitoring of exhaled volumes and other parameters all within a closed circuit.	Weaning mode; used to evaluate patient potential for extubation
PC	Set rate, FiO$_2$, PEEP, and pressure. Pressure is set; tidal volume varies with each breath.	Potential use in restrictive disease (ARDS, ILD, pulmonary fibrosis); reduced risk of barotrauma
APRV Bilevel (Puritan Bennett) Bi-vent (Siemens)	Set FiO$_2$, inspiratory pressure and time, expiratory pressure and time (No set rate, tidal volume). Provides high level of CPAP used for lung recruitment with a brief expiratory release period. Patient breathes spontaneously.	Used most commonly for ARDS. Allows patient spontaneous breathing, which reduces need for heavy sedation or chemical paralysis Increases mean airway pressure for lung recruitment.
DUAL-CONTROL MODES		
PRVC	Can switch between PC and VC during the respiratory cycle. Can deliver a set volume while regulating the pressure with each breath. Adjusts to compliance and resistance of the lungs. Minimum respiratory rate, target volume, and upper pressure limit are set. Patient can breathe above the set rate.	Used as an initial ventilation mode. Lung protective mode with targeted volume and regulated pressure.

A/C, assist control; APRV, airway pressure-release ventilation; ARDS, acute respiratory distress syndrome; CMV, controlled mandatory ventilation; CPAP, continuous positive airway pressure; ILD, interstitial lung disease; PC, pressure control; PEEP, positive end-expiratory pressure; PRVC, pressure-regulated volume control; SIMV, synchronized intermittent mandatory ventilation; VC; WOB, work of breathing.

TABLE 7.10 ABCDEF BUNDLE

BUNDLE ELEMENT	KEY POINTS
A Assess, prevent, and manage pain	Assess pain using valid tool. Treat pain first, then sedate.
B Both spontaneous awakening and spontaneous breathing trials	Coordinate timing of awakening and breathing trials.
C Choice of analgesia and sedation	Use a valid sedation/agitation scale. Titrate medication to light level of sedation. Interrupt sedation daily; restart at half dose.
D Delirium: assess, prevent, and manage	Monitor for delirium (CAM-ICU). Reduce unnecessary deliriogenic drugs. Promote sleep enhancement.
E Early mobility	Assess activity tolerance. Gradually increase activity.
F Family engagement/empowerment	Support family presence in the ICU.

CAM-ICU, Confusion Assessment Method for the ICU.

Source: From Balas, M. C., Pun, B. T., Pasero, C., Engel, H. J., Perme, C., Esbrook, C. L., … Stollings, J. L. (2019). Common challenges to effective ABCDEF bundle implementation: The ICU liberation campaign experience. *Critical Care Nurse, 1*(39), 46–60.

- Elevate HOB and suction airway if indicated. Hyperoxygenate prior to removal of ET.
- Completely deflate ET cuff and remove the airway. Apply oxygen immediately.
- Monitor patient response following extubation. Assess pulmonary status, oxygenation, and airway clearance ability. Assess for complications such as aspiration, bronchospasm, tracheal damage, or stridor. Treatment for stridor: 2.5% racemic epinephrine via aerosol.
- Consider aspiration risk. Identify plan for safe swallow assessment or evaluation as needed (Koser, 2017).

ACUTE RESPIRATORY DISTRESS SYNDROME

ARDS is characterized by noncardiac pulmonary edema caused by excessive alveolar–capillary membrane permeability. Interstitial and alveolar edema leads to V/Q mismatch, severe hypoxemia, and decreased lung compliance. The recent Berlin definition of ARDS is as follows: "The presence within 7 days of a known clinical insult or new or worsening respiratory symptoms of a combination of acute hypoxemia (PaO_2/FiO_2 ≤300 mmHg) in a ventilated patient." The Berlin definition further categorizes ARDS as mild, moderate, or severe as follows:

- Mild ARDS—(200 < P/F ratio [ratio of arterial oxygen partial pressure to fractional inspired oxygen] ≤300)
- Moderate ARDS—(100 < P/F ratio ≤200)
- Severe ARDS—(P/F ratio ≤100)

Etiology

- Primary causes are as follows:
  - Aspiration, pneumonia, smoke inhalation, pulmonary contusion, near drowning
- Secondary causes are as follows:
  - Trauma, sepsis, pancreatitis, fat emboli, disseminated intravascular coagulation (DIC), hypovolemic shock, massive transfusion

Diagnostic Tests

- CXR—Uniform bilateral airspace opacification (white out) without evidence of cardiomegaly
- PaO_2/FiO_2 ratio ≤ 300
- Static compliance < 40 mL/cm H_2O (TV/plateau pressure —PEEP)

Interventions

Treatment involves supportive care and preventing complications (Morton & Fontaine, 2018; Papazian et al., 2019).

Mechanical Ventilation

The goals of mechanical ventilation are to improve oxygenation/gas exchange via alveolar recruitment while preserving lung function.

- Plateau pressure < 30 cm H_2O
- PEEP > 5 cm H_2O
- High PEEP indicated: P/F ratio < 200
- Tidal volume: 6 mL/kg of PBW to keep plateau pressures ≤30 cm H_2O
- Pronation therapy applied >16 hr/d: P/F ratio < 150
- Neuromuscular blockade: P/F ratio < 150
- ECMO: P/F ratio < 80

Ventilator-Induced Lung Injury

Ventilator-induced lung injury (VILI) is lung injury affecting the airways and parenchyma that is caused by or worsened by mechanical ventilation. Inappropriate use of mechanical ventilation can lead to multisystem organ failure and lung injury similar to ARDS. Lung protective ventilation strategies have been shown to decrease the incidence of VILI.

Lung-Protective Strategies

Lung-protective strategies employ lower, more physiologic TVs, avoidance of high plateau pressures and appropriate levels of PEEP (Table 7.11; Fan et al., 2017; Papazian et al., 2019).

VENTILATOR-ASSOCIATED EVENTS: PREVENTION

OVERVIEW

VAE are associated with prolonged mechanical ventilation, longer ICU stays, and increased mortality. Complications associated with mechanical ventilation include VAP, sepsis, ARDS, PE, barotrauma, and pulmonary edema. Evidence-based interventions have been developed to improve the care of mechanically ventilated patients and reduce the risk of these serious complications.

TABLE 7.11 LUNG-PROTECTIVE VENTILATION STRATEGIES

VENTILATOR PARAMETER	RATIONALE
TV limits 4–8 mL/kg PBW	Reduces lung strain
Plateau pressure < 28 cm H_2O	Plateau pressure determines level of overdistention of alveoli
PEEP adjustment is based on patient pathophysiology and respiratory mechanics	Prevents de-recruitment and reduces volutrauma
Driving pressure <15 cm H_2O	Driving pressure = Plateau pressure – PEEP High driving pressures are associated with higher mortality
FiO$_2$ to maintain: PaO$_2$ between 55 and 80 mmHg SpO$_2$ between 88% and 95% mmHg	Maintain oxygen delivery to prevent tissue hypoxia

PBW, predicted body weight; PEEP, positive end-expiratory pressure; TV, tidal volume.

VAE prevention interventions include the following:

- HOB elevated at least 30° unless contraindicated
- Oral hygiene, subglottal suctioning
- Early mobility
- Subglottal suctioning prior to ETT repositioning
- Reposition ETT to prevent device-related pressure injuries
- Assess, prevent, and manage delirium:
  See www.icudelirium.org/medical-professionals/delirium-assess-prevent-and-manage
- Reduce long-term consequences of critical illness: ICU Liberation Bundle—www.sccm.org/ICULiberation/ABCDEF-Bundles
- Deep vein thrombosis and peptic ulcer prophylaxis are not considered evidence-based interventions yet remain a part of VAE prevention measures in some facilities.

Management Strategies to Prevent Complications of Mechanical Ventilation

- ETT cuff pressure should be maintained at 25 cm H_2O.
- Suctioning is performed *according to patient need* using sterile technique.
- Ensure the ventilator circuit is maintained as a closed system.
- Monitor vital signs: blood pressure, mean arterial pressure, heart rate and rhythm, respiratory rate, saturations, EtCO$_2$.
- Monitor ventilator settings and ventilator synchrony in collaboration with the interprofessional team.
- Start postpyloric feedings as soon as the patient is hemodynamically stable.
- If gastric decompression is necessary, consider oral-gastric tube placement to decrease the incidence of sinusitis.
- Maintain IV access through the least invasive technique.
- Deescalate indwelling urinary catheters as soon as hemodynamically stable. Consider exdwelling devices for accurate intake and output.
- If neuromuscular blockade is indicated (ventilator synchrony or to decrease oxygen demand), the patient must have sedation and pain adjuncts *prior* to paralysis (Morton & Fontaine, 2018; Weigand, 2017).

NONINVASIVE VENTILATION

OVERVIEW

Noninvasive ventilation (NIV) is the delivery of positive pressure ventilation via the upper respiratory tract, without the use of an invasive artificial airway, to stent open the alveoli and provide improved oxygenation. The purpose is to reduce alveolar dead space and maximize gas exchange while avoiding the serious risks associated with intubation.

Indications

The goal of therapy is to provide symptom relief for breathlessness that is associated with hypoventilation, COPD exacerbation, acute pulmonary edema, asthma exacerbation, respiratory failure, and postextubation management.

Contraindications

The following represents exclusionary factors related to high risk for complication or conditions requiring emergent intubation:

- Cardiopulmonary arrest
- Hemodynamic instability
- Unable to maintain airway and clear secretions
- Impaired consciousness: Glasgow Coma Scale (GCS) less than 8
- Facial trauma, surgery, burns, or deformity
- High aspiration risk
- Prolonged mechanical ventilation projected secondary to severity of illness or trauma
- Esophageal anastomosis

Nursing Considerations for Noninvasive Ventilation

Nurses should maintain heightened awareness of the following:

- Pressure injury risk is related to the nasal–oral face mask. Pressure ulcer preventions devices should be used with the masks at high-risk areas such as the nasal bridge and the chin. Interventions also may include alternating the type of NIV mask using a full face mask or nasal prongs as the patient tolerates.
- NVHAP is the number one hospital-acquired infection. The oral cavity harbors bacteria. Bacteria replication occurs every 4 to 6 hours in the absence of oral hygiene. Evidence-based prevention measures include brushing and moisturizing of the teeth, gums, and tongue.
- Collaborate with respiratory therapy to coordinate the timing of oral care, nebulization therapy, and pressure reduction techniques. Limit the time off NIV to reduce feeling of breathlessness.
- Positive pressure ventilation may insufflate the GI tract. Careful assessment and pharmacologic interventions to prevent nausea and emesis must be in place to avoid aspiration.
- LOC must be closely monitored. The patient should be free to remove the face mask in the event of emesis. Restraints may pose a safety risk to patients with elevated CO$_2$ levels as movement and manual hand dexterity may be impaired and limit the ability to remove the face mask in case of vomiting (Table 7.12).

TABLE 7.12 MODES OF NONINVASIVE VENTILATION

MODE OF NIV	INDICATION	THERAPY SETTINGS	SAFETY CONSIDERATION	PATIENT CONSIDERATIONS
CPAP	Sleep-related breathing disorders, cardiogenic pulmonary edema, obesity-related hypoventilation	FiO_2 to keep saturations > 92% Start at 4 cm H_2O and titrate by 2 cm H_2O until goal obtained Adjust pressure as needed to ensure snoring is not present	Monitor blood pressure Monitor skin breakdown over bony prominences Watch for decreased cardiac output Watch for signs of pneumothorax	■ Local skin damage ■ Eye irritation ■ Gastric distention ■ Mask requires a snug fit and may not be appropriate for all patients ■ Maintain saturations; saturations greater than 92% on the lowest FiO_2 is preferred ■ Small air leak is permissible ■ Keep HOB >30° ■ Allow 20–30 minutes of therapy and recheck ABG
Bi-PAP	COPD, Sleep apnea, cardiogenic pulmonary edema, and hypoventilation	Inspiratory positive pressure 8 cm H_2O and titrate to achieve an exhaled tidal volume of 5–7 mL/kg and respiratory rate less than 30 Expiratory positive airway 1–2 cm H_2O maximum of 8 cm H_2O Backup rate FiO_2 as ordered to achieve saturations >92%	Monitor blood pressure Monitor for skin breakdown on bony prominences Watch for decreased cardiac output Watch for signs of pneumothorax	■ Local skin damage ■ Eye irritation ■ Gastric distention ■ Mask requires a snug fit and may not be appropriate for all patients ■ Maintain saturations; saturations greater than 92% on the lowest FiO_2 is preferred ■ Small air leak is permissible ■ Keep HOB >30° ■ Allow 20–30 minutes of therapy and recheck ABG

ABG, arterial blood gas; Bi-PAP, bilevel positive airway pressure; COPD, congestive obstructive pulmonary disease; CPAP, continuous positive airway pressure; HOB; NIV, noninvasive ventilation.

Management

■ Successful NIV is associated with patients who are or have younger age, lower illness acuity, more cooperative, moderate hypercarbia $PaCO_2$ >45, moderate acidemia pH < 7.20–7.35, and intact dentation (less air leaks).
■ Initiate NIV as soon as indicated. Patients who fail NIV intervention after 0.5 to 2 hours of therapy should be intubated in a controlled setting if resuscitation status indicates so (Burns & Delgado, Hyzy & McSparron, 2019).

MANAGEMENT OF THE PATIENT WITH AN ARTIFICIAL AIRWAY

OVERVIEW

The ETT is the standard of care and most common advanced airway. In the prehospital, ED, and ICU settings, endotracheal intubation is the most effective way to control the airway and prevent aspiration of gastric contents (Edwards, 2005; High, 2006).

Indications for endotracheal intubation include the following:

■ Apnea ■ Upper airway obstruction ■ Altered LOC (airway protection) ■ Increased ICP	■ Respiratory insufficiency ■ Impending airway compromise (e.g., facial burns) ■ Shock, hemodynamic instability

ICP, intracranial pressure; LOC, level of consciousness.

Rapid Sequence Intubation

Rapid sequence intubation (RSI) is considered the standard of care to achieve endotracheal intubation. RSI is a seven-step process to achieve intubation in a timely and controlled fashion.

■ Preparation
■ Preoxygenation
■ Pretreatment
■ Paralysis
■ Placement
■ Placement verification
■ Post intubation management

Medications associated with RSI include but are not limited to the following:

■ Sedatives (midazolam)
■ Analgesia (fentanyl)
■ Protective agent (lidocaine)
■ Anesthesia (etomidate, ketamine, propofol)
■ Paralytics (rocuronium, vecuronium)

Some facilities may use succinylcholine; however, with heightened awareness of malignant hyperthermia, some facilities have chosen to move away from the use of succinylcholine.

■ Appropriate ETT size:
  ● Adult female = 7.0 mm
  ● Adult male = 8.0 mm
  ● One size larger and smaller should be available prior to intubation.
■ Intubation should be performed in an emergent situation by the most skilled practitioner.
■ Video laryngoscopy may be used to verify that the ETT has passed successfully through the vocal cords.

- Use a commercial tube holder to secure ETT. Device-related pressure ulcer prevention initiatives should be instituted as soon as feasible.
- Documentation of success should include primary and secondary confirmation.
  - *Primary confirmation*—Visualization of the ETT passing through the vocal cords (video laryngoscopy is helpful), equal bilateral breath sounds, rise and fall of the chest, absence of gastric insufflation, misting of the ETT, improved skin color.
  - *Secondary confirmation*—End-tidal CO_2 colorimetric; $EtCO_2$ capnography (preferred); confirmation of rising oxygen saturation.
  - Postintubation chest x-ray to ensure the ETT is 2 to 3 cm above the carina.
- Postintubation management intervention should include sedation, pain management, $EtCO_2$ monitoring, and ventilator compliance (Edwards, 2005; High, 2006; Mechlin & Hurford, 2014).

END-TIDAL CO_2 MONITORING

End-tidal CO_2 ($PetCO_2$) is a continuous noninvasive measurement of exhaled carbon dioxide that is indicative of ventilation status. $PetCO_2$ can be trended to evaluate the $PaCO_2$ as the relationship between the two values is close under normal V/Q conditions. $PetCO_2$ waveform depiction during each respiratory cycle and the corresponding digital display of $PetCO_2$ concentration is called capnography.

Clinical uses of $PetCO_2$ include the following:

- ETT placement after intubation
- Gastric or small bowel tube placement
- Pulmonary blood flow
- Alveolar ventilation
- Monitoring of CPR quality
- Monitoring of patient response to ventilator changes and weaning

The $PetCO_2$ sensor can be placed directly onto a mechanical ventilator circuit or via a special nasal cannula for nonintubated patients. Nonintubated uses of $PetCO_2$ include monitoring patients with OSA, COPD, and asthma and patients receiving opioids or other central nervous system–depressant medications (St. John & Seckel, 2019).

MULTIMODAL OXYGEN THERAPY

Patients with increased metabolic, respiratory, and/or cardiac requirements need oxygen administration. Oxygen administration can occur in any inpatient or outpatient setting. Individual requirements determine the mode of therapy to utilize. Oxygen administration should be titrated to the lowest possible setting to restore blood oxygen levels and relieve symptoms of breathlessness. Oxygen administration reduces ventilator effort, decreases myocardial workload, and increases the oxygen-carrying capacity at the cellular level. Table 7.13 can be used to determine the best intervention for each patient (Ashraf-Kashani & Kumar, 2017; Taylor, 2015).

MANAGEMENT OF THE PATIENT WITH CHEST TUBES

OVERVIEW

Chest tubes are under water sealed drains inserted into the pleural space used to drain air, blood, or fluid, and to restore negative pressure.

Indications

- Drain air, blood, or fluid from the pleural space.
- Occurs with pleural effusion, pneumothorax, hemothorax, chylothorax, thoracostomy.

Chest Tube Placement

- *Air removal*—Second intercostal space, mid-clavicular line
- *Fluid/blood removal*—Fifth or sixth intercostal space, mid-axillary line
- *Thoracostomy*—Mediastinum below xyphoid process, postoperative drainage

Chest Drainage Systems

Chest tubes are placed to a closed drainage system immediately following insertion. Chest drainage systems use gravity or negative suction pressure to drain fluids and restore negative pressure in the pleural space. Closed drainage systems contain a water seal that acts as a one-way valve to prevent atmospheric air from entering the pleural space. Chest drainage systems may be water suction systems or dry suction systems.

- *Wet suction control systems*—The amount of suction pressure is regulated by the height of the column of water in the suction control chamber, not the level of vacuum set on regulator.
- *Dry suction control systems*—The amount of suction pressure is regulated mechanically.

Management of Chest Tubes and Chest Drainage System

- All tubing connections must be secure and air tight.
- Check tube patency—Avoid kinking or dependent loops of tubing.
- Check for clot formation in tubing—gently squeeze tubing to move clots toward the drainage unit.
- Keep drainage system below chest level.
- Monitor drainage amount and type.
- Maintain water levels in suction and water-seal chambers.
- *Tidaling* refers to fluctuations in the water-seal chamber with respirations (when not attached to external suction) are a normal finding.
  - Absence of tidaling indicates the following:
    - Tubing kinked or clamped
    - Complete lung reexpansion
    - Mediastinal tubes—There is no tidaling with tubes in the mediastinal space
- Intermittent bubbling in water-seal chamber—air leak from pleural space
- Continuous bubbling in water-seal chamber—air leak in the system

Patient Assessment and Management

- Focused pulmonary assessment and monitoring.
- Assess for subcutaneous air around chest tube site.
- Assess occlusive chest tube dressing.
- Assess volume and nature of drainage; be aware of the expected volume given the clinical condition; postoperative drainage type should move from sanguineous to serosanguineous to serous.
- Analgesia for comfort and to facilitate deep breathing and mobility.
- Frequent position changes, coughing, deep breathing help reexpand the lung and promote fluid drainage (Burns & Delgado, 2018; Waters, 2017).

TABLE 7.13 MODES OF THERAPY

MODE OF NIV	RANGE	ADVANTAGES	DISADVANTAGES	ADMINISTRATION GUIDELINES
Nasal cannula	0.5–6 L/min	Safe Simple to deliver Adapts to all facial structures Good for low oxygen concentrations Portable Allows for ADL Lower cost	Cannot deliver >40% Nasal obstruction Caused dry mucous membranes in high flow	■ Titrate to lowest oxygen level required to keep SpO_2 >92%. Chronic COPD SpO_2 may be >88%. ■ Do not place straps and tubing tightly around ears or chin. Device-related pressure injury may occur. ■ Flow at greater than 4 L/min should have humidification. ■ Consider alternative therapy for mouth breathers.
Simple mask	35%–50% FiO_2	Higher concentration of oxygen Delivers more consistently for mouth breathers or post sedation	May create a sense of claustrophobia Tight seal may irritate eyes Unable to complete ADL Not for long-term therapy	■ Select mask size to fit over nose, mouth, and chin; then mold metal edge over nose. Assess for device related pressure injuries. ■ Airtight seal not possible with all facial structures. ■ Keep oxygen saturation > 92%. ■ Minimum of 5 L/min flow is needed to expel CO_2 from mask so the patient does not rebreathe.
Nonrebreather	Highest concentration possible 60%–90%	Indicated when > 40% FiO_2 is desired for acute desaturation Highest flow possible short of mechanical ventilation or NIV Conversion to partial NRB is possible Short term	Requires a tight seal, which effects FiO_2 Irritation of eyes and skin possible Interferes with ADL Not appropriate for long-term therapy	■ Ensure snug fit, fully inflated rebreather bag, and intact side valves. ■ Requires a minimum flow rate of 10 L/min. ■ Valve malfunction can cause CO_2 buildup and subsequent decrease in level of consciousness.
Transtracheal oxygen	FiO_2 concentration is product dependent	Efficient delivery of oxygen directly into the trachea. Works well for home and ambulatory patients Humidification is necessary O_2 flow occurs throughout respiratory cycle Can be concealed by shirt or scarf	Not suitable if bronchospasm or bleeding Uncompensated respiratory failure other interventions are necessary	■ Monitor the patient for bleeding, respiratory distress, pain, coughing, and hoarseness. ■ Follow facility guidelines for trach care. ■ Ensure backup supplies are present in the case of decannulation.
Venturi mask	FiO_2 concentration is variable 2–12 L/min	Delivers a more accurate concentration because the same amount of air is always entrained FiO_2 delivery remains consistent even with variable respiratory rate Doesn't dry mucous membranes Humidification or aerosol treatment can easily be applied	Feeling of claustrophobia Irritating to eyes and skin if ill-fitting mask Interferes with ADL	■ Ensure flow rate is set for specific Venturi mask. ■ Adjust FiO_2 to keep SpO_2 >92%.
High-flow nasal cannula	Up to 60 L/min flow with inspired oxygen concentration up to 100%	Precise FiO_2 delivery High flow flushes expired gas from upper airway, reducing dead space Not as drying and tight fitting as other alternatives Not invasive Does not cause claustrophobia Easier to mobilize patient Can be used postoperatively to prevent respiratory failure	Different manufacturers Device-related pressure injuries potential on ears, nose, and upper lip Warmed humidification has historically been associated with bacteria harboring	Nasal prongs and high flow create a positive pressure environment: ■ Consider intermediate oral care interventions. ■ Titrate to prescribed SpO_2. ■ Keep HOB up at least 30–45°. ■ Ensure condensation drains away from the patient.

ADL, activities of daily living; COPD, congestive obstructive pulmonary disease; HOB, head of bed; NIV, noninvasive ventilation; NRB, nonrebreather.

Indications for Removal

- Lung has reexpanded per chest x-ray; remains expanded on water-seal (no suction)
- Decreased drainage (usually <100 mL/24 hours)
- Resolution of air leak

Chest Tube Removal Procedure

- Educate patient about steps of chest tube removal procedure and rehearse breathing technique.
- Administer pain medication prior to the procedure.
- Discontinue skin surface securement/suture.
- Place and hold sterile dressing over the chest tube insertion sites.
- Instruct patient to exhale and hold the breath (Valsalva maneuver or bearing down). Chest tubes should be removed at end expiration in one smooth motion while maintaining dressings over the chest tube insertion sites.
- Instruct patient to breathe normally.
- Secure an occlusive dressing.
- Assess patient tolerance of procedure (Kirkwood, 2017).

REVIEW QUESTIONS

1. A 64-year-old patient with chronic obstructive pulmonary disease (COPD) presents to the ED with sudden onset of shortness of breath. Chest x-ray demonstrates a pneumothorax. What type of pneumothorax is most likely to have occurred for this patient?
   A. Primary spontaneous pneumothorax
   B. Secondary spontaneous pneumothorax
   C. Traumatic pneumothorax
   D. Tension pneumothorax

2. A chest tube/drain may be removed
   A. after discussion of the CXR, chest tube drainage, chest tube air leak and patient status with the physician,
   B. per bedside RN request,
   C. per the confused patient's request and family agreement,
   D. only in the operating room.

ANSWERS

1. **Correct answer: B. Rationale:** Patients with preexisting medical conditions, such as COPD or asthma, are most likely to present with a secondary spontaneous pneumothorax. Primary pneumothorax typically occurs in young male smokers. Tension pneumothorax was not demonstrated on x-ray. This patient had no history of trauma to indicate traumatic pneumothorax.

2. **Correct answer: A. Rationale:** Removing a chest tube is a team decision and requires a chest x-ray and other assessment data. The bedside RN and patient and family are not qualified to make the decision but can help support the assessment. A chest tube can be removed in other areas outside of the operating room.

REFERENCES

The complete reference and additional reading lists appear in the digital version of this chapter, at https://connect.springerpub.com/content/book/978-0-8261-7417-8/part/part01/chapter/ch07

Endocrine System

Stacey Seggelke and Matthew J. Wren

OVERVIEW OF THE ENDOCRINE SYSTEM

The endocrine system consists of glands that produce **hormones**, important for the regulation of metabolism, growth and development, tissue function, sexual function, and reproduction, in addition to others.

- There are three general classifications of hormones based upon their chemical structure.
  - Amino acid derivative hormones (end in "-ine")
    - *Examples:* Epinephrine, norephedrine, thyroxine
  - Peptide hormones
    - *Examples:* Insulin, glucagon
  - Lipid derivative hormones
    - Primarily steroid hormones (ending in "-ol" or "-one")
    - *Examples:* Estradiol, testosterone, aldosterone, and cortisol

DIABETES MELLITUS

OVERVIEW

Diabetes mellitus is an umbrella term encompassing similar yet different autoimmune and metabolic disorders. Nomenclature regarding these disorders has been shifting in recent years owing to evolving knowledge of the disorders and to allow for the overlap between them. With this in mind, as we discuss type 1 diabetes mellitus (T1DM) and type 2 diabetes mellitus (T2DM); remember that there may be significant overlap between the two classical definitions in patients.

Definition

T1DM has historically been defined as an autoimmune process resulting from the destruction of insulin-producing cells and leading to severe and absolute insulin deficiency that requires exogenous insulin administration. T2DM has historically been defined as a metabolic process with multiple disposing factors that results in concurrent insulin resistance and relative insulin deficiency. Treatment for T2DM may span the spectrum from diet control and exercise to exogenous insulin administration (American Diabetes Association [ADA], 2018a).

Pathophysiology

Type 1 Diabetes Mellitus

- Causes immune-mediated destruction of the insulin-producing beta cells in the pancreas.
- T1DM is caused by an absolute insulin deficiency.

- Insulin deficiency leads to inability to transport serum glucose into the cell
- Lack of intracellular glucose triggers fat metabolism for energy
- Increased ketoacid by-products of fat metabolism in conjunction with insulin deficiency causes an elevated anion gap metabolic acidosis (Atkinson et al., 2015)

Type 2 Diabetes Mellitus

- Impaired insulin secretion
- Increased insulin resistance
- **Relative** insulin deficiency
  - Degree of insulin deficiency may progress throughout lifespan to near absolute.

Patients who develop near absolute insulin deficiency become insulin dependent. These patients present as and need to be treated very similarly to patients with T1DM (Coope et al., 2016).

Etiology

Type 1 Diabetes Mellitus

- Patients are typically genetically predisposed.
- Environmental agents trigger autoimmune processes:
  - Coxsackie B virus
  - Enteroviruses
  - Elements of albumin and proteins in cow's milk
  - High nitrate concentration in drinking water
- The immune system destroys beta cells in the islets of Langerhans.
- Destruction typically occurs over months to years (Atkinson et al., 2015).

Type 2 Diabetes Mellitus

- A constellation of hypertension, hyperlipidemia, and obesity; referred to as the *metabolic syndrome*.
- Inherited gene transcriptions and environmental factors determine risk.
- Factors from metabolic syndrome cause increased insulin resistance, leading to increased insulin secretion and hyperinsulinemia.
- Insulin need overtakes ability of body to produce insulin, resulting in relative insulin deficiency.

Risk Factors

Type 1 Diabetes Mellitus

- Close family relative with T1DM
- Ethnicity
  - Caucasians and African Americans have highest prevalence (Atkinson et al., 2015).

The complete reference and additional reading lists appear in the digital version of this chapter, at https://connect.springerpub.com/content/book/978-0-8261-7417-8/part/part01/chapter/ch08

Type 2 Diabetes Mellitus
- Nonmodifiable risk factors
  - Family history of T2DM
  - Ethnicity
    - Highest prevalence in Native Americans and African Americans
- Modifiable risk factors
  - Obesity
  - Sedentary lifestyle
  - Smoking
  - Poor diet (Coope et al., 2016)

Assessment
Patients may not present with any particular signs or symptoms, unless they have chronic diabetic complications or are acutely hypoglycemic or hyperglycemic. Thus, assessment for the diabetic patient revolves around a standard physical assessment, review of relevant diagnostics, and review of blood sugar trends, which may indicate a need for change in the medication regimen. For particular information on assessment of patients in hyperglycemic crisis, see the sections Diabetic Ketoacidosis and Hyperglycemic Hyperosmolar State.

Presentation
Patients may exhibit an extremely wide range of presentations owing to comorbid conditions, degree of hypoglycemia or hyperglycemia, existence of other primary complaints, and relationship between diabetes and their other conditions.

Relevant Diagnostics
- Hemoglobin A1c
  - Indicator of glycemic control over previous 90 days
- Blood glucose
- Serum ketones
  - Positive serum ketones are used in the diagnosis of diabetic ketoacidosis (DKA) and may be trended during treatment to assess therapy.
- Renal function indices
  - Elevated blood urea nitrogen (BUN) and creatinine and decreased glomerular filtration rate (GFR) may alter fluid management and cause the clinician to consider more conservative glycemic targets.
- Anion gap
  - May be used in the diagnosis of DKA and then trended during treatment and used as an indicator for readiness to transition from intravenous (IV) to subcutaneous insulin therapy.
- Serum osmolality
  - Elevated serum osmolality in conjunction with severely elevated glucose and absence of acidosis is used to diagnose hyperglycemic hyperosmolar state (HHS).
- C-peptide
  - Indicates level of endogenous insulin production. It is helpful in the differential diagnosis of hypoglycemia without a clear cause.

Treatment
Treatment for T1 and T2DM in the hospital setting has many similarities. Treatment goals for both are generally the same.
- Minimize severe hyperglycemia.
- Avoid hypoglycemia.
- Avoid iatrogenic hyperglycemic crisis (i.e., DKA and HHS).

Type 1 Diabetes Mellitus
A hallmark of T1DM treatment should be the recognition that the patient has an absolute insulin deficiency. Recognition of this fact should lead to the knowledge that the patient will require endogenous insulin to meet basal, prandial, and correctional needs (Table 8.1). Withholding of basal insulin in this population causes complications that negatively impact morbidity, mortality, and hospital length of stay.

Type 2 Diabetes Mellitus
T2DM exists on a continuum from extremely minor insulin deficiency, which can be controlled through diet and exercise, to near absolute insulin deficiency, which necessitates multimodal insulin therapy.

Medication Therapy
Many patients with T2DM are placed on one or multiple oral antidiabetic agents. Continuation of oral antidiabetic agents in the inpatient setting is generally not advised for the following reasons:
- Limited data on use in the inpatient population
- Increased risk of hypoglycemia with some classes of oral antidiabetic agents
  - Sulfonylureas
  - Meglitinides
  - Thiazolidinediones
- Slow onset of action precludes rapid titration for an inpatient with changing glycemic needs.

It is generally advised to start these patients on multimodal insulin therapy while in the hospital and transition back to their home oral antidiabetic agents upon discharge (Draznin, 2016b, pp. 336–350).

Hyperglycemia
Causative Factors

■ Decreased physical activity ■ Excessive carbohydrate intake ■ Omitted insulin doses ■ Glucocorticoid administration ■ Vasopressor administration ■ Sepsis	■ Decreased insulin sensitivity during cooling phase of targeted temperature management ■ Faulty insertion set or tubing in insulin pump users ■ Surgical stress

Signs and Symptoms
- Polyuria
- Polydipsia
- Lethargy (ADA, 2018c)

Hypoglycemia
Contributing Factors
- Increased physical activity
- Decreased carbohydrate intake or NPO status
- Inappropriately high dose of insulin
  - Insulin not adjusted during steroid wean
  - Intentional self-harm
  - Dosage error
- Mistiming of insulin administration
- Recovery of insulin sensitivity during rewarming phase of targeted temperature management

- Insulin "dose stacking" in patients with renal insufficiency
- Interruption in enteral and parental nutrition
- Advanced age
- Underweight
- Critical illness (Cryer, 2016a, pp. 111–115)

Signs and Symptoms

- Sweating*
- Palpitations*
- Tremors*
- Anxiety*
- Tachycardia*
- Confusion **
- Decreased level of consciousness**
- Seizures**

*These signs and symptoms are mainly mediated by release of epinephrine and norepinephrine. Beta-adrenergic blocking agents will blunt this response, so clinicians may need to have a higher index of suspicion for hypoglycemia with fewer and more vague symptoms in patients receiving any medications in that class.

** These are late signs that are typically associated with severe hypoglycemia. Failure to recognize and promptly treat severe hypoglycemia can result in cardiac arrest (Cryer, 2016b).

MANAGEMENT OF THE PATIENT WITH GLYCEMIC ABNORMALITIES

Nonpharmacological Therapy

All patients with diabetes should be encouraged to follow a healthy diet. There is no specific diet endorsed for the treatment of diabetes. The diet should focus on portion sizes with a goal of achieving or maintaining a healthy body weight. Physical activity is an essential part of diabetes management. Patients should be encouraged to participate in 150 minutes or more of moderate-to-vigorous intensity aerobic activity per week. However, this goal may not be achievable for all patients due to other health factors. Emphasis should then be placed on decreasing the amount of sedentary time (ADA, 2019f).

TABLE 8.1 INSULIN THERAPY

GOAL	INSULIN TYPE
Basal insulin	Insulin glargine, insulin detemir, insulin degludec, insulin isophane
Prandial insulin	Insulin lispro, insulin aspart, insulin glulisine, insulin regular, insulin regular U-500
Correctional insulin	Insulin lispro, insulin aspart, insulin glulisine, insulin regular, insulin regular U-500
Continuous subcutaneous insulin infusion (insulin pump)	Insulin lispro, insulin aspart, insulin glulisine, insulin regular, insulin regular U-500
IV insulin infusion	Insulin regular

IV, intravenous.
Source: From American Diabetes Association. (2018b). Pharmacologic approaches to glycemic treatment: Standards of medical care in diabetes—2019. *Diabetes Care, 42*(Suppl. 1), S90–S102.

Noninsulin Medications

Oral and injectable noninsulin are the mainstay of treatment for patients with T2DM (Table 8.2). Insulin may need to be initiated as add-on therapy with progression of the disease. The approach to treating patients with T2DM should be individualized based upon comorbidities, age, body weight, cost, and patient preference.

Prescribing and Management

- Using extended-release metformin may reduce gastrointestinal (GI) side effects.
- Due to their low side effect profile, dipeptidyl peptidase-4 (DDP4) inhibitors are a good choice for older patients.
- Most oral medications are held in the inpatient setting.

Initiating Insulin

Different strategies exist for initiating insulin for hospitalized patients. Use of a specific strategy depends on provider preference and whether or not the patient was already on antidiabetic medications prior to hospitalization.

- Continue home insulin regimen for patients already on insulin. Obtain hemoglobin A1c values to assess for the effectiveness of home regimen. Initiate a correctional scale based on the patient's weight or total daily dose of insulin.
- A total daily dose of insulin of 0.4 units/kg—half as basal insulin and half divided into three doses of prandial insulin. Patients with significant insulin resistance may need to be started with a higher total daily dose calculation, up to 1 unit/kg. Initiate a correctional scale based on the patient's weight or total daily dose of insulin (ADA, 2018b).

A target blood glucose range should be chosen that limits hyperglycemia while not being so strict as to encourage hypoglycemia. Current evidence does not support tight glycemic control targets except for certain populations.

- A target glucose range of 140 to 180 is recommended for the majority of patients.
- Tighter target ranges of less than 140 may be utilized in obstetric and cardiothoracic surgical ICUs to prevent fetal and surgical complications. These targets may need to be relaxed if the patient experiences recurrent hypoglycemia (ADA, 2018a)

Insulin Therapy

Patients with T1DM require treatment with insulin due to beta cell destruction leading to absolute insulin deficiency. T2DM is a progressive disease with relative insulin deficiency secondary to insulin resistance. Most patients with T2DM will eventually need insulin therapy (ADA, 2019d).

There are two main types of insulin: basal and bolus (Table 8.3). Basal insulin suppresses hepatic glucose output controlling blood glucose in the fasting and premeal states. Bolus insulin is used to suppress the rise in blood glucose after meals (nutritional) and/or to correct for hyperglycemia (correctional).

There are also combination insulins that contain both basal and bolus insulin in fixed amounts. These may be good options for patients who are averse to multiple daily injections.

Contraindications/Warnings

All insulin is renally metabolized. In patients with renal impairment, there is delayed clearance of insulin, which can promote increased risk for hypoglycemia (Rajput et al., 2017).

TABLE 8.2 NONINSULIN MEDICATIONS

MEDICATION	CLASS	MECHANISM OF ACTION	CONTRAINDICATIONS/ SAFETY	DOSAGE	SIDE EFFECTS	PATIENT EDUCATION
			FIRST-LINE THERAPY FOR ALL PATIENTS			
Metformin (Glucophage)	Biguanides	Decreases hepatic glucose production	*Initial and ongoing monitoring of eGFR:* not recommended if eGFR 30–45 Contraindicated if eGFR < 30 Discontinue metformin before iodinated contrast imaging if eGFR 30–60. Recheck eGFR 48 hours after the procedure and restart metformin if GFR stable Avoid use in patients with active liver disease Lactic acidosis is a rare but serious side effect	500–2,000 mg Take 1–2 times daily with meals	Diarrhea, gas, bloating, and nausea	Take with meals to minimize side effects. Discuss need or possibly hold dose if undergoing contrast testing.
			ADD-ON THERAPY IF KNOWN ASCVD, HF, OR CKD			
Dapagliflozin (Farxiga) Canagliflozin (Invokana) Empagliflozin (Jardiance) Ertugliflozin (Steglatro)	SGLT2 inhibitors	Promotes renal excretion by inhibiting reabsorption of glucose in the proximal tubular	*Initial and ongoing monitoring of eGFR* (dapagliflozin and ertugliflozin not recommended for eGFR <60; canagliflozin and empagliflozin not recommended for eGFR <45.) May increase LDL Should not be used in ketosis-prone T2DM or patients at risk for foot amputation Canagliflozin has demonstrated increased risk for bone loss and low extremity amputations	Take once daily with or without food Dosage is dependent on current eGFR	Dehydration, yeast infections, urinary tract infections, and hypotension	Encourage adequate fluid intake to avoid dehydration. Discuss warning signs of yeast and urinary infections and hypotension. Discuss potential weight loss.
Exenatide (Byetta) Exenatide extended release (Bydureon) Lixisenatide (Lyxumia)		Stimulates glucose-dependent insulin release from the beta cells	*Initial and ongoing monitoring of eGFR* Exenatide or lixisenatide should not be used if GFR <30 mL/ min	BID: Exenatide Daily: Liraglutide and lixisenatide Weekly: Exenatide extended release, dulaglutide, and semaglutide	Nausea, vomiting, diarrhea,	Watch for signs of pancreatitis.

(continued)

	Mechanism	Monitoring/Precautions	Dosing	Common side effects	Warnings
Semaglutide (Ozempic) Dulaglutide (Trulicity) Liraglutide (Victoza)	Inhibits the release of glucagon by the alpha cells Slows glucose absorption into the bloods by reducing gastric emptying	Dose-dependent and treatment duration–dependent thyroid c-cell tumors in rodent models have been seen. GLP-1 RA are contraindicated in patients with a personal or family history of MTC or MEN2 Do not use in patients with a history of pancreatitis	Recommended to start at lowest dose and increase based on tolerability In setting of previous MI or stroke, liraglutide or semaglutide should be favorably considered	Abdominal pain and constipation	Weight loss is common with GLP-1 receptor agonists. Monitor for vision changes with semaglutide as possible increased risk for retinopathy.
ADD ON THERAPY WITHOUT KNOWN ASCVD OR CKD					
Alogliptin (Nesina) Sitagliptin (Januvia) Saxagliptin (Onglyza) Linagliptin (Tradjenta)	Slows the inactivation of endogenous GLP-1	*Initial and ongoing monitoring of eGFR:* Sitagliptin, saxagliptin, and alogliptin require dose adjustment with chronic kidney CKD Do not use saxagliptin or alogliptin in patients with HF	Take once daily with or without food	Cold-like symptoms	Watch for signs of pancreatitis. Watch for severe joint pain (sitagliptin, saxagliptin). Watch for rash/blisters (bullous pemphigoid).
Glipizide (Glucotrol) Glyburide (Micronase) Glyburide (Diabeta) Glimepiride (Amaryl)	Increases insulin production by the pancreatic beta cells	Use caution with renal impairment and start at lowest dose Possible cross-reactivity if allergic to sulfonamides Glyburide is the only sulfonylurea used to treat GDM	Take once or BID before or with meal	Hypoglycemia	Take with meal to avoid hypoglycemia.
Pioglitazone (Actos) Rosiglitazone (Avandia)	Increase insulin sensitivity in muscle and liver	*Initial and ongoing LFT monitoring* Not recommended for patients with symptomatic HF, NYHA class III or IV HF, active bladder cancer, active liver disease (>3 times upper reference limit)	Recommended to start at lowest dose and titrate as needed Typically takes 4–6 weeks to see an effect on blood glucose	Weight gain, fluid retention, cold-like symptoms	Watch for signs of heart failure (edema, dyspnea, weight gain). Watch for signs of liver injury (jaundice, dark urine). May improve HDL and triglycerides.

ASCVD, atherosclerotic cardiovascular disease; CKD, chronic kidney disease; DPP-4, dipeptidyl peptidase-4; eGFR, estimated glomerular filtration rate; GDM, gestational diabetes mellitus; GFR, estimated glomerular filtration rate; GLP-1 RA, glucagon-like peptide-1 receptor agonist; HDL, high-density lipoproteins; HF, heart failure; LDL, low-density lipoproteins; LFT, liver function test; MEN2, multiple endocrine neoplasia syndrome type 2; MI, myocardial infarction; MTC, medullary thyroid cancer; NYHA, New York Heart Association; SGLT2, sodium–glucose cotransporter 2; T2DM, type 2 diabetes mellitus.

TABLE 8.3 INSULIN THERAPY

BASAL INSULINS	
Long acting: Detemir (Levemir), glargine (Lantus), degludec (Tresiba), intermediate acting: NPH	Control blood glucose in the fasting and pre-mail state through suppression of hepatic glucose output
BOLUS INSULINS	
Rapid-acting insulins: Aspart (Novolog), glulisine (Apidra), lispro (Humalog)	Nutritional (prandial) insulin: Diminishes the rise in BG following nutritional intake (meals, enteral;/parenteral nutrition)
Short-acting insulins: Regular	Correctional insulin: Corrects hyperglycemia

BG, blood glucose; NPH, natural protein Hagedorn.

Prescribing and Management

- Insulin injection techniques should be practiced with all patients prior to the start of insulin therapy.
- Basal insulin dosages are assessed by bedtime and fasting glucose levels. Glucose levels should remain steady overnight. If there is a significant rise or decrease in glucose levels overnight, the basal dose should be adjusted appropriately.
- Bolus insulin dosages are assessed by prelunch, predinner, and bedtime glucose levels. If the glucose levels are rising during the day at these times, the bolus insulin dose should be increased. If there is hypoglycemia at these times, the bolus dose should be decreased.

Steroid-Induced Hyperglycemia

- Glucocorticoids are commonly used medications due to their antiinflammatory and immunosuppressive effects. However, in patients at risk for hyperglycemia, glucocorticoids can induce steroid-induced hyperglycemia. This hyperglycemia is attributed to increased insulin resistance leading to glucose intolerance and increased hepatic glucose production.
- The treatment of steroid-induced hyperglycemia is dependent upon the type and duration of action of the steroid used. Short-acting steroids, such as daily hydrocortisone, prednisone, or methylprednisolone, generally have a peak effect on glucose in about 6 to 8 hours. Using an intermediate-acting insulin, such as neutral protein Hagedorn (NPH), given at the time of the steroid administration, can counteract the glycemic effect. For longer-acting steroids, such as dexamethasone, or multiple daily dosing of short-acting steroids, a long-acting basal insulin would be the preferred treatment. If there is prolonged steroid treatment or the doses of steroids are remarkably high, as seen during chemotherapy treatment, the doses of bolus insulin may need to be increased also (ADA, 2019f).

Hyperglycemia
Prevention

- Use basal, prandial, and correctional scale insulin.
- Compliance with carbohydrate-controlled diet.
- Avoid inappropriately holding doses of insulin, particularly basal insulin.

Treatment

- Rapid-acting insulin (i.e., insulin lispro, aspart, or glulisine) subcutaneously.

- Correctional scale insulin should not be given any more frequently than every 3 hours.
  - This practice prevents "insulin stacking" (i.e., a second dose given during the duration of effect of a first dose).
  - This window may need to be extended longer for patients with significant renal disease as insulin has a longerthan normal duration of effect in these patients.

Insulin Adjustment

- First, assess basal insulin effectiveness through fasting blood glucose.
  - If blood glucose is less than 140 mg/dL and greater than 100, no changes are needed.
  - If blood glucose is 141 to 160 mg/dL, increase basal by 2 to 3 units.
  - If blood glucose is 160 to 180 mg/dL, increase basal by 4 to 5 units.
  - If blood glucose is 180 to 200 mg/dL, increase basal by 6 to 7 units.
  - If blood glucose is greater than 200 mg/dL, increase basal by 8 units.
  - For patients with increased insulin sensitivity, smaller adjustments may be appropriate.
- Next, assess prandial insulin effectiveness. Blood glucose greater than 180 mg/dL at lunch, dinner, or evening time, with adequate basal insulin, indicates that the patient does not have enough prandial insulin. Increase prandial insulin dose for the meal prior to the hyperglycemia (Draznin, 2016c).

Hypoglycemia
Prevention

- Avoid using only sliding scale correctional insulin—this exposes patients to risk for both hyperglycemia and hypoglycemia.
- Hold prandial insulin when patient is NPO.
- Initiate an IV dextrose solution when patient is NPO.
- Follow day-to-day trends of blood glucose and adjust insulin therapy as needed.

Treatment

- If blood glucose is less than 70 mg/dL, give 20 g of simple carbohydrates (i.e., fruit juice, glucose tablets, etc.).
- Repeat blood glucose and treatment every 15 minutes until blood glucose is greater than 100 mg/dL.
- If patient is unable to tolerate oral treatment, give 25 mL D50 IV (Cryer, 2016b).

TABLE 8.4 PHARMACOKINETICS OF INSULIN

	ONSET	PEAK	DURATION	COMMENTS
RAPID ACTING				
Lispro (Humalog U-100, Humalog U-200)	10–15 min	1–2 hr	3–5 hr	Can take up to 15 minutes before meal.
Glulisine (Apidra)	10–15 min	1–2 hr	3–5 hr	
Aspart (Novolog)	10–15 min	1–2 hr	3–5 hr	
Aspart (Fiasp)	3–5 min	1–2 hr	3–5 hr	
Inhaled insulin (Afrezza)	Seconds	12–17 min	2–3 hr	Before starting Afrezza, patients need to undergo a spirometry test. Do not use in chronic lung disease or patients who smoke.
SHORT ACTING				
Regular	30–60 min	2–3 hr	5–8 hr	Increased risk for hypoglycemia if taken at meal time. Needs to be taken 30 minutes prior to meal.
INTERMEDIATE ACTING				
NPH	2–4 hr	6–10 hr	10–16 hr	Cloudy insulin that needs to be mixed before use; can be combined in same syringe with rapid/short acting insulin; generally, BID dosing.
Regular U-500	30–60 min	8–12 hr	12–18 hr	Should be used in insulin pen or with U-500 insulin syringes to avoid dose confusion; BID or TID dosing.
LONG ACTING				
Insulin glargine (Lantus, Basaglar)	1–2 hr	Limited	20–24 hr	Daily or BID dosing
Insulin glargine U-300 (Toujeo)	1–2 hr	None	24–26 hr	Daily
Insulin detemir (Levemir)	1–2 hr	6–8 hr	18–24 hr	Daily or BID dosing
Insulin degludec (Tresiba)	1–2 hr	None	36 hr	Daily dosing, once steady state is achieved (~ 5 days), can be taken at any time of day
MIXED INSULINS				
NPH/regular (Humulin 70/30, Novolin 70/30)	30–60 min	Dual	10–16 hr	Generally, BID dosing; cloudy insulin that needs to mixed before use
NPH/lispro (Humalog 75/25, Humalog 50/50)	10–15 min	Dual	10–16 hr	
NPH/aspart (Novolog 70/30)	10–15 min	Dual	10–16 hr	

NPH, natural protein Hagedorn.

Insulin Adjustment

- Assess basal insulin effectiveness through fasting blood glucose.
  - Fasting blood glucose less than 100 mg/dL indicates too much basal insulin. Basal should be decreased 10% to 20%.
- Assess prandial insulin effectiveness through postprandial blood glucose.
- Blood glucose less than 70 mg/dL at lunch, dinner, or evening blood glucose with a normal fasting blood glucose indicates that the patient's prandial insulin dose at the previous meal was too high. Decrease the prandial insulin dosage for that meal (Draznin, 2016c).

Common Errors in Diabetes Mellitus Treatment in the Hospital

- Not initiating basal/bolus/prandial insulin therapy in T1DM
  - Remember that patients with T1DM have an absolute deficiency of insulin and require endogenous insulin administration for all basal, prandial, and correctional needs. The practice of placing all diabetic patients on correctional sliding scale insulin alone predisposes insulin-dependent patients to developing DKA.
- Holding basal insulin for NPO patients
  - In an appropriate insulin regimen, basal insulin accounts for the insulin needs of the body between meals and overnight. Prandial and correctional insulin account for the insulin needs due to nutrient intake and other causes of glycemic excursions. Prandial insulin should be held while the patient is NPO, and basal insulin continued with small reductions made if the patient is at risk for hypoglycemia. Complete holding of basal insulin is not advised and can put the patient at risk for both hyperglycemic crisis and hypoglycemic events if an aggressive correctional sliding scale is used during the NPO period.
- Removing insulin pumps for procedures without an alternate treatment strategy in place
  - Insulin pumps utilize a near continuous infusion of short-acting insulin to cover basal insulin needs. Short-acting insulin has an approximately 4-hour duration of effect, as compared to the 20 to 24 hour duration of effect of common basal insulins. For patients on insulin pumps, this means that they can be reduced to no active insulin in the body in a few short hours after the insulin pump is stopped. In the absence of an alternate subcutaneous or IV insulin regimen while off of the pump, these patients are at high risk of developing hyperglycemic crisis.
- Choosing a correctional scale based on the degree of hyperglycemia
  - Correctional sliding scale insulin should be chosen based upon insulin sensitivity, not on the severity of hyperglycemia. An insulin sensitivity factor may be calculated if the patient's total daily dose of insulin is known. Insulin sensitivity may also be approximated based on total daily dose or the patient's weight. Insulin sensitivity has an inverse correlation with total daily dose and weight. As total daily dose or weight increases, insulin sensitivity will decrease, and more correctional insulin is needed for any given blood glucose above target.
- Transitioning from IV to subcutaneous insulin in patients with DKA prior to closing of the anion gap
  - Patients may develop euglycemia prior to resolution of anion gap metabolic acidosis. In these patients, it is important to deliver enough maintenance IV dextrose to allow the insulin infusion to continue so as to continue to correct the anion gap metabolic acidosis. Studies have shown an increase in length of stay when patients are transitioned from IV to subcutaneous insulin prior to the resolution of the anion gap metabolic acidosis.
- Immediately stopping IV insulin when giving a transition dose of basal subcutaneous insulin
  - Currently available basal insulins do not have an immediate onset of action and need to be overlapped with IV insulin in order to prevent reoccurrence of DKA. It is generally advisable to continue the IV insulin infusion for 2 to 4 hours from the time that the transition dose of basal subcutaneous insulin is administered, depending on which basal insulin is used.
- Excessively tight glycemic control in patients with risk factors for insulin sensitivity and hypoglycemia
  - Severe hypoglycemia has a more deleterious effect than mild hyperglycemia. Patients who are known to be highly insulin sensitive or who have had recurrent severe hypoglycemia should have their blood glucose target relaxed to avoid future hypoglycemic events.
- Not making day-to-day adjustments according to glucose trends and amount of correctional insulin received in previous day
  - Patients' insulin needs will often change from day to day. Making adjustments every day helps to prevent hypoglycemia or hyperglycemia due to insulin dosing that is no longer appropriate for the patient's clinical situation.
- Titrating the wrong insulin (basal versus prandial) based on glucose trends
  - Providers must assess both fasting and nonfasting blood glucose results when evaluating whether or not to make insulin adjustments and which type of insulin to adjust. Fasting blood glucose results are the best indicator of basal insulin effectiveness. This is generally either a prebreakfast or early-morning-hour blood glucose result. Prandial insulin effectiveness may be assessed by review of glucose results from the next blood glucose after each prandial dose. For example, this means that breakfast prandial dosing is evaluated by review of lunch blood glucose.
- Not providing supplemental parenteral dextrose for patients that are NPO
  - Diabetic patients are at increased risk for hypoglycemia. Withholding oral glucose intake for long durations without an enteral or parenteral replacement will cause hypoglycemia in most diabetic patients (Draznin, 2016).

Management of the Patient With an Insulin Pump

Insulin pumps are designed to deliver insulin through a flexible cannula into the subcutaneous space. A basal rate of insulin is given continuously, and the patient uses the pump interface to deliver bolus doses for prandial and correctional needs. Insulin pumps generally allow for tighter glycemic control in the outpatient setting but can be troublesome for clinicians who do not have experience with them.

Insulin Pump Settings
Target Range

- Refers to a desired blood glucose range in any given period of time.
- Used in bolus calculations.
- Some insulin pumps use the midpoint of range for calculations; others use the end point.
  - For target range of 100 to 140, either 120 or 140 might be used for calculation depending on the type of insulin pump.
- Target range may change throughout the day.
  - It is common to see higher target range in evening and early morning hours to avoid nocturnal hypoglycemia.

Basal Rate

- Refers to the hourly infusion rate of insulin to cover basal needs.
- Expressed as "X" units of insulin per hour.

- Is similar to the function of basal insulin (i.e., insulin glargine, detemir, degludec, or NPH) in multimodal injection regimens.
- Equal portions of this hourly amount are infused every 3 minutes.
- Basal rates can be programmed to vary to account for changes in basal insulin need throughout the day.

Insulin Sensitivity Factor

- Refers to how much 1 unit of insulin will decrease blood glucose.
- Expressed as 1 unit: "X" mg/dL.
- Used in blood glucose correction calculations as follows: (blood glucose – target) / Insulin sensitivity factor.
- For an insulin sensitivity factor of 1:30, a blood glucose of 240, and a target glucose of 120, the patient would take 4 units of rapid acting insulin:
  - $(240 – 120)/30 = 4$ units

Carbohydrate Factor

- Refers to how many grams of carbohydrates will be covered by 1 unit of insulin.
- Expressed as 1 unit : "X" grams carbohydrates.
- Used in meal bolus calculations as grams of carbohydrates/ carbohydrate factor.
- For a carbohydrate factor of 1:10 and a meal containing 60 g of carbohydrates, the patient would take 6 units of rapid acting insulin:
  - $60/10 = 6$ units

Insulin on Board

- Refers to the amount of active insulin remaining in the body after any given bolus.
- Serves to prevent insulin stacking if a blood glucose correctional bolus is given in close proximity to a previous meal or blood glucose correction bolus.
- Any insulin currently on board is subtracted from the suggested bolus dose.

Example Insulin Bolus Calculation

- Target range: 115 to 125
- Insulin sensitivity factor 1 unit : 25 mg/dL
- Carbohydrate factor 1 unit : 12 g carbohydrates
- Insulin on board currently "0 units"
- Patient's preprandial blood glucose is 195 and patient plans to eat a meal with 60 g of carbohydrates
- Bolus dose = $([195 – 120]/25) + (60/12) = 8$ units (3 units correctional and 5 units prandial)

Important Considerations of Insulin Pump Management

Facilities should have robust policy and procedure governing the care of the patient with an insulin pump. There are several baseline elements that should be addressed in these documents.

- Patients must be able to self-manage their own insulin pump.
- Patients should consent to point-of-care capillary glucose monitoring to provide the basis for treatment decisions.
- In the event that patients become unable to self-manage the insulin pump, a procedure must be in place to obtain alternate therapy (i.e., multimodal subcutaneous insulin or IV insulin infusion).
- Patients must communicate to the care team: all boluses given from the pump and any changes made to the pump settings.
- Where available, consultation with endocrine services is recommended while the patient is hospitalized.
- Patients must be able to supply infusion sets and insulin cartridges.

The clinician should remember the following important elements when caring for a patient with an insulin pump.

- The care team needs to plan ahead for times when the patient needs to be off of the insulin pump.
  - The insulin pump must not be exposed to certain forms of radiation or imaging. The pump should be shielded for patients undergoing an x-ray or CT scan. Under no circumstances can the insulin pump be placed in an MRI. MRI will corrupt the operating system of the insulin pump.
- If the patient were to need to transition from the insulin pump to multimodal subcutaneous insulin therapy, the clinician can use settings and data from the insulin pump to guide multimodal dosing.
  - Basal insulin may be dosed based on total daily basal insulin from insulin pump.
  - Prandial insulin may be dosed based on the patient's carbohydrate factor and the amount of carbohydrates in their ordered diet.
  - A personalized correctional scale may be dosed based on the patient's insulin sensitivity factor and their ordered target range.
  - An institutional correctional scale may be chosen based on the patient's total daily dose from the insulin pump.
- For recurrent unexplained hyperglycemia, the patient should change their infusion set. If no new infusion sets are available, the patient should be transitioned to alternate insulin therapy (Draznin, 2016d, pp. 311–323).

Continuous Glucose Monitoring

Some patients with an insulin pump may also present with a continuous glucose monitoring (CGM) system. As with insulin pumps, there are several different manufacturers, and each device may look slightly different, but general concepts remain the same.

Continuous Glucose Monitoring System Components

- Sensor
  - Inserted under the skin and reads interstitial glucose every 5 minutes
- Transmitter
  - Connects to sensor and transmits interstitial glucose readings to receiver
- Receiver
  - Receives glucose readings from transmitter. This may be a standalone receiver, a smartphone, or an insulin pump.

Continuous Glucose Monitoring Principles

- Due to diffusion of glucose, there is usually a lag time between changes in capillary blood glucose (i.e., fingerstick blood glucose) and interstitial glucose (i.e., sensor glucose).
- Medications containing acetaminophen decrease the accuracy of interstitial glucose readings.
- No commonly used CGM systems are currently FDA approved for use in inpatients.

- Even if patient continues to use personal CGM while in the hospital, all treatment decisions should be based on point-of-care capillary blood glucose testing (Draznin, 2016a, pp. 323–335).

Clinical Practice Guidelines

Refer to the American Diabetes Association's "Standards of Medical Care in Diabetes—2019" for detailed guidelines on the care of patients with diabetes mellitus (ADA, 2018c).

Gestational Diabetes Mellitus

- Gestational diabetes mellitus (GDM) is diabetes that is diagnosed in the second or third trimester of pregnancy. It is transient in that blood glucose levels return to normal after delivery (ADA, 2019a).

Pathophysiology

Excretion of hormones by the placenta, such as placental lactogen hormone, required for fetal development, cause insulin resistance. If the pancreas is unable to sustain higher levels of insulin production, hyperglycemia will occur. Risks factors for the development of GDM are like those of T2DM. GDM-induced hyperglycemia during pregnancy can increase fetal risk for macrosomia, shoulder dystocia, and fetal demise and maternal increase in risk for preeclampsia and need for Cesarean delivery. After delivery, when placental hormones are no longer present, glucose levels return to normal. However, women with GDM are at increased risk to develop T2DM and should be monitored closely (ADA, 2019e).

Blood Glucose Treatment Targets

- *HbA1c:* A general goal is <6%.
- Blood glucose goals:
  - Fasting <95 mg/dL
  - One-hour postprandial <140 mg/dL
  - Two-hour postprandial <120 mg/dL (ADA, 2019e)

Specific Types of Diabetes Due to Other Causes

- Monogenic diabetes syndromes (maturity-onset diabetes of the young)
- Exocrine pancreas disorders (cystic fibrosis, chronic pancreatitis, surgical treatment for pancreatic cancer)
- Endocrine disorders (Cushing's disease, acromegaly, pheochromocytoma)
- Drug induced (nicotinic acid, glucocorticoids, transplant antirejection medications; ADA, 2019a)

CHRONIC COMPLICATIONS OF DIABETES

OVERVIEW

Hyperglycemia can lead to a myriad of complications affecting all parts of the body. These complications are generally broken down into two types: macrovascular and microvascular.

Macrovascular Complications (Large-Vessel Damage)

- *Atherosclerosis* is the main cause of macrovascular complications.
- *Cardiovascular disease (CVD)* leads to increased risk for myocardial infarction.

- *Cerebral artery disease* leads to increased risk for cerebral infarct.
- *Peripheral vascular disease (PVD)* leads to poor circulation and increased risk of infection (ADA, 2019b).

Microvascular Complications (Small Vessel Damage)

- *Retinopathy*
  - Background retinopathy: Small hemorrhages, dot hemorrhages, and microaneurysms appear in the retina. Additional microvascular leakage may cause swelling and macular edema around the retina.
  - Proliferative retinopathy refers to the growth of new blood vessels and neovascularization of the retina that may lead to vitreous hemorrhage or retinal detachment, resulting in blindness.
- *Nephropathy* is a leading cause of kidney disease. Thickening glomerular basement membrane and glomerular sclerosis lead to the loss of high amounts of protein in the urine, which is the hallmark diagnostic criteria.
- *Neuropathy* is caused by a combination of nerve ischemia due to poor circulation and alterations in nerve fiber transmission.
  - Peripheral neuropathy affects the periphery of the body. Distal symmetric polyneuropathy is the most common form of peripheral neuropathy. With this neuropathy, patients may experience a burning or tingling sensation in their hands and feet. This pain is generally worse at night when at rest. In some cases, patients present with painless numbness of their extremities. This numbness is especially dangerous as injuries may occur without detection.
  - Autonomic neuropathy affects a vast range of organs that are regulated by the autonomic nervous system.
    - *Head, eyes, ears, nose, throat:* Keratoconjunctivitis sicca (dry eye); presbycusis (hearing loss)
    - *Cardiovascular:* Resting tachycardia and orthostatic hypotension
    - *Respiratory:* Exercise intolerance
    - *Sudomotor:* Anhidrosis of the lower extremities
    - *Gastrointestinal:* Gastroparesis
    - *Genitourinary:* Cystopathy (neurogenic bladder), erectile dysfunction, female sexual dysfunction

Patients with diabetes also have an increased risk for (ADA, 2019c; Brutsaert, 2019)

- Nonalcoholic fatty liver disease,
- Cognitive decline and dementia,
- Cancer (liver, pancreas, endometrium, colon/rectum, breast, and bladder),
- Osteoporosis,
- Pancreatitis,
- Obstructive sleep apnea,
- Periodontal disease, and
- Anxiety/depression.

ACUTE COMPLICATIONS OF DIABETES: DIABETIC EMERGENCIES

OVERVIEW

The acute complications of diabetes are due to acute hyperglycemia or hypoglycemia.

Diabetic Ketoacidosis

DKA is triggered by the absolute or relative deficiency of insulin (Figure 8.1). This lack of insulin leads to an increase in counter-regulatory hormones (glucagon, cortisol, epinephrine, growth hormone), resulting in increased hepatic glucose output (gluconeo-genesis) and breakdown of fat (lipolysis) to use for energy. Free fatty acids, a by-product of lipolysis, lead to the production of ketones by the liver-producing metabolic acidosis (Fayfman et al., 2017).

Laboratory Diagnosis

Patients with DKA will have an elevated blood glucose, positive ketones or beta-hydroxybutyrate, and an anion gap (>13 mEq/L; Table 8.5). The anion gap can be calculated by

$$\text{Anion gap} = \text{Sodium mEq/L} - (\text{chloride mEq/L} + \text{bicarbonate mEq/L})$$

Hyperglycemic Hyperosmolar State

HHS is triggered by relative insulin deficiency and occurs in patients with T2DM. Because insulin is still present, acidosis is not seen. Instead, glucosuria leads to profound dehydration (osmotic diuresis) and hyperosmolality (Fayfman et al., 2017).

Laboratory Diagnosis

Patients with HHS have profoundly elevated blood glucose (>600 mg/dL), negative ketones and beta-hydroxybutyrate, normal pH, and elevated serum osmolality (>320 mOsm/L) (Grotzke & Jones, 2013b). The serum osmolality calculation is as follows:

$$\text{Serum osmolality} = 2 \times (\text{sodium} + \text{potassium}) + (\text{BUN/2.8}) + (\text{glucose/18})$$

However, due to the markedly elevated glucose, the serum sodium level may be factitiously low (Grotzke & Jones, 2013b). A corrected serum sodium level can be calculated by the following equation:

$$\text{Corrected sodium} = \text{Measured sodium} + [1.6\,(\text{glucose} - 100)/100]$$

See Table 8.6 for signs and symptoms of DKA and HHS.

Etiology of Diabetic Ketoacidosis and Hyperglycemic Hyperosmolar State

DKA can occur in T1DM or T2DM but the etiology is different. HHS only occurs in T2DM (Table 8.7).

Treatment of Diabetic Ketoacidosis and Hyperglycemic Hyperosmolar State

- **Fluid replacement:** Generally, 0.9% NS at rate of 1 L/hr (use caution in patients with congestive heart failure).
- **Insulin infusion:** 0.1 unit/kg/hr (*Note:* Insulin should not be started until the potassium level (*K*) is >3.3 mEq/L as there is risk for severe hypokalemia as potassium moves into the cells with insulin administration.
- **Potassium:** Give 20 to 30 mEq K/L fluid if K ≤5.2 mEq/L Fayfman et al., 2017).

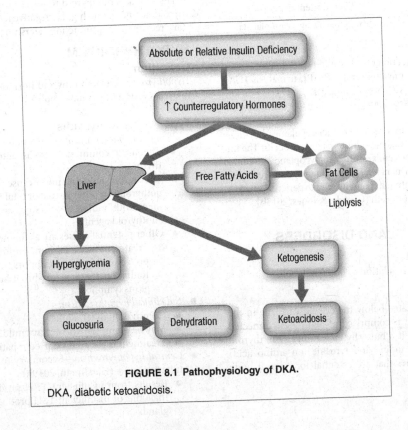

FIGURE 8.1 Pathophysiology of DKA.

DKA, diabetic ketoacidosis.

TABLE 8.5 CLASSIFICATION OF DIABETIC KETOACIDOSIS

	MILD DKA	MODER-ATE DKA	SEVERE DKA
Blood glucose	≥200 mg/dL	≥200 mg/dL	≥200 mg/dL
Venous pH	<7.3	<7.2	<7.1
Serum bicarbonate	<15 mEq/L	<10 mEq/L	<5 mEq/L
Urine/blood ketones	Positive	Positive	Positive
Beta hydroxybutyrate	High	High	High

DKA, diabetic ketoacidosis.

TABLE 8.6 SIGNS AND SYMPTOMS OF DIABETIC KETOACIDO-SIS/HYPERGLYCEMIC HYPEROSMOLAR STATE

	SYMPTOM	PHYSICAL EXAM FINDINGS
DKA	Polyuria Polydipsia Nausea Vomiting Abdominal pain Fatigue	Hypothermia Hypotension Tachycardia Tachypnea (Kussmaul respirations) Acetone sent to breath Altered mental status
HHS	Polyuria Polydipsia Fatigue	Hypothermia Hypotension Tachycardia Altered mental status

DKA, diabetic ketoacidosis; HHS, hyperglycemic hyperosmolar state.

- Treat underlying infection or other etiology (complete blood count [CBC], basic metabolic rate [BMP], urinalysis [UA], EKG, chest x-ray [CXR], blood cultures).
- Once glucose levels are <250 mg/dL switch to a dextrose-containing IV solution.

Hypoglycemic unawareness is a counter-regulatory hormone defect where normal neurogenic symptoms do not occur. The initial symptoms of hypoglycemia are neuroglycopenic symptoms whereby cognitive impairment may prevent appropriate treatment. Without appropriate treatment, patients may experience seizures, unconsciousness, coma, or death (Grotzke & Jones, 2013b).

THYROID GLAND DISORDERS

THYROID GLAND
The primary function is regulation of body metabolism.

Physiology
The thyroid gland is located below the cricoid cartilage in the anterior neck. The gland is comprised of two lobes connected with an isthmus, giving it a butterfly appearance. The thyroid gland combines dietary iodine and tyrosine (an amino acid) to produce two hormones that are essential for normal body metabolism:

- Thyroxine (T4)
- Triiodothyronine (T3)

TABLE 8.7 ETIOLOGY OF DIABETIC KETOACIDOSIS/ HYPERGLYCEMIC HYPEROSMOLAR STATE

DKA	HHS
Noncompliance with medical treatment or monitoring **Infection is the most common precipitating factor** Other stressors that can be associated with DKA include the following: Alcohol/cocaine Cardiovascular event Trauma Corticosteroids, antipsychotic medications Acute GI disease (e.g., pancreatitis)	Noncompliance with medical treatment or monitoring Infection is the most common precipitating factor (sepsis) Other stressors that can be associated with HHS include the following: CHF Renal dysfunction Alcohol/cocaine Cardiovascular event Trauma Corticosteroids, antipsychotic medications Acute GI disease (e.g., pancreatitis)

CHF, congestive heart failure; DKA, diabetic ketoacidosis; GI, gastrointestinal; HHS, hyperglycemic hyperosmolar state.

The secretions of these hormones are regulated by the hypothalamic–pituitary–thyroid axis. When thyroid hormone (T3 and T4) levels are low, the hypothalamus secrets thyrotropin-releasing hormone (TRH), which stimulates the pituitary to release thyroid stimulating hormone (TSH) (Table 8.8). TSH stimulates the thyroid to release thyroid hormones. When thyroid hormones are high, a negative feedback loop to the pituitary reduces TSH production (Hershman, 2019a).

HYPOTHYROIDISM
Definition
Hypothyroidism refers to thyroid hormone deficiency, resulting in excess TSH and hypometabolism.

Types of Hypothyroidism
- *Primary hypothyroidism* (Hershman, 2019b)
  - The most common cause is autoimmune, Hashimoto thyroiditis.
  - The second most common cause is post-therapeutic hypothyroidism (after partial or total thyroidectomies, treatment with radioactive iodine, and overtreatment with antithyroid agents).
  - Other potential causes are as follows:
    - Treatment with lithium, amiodarone, interferon-alpha, or checkpoint inhibitors
    - Radiation therapy for throat/larynx cancer or Hodgkin's lymphoma
- *Subclinical hypothyroidism*
  - Common in older adults
  - May be asymptomatic or have mild symptoms
  - Treatment is generally started if patient is symptomatic
- *Central hypothyroidism*—Secondary to hypothalamic or pituitary disease (Hershman, 2019b)
  - Results from insufficient TRH production by the hypothalamus or insufficient TSH production by the pituitary gland.

Signs and Symptoms

■ Weight gain	■ Hair loss
■ Cold intolerance	■ Dry skin
■ Paresthesia of extremities	■ Depression
■ Depression	■ Constipation
■ Forgetfulness	■ Amenorrhea

Physical Exam Findings

■ Slowed deep tendon reflex	■ Bradycardia
	■ Hypertension
■ Periorbital swelling	

TABLE 8.8 LABORATORY DIAGNOSTIC CRITERIA OF HORMONE DISORDERS

DISORDER	SERUM TSH	SERUM FREE T4	SERUM T3
Subclinical hypothyroidism	High	Normal	Normal
Primary hypothyroidism	High	Low	Normal or low
Central hypothyroidism	Normal, low, or slightly high	Low	
Subclinical hyperthyroidism	Low	Normal	Normal
Hyperthyroidism	Low	Normal or high	High

TSH, thyroid stimulating hormone.

Diagnosis

■ Diagnosis is made based on laboratory finds and clinical symptoms.

Additional Potential Laboratory Findings

■ In addition to the thyroid hormone abnormalities mentioned previously, patients with hypothyroidism may present with hypercholesteremia, macrocytic anemia, elevated creatinine kinase, and hyponatremia (Weber & Haugen, 2013).

Treatment

The goal of treatment with hypothyroidism is to achieve a euthyroid state using synthetic thyroxine (T4), known as *levothyroxine*. Euthyroid states are determined by laboratory measurement of TSH and resolution of clinical manifestations (Table 8.9).

Prescribing and Management

■ Steady-state TSH concentrations are not achieved for at least 6 weeks.
  ● Serum TSH should be measured at 6 weeks to assess effective therapeutic intervention. If the TSH remains above goal, the dose of T4 can be increased by 12 to 25 mcg/d.
■ When the euglycemic state has been achieved, the serum TSH should be checked at least annually or more often if there is an abnormal result or a change in the patient's status is noted.
■ The goal is to keep TSH within the normal reference range (approximately 0.5–5 mU/L).
■ Increases in dose may be required with
  ● pregnancy,
  ● Weight gain of more than 10% of body weight, or
  ● Diminished thyroid hormone absorption.
■ Decreases in dose may be required with
  ● Normal aging,
  ● Weight loss of roughly more than 10% of body weight, or
  ● Initiation of androgen therapy.

TABLE 8.9 LEVOTHYROXINE TREATMENT

LEVOTHYROXINE*				
BRAND NAME	DOSAGE FORMS	CONTRAINDICATIONS	SIDE EFFECTS	SAFETY/PATIENT EDUCATION
Levothroid Levoxyl Synthroid	Tablet, capsules, powder for injection	Contraindicated in uncorrected adrenal insufficiency	If T4 dose is too high: CVD: cardiac arrhythmia, cardiac failure, flushing, increased blood pressure, increased pulse Nervous system: anxiety, emotional lability, fatigue, headache, heat intolerance, hyperactivity, insomnia	T4 should be taken on an empty stomach with water, ideally an hour before breakfast or 2 hours after dinner at bedtime.
INITIAL DOSING				
Healthy young adults	1.6 mcg/kg/d			
Older adults Adults with: Coronary heart disease	25–50 mcg daily			

*Prohormone that is deiodinated in peripheral tissues to form T3.
CVD, cardiovascular disease.

Hypothyroid Emergency—Myxedema Coma

- Myxedema coma is a life-threatening complication triggered by a combination of long-term untreated hypothyroidism and a precipitating incident such as prolonged exposure to cold, trauma, surgery and/or central nervous system–depressive medications (McDermott, 2013a).

Presentation

- Coma
- Hypothermia
- Seizures
- Respiratory depression
- Bradycardia

Treatment

- IV T4
- Stress dose glucocorticoids
- Treatment of underlying precipitating cause

HYPERTHYROIDISM

Definition

Hyperthyroidism refers to thyroid hormone excess, resulting in low TSH levels and hypermetabolism.

Types of Hyperthyroidism

- *Graves' disease* (Hershman, 2019c)
  - Autoimmune disease; thyroid-stimulating immunoglobulins (TSIs) bind to thyroid receptors and increase production of TSH.
  - Patients with Graves' disease usually also develop the following:
    - Exophthalmos (protrusion of the eye anteriorly)
    - Infiltrative dermopathy (pretibial myoedema): Non-pitting dermatologic manifestation of scaly thickening of the skin with papules or nodules
- *Toxic multinodular goiter (MNG)*
  - Enlarged thyroid (goiter) with multiple nodules (multi-nodular) that autonomously produce extra TSH (toxic)
  - Generally due to an iodine deficiency but is also genetic
- *Thyroiditis (inflammation of thyroid tissue;* Chindris & Smallbridge, 2013)
  - Autoimmune disease caused by antithyroid antibodies, acute infection, or treatment with interferon or amiodarone

Signs and Symptoms

Tachycardia	Heat hypersensitivity
Weight loss	Fatigue
Nervousness	Insomnia

Physical Exam Findings

Hyperactivity	Hair is fine/thin
Rapid speech	Tremors
Eyelid retraction (stare)	Hyperreflexia

Diagnosis

- Laboratory testing
- *Radioactive iodine uptake:* The patient ingests a small radioactive iodine pill. Images are taken 4 to 6 hours after initial ingestion and 24 hours later (McDermott, 2013c)
  - High or normal uptake is indicative of Graves' disease or toxic MNG

- Low or absent uptake is indicative of thyroiditis or iodine overload

Treatment (Hershman, 2019c)

- *Methimazole and propylthiouracil:* Antithyroid drugs that decrease thyroid hormone production.
- *Beta blockers:* Relieve signs and symptoms related to adrenergic stimulation.
- *Radioactive iodine:* Radioactive form of iodine I-131; circulates through the body and is picked up by thyroid cells, causing cell death. Most patients develop hypothyroidism after treatment.
- *Surgery:* Usually reserved for patients who do not respond to antithyroid medications or do not want to undergo I-131 treatment. For a solitary thyroid nodule, a partial (1/2 the glad) thyroidectomy is performed. For Graves' disease or MNG, a near total thyroidectomy is performed.

Hyperthyroid Emergency—Thyroid Storm

- Thyroid storm is a life-threatening complication trigged by long-term untreated hyperthyroidism and a precipitating incident such as infection, surgery, trauma, or preeclampsia (McDermott, 2013a). It occurs in patients with Graves' disease or MNG.

Presentation

- Cardiogenic shock
- Fever
- Restless
- Emotional lability
- Confusion/psychosis
- Nausea, vomiting, diarrhea

Treatment

- *Beta blocker:* Relieves signs and symptoms related to adrenergic stimulation
- Antithyroid medication
- *Iodine:* Used to block the release of thyroid hormone
- Stress-dose glucocorticoids

Thyroid hormone levels in critically ill patients may be low due to a condition called euthyroid sick syndrome related to circulating inflammation mediators. This is thought to be a protective mechanism to reduce tissue metabolism (McDermott, 2013b).

REVIEW QUESTIONS

1. What are the blood glucose level goals for inpatient treatment of diabetes/hyperglycemia?
   A. Premeal: 80 to 130 mg/dL; random <180 mg/dL
   B. 80 to 110 mg/dL
   C. 140 to 180 mg/dL
   D. 100 to 150 mg/dL

2. The clinical nurse specialist (CNS) is assisting a bedside nurse taking care of a patient with diabetic ketoacidosis (DKA) who has been admitted from the ED. The patient is currently on a normal saline intravenous (IV) infusion at 500 mL/hr. The patient complains of fatigue, nausea, vomiting, and abdominal pain. The lab results return and show the following: blood glucose of 325 mg/dL; venous pH of 7.13; CO_2 of 6 mEq/L, and K^+ of 3.1 mEq/L. What is the most appropriate next step?
   A. Start the insulin infusion.
   B. Give 20 mEq K^+ IV over 60 minutes.
   C. Give 40 mEq K^+ PO.
   D. Switch to dextrose 5% in 0.45% saline IV solution.

ANSWERS

1. **Correct answer: C. Rationale:** A range of 140 to 180 mg/dL reflects current guidelines for inpatient treatment of hyperglycemia. Levels of 80 to 130 mg/dL premeal and random <180 mg/dL represent outpatient blood glucose goals. A range of 80 to 110 mg/dL is too tight (narrow) for inpatient hyperglycemia. A range of 100 to 150 mg/dL does not correlate with any of the current guidelines.

2. **Correct answer: B. Rationale:** Potassium needs to be replaced prior to starting the insulin infusion. The serum potassium is too low to start insulin as it will result in severe hypokalemia as insulin pushes potassium intracellularly. Oral potassium is not an appropriate route for a patient with continued nausea and vomiting. Dextrose IV solution should not be initiated until blood glucose levels are <250 mg/dL.

REFERENCES

The complete reference and additional reading lists appear in the digital version of this chapter, accessible at https://connect.springerpub.com/content/book/978-0-8261-7417-8/part/part01/chapter/ch08

Hematopoietic System

Robina Kitzler, Melissa Craft, and Angie Malone

ANEMIA

OVERVIEW

Definition

A reduction in the red blood cell (RBC) volume, the concentration of hemoglobin, or the number of erythrocytes in the blood. As oxygen delivery decreases, tissue hypoxia occurs. Anemia is diagnosed when hemoglobin <13.5 g/dL in men or <12.0 g/dL in women is noted (Camp-Sorrell & Hawkins, 2016; Staff et al., 2016; Yarbro et al., 2018).

Normal Red Blood Cell Production

- Erythropoiesis—Low oxygen stimulates RBC production.
- RBC production triggers release of erythropoietin.
- Erythropoietin activates the bone marrow to produce RBCs.

Pathophysiology

The underlying mechanisms of anemia in patients with cancer are numerous but originate from the following:

- Blood loss
- Inadequate production
- Excessive destruction

Classification of Anemia

Anemia can be divided into three categories based on the size of the RBC (determined by mean corpuscular volume [MCV]; normocytic, microcytic, and macrocytic) and the reticulocyte count (RC). The three categories of anemia are as follows:

- **Low reticulocyte count**: Indicates a state of decreased RBC production. A low MCV indicates that RBCs are small, or **microcytic**. Possible causes include iron-deficiency anemia (most common), anemia of chronic disease, B_{12} deficiency, or folate deficiency.
- **Normal reticulocyte count**: Anemia with a normal MCV is known as *normocytic anemia*. Possible causes include blood loss, kidney failure, hemolytic anemia, bone marrow failure, nutritional deficiencies, drug induced, and transfusion reaction.
- **High reticulocyte count**: A high MCV indicates that the RBCs are larger than normal, or **macrocytic**. Possible causes include vitamin B_{12} deficiency, megaloblastic anemia (both vitamin B_{12} and folate deficiency), liver disease, alcoholism, hypothyroidism, chemotherapy drugs, and retroviral therapies for HIV. See Table 9.1 for anemia types and causes.

Symptoms

- Shortness of breath
- Constipation
- Dizziness when moving from a sitting to a standing position
- Irritability

TABLE 9.1 ANEMIA TYPES AND CAUSES

ANEMIA TYPE	CAUSE
Iron-deficiency anemia	Most common form. Usually due to blood loss but occasionally due to poor absorption of iron.
Vitamin-deficiency anemia	May result from low levels of vitamin B_{12} or folate (folic acid). Pernicious anemia is a condition in which the vitamin cannot be absorbed in the GI tract.
Aplastic anemia	Bone marrow failure disorder. Bone marrow stops making enough blood cells, due to destruction or deficiency of blood-forming stem cells.
Hemolytic anemia	Occurs when RBCs are broken up in the bloodstream or spleen. May occur due to heart valve issues, infections, autoimmune diseases, thalassemia, or glucose-6 phosphate dehydrogenase deficiency.
Sickle cell	An inherited hemolytic anemia in which the hemoglobin protein is abnormal, causing the RBCs to be rigid and obstruct the circulation.
Anemias caused by other diseases	Renal disease results from insufficiency of erythropoietin; chemotherapy.

GI, gastrointestinal; RBC, red blood cell.

- Headache
- Hypotension
- Tachycardia
- Fatigue
- Pale skin
- Sores in the mouth
- Edema in the legs or feet
- Decreased bowel sounds/paralytic ileus
- Shortness of breath
- Spleen enlargement
- Chest pain/angina

Diagnostic Testing
- Complete blood count (CBC)

Management

- Treat underlying cause
- RBC transfusion for hemoglobin <8 g/dL, active bleeding, or symptomatic anemia
- Erythropoietin administration
- Iron supplements

See Table 9.2 for anemia grade and severity and Table 9.3 for anemias related to disease treatment.

TABLE 9.2 ANEMIA GRADE AND SEVERITY

HEMOGLOBIN (G/DL)	GRADE	SEVERITY
WNL	0	Normal
WNL–10	1	Mild
<10–8	2	Moderate
<8–6.5	3	Severe
<6.5	4	Life-threatening

WNL, within normal limits.

TABLE 9.3 ANEMIAS RELATED TO DISEASE OR TREATMENT

DISEASE RELATED	TREATMENT RELATED
<ul><li>GI bleed, varices</li><li>Tumor infiltration, primary cancers of the bone marrow</li><li>Acute renal failure, chronic renal failure, hemolysis</li></ul>	<ul><li>Chemotherapy: Destroys rapidly dividing hematopoietic cells</li><li>Radiation: Destroys RBC precursors in the field</li><li>Nephrotoxic agents</li><li>Drugs that inhibit RBC production</li></ul>

GI, gastrointestinal; RBC, red blood cell.

OVERVIEW OF COAGULOPATHIES OF CANCER

VENOUS THROMBOEMBOLISM

Venous thromboembolism (VTE) is a blood clot that begins in a vein (Figure 9.1). It is associated with high mortality and morbidity in patients with cancer, who are at greater risk for VTE and bleeding complications associated with anticoagulation treatment when compared to patients without cancer. Increased risk for VTE is related to the thrombophilia of malignancy and the nature of certain cancer treatments. The management of anticoagulation treatment in patients with cancer presents the unique challenge of managing drug interactions with chemotherapeutic agents (Linden et al., 2012).

The two types of VTE are as follows:

- Deep vein thrombosis (DVT): See Chapter 6.
- Pulmonary embolism (PE): See Chapter 7.

DISSEMINATED INTRAVASCULAR COAGULATION

Definition

Disseminated intravascular coagulation (DIC) is an oncological emergency characterized by overstimulation of normal coagulation that causes a paradoxical disorder of diffuse clotting and profuse hemorrhage (Figure 9.2). In patients undergoing treatment for cancer, specific malignancies and treatment modalities can place a patient at a higher risk for DIC. There are two types: acute and chronic. Acute malignancy occurs over hours or days.

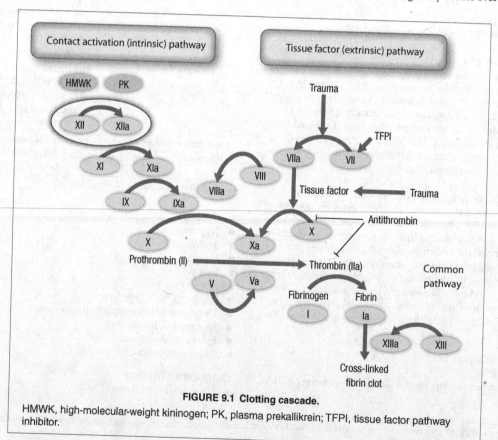

FIGURE 9.1 Clotting cascade.

HMWK, high-molecular-weight kininogen; PK, plasma prekallikrein; TFPI, tissue factor pathway inhibitor.

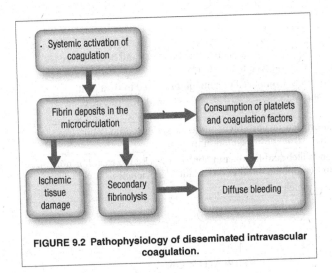

FIGURE 9.2 Pathophysiology of disseminated intravascular coagulation.

Chronic malignancy causes excess clotting but usually doesn't lead to bleeding.

Etiology
Cancer is the most common cause of chronic DIC. The most common clinical condition associated with DIC is sepsis.

Pathophysiology

- Tissue damage
- Clotting stimulated
- Initial microvascular thrombi
- Fibrinolytic mediators released
- Hematopoietic pandemonium (chaos)
- Lysis of all clots
- Ability to clot is lost
- Bleeding starts

Assessment
- Bleeding is usually the first and most obvious sign: oozing from body orifices, surgical wounds, and/or venipuncture sites; gingival bleeding; epistaxis; hemoptysis; blood in urine or stool; vaginal bleeding; petechiae.

TABLE 9.4 LABORATORY FINDINGS IN DISSEMINATED INTRA-VASCULAR COAGULATION

TEST	ELEVATED	DECREASED
Hemoglobin		X
Hematocrit		X
Platelets		X
PT	X	
Fibrinogen		X
Fibrin degradation products, FSP	X	
D-dimer	X	
Partial thromboplastin time	X	

FSP, fibrin split products; PT, prothrombin time.

- Intracranial, gastrointestinal (GI), pleural, and pericardial bleeding can occur in extreme cases.
- Assessment data includes analysis of laboratory studies as outlined in Table 9.4.

Treatment of Disseminated Intravascular Coagulation

- Supportive treatment of primary problem
- Early recognition
- Decrease bleeding risk
- Treat pain
- Transfusion
- Vitamin K
- Heparin
- General management

MANAGEMENT OF PATIENTS RECEIVING BLOOD AND BLOOD PRODUCTS

INDICATIONS
Transfusion therapy is an integral part of cancer therapy. Patients with a history of transfusion reaction may require premedication at the discretion of the provider. Premedication should be administered 30 minutes prior to initiation of blood transfusion (Tables 9.5–9.8; Camp-Sorrell & Hawkins, 2016; Staff et al., 2016; Watkins et al., 2015; Yarbro et al., 2018).

TABLE 9.5 TRANSFUSION PREMEDICATION

REACTION	PREMEDICATION
Mild allergic reaction (hives to platelets)	Antipyretics
Mild allergic reaction (hives to platelets)	Antihistamines
More severe allergic reactions	Steroids can be considered

TABLE 9.6 ABO COMPATIBILITY

PATIENT ABO GROUP	DONOR Red Blood Cells	DONOR Plasma	DONOR Platelets
O	O	O A B AB	O A B AB
A	A O	A AB	O A B AB
B	B O	B AB	O A B AB
AB	AB A B O	AB	O A B AB

TABLE 9.7 TYPES OF TRANSFUSIONS AND INDICATIONS

BLOOD PRODUCT	INDICATIONS
Fresh whole blood	More common in disaster settings, where blood components may be scarce and hemorrhage is common. Composed of RBCs, plasma, cryoprecipitate, and platelets.
Packed red blood cells	Most commonly transfused of all products. Composed of hemoglobin. Used to treat acute and chronic anemias that are not caused by deficiencies in iron, vitamin B_{12}, folic acid, or erythropoietin.
Fresh frozen plasma	Contains albumin multiple coagulation factors, fibrinolytic proteins, and immunoglobin. Used for massive hemorrhage or complications from anticoagulation therapy.
Cryoprecipitate	Contains factor VIII, fibrinogen, von Willebrand factor, and fibronectin. Used to treat fibrinogen deficiency and control bleeding in hemophilia or other coagulation deficiencies.
Platelets	Used for low platelet counts or to treat platelet dysfunction.

RBC, red blood cell.

TABLE 9.8 POTENTIAL COMPLICATIONS OF BLOOD TRANSFUSION

COMPLICATION	TIME	SYMPTOMS	EXPLANATION
Acute hemolytic transfusion reaction	Immediately, or within 24 hours	<ul><li>Increased temperature</li><li>Increased HR</li><li>Chills</li><li>Dyspnea</li><li>Chest or back pain</li><li>Abnormal bleeding or shock</li><li>Hemoglobinuria</li><li>Epistasis</li><li>Oliguria or anuria</li><li>DIC</li><li>Pain or oozing at IV site</li></ul>	Follow the protocol for any acute transfusion reaction:<ul><li>Stop the transfusion.</li><li>Notify provider.</li><li>Send the blood to blood bank.</li><li>Maintain a patent IV line.</li><li>Reassess patient every 5–15 minutes. Observe for signs of coagulopathy and renal failure.</li></ul>
Febrile nonhemolytic transfusion reaction	Usually occurs during or shortly after transfusion	Unexplained rise in temperature of 1 °C (1.8 °F)	Relatively common; may treat with antipyretics.
Allergic and anaphylactic reaction	Usually occurs within 4 hours	Ranges from mild urticaria or wheezing responsive to antihistamines to severe systemic reactions including bronchospasm, hypotension, and tachycardia	Occurs most often with plasma-containing components. Treatment includes supportive care with antihistamines, epinephrine, and, if needed, BP and ventilatory support.
TACO	Usually occurs within 6 hours of transfusion	New onset or exacerbation of at least three of the following:<ul><li>Acute respiratory distress</li><li>Elevated BNP</li><li>Elevated CVP</li><li>Positive fluid balance</li><li>L-sided heart failure</li><li>Pulmonary edema</li></ul>	Life-threatening; close monitoring, supplemental oxygen, nitrates, and noninvasive positive PEEP ventilation needed. At-risk patients should receive blood products at a slow rate.
TRALI	Usually occurs within 6 hours of blood transfusion	Acute onset of the following:<ul><li>Respiratory distress</li><li>Hypoxemia</li><li>Noncardiogenic pulmonary edema</li></ul>May also have the following:<ul><li>Fever</li><li>Tachycardia</li><li>Hypothermia</li><li>Hypotension</li></ul>	Usually self-limiting; treatment includes aggressive respiratory support and possible diuretics, fluid restriction, and extracorporeal membrane oxygenation.
Delayed hemolytic reaction	Can occur days to weeks after transfusion	<ul><li>Low-grade fever</li><li>Mild jaundice</li><li>Low hemoglobin levels</li><li>Elevated lactate dehydrogenase</li></ul>	Direct antiglobulin testing may be positive. In the absence of active hemolysis, no treatment is required.

(continued)

TABLE 9.8 POTENTIAL COMPLICATIONS OF BLOOD TRANSFUSION (*continued*)

COMPLICATION	TIME	SYMPTOMS	EXPLANATION
TA-GVHD	Occurs within 2 weeks of transfusion	■ Fever ■ Rash ■ Diarrhea	Occurs primarily in immunocompromised patients receiving allogenic stem cell transplants. Often fatal. May be prevented by irradiating donor lymphocytes prior to transfusion.
Posttransfusion purpura	May occur 1–3 weeks after transfusion	Thrombocytopenia	Often resolves itself. Patients at risk for bleeding are treated with IV immunoglobins, plasmapheresis, or platelet transfusion.

BNP, brain natriuretic peptide; CVP, central venous pressure; DIC, disseminated intravascular coagulation; HR, heart rate; PEEP, positive end-expiratory pressure; TACO, transfusion-associated circulatory overload; TA-GVHD, transfusion-associated graft versus host disease; TRALI, transfusion-related acute lung injury.

MYELOSUPPRESSION

OVERVIEW
Definition
Myelosuppression is a reduction in the functional ability of the bone marrow, reducing the production and maturation of RBCs, white cells, and platelets. *Myelosuppression* refers to a process that disrupts stem cells and results in **leukopenia, thrombocythemia,** and **anemia.** Greater than 50% of patients with cancer experience myelosuppression. Myeloablation is a severe form of myelosuppression in which no blood cells are made.

Pathophysiology
Suppression of bone marrow secondary to malignancy
■ Dysfunction of cells in bone marrow
■ Infiltration of marrow from tumor cells
■ Depletion of marrow reserves

Manifestation
■ WBC/neutrophils (leukopenia/neutropenia)
■ RBC/erythrocytes (anemia)
■ Platelets (thrombocytopenia)
■ In all three counts (pancytopenia)

Prolonged myelosuppression leads to:
■ Infection
■ Bleeding
■ Fatigue
■ Cardiopulmonary distress

LEUKOPENIA
Definition
Leukopenia is a deficiency in white blood cells (WBCs) carrying the resultant potential increased risk for infection. The major types of circulating WBCs are basophils, eosinophils, lymphocytes (T cells and B cells), monocytes, and neutrophils. **Neutrophils** are the first line of defense against infections caused by bacteria, viruses, fungi, and cancer cells.

Etiology
Cancer, Chemotherapy, and Radiation
■ Chemotherapy-induced bone marrow suppression. Chemotherapy kills off rapidly dividing cells.
■ Cancers of the bone marrow such as leukemias, lymphomas, myeloma, and metastatic cancer to the bone marrow.
■ Deliberate myelosuppression/myeloablation in preparation for a bone marrow transplant or peripheral blood stem cell transplant (Table 9.9; Camp-Sorrell & Hawkins, 2016; Staff et al., 2016; Watkins et al., 2015; Yarbro et al., 2018)

Risk Factors

■ Age >65 years	■ Gastrointestinal disorders
■ Poor nutrition	■ Liver disease
■ Autoimmune disorders	■ Hematologic disorder
■ Diabetes mellitus	

NEUTROPENIA
Definition
Indicates a decreased number of circulating neutrophils.

Pathophysiology
The bone marrow constantly produces neutrophils in a healthy person. The normal life span of a neutrophil is 7 to 12 days. Cytotoxic agents suppress bone marrow and damage stem cells. As a result, the neutrophil count decreases as mature neutrophils die and cannot be replaced.

■ First line of defense against bacterial infection
■ Normal range 2,500 to 6,000 cells/mm^3
■ Of total WBCs, 50% to 60% of total WBC's are neutrophils (Table 9.10)

WBC, white blood cell.

The **absolute neutrophil count (ANC)** is determined by the product of the WBC count and the fraction of neutrophils among the WBCs as determined by the WBC differential analysis (Table 9.11).

(% neutrophils + % of bands) × (WBC)

Risk Factors

■ Older clients >65	■ Advanced cancer
■ Comorbidities such as diabetes and congestive obstructive pulmonary disease	■ Leukemia and lymphoma
	■ Specific chemotherapeutic agents
■ Poor nutrition	■ Concurrent radiation to marrow producing bones
■ Bone marrow involvement in disease	

FEBRILE NEUTROPENIA
Definition
Single temperature greater than 38.3°C or 38°C for more than 1 hour, and an ANC of <500 or a predicted decline to <1,000 in the next 48 hours.

TABLE 9.9 CYTOPENIA

MECHANISM OF CYTOPENIA	DIAGNOSIS	CYTOPENIA	OTHER BLOOD TESTS	BONE MARROW FINDINGS
Myelosuppression	Aplastic anemia	Pancytopenia	Reticulocytopenia	Marked hypocellularity
	Pure red cell aplasia	Anemia, normal WBC, and platelets	Reticulocytopenia	Cellular, absent erythropoiesis
	Megaloblastic anemia	Anemia, sometimes leucopenia, thrombocytopenia	Macrocytosis, reticulocytopenia	Hypercellular, megaloblastic erythropoiesis
	Sideroblastic anemia	Anemia	Reticulocytopenia	Cellular, ring sideroblasts prominent
Myelosuppression or peripheral cell destruction	Agranulocytosis	Severe neutropenia, rapid onset	Normal Hb, platelets	Variable granulocyte representation, absent neutrophils
	Autoimmune neutropenia	Neutropenia, slower onset	Normal Hb, platelets	Left-shifted granulocyte maturation
Peripheral cell destruction	Autoimmune hemolytic anemia	Anemia	Reticulocytosis, hyperbilirubinemia, positive direct antiglobulin (Coombs) test	Hypercellular, erythroid hyperplasia
	Immune thrombocytopenia	Thrombocytopenia	Normal Hb, WBC	Cellular, abundant megakaryocytes

Hb, hemoglobin level; WBC, white blood cell count.

Source: From Carey, P. J. (2003). Drug-induced myelosuppression. *Drug Safety, 26*, 691–706. https://doi .org/10.2165/00002018-200326100-00003

TABLE 9.10 WHITE BLOOD CELL COUNT AND DIFFERENTIAL

WBC TYPE	RELATIVE VALUE (%)	ABSOLUTE VALUE (MM^2)
Neutrophils (total)	50–70	2,500–7,000
Polys	50–65	2,500–6,000
Bands	0.5	0–500
Eosinophils	0–5	0–500
Basophils	0.4–1	100–300
Monocytes	4–6	200–600
Lymphocytes	25–35	1,700–3,500

WBC, white blood cell.

TABLE 9.11 ABSOLUTE NEUTROPHIL COUNT INTERPRETATION

ANC CALCULATION RESULT	INTERPRETATION OF RESULTS
>1,500/mm^3	Normal ANC
1,000–1,500/mm^3	Minimal increased risk of infection
750–1,000/mm^3	Moderate increased risk of infection
500–750/mm^3	Severe risk of infection
<500/mm^3	Severe risk of overwhelming infection

ANC, absolute neutrophil count.

Consequences of Neutropenia

- Increased risk of mortality
- Sepsis is lethal in 47% of patients with ANC <1,000
- Chemotherapy dose reductions or delays
- Decrease in overall cancer survival rates
- Impaired quality of life
- Hospitalization

ANC, absolute neutrophil count.

Chemotherapy Regimens With High Risk of Febrile Neutropenia

- Breast: Dose dense AC-T, TAC, A taxotere
- Small cell lung: Topotecan
- Sarcoma: MAID
- Bladder: MVAC
- Esophagus: DOC/cisplatin/5FU (flurouacil)

DOC docetaxel; 5FU, flurouacil.

Management of Neutropenia

- Obvious signs may not be present
- Fever may be the only symptom
- Look for trends in lab values
- Know nadir* times
- Calculate ANC
- CBC with differential and CMP
- Blood cultures
- Chest X-ray (pneumonia)
- Colony-stimulating factors
- Broad spectrum antibiotic coverage
- Antifungals
- Growth factors
- Corticosteroid therapy

*Point at which WBC counts are likely to be at their lowest, approximately 7 to 12 days after treatment.

ANC, absolute neutrophil count; CBC, complete blood count; CMP.

Neutropenic Precautions

■ Frequent handwashing ■ CSF ■ Antibiotic prophylaxis if appropriate ■ Avoid exposure to infectious situations ■ Avoid ill individuals	■ Restrict fruits and vegetables in diet and fresh flowers ■ Avoid those recently vaccinated with live vaccine ■ Use caution with pet care ■ Flu shot to prevent communicable infection

CSF, colony-stimulating factors.

Patient Education

■ Daily temperature
■ Report temperature elevations
■ Report chills, redness, or edema in any body area, including IV sites

THROMBOCYTOPENIA

Definition

Decrease in number of circulating platelets, below 100,000 (Table 9.12). Normal platelet count is 150,000 to 400,000 per microliter of blood. Life span of platelets is 8 to 10 days.

Causes of Thrombocytopenia in Malignancy

Disease-related causes
■ Idiopathic
■ Hypocoagulation disorders
■ Hypercoagulation disorders
■ Invasion of malignant cells into the bone marrow
■ Malignancy involving the bone marrow
Treatment-related causes
■ Chemotherapy
■ Radiation
■ Medications: Aspirin, heparin, dilantin, Bactrim (sulfamethoxazole/trimethoprim)

Symptoms of Thrombocytopenia

■ Bleeding from rectum, nose, oral cavity
■ Petechiae
■ Conjunctival hemorrhage
■ Ecchymosis, purpura
■ Blood in urine, stool, vomitus
■ Very heavy menstrual period

Assessment

Lab values: Platelet count and coagulation values

TABLE 9.12 THROMBOCYTOPENIA GRADE AND RISK OF BLEEDING

PLATELET COUNT	GRADE	RISK OF BLEEDING
WNL	0	No risk
WNL–75,000/mm^3	1	No significant risk
<75,000–50,000/mm^3	2	Minimal risk
<50,000–25,000/mm^3	3	Moderate risk
<25,000/mm^3	4	Severe risk

mm^3 = 1 mm × 1 mm × 1 mm = microliter of blood.

WNL, within normal limits.

Management of Thrombocytopenia

■ Consider transfusing if actively bleeding and/or going for an invasive procedure.
■ Platelet transfusion: Usually transfuse when platelets <10,000 cells/mm^3.
■ One unit of platelets should increase the platelet count by 10,000 mm^3.
  ● Hormonal agents (menstrual bleeding).
  ● Avoid constipation laxatives, stool softeners.
  ● Minimize occurrence of bleeding.

CANCER

OVERVIEW

Cancer is defined as a group of malignant diseases, exhibiting a multitude of characteristics, caused by genetic alterations and defective cell function (Eggert, 2010). Cancers are classified according to the tissue or cell from which they originate. Cancer cells have the following characteristics, which allow them to survive and grow (Eggert, 2010):
■ Abnormal cell proliferation caused by cellular or genetic alterations
■ Lack of controlled growth or cell division
■ Ability to spread or metastasize to distant sites and establish secondary tumors
■ Ability to involve any tissue of the body and evade programmed cell death (apoptosis)

Risk Factors

■ *Extrinsic:* Exposure to radiation and/or chemicals and viruses/bacteria
■ *Intrinsic:* Hereditary, dietary, and hormones

Cell Cycle

The *cell cycle* refers to the interval between each cell division and causes cells to repair, rest and replicate. There are two main checkpoints in the cell cycle that allow for defects in DNA to be repaired (G1-S, G2-M; Eggert, 2010; Temple, 2016). Inhibitory proteins, such as p53, prevent the progression of the cell cycle when damage is detected. *Example*: p53 Inhibitory protein p53 will arrest the cell cycle and cause apoptosis.

The five-stage cell cycle process plays an important role in the development of cancer. Many events need to occur for a normal cell to transform into a cancer cell, and these events occur in different phases of the cell cycle (Eggert, 2010).
Five-Stage Process (Temple, 2016)
■ G0 (resting phase)
■ G1 (postmitotic phase)
■ S (synthesis)
■ G2 (premitotic phase)
■ M (mitosis)

Cell Cycle Time

This is the amount of time required for a cell to move from one mitosis phase to the next (Temple, 2016):
■ Length of time depends on type of cell.
■ Shorter cell cycle time equals higher cell kill when exposed to cytotoxic cell cycle-specific agents.
■ Continuous infusion of cytotoxic cell cycle–specific agents results in greater number of cells exposed and a higher cell kill for tumors that have a shorter cell cycle time.

Growth Fraction

The percentage of cells that are actively dividing at any point in time (Temple, 2016):

- Higher growth fraction will result in a higher cell kill when exposed to cytotoxic cell cycle–specific agents.
- Greater fraction of cells in G0 phase have higher sensitivity to cytotoxic cell cycle–specific agents.

Tumor Burden

The amount or volume of cancer that is present (Temple, 2016):

- Small tumor burden results in more sensitivity to antineoplastic agents.
- If the tumor is large or there is a large volume of cancerous cells, the tumor will grow at a slower rate and there will be fewer cells dividing. Cancer is a condition of rapidly dividing mutated cells, the division of cells is decreased when there is a larger volume of tumor present.
- Higher tumor burden increases the likelihood of drug resistance.

APPROACHES TO CANCER TREATMENT

Single-Agent Therapy

- Single agent used for treatment (Polovich et al., 2014; Temple, 2016).
- Agents have a proven efficacy when given alone.
- Side effect profile is identified and can be predicted.

Combination Therapy

- Use of multiple agents for treatment of cancer.
- Creates more exposure of the cancer cells.
- Results in higher tumor cancer cell kill.
- Typically uses agents with different mechanism of actions; this increases proportion of cells destroyed at a time.
- Uses principle of synergy or maximizing the effects of another drug.
- Rate of tumor cell proliferation and timing of the drug administration can impact the synergy. One drug potentiates the cytotoxic effects of another drug.
- Allows access to sanctuary sites in the body where tumors may reside
- When possible, avoid using drugs with similar toxicities (Polovich et al., 2014; Temple, 2016)

Criteria for Selecting Agents for Combination Therapy

- Demonstration of cytotoxic activity when used alone to treat specific cancer
- Different, nonoverlapping toxicities
- Toxicities occur at different points of time after treatment
- Biologic effect that can enhances cytotoxicity (Temple, 2016)

Regional Therapy

Delivers doses of antineoplastic agents to specific sites of tumor and reduces the intensity of systemic toxicity (Polovich et al., 2014; Temple, 2016).

- Liver
- Bladder
- Peritoneal cavity
- Pleural space

High-Dose Therapy

This is the use of high doses of chemotherapy to achieve a cure or enduring response (Polovich et al., 2014). Supportive therapy, such as CSF, antidotes, and transfusion, is required due to the severity of toxicities, such as myelosuppression. Other toxicities that can occur with high-dose treatment include cardiotoxicity and cerebellar toxicity (Polovich et al., 2016).

Factors Influencing Response to Treatment

- Location
- Tumor burden (size)
- Growth rate
- Resistance to drug therapy
- Ratio of sensitivity of malignant cells and normal cells affected
- Molecular characteristics or hormonal status
- Adequate blood supply with adequate drug uptake (Temple, 2016)

CANCER TREATMENT OPTIONS

ANTINEOPLASTICS

Antineoplastics are a specialized high-alert group of medications used in the treatment of cancer. They are considered high risk due to the very narrow therapeutic range between maximum benefit and severe side effects, with a high potential for serious and life-threatening toxicities (Gaguski & Karcheski, 2011).

Antineoplastic medications are also known as *cytotoxic chemotherapy*, a systemic treatment that circulates throughout the body. This therapy results in increased cancer cell kill throughout the body by treating circulating cells and cells growing in multiple sites. Cell damage depends on the type of antineoplastic agent used. This therapy attacks not only the cancer cells but normal cells as well, which in turn creates side effects. Cellular replication is prevented by interfering with DNA, RNA, and vital cellular proteins.

Goals of Therapy

- *Cure*: Absence of disease
- *Control*: No further growth of tumor
- *Palliation*: Focus is quality of life and comfort; approach is to shrink tumor to provide symptom relief

Dosing

Antineoplastics have a narrow therapeutic index and wide interindividual variability (Gaguski & Karcheski, 2011). It is important to have safety efforts in place to ensure accurate dosing and reduce harm. Safety efforts include structured processes for ordering, independent check of indications and dosing, and review and recording of laboratory values.

Factors for Appropriate Dosing

- Actual accurate height and weight
- Type of dosing
- Pharmacokinetics
- Patient age and gender
- Genotyping and phenotyping (Gaguski & Karcheski, 2011)

Types of Dosing

- Fixed doses
  - Set dose in milligrams
- Weight-based doses
  - Amount of drug is based on body weight, mg/kg
- It is important to have accurate and current height and weight; current weight should be assessed on day of treatment
- Body surface area (BSA) doses
  - Applicable to a majority of IV-infused chemotherapies and/or biotherapies
  - BSA represents total area of body covered by skin (mg/m²).

- Area under the curve (AUC) doses
  - Primarily used for carboplatin dosing
  - The amount of drug concentration in the blood over a specific amount of time
  - Renal function is part of the calculation; drug clearance of carboplatin is associated with renal function
  - Calvert formula used to determine estimated creatinine clearance

Classification of Antineoplastic Agents

Agents are classified according to the pharmacologic action, mechanism of action, biochemical structure, and physiologic action of the drug (Polovich, 2014). There are two main points of classification for these agents based on the phase of the cell cycle during which they are most effective. These are referred to as *cell cycle-specific* and *cell cycle- nonspecific agents*.

Cell Cycle-Specific Agents
- Exert their maximum effect in a specific phase of cell cycle.

Cell Cycle-Nonspecific Agents
- Exert their maximum effect in all phases of cell cycle, including resting phase.

  See Table 9.13 for specific details and characteristics of cell cycle-specific and cell cycle-nonspecific antineoplastic agents.

Drug Classes of Antineoplastic Agents

See Table 9.14 for drug classes of antineoplastic agents.

Alkylating Agents

Alkylating agents are most active in the resting phase and are considered cell cycle nonspecific. There are dose-limiting toxicities associated with this class of drugs, specifically oxaliplatin (Wilkes, 2009). Oxaliplatin can induce an uncommon manifestation known as *pharyngolaryngeal dysesthesia*, which can be very frightening for the patient (Wilkes, 2009). This is a condition in which the patient experiences a sense that no air is moving into the lungs. Assessment is key to rule out a hypersensitivity reaction.

TABLE 9.13 CHARACTERISTICS OF CELL CYCLE–SPECIFIC/ NONSPECIFIC AGENTS

CELL CYCLE–SPECIFIC AGENTS	CELL CYCLE–NONSPECIFIC AGENTS
The greatest tumor kill occurs when given in divided doses or as continuous infusion with short cycle time.	Exert greatest effects in all phases of the cell cycle including the resting phase.
Allow for maximum number of cells to be exposed to the drug at a specific time in their life cycle.	Agents are effective in treating tumors with fewer and/ or slower dividing cells.
Act on rapidly growing and dividing cells. Patients receiving these drugs should be on a regular schedule of treatment.	Agents are dose dependent and most effective when administered by bolus doses. The cell kill is directly proportional to the amount of drug that is administered.
Cytotoxic effects occur during cell cycle and are expressed when the cell repair or division is attempted.	When the cancer is sensitive to the drug administered, then that drug is incorporated into the cell.
	Cell kill may not be instant but rather when the cells try to divide.

Sources: Adapted from Polovich, M., Olsen, M., & LeFebvre, K. B. (2014). Principles of biotherapy. In *Chemotherapy and biotherapy guidelines and recommendations for practice* (5th ed., pp. 51–96). Oncology Nursing Society; Wilkes, G. M. (2009). Chemotherapy and biotherapy. In B. H. Gobel, S. Triest-Robertson, & W. H. Vogel (Eds.), *Advanced oncology nursing certification review and resource manual* (pp. 149–185). Oncology Nursing Society.

TABLE 9.14 DRUG CLASSES OF ANTINEOPLASTIC AGENTS

CLASSIFICATION	DRUGS	INDICATIONS	MECHANISM OF ACTION
Alkylating agents (nitrosoureas, nitrogen mustards)	Cyclophosphamide Dacarbazine Ifosfamide Mechlorethamine Melphalan Oxaliplatin Temozolomide Thiotepa	Leukemia Lymphoma Hodgkin's disease Multiple myeloma Sarcoma Lung Breast Ovarian	Interferes with DNA replication through cross-linking DNA strands, breaking DNA strands, and abnormal base pairing of proteins.
Antimetabolites (folic acid antagonists, pyrimidine analogs, guanosine analogs)	Methotrexate 5-Fluorouracil Cytarabine Nelarabine	Leukemia Breast Ovarian Intestinal tract Pancreatic	Inhibits protein synthesis, substitutes erroneous metabolites or structural analogues during DNA synthesis, and inhibits DNA synthesis.
Antitumor antibiotics (anthracyclines, alkylating like, miscellaneous)	Daunorubicin Doxorubicin Idarubicin Mitomycin Dactinomycin Bleomycin	AML ALL NHL Solid tumors of every major organ	Inhibits DNA and RNA synthesis.

(continued)

TABLE 9.14 DRUG CLASSES OF ANTINEOPLASTIC AGENTS (continued)

CLASSIFICATION	DRUGS	INDICATIONS	MECHANISM OF ACTION
Plant alkaloids (epipodo-phyllotoxins, camptoth-ecins, taxanes, and vinca alkaloids)	Docetaxel Paclitaxel Etoposide Irinotecan Topotecan Vincristine Vinblastine Vinorelbine	Lung Breast Ovarian Prostate colorectal Testicular cervical	Acts late in the G2 and S phases as well as in the M phase, interferes with topoisomerase II enzymes; stabilizes microtubules and inhibits cell division.
Miscellaneous (platinum compounds)	Carboplatin Cisplatin Oxaliplatin	ALL Renal cell carcinoma Breast Melanoma Ovarian	Inhibits protein synthesis; Acts as an antimetabolite in the S phase; inhibits protein, RNA, and DNA synthesis.

ALL, acute lymphoblastic leukemia; AML, acute myeloid leukemia; NHL, non-Hodgkin's lymphoma.

Antimetabolites

Antimetabolite drugs are very similar to normal substances used within the cell for DNA and RNA synthesis (www.chemocare.com/chemotherapy). This class of drugs was one of the first effective antineoplastic agents discovered; these drugs areclassified according to the substance they interfere with (www.chemoth.com/types/antimetabolites). These classifications are folic acid antagonist, pyrimidine antagonist, and purine antagonist. Pyrimidine and purine are the building blocks for DNA and RNA synthesis within the cell. Antimetabolites work most effectively in the S phase of the cell cycle.

Antitumor Antibiotics

Antitumor antibiotics are made from natural products that are produced by species in the soil fungus, namely, *Streptomyces* (https://chemoth.com/types/antimetabolites). Drugs in this class are considered vesicants (drugs that cause tissue damage when extravasated), except for bleomycin (Wilkes, 2009). They are considered cell cycle specific, with the exception of bleomycin, which is the only drug that works in a specific phase of the cycle.

Plant Alkaloids

Plant alkaloids are cell cycle–specific drugs that are derived from certain types of plants. There are several subcategories, which include vinca alkaloids (made from periwinkle plant), taxanes (made from the bark of Pacific Yew tree), and camptothecins (www.chemocare.com/chemotherapy). Antimicrotubule agents, such as vinca alkaloids and taxanes, work by stabilizing the microtubules in cells, which prevents transition into the M phase, and thus blocking cell division. Vinca alkaloids are considered fatal if given intrathecally, and taxanes have potential to cause cardiotoxicity.

Miscellaneous

These agents have various actions dependent upon the drug. Some drugs in this category act as an antimetabolite and work in the S phase of the cell cycle. These drugs also inhibit protein, DNA, and RNA synthesis and can in some cases trigger apoptosis (Wilkes & Barton-Burke, 2014). A few drugs in this class include procarbazine, hydroxyurea, asparaginase, and arsenic trioxide (Wilkes, 2014).

Common Toxicities

Drug toxicity remains one of the most significant problems associated with cancer chemotherapy. The most common toxicities affecting specific body systems are noted in Table 9.15.

TABLE 9.15 COMMON TOXICITIES OF ANTINEOPLASTIC AGENTS BY BODY SYSTEM

BODY SYSTEM	COMMON TOXICITIES	
Hematopoietic	Neutropenia Thrombocytopenia	Anemia
Gastrointestinal	Anorexia Nausea/vomiting Mucositis Stomatitis	Diarrhea Constipation Pancreatitis Hepatic toxicity
Integumentary	Dermatitis Hyperpigmentation Alopecia Nail changes	Radiation recall Photosensitivity Rash, urticaria
Genitourinary	Cystitis Hemorrhagic cystitis	Acute renal failure Chronic renal insufficiency
Cardiovascular	Decreased ejection fraction Altered cardiac conduction Angina	Phlebitis Extravasation Venous fibrosis
Neurologic	Cerebellar or central neurotoxicity Ototoxicity	Metabolic encephalopathy Peripheral neuropathy
Pulmonary	Fibrosis Pneumonitis	Edema
Reproductive	Infertility Changes in libido Erectile dysfunction	Dyspareunia Amenorrhea
Mood alterations	Anxiety Depression	Euphoria
Metabolic alterations	Hypocalcemia Hypercalcemia Hypoglycemia Hyperglycemia Hyperphosphatemia	Hyperuricemia Hypokalemia Hyperkalemia Hypomagnesemia
Latent effects	Cognitive dysfunction Learning disabilities	Changes in memory
Secondary malignancies	Varies with agent used	
Other	Hypersensitivity Fatigue	Ocular toxicity

MANAGEMENT OF PATIENTS WITH CANCER TREATMENT SYMPTOMS

ANOREXIA
Definition
Loss of appetite accompanied by decreased food intake. Symptoms include weight loss, weakness, and fatigue.

Etiology
- Nausea/vomiting
- Early satiety, dysphagia, mucositis, ascites, taste changes
- Side effects of medications
- Electrolyte disturbances
- Anxiety, fear, depression
- Loss of pleasure of eating

Management
- Early detection and ongoing evaluation of nutritional state
- Correct underlying cause
- Nutritional supplements

Interventions
- Consume nutritionally dense foods: puddings, cottage cheese, mashed potatoes
- Small frequent meals
- Maximize food preferences and favorite foods
- Vitamin supplements, megace, corticosteroids
- Oral care
- Pleasant environment

MUCOSITIS
Definition
Mucositis is a general term describing painful inflammation and ulceration of the mucous membranes lining the digestive tract. Mucositis can occur anywhere along the GI tract, from the mouth to the rectum, and is associated with chemotherapy and radiation treatment. Symptoms include pain, dysphagia, and diarrhea. The ulcerative lesions produced by mucotoxic chemoradiotherapy restrict oral intake and act as sites of secondary infection and portals of entry for endogenous oral flora (Table 9.16). Mucositis is associated with increased risk of bacteremia and sepsis.

Etiology and Incidence
- Chemotherapeutic agents interfere with DNA, RNA synthesis and cause destruction of cells that are rapidly dividing.
- Damage is greater as bone marrow function becomes suppressed.
- Occurs in about 40% of patients receiving standard doses.

TABLE 9.16 WORLD HEALTH ORGANIZATION SCALE FOR ORAL MUCOSITIS

Grade 0	None
Grade 1	Erythema plus pain
Grade 2	Ulceration, ability to eat solid foods
Grade 3	Ulceration, ability to eat liquids
Grade 4	Ulceration, nothing by mouth

Treatment Guidelines
- Meticulous oral hygiene.
- Stay hydrated.
- No alcohol or alcohol-based oral hygiene products.
- Oral moisturizers (artificial saliva).
- If pain develops, use systemic analgesics.

TASTE ALTERATIONS
Definition
Taste alterations refer to changes in the nature of taste, change in taste, or loss of the ability to taste food. Taste alterations occur frequently in patients receiving chemotherapy and can negatively affect appetite and nutritional status in patients with cancer.
- *Hypogeusesthesia*: Decrease in acuity of taste
- *Dysgeusia*: Unusual or unpleasant taste
- *Ageusia*: Absence of taste

Risk Factors
- Disease related, treatment related, life style related

Management
- Nutritional supplements
- Meticulous oral care
- Increase fluid intake
- Experiment with spices and flavorings
- Increase salivation (artificial saliva)

CONSTIPATION
Definition
Infrequent hard passage of stool that may be associated with abdominal cramping and rectal pain. May be a presenting symptom, a side effect of therapy, or a result of tumor progression.

Risk Factors
- Decreased motility due to drug therapy
- Opioids: the primary cause of medication-induced constipation by drugs
- Low-fiber diets
- Decreased mobility
- Dehydration

Assessment
- Diet
- Activity
- Pain/cramping
- Medication use
- Lab results
- X-ray to rule out obstruction
- Physical exam: abdominal and rectal

Management
- Encourage fluids, fiber, and physical activity.
- Develop a regular bowel program.
- Laxatives, lubricants, suppositories.

Complications
- Abdominal pain/discomfort
- Nausea/vomiting
- Anorexia
- Impaction
- Ileus

- Anal fissures/hemorrhoids
- Ruptured bowel

DIARRHEA

Definition

Refers to loose or watery stools. An increase in the frequency, quantity, or fluid content in stools that is different from the usual pattern (Table 9.17; Camp-Sorrell & Hawkins, 2016; Linden et al., 2012; Schmaier et al., 2018; Staff et al., 2016; Yarbro et al., 2018).

Treatment

- Hydration
- Electrolyte replacement if indicated
- Small amounts of soft, bland foods
- High-protein diet
- Low-fiber foods
- Sitz baths
- Imodium
- Sandostatin

HOT FLASHES

Definition

A sudden wave of mild or intense body heat that can sometimes alternate with episodes of feeling cold. A hot flash may cause perspiration, anxiety, tachycardia, and profuse flushing. These episodes may occur multiple times a day and during the night. Hot flashes can disrupt sleep and interfere with activities of daily living. Both men and women can have hot flashes. In patients with cancer, hot flashes and night sweats may be caused by the tumor, its treatment, or other conditions (Camp-Sorrell & Hawkins, 2016; Schmaier et al., 2018; Watkins et al., 2015; Yarbro et al., 2018).

Etiology

The exact cause of hot flashes is not known. Cancer treatments can cause hot flashes by altering the body's level of sex hormones. In women, the hormone is estrogen and in men testosterone. The reaction is often caused when hormone levels drop. That change affects the hypothalamus, the part of the brain that controls body temperature and other functions, causing it to misread the signal as a sign that the body is too hot. Epinephrine, the nervous system's message carrier, transmits that message instantly throughout the body. Hot flashes are the body's attempt to get rid of the heat, quickly. The heart starts to pump faster, blood vessels in the skin dilate to release heat, and the skin starts to sweat to cool the body off (Camp-Sorrell & Hawkins, 2016; Schmaier et al., 2018; Watkins et al., 2016; Yarbro et al., 2018).

Treatment

WOMEN	MEN
<ul><li>Hormone replacement therapy if applicable</li><li>Antidepressants</li><li>Anticonvulsants</li><li>Clonidine</li></ul>	<ul><li>Hormone replacement therapy</li><li>Antidepressants</li><li>Anticonvulsants</li></ul>

Other Interventions

- Avoid spicy foods, caffeine, and alcohol.
- Avoid going out in hot, humid weather if possible.
- Dress in layers so that it is easy to take a layer off or put one on.

LYMPHEDEMA

Definition

Lymphedema is caused by obstruction of the lymphatic drainage system that causes fluid to collect in the interstitial spaces. This buildup causes edema, most often in the arms or legs. Lymphedema can also affect the face, neck, abdomen, and genitals, depending on the body part that was treated. Lymphedema may be acute or chronic in nature.

- **Acute lymphedema** can occur a few days or weeks after surgery or radiation treatment. This type of lymphedema usually resolves.
- **Chronic lymphedema** can occur shortly after surgery or years afterward. This type of lymphedema can become a lifelong issue.

Etiology

The most common causes of lymphedema in patients with cancer are surgery to remove the lymph nodes and radiation treatment. Lymphedema can also be caused by an infection or by a tumor that grows or spreads near a lymph node.

Assessment and Diagnosis

- Edema, warmth, redness, and tenderness in the arm or leg
- Measuring the circumference of the extremity
- Ultrasound
- CT scan/MRI

Treatment

- Treatment is symptomatic
- Compression garments
- Exercise and strength training
- Elevation
- Skin care
- Early identification and treatment can result in a cure
- Avoid blood draws and blood pressure on the affected extremity

CHEMOTHERAPY-INDUCED PERIPHERAL NEUROPATHY

Definition

A serious dose-limiting side effect that is a major source of pain and debilitation. Impairment occurs from inflammation, injury, or degeneration of the peripheral nervous system. Some cases resolve after treatment is discontinued. In most of the cases, chemotherapy-induced peripheral neuropathy (CIPN) will only partially resolve and sometimes become permanent.

TABLE 9.17 MECHANISMS OF CHEMOTHERAPY-INDUCED DIARRHEA

OSMOTIC DIARRHEA	SECRETORY DIARRHEA	EXUDATIVE DIARRHEA
Related to injury to the gut, dietary factors, or problems with digestion <ul><li>Lactose</li><li>Enteral tube feedings</li><li>Intestinal hemorrhage</li></ul>	Intestinal mucosa secretes excessive amounts of fluid and electrolytes <ul><li>Laxatives</li><li>*Escherichia coli* or *Clostridium difficile*</li><li>Neuroendocrine tumors</li></ul>	Caused by changes in mucosal integrity <ul><li>Chemo drugs</li><li>Graft versus host disease</li><li>Radiation</li><li>Irritable bowel disease</li></ul>

Pathophysiology

Exact mechanism is unknown. Associated with numerous pathologic processes that can affect the nerve cells and nerve fibers.

Symptoms

■ Inability to feel where your feet and hands are ■ Tripping, falling, or having trouble walking ■ Dropping things ■ Numbness, tingling, or burning in the fingers, hands, arms, toes, feet, and legs ■ Difficulty picking up small objects	■ Changes in response to touch or dull pain ■ Changes in response to feeling hot or cold temperatures ■ Constipation ■ Urinating less than usual ■ Changes in vision and hearing

Treatment

■ Discontinuation of the medication can reverse symptoms. ■ Address any physical cause such as vitamin deficiency, malnutrition, diabetes mellitus. ■ Reduce neuropathic pain with anticonvulsants, tricyclic antidepressants, and topical agents. ■ Avoid extreme temperatures.	■ Protect hands and feet in cold weather. ■ Wear gloves when washing dishes or gardening. ■ Remove throw rugs. ■ Frequently examine extremities for injury.

DYSPNEA

Definition

Dyspnea is the sensation of difficult or uncomfortable breathing. This symptom is highly prevalent among patients with cancer with and without direct lung involvement.

Etiology in Patients With Cancer

■ Lung cancer ■ Pleural effusions ■ Superior vena cava syndrome ■ Bleeding ■ Anemia ■ Pulmonary embolism	■ Ascites ■ Prior lung surgery ■ Radiation fibrosis ■ Chemotherapy-related lung injury ■ Pneumonia ■ Anxiety

Treatment
Pharmacologic

- Bronchodilators
- Morphine sulfate
- Anxiolytics
- Lasix
- Steroids
- Oxygen/correction of anemia

Nonpharmacologic

- Positioning
- Pacing of activities
- Pursed lip breathing
- Fan blowing on face
- Provide emotional comfort and reassurance
- Allow family to stay with patient

See also Chapter 18 for information related to dyspnea as a symptomatic response to illness.

FATIGUE
Definition

Fatigue refers to extreme tiredness from mental and/or physical exertion or illness. Cancer fatigue is one of the most common adverse effects of both the disease process and the treatment. The exact cause is unknown, and levels of severity vary among patients. One hundred percent of patients receiving active treatment have subjectively reported experiencing fatigue.

Etiology in Patients With Cancer

- The release of cytokines or altering hormones
- Tumor cells competing for nutrition
- Some cancers increase the body's need for energy, weaken muscle, and damage essential organs
- Chemotherapy
- Radiation
- Biologic therapy
- Bone marrow transplant
  See also Chapter 18 for information related to fatigue as a symptomatic response to illns

NAUSEA AND VOMITING
Definition

Nausea is a subjective, unobservable phenomenon of an unpleasant sensation in the back of the throat and the epigastrium that may or may not result in vomiting. Vomiting is a somatic process performed by respiratory muscles causing forceful evacuation of gastric, duodenal, or jejunal contents through the mouth.

Etiology

Primary or metastatic central nervous system tumors and side effects of antineoplastic agents, opioids, and antibiotics are among the causes of nausea and vomiting in patients with cancer.

Risk Factors That Influence the Vomiting Center

- Younger age <50 years/has increased incidence
- Female sex
- Anxiety
- Noxious odors
- Anticipatory response to previous cancer treatments
- History of motion sickness

Treatment

See Table 9.18 for management guidelines for chemotherapy-induced nausea and vomiting. See also Chapter 18 for information regarding nausea as a symptomatic response to illness.

PAIN

Pain is one of the most common concerns and most feared symptoms associated with cancer and cancer treatments. Causes of pain unique to patients with cancer include oral mucositis and radiation fibrosis.

See Chapter 18 for pharmacologic and nonpharmacologic management of pain and pain as a symptomatic response to illness. See Chapter 19 for analgesic medication guidelines.

ANXIETY

Anxiety is a feeling of worry, nervousness, or unease, typically about an imminent event or something with an uncertain

TABLE 9.18 MANAGEMENT GUIDELINES FOR CHEMOTHERAPY-INDUCED NAUSEA AND VOMITING

CINV TYPE	TREATMENT
Acute emesis and highly emetogenic therapy	5-HT, receptor antagonists with dexamethasone, and NK$_1$ receptor antagonists
Acute emesis and moderately emetogenic therapy	Dexamethasone and 5-HT$_3$ receptor antagonist
Low emetic risk	Prochlorperazine, domperidone, metoclopramide, or dexamethasone alone
Anticipatory emesis	Lorazepam for its amnesic, sedative, and anxiolytic effects
Delayed emesis	Dexamethasone alone, with or without oral metoclopramide; prochlorperazine; 5-HT$_3$; or NK$_1$ receptor antagonists

CINV, chemotherapy-induced nausea and vomiting; 5-HT, 5-hydroxytryptamine. NK, natural killer.

outcome, and is often experienced by patients with cancer. Anxiety can be mild, moderate, or severe. The highest levels of anxiety are reported in lung, gynecologic, and hematologic cancers (Camp-Sorrell & Hawkins, 2016; Linden et al., 2012; Staff et al., 2016; Yarbro et al., 2018).

Events that can cause anxiety in patients with cancer:

- Noticing a worrisome sign or symptoms
- Testing to find out the cause of a symptom
- Being diagnosed with cancer
- Awaiting cancer treatment
- Side effects of treatment
- Finishing treatment

See Chapter 18 for anxiety as a symptomatic response to illness, and Chapter 15 for the pathophysiology and management of anxiety disorders and for psychiatric medication guidelines.

DEPRESSION

Depression is a common comorbidity in patients with cancer. A cancer diagnosis is life changing and is a source of psychologic and emotional stress.

See Chapter 15 for the pathophysiology and management of mood disorders, including depression and for psychiatric medication guidelines.

BIOTHERAPY/IMMUNOTHERAPY

OVERVIEW

The National Cancer Institute defines *biotherapy* as a treatment used to boost or restore the ability of the immune system to fight cancer, infections, and other diseases (Polovich, 2014). Biotherapy, also referred to as *immunotherapy*, can also be used to help alleviate or lessen side effects of cancer treatments. These agents utilize the body's own immune system to elicit a biologic response to fight cancer. They are biologically derived substances that are created by the body or in a lab to improve or restore the immune system function (www.cancer.net/navigating

-cancer-care/how-cancer-treated/immunotherapy-and-vaccines/understanding-immunotherapy; Temple, 2016).

These therapies alter the immune system with either a stimulatory or a suppressive effect, providing a targeted approach to cancer treatment. These agents can be used alone or in combination with other therapies such as antineoplastic agents and/or radiation. Most of these agents are fetotoxic and embryotoxic; therefore, pregnancy and breastfeeding should be avoided. Mandatory monitoring may be required for some agents, to prevent pregnancy (Wilkes, 2009).

Immune Surveillance Theory

The theory of immune surveillance indicates that the process of a normal cell converting to a cancer cell can take years. As the cells differentiate, they produce proteins or antigens that are attached to the surface of the cells. The immune system will elicit a response to attack these foreign substances. However, in some instances, the immune system does not recognize these antigens as foreign. Biotherapy works in the following ways to boost the immune system to recognize and attack these foreign antigens (Polovich, 2014).

- Enhances the body's own immune system
- Alters the environment the cancer cells are growing in by modifying normal cell action
- Increases cancer cell vulnerability to the body's immune system
- Alters the pathways in which normal cells transform into malignant cells; this is a preventive measure
- Prevents the cancer cell from metastasizing or spreading to other parts of the body or tissue
- Enhances the repair capabilities of normal cells that may have been damaged by treatment
- Alters the cancer cells so that they behave as a healthy normal cell

Biotherapy Categories

There are several biotherapy agents that include monoclonal antibodies, growth factors, and vaccines (Polovich, 2014).

Cytokines

Cytokines are small protein molecules that provide communication between the cells of the immune system (Table 9.19). These molecules are activated when certain receptors on the cancer cell are present. This response can be an activation or inhibition of a process that will in turn alter the immune effector function of the cell (Polovich, 2014). Cytokines affect the growth and differentiation of WBCs and regulate the immune and inflammatory responses. Because cytokines may secrete additional cytokines, this can enhance the cytotoxic activity of the drug and will thus enhance the immune system response. Cytokines have proinflammatory, antiinflammatory, and regulatory functions in the immune system. They are also responsible for the production of antibodies, the functions of B and T cells, and interacting with antigen-presenting cells and NK cells (Polovich, 2014).

Monoclonal Antibodies

These are antibodies derived from human antibodies, mouse antibodies, or a combination of both (Polovich, 2014). These drugs are a type of targeted biotherapy that focuses on specific antibodies/antigens on the surface of the cancer cell. Monoclonal antibodies inhibit the binding of growth factors by recognizing

TABLE 9.19 CYTOKINES

EXAMPLES OF CYTOKINES	SPECIFIC AGENTS
Colony-stimulating growth factors	Darbepoetin alfa Epoetin alfa Filgrastim Pegfilgrastim Sargramostim
IFNs	IF-alpha-2a IF-alpha-2b
ILs	Aldesleukin

IF, interferon; IFNs, interferons; ILs, interleukins.
Source: Adapted from Wilkes, G. M. (2009). Chemotherapy and biotherapy. In B. H. Gobel, S. Triest-Robertson, & W. H. Vogel (Eds.), *Advanced oncology nursing certification review and resource manual* (pp. 149–185). Oncology Nursing Society.

Box 9.1 Unconjugated/Conjugated Antibodies

Unconjugated Antibodies
    Rituximab: Targets CD20
    Trastuzumab: Targets HER2
    Cetuximab: Targets EFGR
    Bevacizumab: Targets VEGF
    Ipilimumab: Targets anti CTLA-4
Conjugated Antibodies
    Ibritumomab tiuxetan (Zevalin)
    Iodine-131 tositumomab (Bexxar)

and binding to specific antigens. The major mechanism of action for this group of drugs is a three-step process (Polovich, 2014):

- Antibody binds to tumor cell antigen. Example: rituximab, which targets CD 20 receptors on lymphocytes.
- NK cells recognize the antibody-covered tumor cells.
- Cytotoxic proteins are released, and the tumor cells are destroyed.

Infliximab (Remicade), is an example of a chimeric monoclonal antibody medication. Infliximab is used to treat a number of autoimmune diseases, including Crohn's disease, ulcerative colitis, rheumatoid arthritis, psoriasis, and psoriatic arthritis.

Unconjugated/Conjugated Antibodies

There are two subcategories of monoclonal antibodies: unconjugated antibodies and conjugated antibodies (Box 9.1). Unconjugated antibodies do not have cytotoxic agents or radioisotopes attached to them (Polovich, 2014). Conjugated antibodies have antibodies that are physically attached to the antitumor agent such as radioisotopes, chemotherapy, toxins, or other biologic agents (Polovich, 2014).

There are numerous side effects associated with biotherapy. Table 9.20 highlights some of the more common agents and the potential side effects associated with them.

Targeted Therapy

Targeted therapies use drugs to block the growth and spread of cancer by interfering with specific molecular targets that are involved in the tumor's growth and progression (Keith & Abueg, 2019). These agents target specific genes, proteins, or tissue contributing to tumor growth and involved in cell-signaling pathways. Targeted therapies are cytostatic, blocking tumor cell proliferation, and are deliberately designed to interact with their specific target. Patients must exhibit positive testing for

TABLE 9.20 BIOTHERAPY AGENTS AND COMMON TOXICITIES

BIOTHERAPY AGENTS	COMMON TOXICITIES
Rituximab	Hypersensitivity reactions that can include anaphylaxis during the infusion Fever, chills, rigor Tumor lysis syndrome in patients with a high tumor burden (large amount of tumor)
Alemtuzumab	Infusion reactions that include rash, rigors, fever, and hypotension Myelosuppression Pain Asthenia Peripheral edema
Gemtuzumab	Acute hypersensitivity reactions that include anaphylaxis, pulmonary edema Fever Neutropenia, thrombocytopenia Nausea/vomiting Chills Headache Dyspnea
Bevacizumab	Hypertension Bleeding Delayed wound healing; do not give within 28 days of major surgery
Cetuximab	Sterile, inflammatory rash that can be severe Severe hypersensitivity reaction (90% occur during first infusion) Nausea/vomiting Diarrhea
Trastuzumab	Cardiomyopathy (increased risk when receiving anthracycline agents as well) Infusion reactions (can be severe with dyspnea and hypotension) Anemia and neutropenia risk increased when receiving chemotherapy
Ibritumomab tiuxetan	Severe cutaneous and mucosal reactions Rare but fatal infusion reactions within 24 hours of rituximab infusion Contraindicated if >25% of bone marrow shows lymphoma or impaired bone reserve Hypersensitivity reaction to murine antibody
Iodine-131 tositumomab	Hypersensitivity reactions that can include anaphylaxis Nausea/vomiting Diarrhea Rash Fetotoxicity (avoid pregnancy) Hypothyroidism Secondary malignancy (MDS, AML) Contraindicated if hypersensitivity to murine antibody

AML, acute myeloid leukemia; MDS, myelodysplastic syndrome.

Source: Adapted from Wilkes, G. M. (2009). Chemotherapy and botherapy. In B. H. Gobel, S. Triest-Robertson, & W. H. Vogel (Eds.), *Advanced oncology nursing certification review and resource manual* (pp. 149–185). Oncology Nursing Society.

specific cells or enzymes in order for the therapy to be effective. These new therapies are the cornerstone for precision medicine, which uses information about a patient's genes and proteins to diagnose and treat disease. There are several different targeted therapies approved for cancer treatment. Table 9.21 provides information on the categories of therapy and mechanism of action (Wilkes, 2009; www.cancer.net/navigating-cancer-care/how-cancer-treated/personalized-and-targeted-therapies/understanding-targeted-therapy).

Targeted therapies are considered less toxic than traditional antineoplastic agents but can still have substantial side effects. Some side effects, however, are considered a beneficial consequence of treatment and have been linked to better outcomes.

TABLE 9.21 CATEGORIES OF TARGETED THERAPY

CATEGORY	MECHANISM OF ACTION
Hormone therapies	Slow or stop growth of hormone-sensitive tumors. Prevent the body from producing the specific hormones required by the tumor for growth. Approved for both breast and prostate cancers.
Signal transduction inhibitor	Block the activities of molecules involved in the signal transduction. Once the cell has received the signal, it is relayed within the cell to produce appropriate responses. In some cancers, malignant cells divide continuously and avoid apoptosis; these inhibitors interfere with this inappropriate signaling.
Gene expression modulators	The function of proteins that are integral in controlling gene expression are modified.
Apoptosis inducers	Cancer cells have ways to avoid apoptosis (programmed cell death). These inducers interfere with the cancer cell's strategies and cause the cell death to occur.
Angiogenesis inhibitors	Tumors require blood supply to carry oxygen and nutrients and can create their own blood supply through a process called angiogenesis. These inhibitors interfere with angiogenesis to block tumor growth.
Immunotherapies	Trigger the immune system to attack and destroy cancer cells. These are considered targeted immunotherapy because of these agents target specific antigens or antibodies on the cancer cell to assist with the destruction of the cancer cell.
Monoclonal antibodies with toxic molecules	Also considered a biotherapy, these agents have toxic molecules attached to them that link to the antibody on the cancer cell. The toxin will be taken up by the cell and ultimately result in cell kill. These agents do not affect cells that do not exhibit the target antibody or antigen.

For example, patients who develop an acneiform rash while being treated with a signal transduction inhibitor tend to respond better than those who did not develop the rash.

MANAGEMENT OF PATIENTS WITH IMMUNOSUPPRESSION THERAPY

IMMUNOSUPPRESSION THERAPY

Immunosuppressive medications may require long-term use and have significant side effects. Many of these drugs require long-term use with the potential for major side effects of chronic immunosuppression, including increased risk of infection and cancer. Within each class are other additional side effects that need to be considered when managing these patients.

Immunosuppressive Drug Classes and Indications

For prevention and treatment of tissue rejection:
- Calcineurin inhibitors (CNIs)
- mTOR inhibitors
- Cytotoxic agents
- Glucocorticoids
- Monoclonal antibodies

For the treatment of diseases arising from autoimmune processes:
- Sphingosine-1-phosphate receptor (SIP-R) modulators
- Inhibitors of costimulatory molecules of T-cell activation
- Cytotoxic agents
- Glucorticoids
- Monoclonal antibodies

For the treatment of nonimmune inflammatory diseases, such as allergic asthma:
- Glucocorticoids

For the treatment of Rh hemolytic disease of the newborn:
- Rho D immune globulin

Dose-Limiting Toxicity

This refers to side effects of a drug that are serious enough to prevent an increase in dose or level of that treatment.

Common Major Side Effects and Management

- *Nephrotoxic effects of CNIs:* Dose-limiting toxicity for CNIs. Toxicity can be reduced by delaying administration of CNIs after transplant by using an induction regimen with other less nephrotoxic agents. Other interventions to reduce risk and severity of nephrotoxicity are careful monitoring of the dose, maintaining adequate hydration, and avoiding other drugs capable of causing nephrotoxicity. Patients must be monitored for acute and chronic renal failure. For patients with preexisting renal insufficiency, other agents should be considered (Holt, 2017).
- *Neurotoxic effects of CNIs:* Another dose-limiting toxicity for CNIs. Lowering the dose may decrease or reverse these symptoms. The neurologic effects range from headache to seizure with reported incidence as high as 28%.
- Cardiovascular effects of immunosuppressive therapy: This is due in part to increasing the risk of the following:
  - Hyperlipidemia
  - Hyperglycemia
  - Hypertension

Monitor patients at risk for these side effects and treat accordingly. Encourage healthy lifestyle changes. It is helpful to note that cyclosporin may increase statin concentration and toxicity such as myopathy. For this reason, start patients slow and on the lowest dose possible while monitoring for toxicity (Khan, 2016).

- *Infection due to immunosuppression:* Early posttransplant management of infection risk is focused on prophylaxis of opportunistic infections. The risk increases with the degree of immunosuppression and includes such organisms as *Pneumocystis jirovecii, Nocardia, Aspergillus,* and *Cryptococcus.* Patients who are severely immunocompromised are also at risk for reactivation of varicella zoster, herpes simplex, cytomegalovirus, hepatitis B, hepatitis C, and tuberculosis. A thorough history of the patient's past immunizations and illnesses may help identify specific infections requiring prophylaxis or increased surveillance. Further from transplant, less immunosuppression for rejection is needed so prophylaxis is not necessary (Khan, 2016).
  - Overall, the prevalence and incidence of infection creates a need for close monitoring of clinical signs and symptoms and appropriate diagnostic testing for any suspicion. Infectious organisms may include any of those listed here and may be both nosocomial or community acquired.
  - Bacterial
  - Viral
  - Parasitic
  - Fungal infections
  - Donor-derived infections, such as HIV, West-Nile virus, rabies, Chagas disease, and lymphocytic choriomeningitis virus
- Use of vaccines in patients receiving immunosuppressive medications is receiving much-needed attention with specific recommendations focused on type of vaccine, for example, live, attenuated, or inactivated, and timing of the immunosuppressive treatment. The practitioner should review the newest recommendations related to the specific vaccine they are considering. The Centers for Disease Control and Prevention recommends the influenza vaccine each year and the Tdap vaccine and pneumococcal vaccine for adults with a weakened immune system. See www.cdc.gov/vaccines/schedules (Vaccine Schedules, 2019).
- *Cytokine release syndrome:* More common with biological agents such as monoclonal antibodies. The syndrome is characterized by fever, hypotension, hypertension, tachycardia, dyspnea, urticaria, and rash. Effects are worse with higher rates of infusion. Risk and severity of the reaction is lowered through premedicating with acetaminophen, diphenhydramine, and corticosteroids (Khan, 2016; Schonder, 2011).

- *Cancer:* Due to long-term use of immunosuppressants, the immune system has a weakened defense against neoplastic processes. Cancers most commonly associated with chronic immunosuppression include skin cancer and lymphoproliferative disease (Holt, 2017; Schonder, 2011).

REVIEW QUESTIONS

1. The oncology CNS is scheduled to see a patient with breast cancer undergoing chemotherapy and radiation treatment for symptom management. Based on research evidence, the CNS knows to always be prepared to address which of the following symptoms?
   A. Nausea
   B. Fatigue
   C. Pain
   D. Hot flashes

2. Which of the following patients is at the highest risk for developing chemotherapy-induced nausea and vomiting?
   A. Female sex
   B. Alcohol user
   C. Male sex
   D. Smoker

ANSWERS

1. **Correct answer: B. Rationale:** The incidence of fatigue subjectively reported in patients with cancer undergoing active treatment is estimated to be 100%. Fatigue is the most common and feared symptom of treatment for cancer. Nausea is not correct because not all chemotherapy drugs cause nausea and this is not a symptom of radiation. Pain is not typically a symptom of treatment but rather the cancer itself. Chemo and radiation are usually given to alleviate pain by shrinking tumors, sometimes referred to as *palliative chemo* or *radiation.* Hot flashes are not a typical sign of either treatment, but may be experienced by patients receiving a few drugs.

2. **Correct answer: A. Rationale:** Females are at a higher risk for developing chemotherapy-induced nausea and vomiting (CINV). Alcohol use, male gender, and smoking history are not high-risk criteria.

REFERENCES

The complete reference list appears in the digital version of this chapter, at https://connect.springerpub.com/content/book/978-0-8261-7417-8/part/part01/chapter/ch09

Gastrointestinal System

10

Tamera Brown, Alyson Keen, K. Denise Kerley, Carmen R. Davis, Jan Powers, and Amy C. Shay

OVERVIEW OF THE GASTROINTESTINAL SYSTEM

OVERVIEW

Physiology
- *Innervation*
  - Parasympathetic—Excites
  - Sympathetic—Inhibits
  - Enteric—Intrinsic secretion and movement, considered "gut brain"; see Figure 10.1.

Organs: Two Categories
- *Alimentary canal*: Nourishes the body
- *Accessory organs*: Break down food

Circulation: 25% to 30% of cardiac output supplies the gastrointestinal (GI) system

Primary Functions
- Provides body with a constant supply of nutrients, water, and electrolytes
- Digestion and absorption

Problems of the Gastrointestinal System
- GI hemorrhage
- Bowel infarction/obstruction/perforation (Table 10.1)
- Gastroesophageal reflux disease (GERD)
- GI infectious disorders
- GI motility disorders (constipation, diarrhea, ileus, gastroparesis; Bielefeldt et al., 2016)

ABDOMINAL ASSESSMENT AND EXAMINATION
- A thorough history is crucial to determine cause of symptoms.

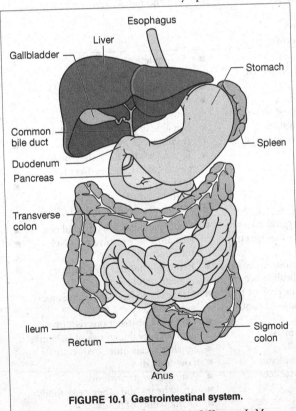

FIGURE 10.1 Gastrointestinal system.

Source: Reproduced from Myrick, K. M., & Karosas, L. M. (2021). *Advanced health assessment and differential diagnosis: Essentials for practice.* Springer Publishing Company.

TABLE 10.1 BOWEL INFARCTION/OBSTRUCTION/PERFORATION

	BOWEL INFARCTION	BOWEL OBSTRUCTION	BOWEL PERFORATION
Definition	Irreversible injury to part of intestine with lost blood flow to the area = tissue death. Medical emergency.	A blockage in the small or large intestine that keeps liquid and/or food from passing through.	A hole through an area of the bowel
Pathophysiology	Infarction occurs when one or more arteries have a narrowing or blockage that supply the intestines.	Impairment of the passage of digested material through the bowel will result in stopping any passage of feces and gas. Blockage causes distention of the proximal intestine with the fluids, solids, and gas and causes pain, tension in the intestinal wall, and increased size of the abdomen.	Perforation causes leakage of the intestinal contents into the abdominal cavity. Can lead to peritonitis: • Fatigue • Passing less stools, gas, or urine • Shortness of breath • Tachycardia • Dizziness
Etiology	▪ Hernia ▪ Adhesions ▪ Blood clots ▪ Narrowing or blocked arteries ▪ Decreased blood pressure from other conditions can cause loss of blood flow to intestinal arteries.	▪ Can be due to mechanical obstructions from a tumor, diverticulitis, or hernia ▪ A result of some medications. ▪ Surgery or nervous system disorders. ▪ Physical obstruction: twisting of the intestines or impaction.	Can occur from different diseases or trauma, such as the following: • Diverticulitis • Appendicitis • Cancer • Crohn's disease • Knife wound • Gunshot wound
Risk factors	▪ Irregular heartbeat ▪ High blood pressure ▪ High cholesterol ▪ Smoking ▪ Poor nutrition ▪ Untreated hernias	▪ Cancer, Crohn's disease, or other IBDs, adhesions from previous surgery and radiation therapy.	▪ Underlying GI disease
Assessment	▪ Abdominal pain ▪ Vomiting and diarrhea ▪ Fever ▪ Elevated WBC ▪ CT scan to show abnormalities in the intestine ▪ Angiogram to show the location	▪ A complete physical exam, especially the abdomen ▪ Cramps/abdominal pain ▪ Vomiting and diarrhea or constipation ▪ Not able to pass gas and abdominal swelling ▪ Blood tests to check electrolytes, blood counts, kidney/liver function ▪ Endoscopy ▪ KUB ▪ CT scan (current standard of care)	▪ Will have sudden and severe stomach pain, tenderness, chills, N/V, and fever ▪ Symptoms of peritonitis ▪ Bowel sounds are quiet to nonexistent ▪ Will need abdominal series x-rays and possibly CT scan (with or without contrast) ▪ Check other labs for any signs of infection
Treatment/ prevention	▪ Immediate surgical intervention to remove that part of the bowel ▪ Temporary colostomy may be needed until healing occurs ▪ Avoid smoking; prompt treatment of hernias and control of risk factors ▪ Heart arrhythmias ▪ Hypertension ▪ Hypercholesterolemia ▪ Healthy diet practices	▪ Stable patients with a partial obstruction may resolve with NG tube decompression ▪ Reducible hernias may require nonemergent surgery ▪ Strangulated hernias require emergency surgery ▪ Complete obstructions require urgent surgery due to risk of ischemia ▪ Smaller meals more frequently ▪ Low-fiber diet ▪ Avoid fatty/greasy foods ▪ Avoid beans and other gassy foods ▪ Drink plenty of fluids	▪ Surgery ▪ IV fluids and antibiotics ▪ NG tube ▪ Monitor urine output

GI, gastrointestinal; IBD, irritable bowel disorder; IV, intravenous; KUB, kidney ureter bladder; NG, nasogastric; N/V, nausea/vomiting; WBC, white blood cell.

Sources: Data from Ozturk, E., van Lersel, M., Stommel, M., Schoon, Y., Broek, R., & van Goor, H. (2018). Small bowel obstruction in the elderly: A plea for comprehensive acute geriatric care. *World Journal of Emergency Surgery, 13*, 48. https://doi.org/10.1186/s13017-018-0208-z

- History should include current medications (prescription and over the counter) and any family history of GI problems (cancer or GI disease) as well as social history (alcohol use, recreational drugs, stress).
  - Bowel changes
  - Nausea and vomiting (N/V)
  - Changes in appetite
  - Weight loss/gain
  - Associated symptoms such as fever, chills, shortness of breath
- The physical assessment must be done in the proper sequence to eliminate any internal interference:
  - Inspection
  - Auscultation
  - Percussion
  - Palpation

GASTROINTESTINAL HEMORRHAGE

Definition

- Acute blood loss from GI tract
- Defined as up to a loss of up to 25% of an adult's circulating volume
  - Upper GI bleed occurs from the esophagus, stomach, or duodenum.
  - Lower GI bleed occurs from the jejunum, ileum, or colon.
  - The Treitz ligament, which is between the duodenum and the jejunum, is what separates an upper GI bleed from a lower GI bleed.

Pathophysiology/Etiology

Upper GI Bleed

- Mallory-Weiss tear (esophageal tears) due to mechanical irritation
  - Aspirin and alcohol abuse
- Erosive lesion from an increase in gastric acid
- Esophageal varices from increased pressure from portal hypertension
  - Liver destruction from backflow of blood
  - Increased intra-abdominal pressure from lifting, coughing, or straining
  - Varices develop
- Hemorrhagic peptic ulcers
- Peptic ulcer disease (PUD)—*Helicobacter pylori* (*H pylori*) bacteria and nonsteroidal antiinflammatory drug (NSAID) use
- Malignancy (https://aneskey.com/gastrointestinal -hemorrhage)

Lower GI Bleed

- Less common than upper GI bleeds
- Hemorrhoids
- Diverticulosis
- NSAIDs
- Ulcerative colitis
- Anticoagulant therapy

Risk Factors

- Older adults
- More frequent in women
- Chronic NSAID use
- *H. pylori* infection
- Mechanical ventilation >48 hours
- Coagulopathies (platelet count <50,000/mm^3 (international normalized ratio [INR] >1.5, or partial thromboplastin time (PTT) >2 times the control value)

- Antiplatelet/anticoagulant therapies
- PUD
  - *H. pylori* infection
  - Stress
  - Excess gastric acid
- Advanced liver failure

Assessment

- Initial primary survey for severity of symptoms and needed resuscitation
- Complete blood count (CBC)
- Drug history or any antiplatelet medications
- Vascular accessibility
- Secondary survey
  - Patient history to include melena, hematemesis, syncope, dizziness, hematochezia, palpitations, or previous history of any GI bleeding
  - Recent trauma
- Lab testing for prothrombin time (PT)/INR, complete metabolic panel (CMP), and possible frequent hemoglobin and hematocrit (H&H)
  - Hematocrit levels typically don't change until 8 to 10 hours later
  - Elevated blood urea nitrogen (BUN) and creatinine levels
  - Increased platelet count
- Current type and crossmatch
- Esophagogastroduodenoscopy (EGD) is considered the gold standard for diagnosing gastroesophageal varices
- Colonoscopy for lower GI bleed is the gold standard

Treatment

Upper GI Bleed

- Triage patient to the level of care needed.
- Order lab tests:
  - CBC
  - Electrocardiogram with cardiac enzymes
- Perform nasogastric lavage prior to endoscopy.
- Consult with gastroenterology.
- Resuscitate fluid; watch for fluid overload.
- Transfuse blood as needed: red blood cells (RBCs), plasma, and platelets.
- Prepare for diagnostic tests; upper endoscopy is the gold standard.
- Start an intravenous proton pump inhibitor (PPI).
- Pantoprazole and esomeprazole are common intravenous medications given BID initially and tapering to once daily. Once the bleeding is controlled, then switch to an oral PPI such as omeprazole.
- Endoscopic therapy:
  - Injection therapy
  - Hemoclips

Lower GI Bleed

- Once the bleeding site has been identified, endoscopic hemoclips or banding can be used to control the bleeding.
- A tagged red cell scan can be performed followed by angiography to infuse a vasoconstriction medication (e.g., epinephrine).
- If bleeding is not stopped, a subtotal or segmental colectomy may need to be done.

Prevention Strategies

- Manage any GERD, PUD, or ulcerative colitis. Take all medications as prescribed.
- Limit the use of NSAIDs.
- Limit intake or don't drink alcohol.
- Do not smoke.
- Maintain a healthy diet and exercise program.

GASTROESOPHAGEAL REFLUX DISEASE

- Reflux of gastric contents into the esophagus

Pathophysiology

- Presence of gastric contents causes inflammation and irritation of the esophagus.
- Weakened esophageal tone results in backflow (reflux) of gastric contents (Pandit et al., 2018).

Etiology/Risk Factors

- *Hiatal hernia*: Weakened diaphragm allows for reflux.
- Obesity can increase pressure on the abdomen.
- Pregnancy due to increased pressure.
- Certain medications, including some asthma medications, calcium channel blockers, antihistamines, sedatives, and antidepressants.
- Smoking and being exposed to second hand smoke.

Assessment

- Heartburn, regurgitation, and belching
- Possibly wheezing or coughing
- Symptoms may worsen while lying down or with exercise
- Can have bad breath or decay

Possible Tests to Diagnose GERD

- Esophageal pH and impedance monitoring
- Upper GI endoscope
- Upper GI series
- Esophageal manometry

Treatment

- PPIs are one of the main treatment options.

Other options include the following (Tables 10.2–10.5):

- H2 blockers
- Antacids
- Prokinetics
- Erythromycin: An antibiotic that helps empty the stomach

Surgical Options

- *Fundoplication*: Suture the top of the stomach around the esophagus
- *Endoscopic procedures*: Endoscopic approach to tighten the sphincter muscle

Prevention

- Avoid overeating.
- Don't eat 2 to 3 hours before bedtime.
- Avoid smoking.
- Maintain a good weight.
- Don't wear tight clothing around the abdomen.
- Sleep slightly elevated.

GASTROINTESTINAL INFECTIOUS DISORDERS

Definition

- Common viral, bacterial, and parasitic pathogens are spread via water, person to person, and food.

Pathophysiology

- Pathogens must be ingested in significant amounts or make it past the host defenses of the upper GI tract and make it to the intestines.
- Pathogens that remain can cause disease by multiplying and producing toxins.
- Pathogens may also invade through the mucosa to reach the bloodstream or lymphatics.

Etiology of Noninfectious Causes of Diarrhea

- Medication side effects
- Gastroenterologic diseases
- Endocrine diseases

Risk Factors

- Weakened immune system
- Young children/older adults
- Travel to foreign countries (food/water pathogens; see Table 10.6)
- Food that is undercooked or left at room temperature too long (Table 10.7)

Assessment

- Thorough history and physical assessment
- Onset, duration, severity, and frequency of symptoms
- Environmental exposure
- Symptoms
  - Loss of appetite
  - N/V
  - Diarrhea
  - Abdominal pains and cramps
  - Blood in the stools
  - Fever
- Diagnosis
  - Stool testing
  - Blood cultures as necessary
  - Abdominal CT
  - Endoscopy if diarrhea persistent

Treatment

- Rehydration—Oral or IV if severe
- Antibiotics in severe cases
- Bismuth subsalicylates may help with traveler's diarrhea
- Loperamide if receiving antibiotics that cause diarrhea (Table 10.8)

Prevention

- Handwashing is the number one preventative measure.
- Disinfect surfaces.
- Follow careful practices with food and fluids when in another country.

GASTROINTESTINAL MOTILITY DISORDERS: CONSTIPATION

Refers to infrequent bowel movements or difficulty passing hardened stools.

Pathophysiology

- Constipation is categorized as either primary or secondary.
  - Primary constipation is further categorized as
    - Normal transit constipation,
    - Slow transit constipation,
    - Obstructed defecation (pelvic floor dysfunction), and
    - Irritable bowel syndrome (IBS).

TABLE 10.2 TYPES OF ANTACIDS

CLASS (GENERIC/ BRAND NAME)	MECHANISM	INDICATIONS, CONTRAINDICATIONS	DOSAGE	COMMON ADVERSE EFFECTS	SAFETY AND PATIENT EDUCATION
Aluminum hydroxide (Amphojel, AlternaGEL)	Neutralizes hydrochloric acid, reduces phosphate levels	Antacid, peptic ulcer disease, hyperphosphatemia	Depends upon indication. For antacid indication: 5–30 mL PO between meals and at bedtime	Constipation; rebound hyperacidity	Use with caution in older adults, renal disease
Magnesium oxide (Mag-Ox)	Neutralizes gastric acid by reacting with hydrochloric acid to form magnesium chloride and water	■ Relief of heartburn, upset stomach, sour stomach, or acid indigestion ■ Renal failure	One 400 mg tablet BID for up to 2 weeks	Diarrhea; usually used with other agents to counteract this affect	Use with caution in patients with renal insufficiency
Combination aluminum hydroxide and magnesium carbonate (Gaviscon)	Neutralizes gastric acid	Acid indigestion	■ Gaviscon: Regular strength suspension: 15–30 mL PO q6h PRN; not to exceed 120 mL/d	Nausea, vomiting, rebound hyperacidity, hypophosphatemia	Aluminum hydroxide binds to certain drugs reducing their effect (e.g., warfarin, digoxin, tetracycline)
Calcium carbonate (Maalox, TUMS, Mylanta)	Neutralizes gastric acid	Acid indigestion	■ TUMS: 2–4 tabs as symptoms occur; maximum 15 tabs/d for 2 weeks ■ Maalox: 10–20 mL up to QID	Hypercalcemia, hypercalciuria	■ May cause constipation; use may result in kidney stones; long duration of antacid action may cause increased gastric acid secretion (hyperacidity rebound) ■ Calcium blocks absorption of tetracyclines. May affect absorption of other drugs
Sodium bicarbonate/ aspirin/citric acid (Alka Seltzer)	Highly soluble; buffers HCl acid; quick onset with short duration	Hypocalcemia, hypochloremia, respiratory alkalosis	2 tablets (dissolved in water) PO q4h PRN; not to exceed 8 tablets/d	Flatulence, rebound hyperacidity, stomach cramps, vomiting	■ May cause metabolic alkalosis; sodium content may cause problems in patients with heart failure, hypertension, or renal insufficiency due to fluid retention ■ Risk of bleeding if used for longer period or at higher doses than recommended

TABLE 10.3 HISTAMINE TYPE 2 (H2) AGONISTS

MECHANISM	Blocks histamine-2 at the receptors of acid-producing parietal cells with decreased production of hydrochloric acid			
INDICATIONS	GERD, duodenal ulcer, gastric ulcer, Zollinger-Ellison syndrome			
GENERIC NAME (BRAND NAME)	**DOSAGES**		**COMMON ADVERSE EFFECTS**	**SAFETY AND PATIENT EDUCATION**
Cimetidine (Tagamet)	Benign gastric ulcer Duodenal ulcer Gastroesophageal reflux disease Heartburn	800 mg PO qHS OR 300 mg PO q6h 800 mg PO qHS OR 400 mg PO q12h OR 300 mg PO q6h 800 mg PO q12h OR 400 mg PO q6h 200 mg PO up to q12h	▪ Headaches, lethargy, confusion, diarrhea ▪ May cause impotence and gynecomastia	▪ H2 antagonists may inhibit the absorption of certain drugs that require an acidic GI environment for absorption. Monitor for renal and liver function impairment. Use with caution in older adults or in patients who are confused/disoriented due to high incidence of CNS side effects. ▪ Take with meals or immediately afterward and at bedtime for best results. Once daily dose is best taken at bedtime. Do not take with antacids.
Famotidine (Pepcid)	Active DU Active gastric ulcer GERD	40 mg once daily; or 20 mg BID up to 8 weeks 40 mg once daily up to 8 weeks 20 mg BID up to 6 weeks	▪ Headaches, lethargy, confusion, diarrhea	
Ranitidine (Zantac)	Duodenal and gastric ulcer GERD Zollinger–Ellison syndrome	150 mg BID or 300 mg once daily 150 mg BID 150 mg BID	▪ Headaches, lethargy, confusion, diarrhea ▪ Prolonged treatment may lead to B12 malabsorption and subsequent vitamin B12 deficiency	

CNS, central nervous system; DU, duodenal ulcer; GERD, gastroesophageal reflux disease.

Constipation originating from the colon or rectum includes:
- Colon obstruction (neoplasm, volvulus, stricture)
- Slow colonic motility
- Outlet obstruction (anatomic or functional)
- Hirschsprung disease in children
- Chagas disease

Factors involved in constipation outside the colon include the following:
- Poor dietary habits (the most common is not enough fiber and fluid intake)
- Medications
- Systemic endocrine or neurologic diseases
- Psychological issues

Etiology
- *Poor diet*: Rich in fat, high sugar, and low fiber.
- *Inadequate fluid intake*: Not drinking enough water or fluids.
- *Caffeine and alcohol*: These can lead to dehydration.

- Overuse of laxatives (Table 10.9) can lead to their inability to continue to work effectively.
- Mechanical problems with rectum or anus.
- Damage to nerves in the spinal cord.
- *Connective tissue disorders*: conditions such as scleroderma and lupus.
- Hypothyroidism
- Age
- Digestive problems:
  - IBS
  - Intestinal obstruction

Assess medications that can cause constipation,

Risk Factors
- Female
- Age 65 or older
- Low income
- Pregnancy
- Postsurgery

TABLE 10.4 PROTON PUMP INHIBITORS

MECHANISM	Blocks acid secretion by combining with K+, H+, and ATPase enzymes in parietal cells. Results in blockage of all gastric acid secretion (gastric pH > 4).			
INDICATIONS	GERD, gastric ulcers, duodenal ulcers, erosive esophagitis, Zollinger-Ellison syndrome			
COMMON ADVERSE EFFECTS	Nausea, diarrhea, constipation, abdominal pain			
GENERIC NAME (BRAND NAME)	**DOSAGES**		**SAFETY**	**SAFETY AND PATIENT EDUCATION**
lansoprazole (Prevacid)	Duodenal ulcer Gastric ulcer GERD Zollinger-Ellison syndrome	15 mg PO daily for 4 weeks 30 mg PO daily for 8 weeks 15 mg PO daily for 8 weeks 60 mg PO daily	Iron, B_{12}, and calcium deficiency; risk of osteoporosis; increased risk of C diff, salmonella, and *Campylobacter* GI infections; increased risk of pneumonia. Cellular hyperplasia with questionable relationship to gastric cancer.	Take 1 hour before meals; do not crush, chew, or open. May be given with antacids; Short-term therapy only; follow up if symptoms last for more than 2 weeks; take with antacids.
Omeprazole (Prilosec)	Duodenal ulcer Gastric ulcer GERD Erosive esophagitis	20 mg PO daily for 4 weeks 40 mg PO daily for 4–8 weeks 20 mg PO daily for 4 weeks 20 mg PO daily		
Esomeprazole (Nexium)	GERD without erosive esophagitis GERD with erosive esophagitis	20 mg PO daily for 4 weeks 20–40 mg PO daily for 4–8 weeks		

GERD, gastroesophageal reflux disease; GI, gastrointestinal.

TABLE 10.5 CYTOPROTECTIVE AGENTS

GENERIC NAME (BRAND NAME)	SUCRALFATE (CARAFATE)
Mechanism	Reacts with hydrochloric acid to form pasty substance that adheres to the gastric mucosa to promote healing
Indication	Duodenal ulcer treatment
Dosage	1 g PO QID
Common adverse effects	Constipation
Safety	May impair absorption of other drugs; binds with phosphate; may be used in renal failure to reduce phosphate levels
Patient education	Do not administer with other medications.

TABLE 10.6 COMMON CAUSES OF TRAVELER'S DIARRHEA

BACTERIAL	VIRAL	PARASITIC
Shiga-toxin producing *Escherichia coli*	Rotavirus	Giardia lamblia
Other *E. coli* types	Norovirus	Cryptosporidium
Salmonella		Cyclospora
Campylobacter		*Entamoeba histolytica*
Shigella		
Aeromonas		
Vibrio		

Source: Adapted from Eslick, G. (2019). *Gastrointestinal diseases and their associated infections*. Elsevier.

TABLE 10.7 COMMON SOURCES OF WATER- OR FOOD-BORNE ILLNESSES

SOURCE	PATHOGEN
Camping, untreated river water	Giardia
Fried rice	*Bacillus cereus*
Raw milk	*Salmonella, Campylobacter, Listeria, STEC*
Seafood	*Vibrio cholerae, Vibrio parahaemolyticus*
Undercooked meat	*Bacillus cereus, Campylobacter, C. perfringens, Listeria, Salmonella, STEC, Staphylococcus aureus, Yersinia*

STEC, Shiga-toxin-producing *E. coli.*

Source: Adapted from Eslick, G. (2019). *Gastrointestinal diseases and their associated infections*. Elsevier.

TABLE 10.8 ANTIDIARRHEAL AGENTS

First-line therapy	Adsorbents such as bismuth subsalicylate (Pepto-Bismol) and attapulgite (Kaopectate)	
Second-line therapy	Diphenoxylate, difenoxin, loperamide	
Patient education	<ul><li>Take medications exactly as prescribed and be aware of fluid intake and dietary changes.</li><li>Take 1 hour before or 2 hours after other medications.</li><li>Notify provider if diarrhea symptoms persist.</li></ul>	
CLASS	**ADSORBENTS**	
Mechanism	Protective coating of intestinal tract; binds to the causative bacteria or toxin, which is then eliminated through the stool	
Indications	Mild diarrhea	
Generic name (brand name) and dosages	Bismuth subsalicylate (Pepto-Bismol)	2 tablets (262 mg/tab) or 30 mL PO every 30 minutes to 1 hour PRN; maximum daily dose: eight regular-strength doses
	Bismuth subsalicylate (Kaopectate)	2 tablespoonfuls every 30 minutes to 1 hour if needed; maximum daily dose 16 tablespoonfuls
Common adverse effects	Rebound constipation; bismuth subsalicylate can turn the tongue and stools gray black.	
Safety	<ul><li>Absorbents decrease the absorption of many agents, including digoxin, clindamycin, quinidine, and hypoglycemic agents. Absorbents cause increased bleeding time when given with anticoagulants. Antacids can decrease effects of antidiarrheal agents.</li><li>Use adsorbents carefully in geriatric patients or those with decreased bleeding time, clotting disorders, recent bowel surgery, confusion.</li></ul>	
CLASS	**OPIATES**	
Mechanism	Decreases bowel motility and relieves rectal spasms; decreased transit time through the bowel, which allows more time for water and electrolyte absorption	
Indications	Acute and chronic diarrhea	
Generic name (brand name) and dosages	Loperamide (Imodium)	Acute diarrhea: 4 mg PO initially then 2 mg after each unformed stool; maximum dose is 16 mg/d
	diphenoxylate (Lomotil)	Acute diarrhea: 5 mg PO QID maximum dose 20 mg/d
Common adverse effects	Drowsiness, sedation, dizziness, lethargy	
Safety	May cause respiratory depression; exceeding maximum dose increases risk of torsades de pointe	
CLASS	**INTESTINAL FLORA MODIFIERS**	
Mechanism	Bacterial cultures of Lactobacillus organisms supply missing bacteria to the GI tract; suppresses growth of diarrhea-causing bacteria	
Indications	Restoration of intestinal flora and post antibiotic diarrhea and prevention of post-antibiotic vulvovaginal candidiasis	
Contraindications	Immunocompromised patients	
Generic name (brand name) and dosages	*Lactobacillus acidophilus* (Lactinex)	1–2 capsules/d PO (1–10 billion CFUs/d) PO divided TID–QID
Common adverse effects	Flatulence	

CFU, colony-forming units; GI, gastrointestinal.

- Getting <20 g to 35 g of dietary fiber each day
- Getting insufficient fluids, which allows stools to dry out
- Sedentary lifestyle
- Avoiding passing bowel movements when you feel the urge
- Taking certain medications, such as opioids
- Having certain diseases or conditions, such as diabetes, lupus, or multiple sclerosis
- Having an intestinal problem—Obstruction, IBS, or a tumor

A patient may be asymptomatic or experience the following:
- Abdominal bloating
- Pain with bowel movements
- Spurious diarrhea
- Low-back pain
- Feeling of fullness
- Fewer bowel movements than what is normal for them

If any of these symptoms are present, further evaluation is needed:
- Rectal bleeding
- Abdominal pain (suggestive of possible IBS with constipation [IBS-C])
- Inability to pass flatus
- Vomiting
- Unexplained weight loss

A complete abdominal assessment and pelvic exam should be done in female patients to rule out serious causes of constipation, such as the following (Chaney, 2017):
- Perianal excoriation
- Skin tags/hemorrhoids
- Anal fissure
- Anocutaneous reflex

TABLE 10.9 LAXATIVES

Indications	Constipation
Contraindications	Bowel obstruction or perforation, acute surgical abdomen, megacolon, toxic colitis. Use with caution in presence of rectal or anal conditions
First-line therapy	Rapid response: Stimulants Slower response: Bulk-forming laxatives
Second-line therapy	Rapid response: osmotic laxatives Slower response: lactulose
Safety and patient education	■ Patients should not take a laxative or cathartic if they are experiencing nausea, vomiting, and/or abdominal pain. ■ Patients should take all laxative tablets with 6–8 oz of water. ■ Patients should take bulk-forming laxatives as directed by the manufacturer with at least 240 mL (8 oz) of water. ■ Laxative tablets should be swallowed whole, not crushed or chewed, especially if enteric coated. ■ Patients should contact their provider if they experience severe abdominal pain, muscle weakness, cramps, and/or dizziness, which may indicate fluid or electrolyte loss. ■ Rapid-acting laxatives best taken in the morning; slower-acting ones best taken at bedtime. ■ Taking laxative on empty stomach with a full glass of water produces more rapid results.

CLASS	**BULK FORMING**	
Mechanism	High fiber absorbs water to increase bulk; distends bowel to initiate reflex bowel activity	
Generic name (brand name) and dosages	Psyllium (Metamucil) Methylcellulose (Citrucel)	2.5–30 g/d in divided doses Start with two 10-mg caplets; increase up to 6 times per day; maximum of 12 caplets per day
Common adverse effects	Impaction	
CLASS	**EMOLLIENT OR SURFACTANTS**	
Mechanism	Stool softeners and lubricants; promote more water and fat in the stools; lubricate the fecal material and intestinal walls, small intestine, and colon	
Generic name (brand name) and dosages	Stool softeners: docusate salts (Colace) Lubricants: mineral oil	50–400 mg PO, 1–4 equally divided doses per day 15–45 mL/d PO, single or divided doses
Common adverse effects	Throat irritation	
CLASS	**STIMULANT LAXATIVES**	
Mechanism	Increases peristalsis via intestinal nerve stimulation	
Generic name (brand name) and dosages	Bisacodyl (Dulcolax) senna (Senokot)	5–15 mg PO once a day as needed for up to 1 week 10 mg (1 suppository) rectally once a day as needed up to 1 week 15 mg PO once daily; not to exceed 70–100 mg/d divided q12h; not for use more than 1 week
Common adverse effects	Urine discoloration, nutrient malabsorption	
CLASS	**SALINE OSMOTICS**	
Mechanism	Increase osmotic pressure within the intestinal tract, causing more water to enter the intestines. Results in bowel distention, increased peristalsis, and evacuation	
Generic name (brand name) and dosages	MOM Magnesium citrate	(400 mg/5 mL): 5–15 mL as needed up to QID; do not exceed 60 mL in 24 hours. 1/2 to 1 bottle (10 fl oz). Drink a full 8-oz glass of liquid with each dose. The dose may be taken as a single daily dose or in divided doses.
Common adverse effects	Magnesium toxicity (with renal insufficiency); fluid imbalance	
CLASS	**HYPEROSMOTICS**	
Mechanism	Increases fecal water content by diffusion of fluid into the intestinal lumen. Results in bowel distention, increased peristalsis, and evacuation.	
Generic name (brand name) and dosages	Glycerin: Fecal impaction Lactulose (Chronulac)	One adult suppository once daily as needed 30–45 mL TID or QID
Common adverse effects	Fluid and electrolyte imbalances	

MOM, magnesium hydroxide.

- Prolapse during straining
- Anorectal masses
- Tone of the internal anal sphincter
- Strength of the external anal sphincter and puborectalis muscle
- Presence of a rectocele (an outpouching usually present in the anterior rectal wall)
- Presence of fecal impaction

Additional assessment:

- Imaging studies are used to rule out acute processes that may be causing chronic constipation or other systemic or intra-abdominal problems.
- Endoscopy, colonic transit study, surface anal electromyography (EMG), defecography, balloon expulsion, and anorectal manometry may be used in the evaluation of constipation.
- Lab workup to determine blood counts, thyroid, and so on.
- X-ray to determine if bowel is full or other radiographic studies.

Treatment/Prevention

- Review current medications that may be causing constipation.
- Increase fluid and fiber intake. Restrict fiber intake at 20 to 35 g/d.
- Increase physical activity if able.
- Pharmacological agents:
  - Milk of magnesia 1 oz BID
  - Bisacodyl suppository once daily
  - Psyllium 1 tbsp 1 to 3× daily
  - Methylcellulose 1 tbsp 1 to 3× daily
  - Docusate sodium 100 mg 1 to 2 daily
  - Metoclopramide (Reglan; see Table 10.10)

  See Table 10.11 for more information on motility disorders.

GASTROINTESTINAL SURGERIES

OVERVIEW

This section provides a brief overview of GI surgeries, including cholecystectomy, bowel resection, fundoplication, and appendectomy.

CHOLECYSTECTOMY

- Surgery involves gallbladder removal through abdominal incision after ligation of the cystic duct and artery; performed for cholecystitis (gallbladder inflammation; Smelter et al., 2010a).

- The laparoscopic approach is the most common (Smelter et al., 2010a).
- An open procedure may be required for complicated or high-risk surgeries, which increases the risk for paralytic ileus and typically requires a longer length of stay (Smelter et al., 2010a).
- A percutaneous approach may be used for poor surgical candidates, involving fine needle aspiration and catheter insertion for decompression (Smelter et al., 2010a).

Key Considerations

- Important to monitor for obstruction of bile drainage or leakage of bile into peritoneum. Assess for jaundice, bile drainage, right upper quadrant pain, nausea/vomiting, clay-colored stools, and vital-sign changes (Smelter et al., 2010a).
- Important to administer analgesia and encourage patient to turn, cough, and deep breathe to promote full lung expansion (Smelter et al., 2010a).

BOWEL RESECTION

Excision of a segment of the small and/or large bowel to remove the portion of the bowel that is affected or damaged and to connect the remaining healthy bowel (Lippincott Advisor, 2018b).

This can be achieved through the following: (a) proximal and distal end anastomosis; (b) temporary loop ostomy in addition to proximal and distal end anastomosis; (c) proximal ostomy and distal mucous fistula, with proximal and distal ends of the bowel exteriorized to abdominal wall; (d) large bowel distal end over-sewn inside abdomen as Hartmann's pouch, wherein proximal large bowel becomes an ostomy (Piercy, 2014).

Key Considerations

- Intestinal leakage is a rare complication in which fecal matter leaks into the abdominal cavity. This complication may require surgery to repair the leak (Lippincott Advisor, 2018b).
- Malabsorption may occur if a significant portion of the bowel is resected. Nutritional supplements may be required for nutrient absorption.
- Depending on the surgical technique used, an ostomy may be created to divert stool through an opening on the abdomen surface, called a *stoma*.

TABLE 10.10 MOTILITY AGENTS

Generic name (brand name)	Metoclopramide (Reglan)	
Mechanism	Dopamine antagonist, enhances lower esophageal tone, stimulates gastric emptying, increases transit time; antiemetic properties	
Indications	Mild to moderate GERD, gastroparesis associated with diabetes, emesis associated with cancer chemotherapy	
Dosage	Diabetic gastroparesis	10 mg PO 30 minutes before meals and at bedtime
	Gastroesophageal reflux disease	10–15 mg PO 30 minutes before meals and at bedtime; not to exceed 80 mg/d
Common adverse effects	Sedation; extrapyramidal symptoms; increased prolactin secretion, which may cause galactorrhea; amenorrhea; gynecomastia; and impotence	
Safety	May cause irreversible tardive dyskinesia. Metoclopramide may cause NMS. Reglan is on the Beers list of potentially harmful drugs for older adults	

GERD, gastroesophageal reflux disease; NMS, neuroleptic malignant syndrome.

OSTOMY

Bowel resection surgery may result in a temporary or permanent ostomy, creating a stoma from the small bowel (ileostomy) or the large bowel (colostomy).

Ostomy and Pouch Care

- Assess for red, moist stoma.
- Empty the ostomy pouch when it is less than half full.
- May need to "burp" the pouch by allowing air to escape.
- Routine change is every 3 to 5 days; may be more frequent if leaking is present.
  - Preserve skin integrity by using skin barrier.
  - Allow skin time to completely dry before adding new appliance.

Nutrition

- Encourage patients to consume soft, high-fiber food to facilitate digestion. Food items such as grapes, apples, and nuts may cause blockages (Lippincott Advisor, 2018b).

Monitoring for Complications

- Assess for signs of infection, increased pain, change in stoma color, rash around stoma, increased or decreased output, and presence of blood in the stool (Lippincott Advisor, 2018b).

FUNDOPLICATION

- A tight lower esophageal sphincter is created by wrapping the upper portion of the stomach around the distal esophagus and suturing in place (Piercy, 2014).
- Performed to treat GERD not responsive to medications, treat reflux that may trigger asthma symptoms, or decrease the risk of long-term problems such as cancer (Lippincott Advisor, 2018c).

Key Considerations

- Preventing aspiration is important post-surgery as patients can have trouble swallowing.
- Ensure oral medications are pea sized or smaller and encourage patients to maintain good posture to avoid additional intra-abdominal pressure.
- Narrowing of the esophagus may require dietary modifications. Advise patient not to eat 3 hours before bedtime to prevent reflux (Lippincott Advisor, 2018c).

TABLE 10.11 OTHER MOTILITY DISORDERS

DISORDER	DEFINITION	RISK FACTORS	ASSESSMENT	TREATMENT
Diarrhea	Increase in frequency and volume of stools. Chronic diarrhea can be caused by infection, or other underlying bowel conditions. Symptoms include loose, watery stools; abdominal cramps; and bloating.	**Etiology** Bacteria: *E. coli*, Salmonella, Shigella Viruses: norovirus and rotavirus Parasites: Cryptosporidium and Giardia lamblia Food allergies Certain medications Intestinal disorders Cancer **Risk factors** Older adults Immunocompromised Children under 3 years old Travel to foreign places Medications	Thorough history taking for travel, food consumption, new medications Stool sample, CBC, CMP May need a colonoscopy Persistent loose, watery stools Dehydration Urgent need to have bowel movement Abdominal cramps and pain Fever Nausea Blood in the stool	Drink plenty of fluids Treat the cause if a pathogen involved Bismuth subsalicylate Lomotil Cipro for traveler's diarrhea Hospitalization if severe enough Prevention: Handwashing, safe handling of food
Ileus	Partial or complete nonmechanical blockage of the small and/or large intestine. **Pathophysiology** An obstruction of the intestine from bowel paralysis. The paralysis need not be complete to cause an ileus, but the intestine must be inactive so food cannot pass through it. Ileus is common after certain surgeries. It can also stem from certain illnesses, drugs, and injuries.	**Etiology** Medicines such as morphine and oxycodone Infections causing gastroenteritis Intestinal cancer Electrolyte imbalances Crohn's disease Abdominal surgery Diverticulitis Parkinson's disease, which affects muscles and nerves in the intestines **Risk factors** Advanced age Digestive disorders such as diverticulitis or IBD Electrolyte imbalances Radiation near the abdomen Intestinal injury Rapid weight loss Sepsis	**Assessment** Abdominal discomfort Loss of appetite Feeling of fullness Constipation Inability to pass gas Bloating Excessive belching Nausea Vomiting **Physical exam and diagnostics** X-ray CT provides more detail than standard X-ray images Ultrasound Air or barium enema	Treatment options for an ileus include waiting for the ileus to resolve, making dietary changes, or adjusting medication use Surgery may be necessary Intravenous fluids to prevent dehydration Nasogastric decompression Pain relief ERAS protocols are being used more and more frequently to decrease the incidence and reduce the duration of postoperative paralytic ileus

(continued)

TABLE 10.11 OTHER MOTILITY DISORDERS (continued)

DISORDER	DEFINITION	RISK FACTORS	ASSESSMENT	TREATMENT
Gastropa-resis	Gastric motility slows down or doesn't work at all, which prevents complete emptying of the contents. **Pathophysiology** Can be caused by damage to the vagus nerve, which regulates the digestive system. A damaged vagus nerve prevents muscles in the stomach and intestine from functioning, which prevents food from moving through properly.	**Etiology** The exact cause is unknown but may be a result from damaged nerves in the stomach. This nerve damage can be from the following: Diabetes Surgeries in the abdomen or esophagus Infections, specifically viral infections Certain medications (narcotic pain medications and antidepressants) Scleroderma Parkinson's disease and MS Hypothyroidism or hyperthyroidism Cancer treatments	Constant nausea and vomiting: especially vomiting undigested food a few hours after eating Feeling full after eating very little Acid reflux or heartburn Abdominal pain and/or bloating Changes in blood sugar levels Lack of appetite Weight loss	There is no cure for gastroparesis. Treatment aims to manage symptoms by treating the underlying cause (Abdalla et al., 2016) **Medication** Medications to stimulate the stomach muscles. Metoclopramide Erythromycin Domperidone Antiemetic medications to control nausea and vomiting. Prochlorperazine Diphenhydramine **Self-care** Maintain proper nutrition Eat foods that are easy to digest Eat well-cooked fruits and vegetables **Medical procedures** Jejunostomy Botulinum toxin Gastric electrical stimulation and pacing (Chen et al., 2017)

CBC, complete blood count; CMP, comprehensive metabolic panel; ERAS, enhanced recovery after surgery; IBD, inflammatory bowel disease; MS, multiple sclerosis.

APPENDECTOMY

Surgical removal of the appendix using laparoscopic or open surgery technique primarily performed to treat appendicitis (Lippincott Advisor, 2018a).

Key Considerations

- Peritonitis is a life-threatening condition that can result from leaking of infectious material into the abdomen due to an appendix rupture (Lippincott Advisor, 2018a). Early identification and treatment of appendicitis is vital.
- Post surgery, one or more drains to allow fluid to escape the abdominal cavity may remain in the incision site (Lippincott Advisor, 2018a).

Gerontologic Considerations
Presentation

- Signs and symptoms may deviate from classic presentation and may include the following (Smelter et al., 2010a, 2010b):
  - Vague symptoms
  - Minimal or absent pain
  - Absence of leukocytosis and fever
- Symptoms of shock may precede or accompany disease presentation (Smelter et al., 2010a).
  - Important to assess for oliguria, mental status changes, tachycardia, tachypnea

Complications

- Presence of other chronic disease and/or more complicated presentation commonly places older patients at higher risk for intraoperative or postoperative complications.
- Delayed presentation with less profound symptoms in older patients can increase risk for complications.

Disease-Specific Concerns

- Cholecystitis is common in older adults due to bile saturation resulting from increased hepatic cholesterol secretion and decreased bile acid synthesis (Smelter et al., 2010a).
- Higher incidence of perforated appendix in older patients because acute appendicitis is uncommon, symptom presentation is atypical, and delays engagement in healthcare (Smelter et al., 2010b).

Preoperative Management

Prepare patient for procedure and postoperative plan including the following:

- Postoperative pain management plan, drains, tubes, incision care, fluids, nutrition, and prevention of complications (Table 10.12)

Potential Complications

- Bleeding
- Blood clots

TABLE 10.12 NURSING INTERVENTIONS

Promote comfort.	■ Provide analgesia and alternative therapies for pain/discomfort. ■ Laparoscopic surgeries may result in abdominal and/or right shoulder pain related to insufflation of carbon dioxide during surgery; ambulation and application of heat can help to relieve discomfort (Smelter et al., 2010a). ■ An abdominal binder may be applied to support the incision and decrease discomfort during position changes and ambulation. ■ A pillow can be used to brace against the abdomen and provide support during coughing, laughing, and/or position changes.
Encourage nutrition and monitor fluid volume.	■ High-protein, low-fat diet ■ Advance diet as tolerated ■ Strict intake and output
Promote skin integrity.	■ Assess surgical site for drainage, redness, tenderness. ■ Encourage or assist with frequent position changes to offload bony prominences.
Promote bowel elimination.	■ Assess for rigidity, rebound tenderness, and increased pain in the abdomen. ■ Ensure patient is passing flatus and bowel movements. ■ Encourage ambulation.
Prevent infection.	■ Monitor for leukocytosis, fever, tachycardia, hypotension. ■ Assess incision and drain sites for purulent drainage, odor, and tenderness.
Prevent pneumonia.	■ Turn, cough, deep breath q2h ■ Incentive spirometry q2h

- Infection
- Pneumonia
- Wound dehiscence
- Paralytic ileus
- Anesthesia complications

Patient Education

Provide time for patient and family/caregiver to return demonstrate and/or teach back the following:

- Care for surgical incision(s), drains, and/or ostomy
- Medication purpose and side effects
- Bowel management strategies
- Nutrition and diet changes
- Turn, cough, deep breath
- Incentive spirometry
- How to splint abdomen with a pillow

Discharge Planning

Involve family or caregivers who will be providing assistance at home in the discharge teaching session, including the following:

- Review dosage, frequency, side effects, and potential adverse effects of prescribed medications. Include teaching regarding weaning strategy for pain medications.
- Review nutrition plan and instruct to advance diet slowly.
- Advocate for importance of frequent activity in short duration with rest periods, advancing as tolerated.
- Review incision, drain, and/or ostomy care: dressing type, technique, and frequency.
- Discuss dates, times, and locations of follow-up appointments.
- Discuss importance of calling their provider with symptoms of the following:
  - Fever greater than 100.4 °F (37.9 °C)
  - Worsening pain, redness, bleeding, swelling, drainage, or bruising at incision site
  - Constipation, diarrhea, nausea, or vomiting
  - Abdominal distension
  - Blood in stool or coughing up blood
  - Uncontrolled pain

Early Recovery After Surgery

Enhanced recovery after surgery (ERAS) is a set of guidelines for pre- and postoperative care designed to achieve early recovery after surgical procedures by optimizing care, improving functioning, and reducing complications after surgery. Key strategies are listed in Table 10.13.

ACUTE PANCREATITIS

OVERVIEW

Acute inflammation of the pancreas is primarily caused by gallstones, alcohol consumption, high triglycerides, bacterial or viral infections, medications, and in some cases postsurgical or interventional complications (Campion et al., 2016; Forsmark & Yadav, 2016; Lindberg, 2009).

Pathophysiology

- Early activation of digestive enzymes (trypsinogen to trypsin) occurs inside the pancreas instead of the intestine, which leads to auto digestion of pancreatic tissue, which in turn leads to inflammation.
- Inflammation may lead to accumulation of fluid in the peripancreatic region and/or necrosis (Vege, 2019a).

Risk Factors

- Daily alcohol consumption >4 drinks for >5 consecutive years causes toxicity of pancreas
- Smoking
- Familial history
- Hypertriglycerides
- Congenital abnormalities and genetic disorders
- Bacterial (mycobacterium, leptospirosis, legionella, mycoplasms)
- Viral (coxsackie; Epstein–Barr; hepatitis A, B, C; HIV; mumps; varicella; rubella)
- Renal disease
- Hypercalcemia
- Patient populations receiving certain medications within immunosuppressive, immunomodulators, antifungal, HIV

TABLE 10.13 GASTROINTESTINAL SURGERY GUIDELINES AND ASSOCIATED NURSING STRATEGIES

ERAS ELEMENT	NURSING STRATEGIES
Risk assessment	<ul><li>Preoperative risk assessment</li><li>Identification of potential complications</li></ul>
Perioperative optimization	<ul><li>Counsel patients on smoking and/or alcohol cessation 4 weeks prior to surgery</li></ul>
Glycemic control	<ul><li>Routine administration of carbohydrates preoperatively (excluding patients with motility/gastric emptying issues)</li><li>Promote glucose stability intraoperatively</li></ul>
Intraoperative hypothermia	<ul><li>Advocate for active warming strategies intraoperatively</li></ul>
Pain management	<ul><li>Promote patient comfort and maximize function</li><li>Implement multimodal (opioid sparing) approaches to analgesia</li><li>Implement nonpharmacologic pain management techniques</li></ul>
Postoperative delirium	<ul><li>Routine screening</li><li>Prevention: promote sleep–wake cycle, promote mobility, avoid benzodiazepines in older adults</li><li>Investigate rationale for delirium symptoms</li></ul>
Prevention and treatment of postoperative ileus	<ul><li>Facilitate multimodal pain management (opioid sparing)</li><li>Mobilization</li><li>Gum chewing</li><li>Early nutrition</li><li>Advocate avoidance of routine nasogastric tube insertion</li></ul>
Early mobilization	<ul><li>Collaborate with interprofessional team on safe patient handling</li><li>Develop and implement daily activity plan</li><li>Advance activity as patient tolerates</li></ul>

Source: Adapted from Feldheiser, A., Aziz, O., Baldini, G., Cox, B. P. B. W., Fearon, K. C. H., Feldman, L. S., Gan, T. J., Kennedy, R. H., Ljungqvist, O., Lobo, D. N., Miller, T., Radtke, F. F., Garces, T. R., Schricker, T., Scott, M. J., Thacker, J. K., Ytreb., L. M., & Carli, F. (2015). Enhanced recovery after surgery (ERAS) for gastrointestinal surgery, part 2: Consensus statement for anaesthesia practice. *Acta Anaesthesiologica Scandinavica, 60*, 289–334. https://doi .org/10.1111/aas.12651

therapy drug classes (Forsmark & Yadav, 2016; Lindberg, 2009; Reese & Glass, 2019; Tenner et al., 2013; Trivedi & Pitchumoni, 2005)

Assessment

- *Pain*: Variable and dependent on patient pain tolerance (Tenner et al., 2013)
  - Obstructive pain is sharper and more acute.
  - Alcoholic causes are dull and generalized.
  - Location of pain—Midepigastric pain radiating between shoulder blades
- Anorexia
- N/V
- Fever >38°C

Abdominal Exam

- Epigastric tenderness
- Guarding on palpation
- Hypoactive bowel sounds (Vege, 2019a)
- Palpable masses in upper abdominal region in the presence of pseudocyst
- Assess for peritoneal hemorrhage (Campion et al., 2016; Vege, 2019a)
  - Grey Turner's sign: Flank ecchymosis
  - Cullen's sign: periumbilical ecchymosis

Diagnosis

Revised Atlanta criteria: Must meet two out of the following three criteria (Crockett et al., 20018):

- Abdominal pain consistent with pancreatitis
- Amylase and/or lipase >3× upper range of lab's normal limit
- Abdominal imaging indicating acute pancreatitis

Diagnostic Findings

Serum Labs

Amylase, Lipase, Triglycerides
Lipase level

- Has greater specificity for pancreatitis

Amylase level

- Rises within 6 hours of acute episode, dropping within 10 hours of peak.
- Some patients may have normal levels (alcoholic and hypertriglyceridemia causes; Vege, 2019a).
- Triglycerides >1,000 mg/dL if no gallstones or history of alcohol.
- Potassium and magnesium decreased.

Other Labs

Imaging Findings
Chest x-ray (present in 30% patients; Vege, 2019)

- Elevated hemidiaphragm
- Pleural effusions
- Pulmonary infiltrates or acute respiratory distress syndrome (ARDS)
- Ground glass opacities if peripancreatic fluid present

Abdominal x-ray

- Negative or ileus

Abdominal ultrasound

- Enlarged pancreas
- Gallstones in gallbladder or common bile duct
- Ileus may not allow visualization of pancreas or gallbladder structures

Abdominal CT

- Enlarged pancreas (localized or diffuse).
- IV contrast does not show necrosis.
- Gas bubbling indicates gas-forming organisms.

Magnetic resonance cholangiopancreatography (MRCP)
- Assists with diagnosis of ductal blockage.

Severity Rating Scales

Different scales are available for determining disease severity and/or mortality. Any tool used should accompany ongoing clinical examination of the patient.
- **American College of Gastroenterology Severity Classification** (Tenner et al., 2013; Vege, 2019a): Disease severity increases with age, body mass index (BMI), comorbid conditions, imaging results, and renal labs (Table 10.14).
- **Modified Glasgow**—Modification of Ranson's criteria. Uses mnemonic **P-A-N-C-R-E-A-S** (Table 10.15). Each item present is given a score of 1 (severe disease if >3 indicators are present during the first 48 hours).
- **Ranson's Criteria**—Each item receives 1 point. Mortality increases with the number of criteria present (Ranson et al., 1974; Table 10.16).

Complications
- *Pre-renal azotemia* due to pancreatic fluid leakage, acute tubular necrosis, and ileus
  - Onset within 24 hours symptoms, lasting 10 days
    - May require renal replacement therapy
- *Fluid collection*: Intervention required if persistent abdominal pain or infection
  - Encapsulated collections—Walled off or pseudocyst: See "Interventions"
- *Necrosis*
  - Predictors
    - **Increase BUN/creatinine at 48 hours**
    - **Hematocrit >44% (indicates hemoconcentration)**
    - **C reactive protein after 48 hours**
- *Organ failure* due to sepsis or ARDS
  - Results from large volume fluid resuscitation.
  - Pancreatic abscesses may cause pleural effusions.

Treatment
- Early and aggressive hydration (Campion et al., 2016; Tenner et al., 2013)
  - *Rationale*
    - Restores fluid losses from anorexia, vomiting, third spacing, and other sources of fluid loss.
    - Reduces pancreatic inflammation and necrosis.
    - Reduces elevated hematocrit and BUN.
    - Promotes perfusion to pancreas and surrounding structures.

TABLE 10.14 AMERICAN COLLEGE OF GASTROENTEROLOGY SEVERITY CLASSIFICATION

MILD ACUTE PANCREATITIS	NO ORGAN FAILURE AND NO LOCAL OR SYSTEMIC COMPLICATIONS
Moderately severe pancreatitis	Transient organ failure resolving within 48 hours onset or <48 hours of local or systemic complication that does not involve continued organ failure
Severe pancreatitis	Persistent failure of one or more organs or Pancreatic necrosis

Source: Tenner, S., Baillie, J., DeWitt, J., & Vege, S. S. (2013). American College of Gastroenterology Guideline: Mangement of acute pancreatitis. *American Journal of Gastroenterology, 108*(9), 1400–1415. Retrieved from https://www.ncbi.nlm.nih.gov/pubmed/23896955

TABLE 10.15 PANCREAS MNEMONIC FOR MODIFIED GLASGOW

	MEANING	SIGNIFICANCE
P	PaO_2	<60; lower PaO_2 increases mortality
A	Age	≥55
N	Neutrophils	WBC ↑
C	Calcium	↓ Calcium or I ionized calcium
R	Renal function	BUN ↑
E	Enzymes	ALT and LDH↑
A	Albumin	↓ Albumin
S	Sugar	Blood glucose >10 mmol/L or >180 mg/dL

ALT, alanine aminotransferase; BUN, blood urea nitrogen; LDH, lactate dehydrogenase; WBC, white blood cell.

- Administer isotonic crystalloids within the first 12 to 24 hours (250–500 mL/hr).
  - Lactated ringers (LR)—preferred to minimize potential electrolyte imbalances
- *Pain control*
  - IV opiates preferred.
  - Morphine may cause sphincter of Oddi spasms.
- *Antibiotics*
  - Use only when infection is present.
  - Prophylactic treatment not recommended.

TABLE 10.16 RANSON'S CRITERIA

NUMBER CRITERIA	0–2	3–4	5–6	7–8
Mortality rate %	1	16	40	100
Admission presentation	48 hours after admission—Changes in labs			
Age >55	Hematocrit drops by 10%			
WBC >16,000	BUN increase by 8 mg/dL			
Glucose >200	Serum Ca++ decreases by 8 mg/dL			
Serum LDH >35 units/L	PaO_2 <60 mmHg			
AST >250 units/L	Base deficit >4 mEq/L			
	Estimated sequestrian fluid >600 mL			

AST, aspartate aminotransferase; BUN, blood urea nitrogen; LDH, lactate dehydrogenase; WBC, white blood cell.

- *Nutrition*
  - Delayed feeding increases the risk for necrosis (Crockett et al., 2018).
  - Early nutrition via the GI route reduces length of stay, mortality. and end organ damage.
  - Early nutrition protects the lining of the GI tract and reduces bacterial translocation (Crockett et al., 2018, Vege et al., 2018).
  - Gastric-route nutrition
    - Mild severity
      - IV hydration and then oral nutrition within 5 to 7 days starting with clear liquids; then advance to low-fat diet as tolerated.
    - Moderate to severe
      - Enteral nutrition if unable to tolerate oral feeding (pain, nausea, vomiting)
      - Weighted enteral tube at jejunum ligament of Treiz preferred
  - Parental-route nutrition
    - **Use in patients with ileus or who are unable to tolerate enteral nutrition.**
- *Alcohol reduction/cessation* counseling needed for individuals who have repeat attacks.

Interventions
Endoscopic Retrograde
Cholangiopancreatography

- Indications
  - Presence of new jaundice
  - Suspected bile duct blockage/stone removal
  - Suspected tumor
    - **Complications**
      - Sepsis
      - Bleeding
      - Reactions to contrast of anesthesia
      - Aspiration
- Necrosectomy
  - **Laproscopic surgical removal of necrotic tissue**
    - Best performed 4 weeks after onset of fluid collection (Crockett et al., 2018)
    - High risk for postoperative complication
  - Endoscopic ultrasound (EUS)—Placement of stents for drainage or endoscopic necrosectomy

CHRONIC PANCREATITIS

OVERVIEW

- Chronic pancreatitis (CP) is the result of repeated injury, inflammation (Freedman et al., 2019) of acinar cells of the pancrease or damage caused by structural blockage (Singh et al., 2019)
- Inflammation causes scarring and calcification leading to atrophy and impaired endocrine and exocrine function of pancreatic tissue (Freedman et al., 2019; Gardner et al., 2020)
- Diagnosis of CP is determined by careful review of patient history, assessment, and risk factors along with diagnositic evaluation (Conwell et al., 2014; Freedman, 2019; Tenner, 2013)
- Progressive pancreatic inflammation associated with fibrotic, calcified damage to pancreatic tissue leading to impaired function of the gland (Freedman, 2019)

Risk Factors

- Acute pancreatitis may progress to chronic pancreatitis.
- The acronym TIGAR is used to help classify risk for chronic pancreatitis (toxic/metabolic, idiopathic, genetic, autoimmune, recurrent pancreatitis, obstructive; Gardner, 2020).
- Similar to acute pancreatitis, risk for chronic pancreatitis occurs in alcoholic patients (>60%).
- Smoking and alcohol consumption contributes to disease progression (Conwell et al., 2013; Freedman, 2019, Singh et al., 2019).

Pathophysiology

- *Initial or sentinel acute pancreatitis*
  - First event of acute pancreatitis creates an inflammatory response that causes injury, leading to fibrosis of the pancreas.
- Recurrent acute episodes
  - Results in chronic pain, which leads to insufficiency of endocrine and exocrine functions
- Excessive protein secretion causes increase in bicarbonate
  - Pancreatic proteins → plugs pancreatic ducts → ductal scarring and obstruction → increases inflammation
- Antioxidant deficiencies
  - Selenium, methionine, vitamin C, vitamin D → stressed cells → increasing free radicals → lipid peroxidation → cell damage (Freedman et al., 2019)

Assessment

- Epigastric pain radiating to back, with onset approximately 20 minutes after eating.
  - Intensity varies by individual and pain may be absent.
  - May have continuous pain for days followed by days or months of pain-free episodes.
- Nausea, vomiting
- Steatorrhea due to fat malabsorption (vitamins A, D, E, K, and B_{12}); occurs late in disease process
  - Loose, foul smelling
  - Increased flatus
- Weight loss
- Symptoms associated with diabetes mellitus
- Jaundice
- Laboratory and imaging tests may be normal due to fibrosis and reduced pancreatic enzymes
  - Abdominal CT, MRI, and ultrasound, MRCP
  - Pancreatogram
    - **Beading in main duct or side branches**
  - Abnormal secretin pancreatic function test
  - Fecal elastase (evaluates exocrine function Conwell et al., 2013; Freedman et al., 2019; Vege, 2019)

Treatment

- Low-fat diet
  - Approximately 50-g low-fat diet may assist with pain control. Avoid greasy and fried foods.
  - Eliminate alcohol consumption.
- Pain control
  - Avoid opioids
  - NSAIDs if not contraindicated
- Tricyclic antidepressants, serotonin uptake inhibitors, gabapentin, or pregabalin
- Pancreatic enzymes (may decrease pain caused by ductal pressure)

- Nerve block
- Steatorrhea (fatty or oily stools)
  - Lipase enzymes
  - Not all patients will benefit from use; osage depends on the degree of remaining pancreatic function
- H2 receptor antagonist, PPI, or sodium bicarbonate reduces lipase inactivation
- H2 blockers or PPIs are beneficial in those using nonenteric-coated enzymes; nonenteric-coated enzymes are deactivated from the acidic pH of the gastric contents (Freedman, 2018)

Surgical Interventions
- Endoscopic stent into pancreatic or biliary ducts for drainage
- Sphincterotomy
- Distal pancreatectomy
- Total pancreatectomy for severe cases

ANATOMICAL OVERVIEW AND FUNCTIONS OF THE LIVER

OVERVIEW
The liver is one of the largest organs in the body. Considered a helper organ of digestion, the liver works with the pancreas, gallbladder, and intestines to produce and process enzymes, fat, protein, and nutrients. The liver is also able to regenerate cells (Heuther, 2010).
- **Glisson capsule:** Layer of fibrous connective tissue covering the liver: contains supply of blood, lymphocytes, and nerve cells.
  - **Diseases of the liver cause swelling to the capsule, which results in pain and leakage into the peritoneum.**
- **Common hepatic duct**
  - Transports bile to gallbladder and duodenum (first part of small intestine)
  - Bile goes from gallbladder back to the hepatic duct

Blood Supply
- The liver is a very vascular organ. It accounts for approximately 13% of the body's total blood supply.
- Blood from stomach and intestine must pass through liver.
  - Hepatic artery
    - **Oxygenated blood comes from the hepatic artery via the abdominal aorta.**
    - **Supplies 25% cardiac output at rate of 400 to 500 mL/min.**
  - Hepatic portal vein (liver's primary blood supply)
    - **Deoxygenated blood comes from both mesenteric and splenic veins.**
    - **Carries 70% to 75% of blood to the liver at a rate of 1,100 mL/min.**
  - Inferior vena cava

Functions of the Liver
- *Supports gastric digestion through secretion of bile.*
  - Hepatocytes create bile, which contains bile salts.
  - Bile is secreted at a daily rate of 700 to 1,200 mL.
  - Bile salts contain cholesterol, bilirubin, electrolytes, and water.
    - **Aids small bowel in digestion and absorption of fat and cholesterol digestion.**
    - **Bile salts form bilirubin, which is a waste product of hemoglobin breakdown.**

- Formed from hemoglobin breakdown of RBC
- Liver stores iron from hemoglobin to produce new RBC
  - Unconjugated bilirubin is the waste product of broken-down red blood cells that are sent to the liver. The end result is a lipid-based product. The unconjugated bilirubin is transported to the liver and conjugates with glucuronic acid to make it water based.
    - Bilirubin that binds to albumin
    - Dissolves in lipids (lipid soluble)
  - Conjugated bilirubin flows through the bile and is excreted through the small intestine.
- *Production of clotting factors*
  - Adequate production of bile is needed for vitamin K absorption.
  - Vitamin K produces clotting factors.
    - **Reduced bile production results in decreased availability of clotting factors, increasing the risk of bleeding.**
  - Liver also produces thrombin, fibrinogen, and clotting factors I, II, VII, IX, and X.
- *Protein and carbohydrate metabolism*
  - Liver enzymes aid in digestion of proteins and carbohydrates.
  - Carbohydrates are metabolized into glycogen.
  - Glycogen converts into glucose to maintain normal blood glucose levels.
- *Vitamin and mineral storage*
  - Stores vitamins A, D, E, K, and B_{12}.
  - Iron is stored as ferritin needed for development of new RBCs.
- *Filtration system*
  - Removes and converts naturally occurring ammonia into urea, which is excreted as urine.
  - Detoxifies internal hormones and external chemicals to prevent retention of these substances, which may cause harmful effects to other organs.
  - Excessive usage of certain chemicals, such as alcohol, and certain substances reduces and weakens the detoxification function of the liver.

SELECTED SCORING CALCULATORS FOR DETERMINING ALCOHOL AND LIVER DISEASE
Several instruments exist to quantify or qualify the extent of liver disease, predict mortality, and determine the best course of treatment (Table 10.17). Automated calculators are available on the internet or as mobile applications, where data can be easily entered and calculated.

NONALCOHOLIC FATTY LIVER DISEASE

OVERVIEW
Nonalcoholic fatty liver disease (NAFLD) is an international health problem related to cardio-metabolic factors such as obesity and metabolic syndrome. Increased amounts of fat within the liver cause oxidative overload due to damaged hepatic mitochondria.

TABLE 10.17 INSTRUMENTS TO QUANTIFY OR QUALIFY LIVER DISEASE

INSTRUMENT/ ACRONYM/AUTHOR	PURPOSE/DESCRIPTION	VARIABLES	SCORING SIGNIFICANCE
AUDIT (Saunders et al., 1993)	Identifies low-risk alcohol consumption from harmful drinking. Scripted 10-item list or self-report; 5 answer choices; scored 0–4.	Three subcategories (# questions) Hazardous alcohol use (3) Dependence symptoms (3) Harmful alcohol use (4)	8–15, medium risk: Brief interventions recommended 16–19, hazardous alcohol use >20, alcohol dependence Counseling, monitoring, and intense intervention are recommended for scores >16
CAGE (Mayfield et al., 1974)	Simple 1-minute alcohol screen to determine problem drinking and alcohol-related problems. Not validated to diagnose alcohol use disorder.	Four yes/no questions about alcohol consumption based on the instrument's acronym C = cut down A = annoyed G = guilty E = eye opener	2 or higher, positive. Follow up is recommended for positive result and if answer to eye opener question is "yes." Note: Alcohol screening is recommended on all populations by National Institute of Alcohol Abuse and Alcoholism.
Child Pugh (Angermayr et al., 2003; Papatheodoridis et al., 2005)	Determines severity of chronic liver disease, mortality, response to treatment, and need for transplantation. Six-item instrument evaluates laboratory data, physical assessment, and diagnosis, scored on a scale of 1–3.	**Lab values** categorized and entered into ranges on instrument. Serum albumin, total bilirubin, INR. **Assessment findings** Ascites and hepatic encephalopathy **Diagnosis of liver disease** Sclerosis cholangitis, biliary cirrhosis or other type	See mortality table below
Discriminant function (Maddrey's Discriminant Function test) (Maddrey et al., 1978)	Determines severity of alcoholic hepatitis, estimated 30-day mortality, and the need for corticosteroid therapy. Instrument has also been used to determine use of pentoxifyline and reduce risk of hepatorenal syndrome.	Patient prothrombin time and bilirubin, laboratory prothrombin control	Score of >32, severe disease and 30-day mortality of 50% or greater; may benefit from corticosteroid therapy Score of <32, mild/moderate disease; mortality rate of 1%; will not benefit from corticosteroids
Lillie Score (Louvet et al., 2007)	Determines estimated 6-month mortality in patients with severe alcoholic hepatitis not responsive to corticosteroid therapy.	Tested on day 7 of corticosteroid therapy using patient's age and **Baseline lab data** for albumin, bilirubin, prothrombin time, and creatinine **Day 7 lab data** for bilirubin	Score <0.45, improvement due to corticosteroid and 85% survival rate Score >0.45, survival rate is 25% and continued use of corticosteroids is ineffective
MELD-Na (Myers et al., 2013)	Determines 3-month mortality and survival due to chronic liver disease. Use to determine urgency for transplant based on UNOS. Considered a more accurate determinant of mortality over original MELD scoring system.	**Serum laboratory results** bilirubin, creatinine, INR, sodium **Renal failure** requiring dialysis	Scores range from 6 to 40. Scores should be calculated after excluding acute and treating reversible causes of liver disease. The higher the score, the greater the need for transplantation.
MELD (Sheth et al., 2002; Singal et al., 2018)	Determines mortality in alcoholic hepatitis and cirrhotic liver disease. May also be used to determine corticosteroid use. This is the original scoring instrument and does not include sodium and dialysis qualifiers.	**Serum laboratory results** Creatinine, bilirubin, INR	MELD score >11 or bilirubin >8 corticosteroids can reduce mortality by 10% MELD >21 corticosteroids treatment can be applied
NAFLD Fibrosis Score (Angulo et al., 2007)	Noninvasive measure, clinical and lab findings to differentiate NAFLD patients with and without progressive disease.	Age, BMI, glucose, AST/ALT ration, platelet count and albumin	Patients identified as lower risk for fibrosis are less likely to undergo liver biopsy.

Child Pugh mortality table:

Score	1-year mortality (%)	2-year mortality (%)
5–6	100	85
7–9	80	60
10–15	45	35

ALT, alanine aminotransferase; AST, aspartate aminotransferase; AUDIT, Alcohol Use Disorder Identification Tool; BMI, body mass index; CAGE, cut down, annoyed, guilty, eye opener; INR, international normalized ratio; MELD, model for end-stage liver disease; Na, sodium; NAFLD, nonalcoholic fatty liver disease; UNOS, United Network for Organ Sharing.

- Increases the risk for development of cardiovascular disease, chronic kidney failure, and colorectal cancer (Diehl & Day, 2017).
- Associated with high mortality when fibrosis is present and is considered the third leading cause of hepatocellular cancer within the United States (Chaney, 2017; Younossi et al., 2018).

Hepatic steatosis (fat) confirmed by CT, MRI, and ultrasound or by liver biopsy eliminates secondary causes for steatosis such as significant amounts of alcohol consumption, medications, infection, or genetic factors (Chalasani et al., 2018; Chaney, 2017).

Significant amounts of alcohol consumption: A drink containing 1 to 1.5 tablespoonfuls of pure alcohol (14 g; National Institute on Alcohol Abuse and Alcoholism, 2019).

- Men >21 standard drinks/wk
- Women >14 drinks/wk (Chalasani et al., 2018)

NONALCOHOLIC FATTY LIVER DISEASE TYPES

There are currently two types of NAFLD. Nonalcoholic fatty liver (NAFL) and nonalcoholic steatohepatitis (NASH). Classification of NAFLD is based on percentage of accumulated fat in the liver and the degree of injury to the hepatocytes in the form of ballooning or fibrosis (Table 10.18). The NAFLD Fibrosis Score indicates the degree of liver scarring present.

NAFLD FIBROSIS SCORE

The NAFLD fibrosis score determines the degree of liver scarring.

- It uses age, hyperglycemia, BMI, platelets, albumin, and aspartate aminotransferase (AST)/alanine aminotransferase (ALT) ratio
- Identifies patient at risk for complications and death related to liver disease
- Levels of severity (see Tables 10.19 and 10.20)

Risk Factors for Nonalcoholic Fatty Liver Disease

Comorbid Risk Factors (Chalasani et al., 2018; Younossi et al., 2018)

- Metabolic syndrome—Risk for NAFLD increases with the presence of metabolic syndrome
- Diabetes mellitus
- Obesity, including childhood obesity
- Hypertension
- Coronary artery disease
- Familial history
- Dyslipidemia (high triglycerides, low high-density lipoproteins [HDL])
- Sleep apnea (in patients with nonalcoholic steatohepatitis [NASH])

Drug-Induced Risk Factors

- Amiodarone
- Steroids
- Valporic acid (Depakote)
- Methotrexate
- Tamoxifen
- Steroids

Dietary Risk Factors

- Starvation
- Consuming soft drinks
- Total parental nutrition

Symptoms

- 80% asymptomatic
- Symptoms appear over time and usually with the onset of cirrhosis

Laboratory Findings

- Increased ratio of AST to ALT >0.8, sometimes at a 2:1 ratio
- Albumin ↓
- Ferritin ↑
- Triglycerides ↑

TABLE 10.18 NONALCOHOLIC FATTY LIVER DISEASE CLASSIFICATION

TYPE	FAT ACCUMULATION (%)	INFLAMMATION	HEPATOCELLULAR INJURY	CIRRHOSIS, LIVER FAILURE, OR CANCER RISK
NAFL	≥5	No	No evidence	Minimal risk
NASH	≥5	Yes	Injury/ballooning present May/may not have fibrosis	May progress to cirrhosis or liver failure; cancer is rare

NAFL, nonalcoholic fatty liver; NASH, nonalcoholic steatohepatitis.

TABLE 10.19 NONALCOHOLIC FATTY LIVER DISEASE SCORE CORRELATED WITH FIBROSIS SEVERITY

NAFLD SCORE	FIBROSIS SEVERITY
<−1.455	F0–F2
−1.455 to 0.675	Indeterminate score
>0.675	F3–F4

NAFLD, nonalcoholic fatty liver disease.

TABLE 10.20 SEVERITY OF FIBROSIS

FIBROSIS SCALE	F0	F1	F2	F3	F4
Fibrosis severity	None	Mild	Moderate	Severe	Cirrhosis

■ Confirmation with (noninvasive) FibroScan or liver biopsy (invasive)

Treatment
- **Lifestyle changes**
  - Weight loss, exercise
    - **Body fat reduction of 3% or more needed to reduce fatty deposits.**
    - **A 10% reduction can improve injury and fibrosis.**
- Dietary modifications (restrict fat) or adopt Mediterranean diet
- Discontinue or reduce alcohol intake
- Consider bariatric surgery if BMI >35
- Liver transplant with advanced NASH cirrhosis

CIRRHOSIS OF THE LIVER

OVERVIEW

Cirrhosis is the end-stage result of injury to hepatocytes over time. Untreated and repeated injury to the liver increases predisposition to cirrhosis (Fowler, 2013; Reese & Glass, 2019). Recurring injury from inflammation causes fibrosis, which substitutes normal regenerating tissue with nodular tissue. This cycle of chronic inflammation leads to successive pathologic processes that affect the overall function of the liver (Goldberg & Chopra, 2019; Reese & Glass, 2019).

- Late stages of liver cirrhosis are typically irreversible; when identified early, treatment may reverse its sequela.
- Disease outcomes are dependent on the extent and etiology of cirrhosis along with associated comorbidities and timing of treatment.
- Most individuals with cirrhosis are susceptible to multiple complications that increase mortality risk and incidence of liver carcinomas (Goldberg & Chopra, 2019).

Causes and Risk Factors
- Hepatitis C is the number one cause of liver cirrhosis followed by alcoholism.

Common Risk Factors
- Chronic viral hepatitis (B, C, D; Goldberg & Chopra, 2018, 2019)
- Alcoholism (Runyon, 2013)
- Drug toxicity (Reese & Glass, 2019)
- Autoimmune and genetic diseases (Goldberg & Chopra, 2018; Reese & Glass, 2019)
- NAFLD (Reese & Glass, 2019)
- Primary biliary cholangitis (Goldberg & Chopra, 2018)
- Primary sclerosing cholangitis
- Having more than one risk factor increases the likelihood of developing cirrhosis (Goldberg & Chopra, 2018, 2019)

Symptoms and Stages of Cirrhosis
Three stages of cirrhosis:
- Compensated
- Compensated with varices
- Decompensated

The majority of symptoms and complications appear in the decompensated stage, whereas subtle nonspecific symptoms occurring in compensated stages may be attributed to nonliver-related conditions (Flamm, 2018; Fowler, 2013; Garcia-Tsao et al., 2017; Goldberg & Chopra, 2018, 2019; Pose & Cardenas, 2017). See Tables 10.21 and 10.22.

Diagnostic Tests (Table 10.23)
Imaging

- *Abdominal ultrasound or CT scan* may reveal nodular, irregular-shaped atrophy or hypertrophy of the liver (Goldberg & Chopra, 2018; Reese & Glass, 2019).
- *Elastography* measures liver stiffness and degree of fibrosis through the application of noninvasive vibrations (Curry & Afdhal, 2018).
- *Surgical and procedural interventions* (Goldberg & Chopra, 2018; Pose & Cardenas, 2017):
  - *Endoscopy* allows visualization, grading, and treatment of varices.
  - *Transjugular intrahepatic portosystemic shunt (TIPS):* Radiologic-guided stent placement to redirect blood flow from the portal vein to one of the three hepatic veins.
    - **Alleviates pressure from veins in the stomach, bowel, and esophagus** (Garcia-Tsao et al., 2017)
  - *Distal splenorenal shunt (DSRS):* Surgical procedure used to control bleeding by connecting splenic vein to the left renal vein.

Management and Prevention of Cirrhosis Complications
- Prevent further complications from cirrhosis (Chaney et al., 2015; Fitzpatrick et al., 2017; Fowler, 2013; Goldberg & Chopra, 2019; Reese & Glass, 2019; Runyon, 2013; Sinha-Hikim et al., 2017).
- Vaccinate against hepatitis A and B along with an annual influenza vaccine.
- Abstain from alcohol and tobacco.
  - Tobacco use with NAFLD has been linked to fibrosis due to cytokine release triggering inflammation that damages liver cell and other organs.
- Diet counseling for uncomplicated cases of cirrhosis.
  - Use low sodium (2–4 g) diet to reduce ascites and peripheral edema.
  - Ingest 60 to 80 g protein to prevent malnutrition.
  - Reduce fat intake and seek dietary consultation for diet planning.
- Avoid hepatotoxins and NSAIDs, including over-the-counter medication and herbal supplements.
  - Reduce prescription medication dosage for hepatic impairment.
- Avoid PPIs as these can increase risk for spontaneous bacterial peritonitis.
- Adhere to prescribed diet and medications focused on reducing hepatotoxic symptoms.
- Referral for liver transplant when complications from decompensated disease are present.

DECOMPENSATED CIRRHOSIS OF THE LIVER: COMPLICATIONS AND TREATMENT

OVERVIEW
Failure to respond to conservative cirrhosis treatment and to avoid hepatotoxins, including alcohol, increases risk for developing complications associated with decompensated liver disease.

TABLE 10.21 PATHOGENESIS AND PATHOPHYSIOLOGY OF CIRRHOSIS AND LIVER FAILURE

ASSESSMENT FINDINGS	PATHOGENESIS	SIMPLE PATHOPHYSIOLOGY
Abdominal pain	Growing size of the liver	Glisson capsule is stretched; presence of ascites
*Ascites	Fluid accumulation in peritoneal cavity	Vasodilation changes hepatic blood flow Loss of compensatory mechanisms to maintain arterial blood flow Causes H_2O and Na+ retention *Precursor to portal HTN, SBP, hydrothorax, and HRS
Asterixis (liver flaps)	Metabolic condition (not specific to liver) Also associated with HE	Abnormal firing and signaling of diencephalon (motor) centers in brain
Bleeding and bruising	Ineffective production of clotting factors	Dysfunctional clotting mechanisms
Hyponatremia	Increased Na+ absorption associated with ascites	High levels of aldosterone from the compensating renal angiotensin aldosterone system increases sodium reabsorption. Increased sodium reabsorption causes **free water retention from reduced serum osmolality**. This results in hyper or hypotonic hyponatremia.
Gastric bleeding and varices	Due to portal hypertension; collateral circulation cannot keep up with demand of portal vein	Obstructed hepatic blood flow $\Rightarrow$ collateral circulation in lower esophagus and stomach $\Rightarrow$ increased venous pressure and enlargement of the esophageal veins. Results in erythema, friability and rupture of the mucosal lining
Hepatic encephalopathy	Liver is unable to clear toxins	Hepatocytes cannot effectively remove accumulated toxins in the blood and results in toxins flowing to the brain.
Hepatorenal syndrome	Renal dysfunction associated with portal hypertension	Splanchnic vasodilation interferes with normal systemic circulation and releases vasoactive mediators that result in arteriolar vasoconstriction.
Hydrothorax	Translocation ascites fluid into lung	Ascites causes liver to grow in size, pushing against diaphragm; eventually weakening a defect (left or right) in diaphragmatic wall.
Jaundice (skin, sclera icterus), dark urine, pruritus, palmar erythema	Rising bilirubin	Ineffective bilirubin metabolism
Muscle wasting, edema, cachexia, hypotension	Low albumin Asterixis may also be associated with hepatic encephalopathy	Hypoalbuminemia due to reduced protein synthesis and blood flow that limits distribution to other organs. Hypoalbuminemia causes capillary leakage resulting in edema.
Nausea, malaise, headache, confusion, lethargy, coma, and seizures	Multiple causes; direct cause of hyponatremia or hepatic encephalopathy	See hyponatremia See hepatic encephalopathy
Portal hypertension	A direct result of ascites Due to reverse blood flow	Vasodilation from ineffective collateral circulation of the portal venous system causes **congestion and reverse flow**. Reverse portal flow causes increase cardiac output, reduced blood flow and high output heart failure
Spontaneous bacterial peritonitis	Translocation of gut microbes into peritoneal cavity	Gut microbes enter peritoneal cavity through lymph system

HE, hepatic encephalopathy; HRS, hepatorenal syndrome; HTN, hypertension; SBP, spontaneous bacterial peritonitis.

Source: Goldberg, E., & Chopra, S. (2019). Cirrhosis in adults: Overview of complications, general management and prognois. In K. M. Robson (Ed.), *UpToDate* (pp. 1–28). Retrieved from https://www.uptodate.com/contents/cirrhosis-in-adults-overview-of-complications-general-management-and-prognosis

- Prognosis and survivability determined by type, severity, and etiology of decompensated disease.
- Individuals with decompensated disease have a 10-fold risk for mortality than those without liver disease and 2-time increased risk compared with those with compensated liver disease.

- Survival rates can be predicted by scoring tools such as the Model for End Stage Liver Disease (MELD-Na) or the Child-Pugh Score (see Table 10.17).
  Once decompensation arises, a referral for liver transplantation is required (Goldberg & Chopra, 2019).

TABLE 10.22 SYMPTOMS AND ASSESSMENT OF HEPATIC CIRRHOSIS

COMPENSATED CIRRHOSIS AND COMPENSATED WITH VARICES	
Subjective findings	May be asymptomatic. Subtle symptoms may include weakness, anorexia and weight loss, muscle cramps, fatigue mild edema.
Objective findings	Minimal at this stage; may present in other conditions. May have slightly enlarged liver and spleen; cachectic appearance, weight reduction. Varices <10 mmHg identified on esophageal gastroduodenal screening.
DECOMPENSATED CIRRHOSIS	
Subjective findings	Skin color or sclera turning yellow is usually noticed by family member; shakiness or tremors, bloating and excessive weight gain, dark urine with decreased output, hematemesis, hematochezia, melena, confusion, excessive sleep, pruritus, seizure
Objective findings	**Neurologic**: Symptoms of hepatic encephalopathy (delayed or inappropriate response to questions, confusion, unresponsiveness, coma, seizures; asterixis; uncoordinated gait). **Skin**: Caput medusa, jaundice, spider angiomas, palmar erythema, scleral icterus, unexplained bruising. **Abdomen**: Abdominal distention/bulging positive fluid wave due to ascites, venous hum, hepatomegaly, and splenomegaly (palpable sharp margins or nodules), abdominal vein distention, dullness on percussion noticeable when 1.5 L ascites present. **Oral exam**: Bleeding in oral cavity noted in posterior pharynx, fetor hepaticus breath (rotten egg/garlic odor present in HE). **Vital signs**: Weight reduction or increase, hypotension

HE, hepatic encephalopathy.

Sources: Data from Reese, K. R., & Glass, C. A. (2019). Cirrhosis of the liver. In J. C. Cash & C. A. Glass (Eds.), *Adult-gerontology practice guidelines* (2nd ed., pp. 293–297). Springer Publishing Company. https://doi.org/10.1891/978082619597.0014; Goldberg, E., & Chopra, S. (2019). Cirrhosis in adults: Overview of complication, general management and prognois. In K. M. Robson (Ed.), *UpToDate* (pp. 1–28). https://www.uptodate.com/contents/cirrhosis-in-adults-overview-of-complications-general-management-and-prognosis

TABLE 10.23 LABORATORY FINDINGS RELATED TO CIRRHOSIS

LAB VARIANCE	SERUM LABORATORY RESULT AFFECTED
Elevated	AST/ALT, ammonia, alkaline phosphate (up to three times normal), creatinine, GGT (higher levels are seen in disease from chronic alcoholism), glucose, PT/INR, total bilirubin, SAAG
Reduced	Albumin, glucose, hemoglobin, platelets, sodium

ALT, alanine aminotransferase; AST, aspartate aminotransferase; GGT, gamma-glutamyl transpeptidase; INR, international normalized ratio; PT, prothrombin time; SAAG, serum albumin to ascites albumin.

The following are major complications associated with decompensated liver cirrhosis.

ASCITES

- *Ascites* refers to the accumulation of fluid in the peritoneal cavity. Over 80% ascites cases are due to cirrhosis, followed by peritoneal malignancy (<10%) and heart failure (Patel & Muir, 2016).
- Ascites increases risk of infection, hyponatremia, progressive decline in renal function, and causes a predisposition to injury, bleeding tendencies, and even death (Cárdenas et al., 2014; Marciano et al., 2019; Patel & Muir, 2016; Runyon, 2013).
- *Type of ascites:* Ascites is graded by the level of severity, which guides the method of management (Table 10.24).

TABLE 10.24 GRADES OF ASCITES

GRADE 1	GRADE 2	GRADE 3*
Identifiable by ultrasound	Moderate and symmetrical abdominal distention	Extensive fluid collection with tense abdomen

*Refractory ascites** is a grade 3 collection that does not respond to medical management modalities.

Source: Adapted from Pose, E., & Cardenas, A. (2017). Translating our current understanding of ascites management into new therapies for patients with cirrhosis and fluid retention. *Digestive Diseases, 35*(4), 402–410.

- Grading system is per the International A-S-C-I-T-E-S Club (**a**scites, **s**epsis, **c**ardiovascular, **i**mpairment, **the**, en**d**, **s**tage liver failure).

Medical Management of Ascites
- *Management of grades 1 to 3*
  - *Diet*: Restrict sodium intake to 2 to 4 g
  - Alcohol cessation
    - **Baclofen may be useful to reduce alcohol cravings** (Runyon, 2013)
- *Grades 2 and 3: Oral diuretic management*
  - Oral diuretic medication management indicated for grades 2 and 3 ascites (Fowler, 2013; Garcia-Tsao et al., 2017; Pose & Cardenas, 2017; Runyon, 2013; Table 10.25).
    - Diuretics, along with dietary restrictions, can reduce >80% ascites volume (Runyon, 2013).
      - Intravenous furosemide should be given in consultation with nephrology as it may cause decline in renal function (Garcia-Tsao et al., 2017).

TABLE 10.25 ORAL DIURETIC MEDICATION DOSING FOR GRADES 2 AND 3 ASCITES

GRADE	MEDICATION CLASS	MEDICATION	ORAL DOSAGE
2 and 3	Aldosterone antagonist	Spironolactone	50–100 mg/d until desired weight loss achieved; dosage increased every 7 days to maximum daily dose of 400 mg
	Loop diuretic	Furosemide oral	20–40 mg daily; maximum increase to 160 mg daily; used if spironolactone unsuccessful and no renal impairment

Source: Adapted from Pose, E., & Cardenas, A. (2017). Translating our current understanding of ascites management into new therapies for patients with cirrhosis and fluid retention. *Digestive Diseases (Basel, Switzerland), 35*(4), 402–410.

- *Grade 3: Refractory ascites management:* Complications include fluid overload, hepatic encephalopathy, hyponatremia, hyperkalemia, and azotemia (Flamm, 2018; Fowler, 2013; Goldberg & Chopra, 2019; Runyon, 2013).
  - *Paracentesis*: Ultrasound-guided procedure to remove small or large volume of ascites fluid from the abdominal peritoneal space using a hollow needle
    - May be added to diuretic and diet therapy.
    - Albumin administered intravenously to replace >5 L paracentesis volume losses.
    - Administer artificial plasma expanders, saline, or albumin to replace <5 L volume losses (Pose & Cardenas, 2017).
  - Midodrine 5 to 7.5 mg TID may increase blood pressure and increase urine output and urine sodium.
  - TIPS procedure should be considered in refractory ascites not responsive to therapeutic paracentesis along with diuretic, sodium restriction, and other medical management.

PORTAL HYPERTENSION AND GASTROESOPHAGEAL VARICEAL BLEEDING

OVERVIEW

Portal hypertension (PH) is a primary result of cirrhosis. PH occurs when the pressure gradient between the portal vein and the inferior vena cava exceeds 10 to 12 mmHg (Garcia-Tsao et al., 2017). Varices are grossly enlarged veins in the lining of esophageal or upper gastric body. Varices that rupture may lead to life-threatening blood losses and mortality (Fowler, 2013).

- *Variceal bleeding* occurs in 30% of cirrhotic cases. Approximately 50% will experience an initial episode of bleeding that resolves without treatment. However, 55% will rebleed in 6 weeks and 20% will die (Brunner et al., 2017; Cárdenas et al., 2014).

Pathophysiology

- Fibrotic changes or obstruction inside the liver obstructs hepatoportal blood flow.
- Hyperdynamic circulation due to an increase in nitric oxide production causes splanchnic vasodilation (Pose & Cardenas, 2017).
- Splanchnic vasodilation causes increased blood flow resistance of the portal or splenic (Berzigotti, 2013) vein, resulting in collateral circulation of the coronary and gastric veins (Garcia-Tsao et al., 2017), which increases portal pressure and backward flow.
  - The collaterals are weak and fragile vessels that become engorged and eventually rupture due to inability to accommodate the blood flow demand of the portal system (Fowler, 2013).

Symptoms

- Hematemesis (most common)
- Melena (may appear without hematemesis)
- Symptoms of cirrhosis
- Noticeable abdominal wall veins (diversion mechanism to move portal blood into the caval system through the periumbilical veins)
- Caput medusa: Spider nevi when touched result in blood flow away from umbilicus

Treatment
Prevent Variceal Rupture

- Nonselective beta blockers (propranolol, nadolol, carvedilol) promote vasoconstriction (Fitzpatrick et al., 2017; Fowler, 2013; Garcia-Tsao et al., 2017).
- Diagnostic endoscopy used to detect and grade varices. Repeat every 2 to 3 years if no varices (Brunner et al., 2017).

Acute Variceal Rupture

- Protect airway and prevent aspiration: endotracheal intubation as indicated.
- Maintain hemodynamic and coagulation status by replacing blood loss with blood products (plasma, platelets, RBCs) and fluids.
  - Limit use of normal saline as this may increase ascites.
  - Transfusion goals are usually for hemoglobin above 7 gm/dL, but may differ from the patient's underlying disease.
  - Administer Vitamin K to correct PT/INR.
- Provide endoscopic ligation or banding of varices.
- Place balloon tamponade device (Minnesota tube or Sengstaken–Blakemore tube) if unable to control blood loss (Garcia-Tsao et al., 2017).

Medications

- Octreotide 50 mcg bolus followed by 50 mcg/hr infusion for 2 to 5 days
- Vasopressin 0.2 to 0.4 units/min continuously for hemodynamic instability
- Terlipressin (not available in the United States)
- Ceftriaxone 1 g q24h for 7 days or sooner if bleeding resolves TIPS if endoscopy does not control bleeding (Garcia-Tsao et al., 2017)

HEPATORENAL SYNDROME

OVERVIEW

Hepatorenal syndrome (HRS) is severe functional (Angeli et al., 2019) vasoconstrictive acute kidney injury (AKI; Francoz et al., 2019) leading to multiorgan failure in the setting of end-stage liver disease (Fisher, 2010). Treatment considerations are made in a case-by-case basis.

- HRS typically occurs after an episode of acute liver decompensation (Amin et al., 2019; Mindikoglu & Pappas, 2018).

- HRS can be precipitated by infection, especially spontaeous bacterial peritonitis (SBP; Amin et al., 2019).
- Many patients with liver disease have some form of chronic kidney disease (CKD; Amin et al., 2019; Davenport et al., 2017). Acute renal failure in cirrhotic patients with CKD is considered non-HRS–AKI. Differentiating HRS–AKI from non-HRS–AKI guides treatment and determines patient outcomes (Amin et al., 2019).
- HRS yields an extremely high mortality rate from its onset. This life-threatening emergency requires prompt diagnosis and early intervention (Davenport et al., 2017).
- Patients diagnosed with HRS should be referred for liver transplant evaluation.

HEPATORENAL SYNDROME ACUTE KIDNEY INJURY

Describes functional intrarenal deterioration in individuals with structurally normal renal tissue. Although HRS AKI can be caused by some form of damage to renal tissue, HRS AKI is *not* an AKI due to other causes (Amin et al., 2019). HRS AKI is characterized by continued renal decline occurring over time; in advanced cirrhosis meeting certain criteria and who are unresponsive to volume expansion (Table 10.26).

Pathophysiology

Cirrhosis and portal hypertension cause neurohormonal changes that signal release of pro-inflammatory cytokines. Cytokine release causes severe vasodilation of splanchnic circulation, which results in reduced cardiac output, renal vasoconstriction, and reduced renal perfusion (Amin et al., 2019; Fisher & Brown, 2010; Mindikoglu & Pappas, 2018).

NONHEPATORENAL SYNDROME ACUTE KIDNEY INJURY

AKI due to other causes, including structural (renal tissue) problems; hypovolemia from blood loss, such as in variceal rupture; overuse of diuretics; early acute tubular necrosis or bile cast nephropathy; decompensation due to heart failure; obstruction or intra-abdominal hypertension.

Pathophysiology

- Translocation of gut bacteria and systemic inflammation
- Abnormally high bilirubin creates bile acids that degrade renal tubules (Amin et al., 2019; Davenport et al., 2017; Fisher & Brown, 2010; Mindikoglu & Pappas, 2018)

Treatment

- Identify and eliminate all contributing factors causing HRS.
- Fluid replacement and expansion are based on immediate hemodynamic need.
- If no progress, administer albumin at 1 g/kg/body weight for 2 days.
- If no response to fluid or expanders, add vasoconstrictive therapy to counteract vasodilation. Vasoconstrictors and albumin therapy should be continued until serum creatinine (sCr) reaches baseline.
- TIPS evaluation may help improve renal function by decreasing portal hypertension and improving cardiac output.
- Renal replacement therapy used as a bridge to transplantation or for reduction in fluid accumulation.
- *Transplantation evaluation and transplant:* Liver transplant or liver kidney transplant. Criteria for candidacy and type of transplantation are center based.

Prevention

- Prevention measures include controlling disease progression in patients with compensated cirrhosis and reversal of causes and complications in individuals with decompensated disease.
  - Treatment for SBP
  - Management and control of ascites with diuretics (if not contraindicated) and diet
  - Avoidance of nephrotoxic agents
  - Control and treat variceal bleeding portal hypertension

HEPATITIS: NONVIRAL AND VIRAL

OVERVIEW OF NONVIRAL HEPATITIS

Nonviral hepatitis is an inflammation of the liver and is classified as autoimmune, toxic, alcohol, or drug induced. This condition is not contagious and can lead to liver cell destruction, fibrosis,

TABLE 10.26 HEPATORENAL SYNDROME ACUTE KIDNEY INJURY: CRITERIA AND EVALUATION

EVALUATION	HRS AKI QUALIFYING CRITERIA
Diagnosis	Cirrhosis with ascites, acute liver failure or acute on chronic liver failure, and acute kidney injury
Serum creatinine or urine	Elevated ≥0.3 mg/dL in 48 hours or increases 50% above baseline in last 7 days If past 7-day serum creatinine unavailable, use lowest sCr in last 3 months or use urine output from urinary catheter less than 0.5 mL/kg/body weight over 6 hours
Unresponsive kidney function	After no diuretic therapy for 2 consecutive days and with the use of albumin dosed at 1 g/kg/body weight
Negative urine studies	No microhematuria (<50) No proteinuria (<50)
Fractionated excreted urine	<0.2%
Other	Not in shock state No recent use of nephrotoxins (ACE inhibitors, NSAIDs, diuretics, antibiotics, etc.) Normal renal ultrasound

ACE, angiotensin-converting enzyme; AKI, acute kidney injury; HRS, hepatorenal syndrome; NSAIDs, nonsteroidal anti-inflammatory drugs; sCr, serum creatinine.

and eventually cirrhosis. Depending upon classification, cause of inflammation may be secondary to alcohol misuse, drugs (e.g., antibiotics, anabolic steroids, hormonal contraceptives, and some cytotoxic agents), cholestatic reactions, hypersensitivity to certain phenothiazine derivatives, or infectious agents (Lippincott Advisor, 2018a).

Risk Factors
- Excessive alcohol use
- Lack of bile excretion
- Metabolic and autoimmune disorders
- Genetic predisposition (autoimmune)
- History of diabetes, renal failure, or acquired deficiency syndrome

Complications
- Liver failure
- Renal disease
- Portal hypertension
- Primary hepatocellular carcinoma
- Esophageal varices
- Malnutrition
- GERD

Assessment
- History and physical
  - Nausea, vomiting, diarrhea, fatigue
  - Anorexia, weight loss
  - Jaundice (or icterus) of sclera or skin
  - Liver tenderness
  - Ascites
  - Dark urine, clay-colored stools

Diagnostic Test Results
Laboratory Data
- Serum AST and ALT are elevated
  - Also known as *serum glutamic oxaloacetic transaminase (SGOT)* and *serum glutamic pyruvic transaminase (SGPT)*, respectively.
  - AST may not be specific for liver injury because these enzymes may be elevated in other conditions; therefore, elevated ALT is more specific for liver injury.
  - AST–ALT ratio of 2.0 or higher may indicate alcohol abuse.
- Gamma- glutamyl transpeptidase (GGT)
  - Enzyme increases with hepatobiliary dysfunction.
- Bilirubin
  - Total and direct bilirubin levels are elevated.
  - Unconjugated (indirect) and conjugated (direct) fractionation measures the proportion of bilirubin that is conjugated.
- Alkaline phosphatase
  - Levels may be elevated to suggest cholangitis but may not be specific because enzyme has widespread distribution outside of the liver, such as small intestine, kidneys, placenta, and especially bone.
- Other laboratory tests
  - PT may be prolonged and antibodies (autoimmune) may be present
  - PTT and INR
  - White blood cell (WBC) and differential are elevated; platelets may be decreased

- Ammonia
  - Levels may be elevated in the presence of hepatic encephalopathy but can be falsely low or high; therefore, they are of limited clinical usefulness.
- Serum proteins and immunoglobulins

Imaging and Diagnostic Procedures
- CT scanning may be used to assess for hepatic lesions.
- MRI may be used to identify tumors.
- Liver biopsy may be used to assess for degree of inflammation and underlying disease process.

Treatment Interventions (Determined by Type of Hepatitis and If Acute or Chronic)
- Remove causative agent and limit further exposure.
- Provide emotional and needed psychosocial support and help to identify ongoing appropriate coping strategies.
- Follow low-sodium, well-balanced diet with adequate fluid intake.
- Activity as tolerated; include daily exercise regimen if appropriate.
- Medications administered depending on causative agent.
  - Acetylcysteine (Mucomyst) for acetaminophen (Tylenol) poisoning
  - L-Carnitine for valproic acid (Depakene) poisoning
  - Corticosteroids (drug induced or autoimmune)
  - Azathioprine (Azasan), mycophenolate (Cellcept), tacrolimus (Prograf), or cyclosporine (Neoral)
- Surgery—Liver transplantation needed for those patients unresponsive to treatment and meet criteria for transplantation.

OVERVIEW OF VIRAL HEPATITIS
Viral hepatitis is an infection and inflammation of the liver caused by one of five types of viruses; it typically progresses through three stages (prodromal, clinical jaundice, and post-icteric; Table 10.27).
- Inflammation is marked by hepatic cell destruction, necrosis, and autolysis, which leads to anorexia, jaundice, and hepatomegaly.
- Recovery is possible, pending complications or worsening symptoms such as edema and hepatic encephalopathy (Lippincott Advisor, 2018b).
- Current viral hepatitis testing includes serological testing followed by virologic testing to help guide treatment decisions (Easterbrook et al., 2017).

Clinical Practice Guidelines
- The National Institute of Diabetes and Digestive and Kidney Diseases (NIDDK) presents more detailed guidelines to assess and manage liver disease (www.niddk.nih.gov/health-information/liver-disease).
- The American Association for the Study of Liver Disease (AASLD) presents more detailed guidelines to assess and manage liver disease (www.aasld.org/publications/practice-guidelines).
- Refer to the Centers for Disease Control and Prevention (CDC) website for more detailed guidelines to assess and manage viral hepatitis (www.cdc.gov/hepatitis/index.htm).

TABLE 10.27 TYPES OF VIRAL HEPATITIS

TYPE	TRANSMISSION	INCUBATION	DIAGNOSIS	DURATION	TREATMENT
A	Fecal–oral route; spread by anal–oral route (ingestion of contaminated food or drink)	Average is 28 days; range is 15–50 days	Serum positive for IgM antibodies	Symptoms typically last <2 months, but it may take 6 months for liver to recover	Receive vaccination for prevention Supportive care, prevent transmission.
B	Parenterally and sexually by contact of contaminated human blood, secretions (saliva and semen), other body secretions and stool	Approximately 75 days (acute); Range is 60–150 days	Serum positive for hepatitis B surface antigens and antibodies	Acute symptoms may last a few weeks up to 6 months. Chronic long-lasting infection, increased risk of cirrhosis, liver failure, or live cancer	Receive vaccination for prevention For acute infection, treatment is supportive For chronic infection there are antiviral medications, along with ongoing supportive care
C	Parenterally, perinatally (uncommon), and sexually via percutaneous exposure to infected blood or plasma	Approximately 8 weeks; range 2–26 weeks	Serum positive for hepatitis C antibodies	Many patients are asymptomatic until either found on routine exam or screened prior to donating blood	Supportive care; goal to clear virus from body, stop, or slow liver damage. *Has the highest risk of cirrhosis and liver cancer*
D	Same as that for hepatitis B	Average 35 days	Serum positive for IgM and IgG antibodies to hepatitis D (*requires the presence of hepatitis B infection*)	Can be acute, short term or transition into chronic, long-term infection Also known as *delta hepatitis*	Same as that for hepatitis B
E	Fecal–oral route (fecally contaminated water)	Average 45 days	Detection of IgM and IgG antibodies to hepatitis E in serum and stool	The duration of symptoms is unknown	Most patients recover completely without any treatment

IgG, immunoglobulin G; IgM, immunoglobulin M.

Source: Data from Centers for Disease Control and Prevention. (2017). *Surveillance for Viral Hepatitis—United States*. https://www.cdc.gov/hepatitis/statistics/2017surveillance/index.htm

NAUSEA AND VOMITING

OVERVIEW

N/V are unpleasant symptoms associated with a variety of conditions and circumstances. Treatment modalities to alleviate symptoms require an understanding of underlying pathogenesis only obtained by a thorough health history and assessment.

Pathophysiology of Nausea and Vomiting

- The vomiting center inside the medulla contains receptors that work with the GI tract to trigger or suppress the urge to vomit (Figure 10.2). Depending on the stimulus, receptors release serotonin, dopamine, histamine, and/or acetylcholine to trigger the N/V response.
- *Role of receptors in nausea and vomiting when activated*
  - Muscarinic receptors or cholinergic (M1) sends signals to vomit.
  - Chemo receptor trigger zone (CTZ) receptors (dopamine and serotonin) located outside the blood–brain barrier cause emesis when exposed to circulating elements (toxins, alcohol).
    - CTZ area is where most antiemetics work.

- The vagus nerve (CNX) houses the gag reflex. When the gag reflex is triggered, the pharynx is stimulated. This causes afferent branches of cranial nerves V, VII to trigger sympathetic pathways within the GI tract, causing cardiovascular responses and reverse peristalsis of vomiting.
- Disturbances in the vestibular center, responsible for balance and motion, can trigger vomiting.
- Stress response from the cerebrum can induce psychologic N/V (Cangemi & Kuo, 2019; Longstreth, 2018).

Nausea

Unpleasant subjective symptom caused by either an environmental or an emotional trigger, caused by ingestion of substances such as medication, or that is the result of a physiologic malfunction.
- Nausea is usually a precursor to vomiting.
- May also be related to slowed or fast gastric emptying.

Retching

Retching is caused by a vagal response, from sympathetic and parasympathetic action.

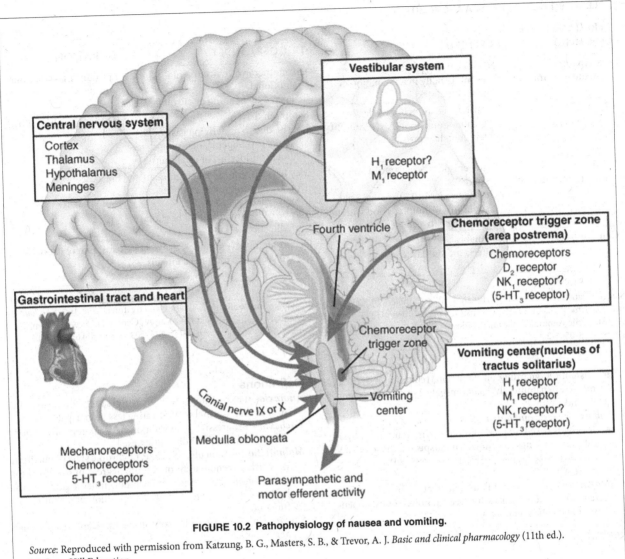

FIGURE 10.2 Pathophysiology of nausea and vomiting.

Source: Reproduced with permission from Katzung, B. G., Masters, S. B., & Trevor, A. J. *Basic and clinical pharmacology* (11th ed.). McGraw-Hill Education.

- *Vagal response*: Begins with deep inspiration → spasm occurs from increased intra-thoracic pressure in the esophageal sphincter after closure of the glottis → spasm causes reverse peristalsis of chyme from the gastric-duodenal into the esophagus.
  - Chyme is not released due to closure of the esophagus.
- Sympathetic action causes increased heart rate and respirations along with diaphoresis.
- Parasympathetic action causes increased gastric salivation and motility of gastric secretions.

Vomiting
- Associated with nausea and follows retching
- Should not be confused with regurgitation (Longstreth, 2018)

Types of Nausea and Vomiting
Classified by onset, duration, and triggers. Triggers listed in Tables 10.28 and 10.29 are common; however, intensity and duration are individualized (Bartoo & Schroeder, 2019; Bhandari et al., 2018; Cash & Glass, 2019; Lacy et al., 2018; Li, 2018).

Assessment
- **Effects of N/V** may include anorexia, dehydration, electrolyte imbalances, metabolic alkalosis, hypotension due to loss of fluids and electrolyte imbalances, dental erosion, and aspiration.
- It is imperative to rule out life-threatening conditions associated with N/V, such as a myocardial infarction; ischemic, perforated, or obstructed bowel; or acute abdomen.

Emesis description: Description of emesis may assist in differential diagnosis (Table 10.30).

Assessment
- *Skin*: Color (pallor, jaundice), tenting
- *Oral mucosa*: Eroded dental enamel (signs of bulimia)
- *Abdominal exam*

TABLE 10.28 TYPES OF NAUSEA AND VOMITING

TYPE/(ACUTE OR CHRONIC)	CRITERIA	TRIGGER/ONSET	DURATION
Anticipatory (Acute or chronic)	N/V occurring prior to or after an event. Usually in anticipation of chemotherapy.	Chemotherapy, environmental, emotional. Triggered by pending or current event.	Episodic; may last hours or days
Chronic (Chronic)	Persistent episodes of N/V lasting greater than 1 month; requires differential diagnosis.	Symptom driven. May be due to underlying gastroenterologic, psychogenic, neurologic, vestibular, endocrine, or renal causes.	Greater than 1 month
Cyclic (Acute and chronic)	Acute episode <7 days and 1 week apart. Three episodes in 12 months; 2 episodes in a 6-month period with no vomiting between episodes	May have an emotional component; pregnancy, migraine, cannabis, menstrual. May be caused by maternal hereditary predilection.	Episodic
Cannabinoid (Acute)	Cannabis. Criteria are similar to cyclic	Occurs after heavy cannabis use or 2–10 years of continued cannabis use.	Cessation of cannabis

N/V, nausea and vomiting.

Sources: Data from Lacy, B. E., Parkman, H. P., & Camilleri, M. (2018). Chronic nausea and vomiting: Evaluation and treatment. *The American Journal of Gastroenterology, 113*(5), 1. https://doi.org/10.1038/s41395-018-0039-2; Bhandari, S., Jha, P., Thakur, A., Kar, A., Gerdes, H., & Venkatesan, T. (2018). Cyclic vomiting syndrome: Epidemiology, diagnosis, and treatment. *Clinical Autonomic Research, 28*(2), 203–209. https://doi.org/10.1007/s10286-018-0506-2.

- Distention, guarding on palpation, rebound tenderness, masses, hepatomegaly, splenomegaly, bowel sounds, aortic aneurysm
- **Laboratory tests and diagnostics**
  - Testing is based on presentation of symptoms and physical exam findings to confirm the suspected cause of N/V (Anderson & Strayer, 2013; Longstreth, 2018; Reese & Glass, 2019).
- **Imaging:** KUB to rule out ileus, pancreatitis, or CT for suspected obstruction to check for free air, bowel loops, appendicitis, pancreatitis; endoscopy.

Treatment
- **Diet**
  - Severe acute: Nothing per os (NPO) status needed.
  - Self-limiting episodes: Abstain from food and sensory triggers.
  - Ingest clear liquids with small amount of dry foods.
- **Geriatric considerations**: Lower dosage in the geriatric population due to reduced metabolism and the higher incidence of neurologic and cardiac side effects.

MALNUTRITION

OVERVIEW
Normal and Altered Metabolism
Carbohydrates, proteins, and fat are required to provide the body with the energy it needs to obtain from food sources. Those sources, such as protein and amino acids, are not stored, whereas carbohydrates may be stored in the muscle and liver as glycogen. When adequate protein is not available, muscle or body protein is then catabolized for energy needs. Long-term energy needs are covered by the dietary fat in the adipose tissue. In disease or injury states, acute and chronic inflammation are important etiologic factors to consider in the pathogenesis of malnutrition (Jensen et al., 2013).

Definitions
Anorexia—Loss of appetite with early satiety or feeling full sooner than normal or after eating less than usual.

Cachexia—Progressive deterioration or weakness of the body due to a multitude of disease states.

Malnutrition—An acute, subacute, or chronic state of nutrition, in which a combination of varying degrees of overnutrition or undernutrition with or without inflammatory activity leads to a change in body composition and diminished function.

Sarcopenia—Refers to a loss of muscle mass and strength and performance.

Etiologies of Malnutrition
There are three classification types (White et al., 2012):
- *Starvation-related malnutrition*: Chronic starvation without inflammation (e.g., anorexia nervosa)
- *Chronic disease-related malnutrition*: Inflammation is chronic and of mild to moderate degree (e.g., organ failure, pancreatic cancer, rheumatoid arthritis, or sarcopenic obesity)
- *Acute disease- or injury-related malnutrition*: Inflammation is acute and of severe degree (e.g., major infection, burns, trauma, or closed head injury)

Risk Factors
- Female
- Depression
- Dementia
- Congestive heart failure
- Decubitus ulcer

Clinical Characteristics for Malnutrition (No Single Parameter Definitive of Malnutrition Diagnosis)
- Insufficient energy intake
- Weight loss
- Loss of muscle mass

TABLE 10.29 NAUSEA AND VOMITING: TRIGGERS, CAUSES, AND FURTHER ASSESSMENT CONSIDERATIONS

TRIGGER, SYMPTOM, OR PRESENTATION	POSSIBLE CAUSES	FURTHER ASSESSMENT
Pre- or postmeal	Bulimia/eating disorders Psychologic	Self-induced trigger Food types Greasy/spicy may be associated with reflux or gallbladder disease Milk-based food may be associated with lactose intolerance Recent diet changes Recent meal at restaurant Food avoidances
Olfactory (hyperosmia)	Central nervous system Pregnancy (first trimester) or seen in hyperemesis gravidarium	Time of day Accompanied with headache? Last menstrual cycle
Medications	New or recent changes in medication Drug withdrawal	Following list is not exhaustive: Chemotherapeutic agents Antiepileptic drugs Antiarrhythmic (digoxin) Antihypertensive Antibiotics Antiviral agents Aspirin Hypoglycemic agents (Metformin) Oral contraceptives Opioids Herbal agents
Neurologic symptoms	Central nervous system tumor, bleeding, hematoma, increased ICP Aura due to migraine headache or seizures Ménière's disease Autonomic dysfunction Head trauma	Accompanying headache, nausea, tinnitus, dizziness, history of seizures or migraine Photosensitivity New onset confusion Recent head trauma
Emesis with undigested food	Mechanical or functional bowel obstruction Constipation	Last BM, quality and frequency of BM Abdominal exam: pain, distension, tenderness Recent medication addition or changes
Early morning/upon awakening	Hypercalcemia Constipation Medications	BMs, medications, illicit drug use, after alcohol consumption (hangover)
Following exposures	Others with gastrointestinal illness or hepatitis Ingestion of chemical Binge drinking Cannabis use Use of illicit street drugs Hepatitis A and E, cholera, parasitic or enterotoxins from food handlers	Health history for exposure to offending agents Recent travel, dining outside of home
Other conditions	Postoperative N/V Food poisoning, gastritis, norovirus	Recent surgery. Inquire type, date of surgery, and type of anesthesia Accompanying diarrhea, dining outside home
Geriatric/older adults	Neurologic, gastrointestinal medication-induced causes	Falls, loss of consciousness, delirium, change in medication, electrolyte disturbance, urinary tract infection, constipation, diarrhea

BM, bowel movement; ICP, increased intracranial pressure; N/V, nausea and vomiting.

TABLE 10.30 EMESIS: DIFFERENTIAL DIAGNOSIS

EMESIS CHARACTERISTICS	POSSIBLE CAUSES
Bilious–green, yellow	Gallbladder
	Pancreatitis
	Small bowel obstruction
Bright red	Variceal bleed
	Peptic ulcer
Coffee ground	Gastric ulcer
	Duodenal ulcer
	Erosive gastritis
Fecal material	Small bowel obstruction
Projectile	Neurologic causes
	Meningitis
	Central nervous system tumor
Undigested food	Gastric outlet obstruction
	Gastroparesis
N/V with abdominal pain	Acute
	Appendicitis
	Cholecystitis
	Bile duct obstruction
	Pancreatitis
	Kidney stone
	Food poisoning
	Gastritis
Upon awakening	Pregnancy
	Uremic syndrome
	Increased intracranial pressure

N/V, nausea and vomiting.

- Loss of subcutaneous fat
- Localized or generalized fluid accumulation (may mask weight loss)
- Decreased functional status (hand grip strength)

Note: Two out of these six clinical characteristics are recommended for diagnosis of either severe or nonsevere malnutrition (Jensen et al., 2013).

Screening Tools and Assessment

Nutrition screening is among the first steps in providing adequate nutrition care and support. Aside from multiple valid and reliable screening tools, other methods of screening may include body fat and lean muscle mass estimation, upper arm circumference, or assessment of food diary and regular intake (Table 10.31).

In the United States, The Joint Commission mandates nutrition screening within 24 hours of admission to an acute care facility. The goal of the nutrition assessment is to identify patient risk or obvious presence of malnutrition (Jensen et al., 2013).

Comprehensive Nutrition Assessment

- Medical, nutrition, and medication histories
- Physical exam
  - Potential presence of clinical diagnostic characteristics such as weight loss/gain, fluid retention, loss of muscle or fat, and other nutrient deficiencies
- Anthropomorphic measurements
  - Height
  - Weight: On admission and frequently throughout length of stay
  - BMI: Weight in kilograms divided by the square of height in meters; strongly correlated with specific metabolic and disease outcomes compared to other direct measures of body fatness (Sun et al., 2010; Table 10.32)
- Laboratory data
  - Use traditional indicators, such as serum albumin, prealbumin, and transferrin, with caution. These serum concentrations are more likely influenced by many disease states rather than nutrient intake.

TABLE 10.31 NUTRITION SCREENING TOOLS

SCREENING TOOL	DESCRIPTION	CLINICAL CHARACTERISTICS USED
SGA (gold standard)	Utilizes a physical assessment and patient history for screening; considered to take increased time to administer compared to other tools.	Muscle and fat wasting and edema History of weight loss and reduced physical function
MST	Utilizes a simple and quick two-question tool for assessment.	Unintentional weight loss Reduced appetite
NRS	Preferred in European settings; uses several clinical characteristics in screening.	Unintentional weight loss Low BMI Disease severity >70 years of age Impaired condition
MUST	A five-step screening tool used primarily in the United Kingdom and Europe.	Unintentional weight loss BMI Disease severity Problems with food intake

BMI, body mass index; MST, Malnutrition Screening Tool; MUST, Malnutrition Universal Screening Tool; NRS, nutrition risk screening; SGA, subjective global assessment.

Source: Adapted from Mueller, C., Compher, C., Ellen, D. M., & American Society for Parenteral and Enteral Nutrition (A.S.P.E.N.) Board of Directors (2011). ASPEN clinical guidelines: Nutrition screening, assessment, and intervention in adults. *Journal of Parenteral and Enteral Nutrition, 35*(1), 16–24. https://doi.org/10.1177/0148607110389335

TABLE 10.32 ADULT STANDARD WEIGHT CATEGORIES AND BODY MASS INDEX

BODY MASS INDEX	WEIGHT
Below 18.5	Underweight
18.5–24.9	Normal or healthy weight
25.0–29.9	Overweight
>30.0	Obese

Source: Adapted from Centers for Disease Control and Prevention. (2019). Healthy weight. https://www.cdc.gov/healthyweight/assessing/bmi/index.html

- Consider other inflammation markers such as C reactive protein, WBC count, blood glucose, and nitrogen balance. These may help determine etiologic-based diagnosis.
- Other testing may include CBC, folate, B vitamins, vitamin D, and thyroid-stimulating hormone. These levels may identify certain anemias, thyroid disease, or other deficiencies.
- Functional assessment
  - Handgrip strength: Weak handgrip is a sign of malnutrition.

Malnutrition Interventions
- Assess environment
- Medication review (to assess for causing anorexia)
- Specialized diets
- Use of snacks and supplements
- Fortification of food
  - Enteral nutrition: Select appropriate enteral access device based on patient needs.

Malnutrition Considerations
- Advocate for optimal adult nutrition and treat via a multidisciplinary, systematic team approach.
- Implement valid and easy-to-use screening tools for nutrition risk and screen early and often.
- There must be a careful review of risk factors, patient's history, and physica and clinical characteristics by appropriate team members in order to make the diagnosis, to determine, and to implement the plan of care and modify as needed to achieve optimal patient outcomes.

Clinical Practice Guidelines
- Refer to the American Society for Parenteral and Enteral Nutrition (ASPEN) for detailed guidelines to assess and manage clinical nutrition (www.nutritioncare.org/Guidelines_and_Clinical_Resources/Clinical_Guidelines/).
- Refer to the European Society for Parenteral and Enteral Nutrition (ESPEN) for detailed guidelines to assess and manage clinical nutrition (www.espen.org/guidelines-home/espen-guidelines).
- Refer to the Canadian Clinical Practice Guidelines for detailed guidelines to assess and manage clinical nutrition (www.criticalcarenutrition.com/resources/cpgs/past-guidelines/2015).

SKILLS/PROCEDURES: DRAINAGE CATHETERS AND TUBES

- Drainage catheters are placed in the GI system for a number of reasons: drainage of excess fluid accumulations, abscess drainage, or drainage of specific areas (e.g., biliary drains or T-tubes).
- Other tubes placed in the GI tract are used for delivery of fluids, medications, and/or nutrition. These tubes can be placed in the stomach or small bowel depending on specific need.

- Understanding the care of patients with drainage catheters or tubes is essential knowledge for the CNS.
- Surgical drains are used to monitor for a postoperative leak or abscess, to collect normal physiologic fluid, or to minimize dead space.
- Nurses should know the location and purpose of drains; however, they should not manipulate surgical drains without input from the surgeon who placed them (Table 10.33).

Key Interventions With Surgical Drains
- Assess tubes for patency and proper functioning (draining or infusions).
- Diligent nursing assessment is imperative to prevent skin injury as a result of the tube and pressure on the skin or excoriation from excessive drainage.
- Assess drain insertion site for signs of leakage, redness, or signs of ooze.
- Ensure drain is located below the insertion site and free from kinks or knots. Note amount and type of drainage.
- Monitor patient for signs of sepsis; if the patient is febrile or has redness, tenderness, or increased ooze at the drain site, this could be a sign of infection.
- Drains should be removed as soon as possible; the longer a drain remains in place, the higher the risk of infection as well as development of granulation tissue around the drain site (causing pain and trauma when removed).

Complications
- Drains can become occluded or clogged, resulting in retained fluid, which can contribute to infection.
- If a drain becomes clogged or occluded, it is usually removed since it no longer provides benefit.

Managing Patients With Enteral Nutrition
- Enteral nutrition is most commonly administered through small-bore flexible feeding tubes. For long-term enteral nutrition, the patient will require a percutaneously inserted gastric tube or jejunal tube (PEG/PEJ).
- In the hospital setting, nasogastric or orogastric sump tubes may be used. It is important to note that these tubes are not indicated for administration of enteral nutrition; they should therefore only be used short term until an appropriate feeding tube can be inserted.

Intolerance
- Monitor patient for any signs of intolerance (abdominal distention, nausea or vomiting).
- Patients may have decreased gastric motility.
- May need to decrease feeding rate or divert to small bowel feedings.

Enteral Access Tube Maintenance
- Prevent clogging of enteral feeding device, which is best accomplished by flushing the tube at least q4h, before and after medication administration and after aspirating from the tube.
- If clogs develop, the first step is to flush with warm water. Do not use carbonated beverages—this actually increases further clogging.
- If this does not work, use pancreatic enzymes.
- Lastly, there are mechanical removal products on the market that can assist with breaking down the clog.
- Medications—Always try to change medications to liquid or elixir forms; if none are available, dissolve completely in warm water before administering. Never crush or give sustained release medications via an enteral feeding tube.

TABLE 10.33 TYPES OF DRAINS, INDICATIONS, COMPLICATIONS, AND NURSING CONSIDERATIONS

SKILL	INDICATIONS	POTENTIAL COMPLICATIONS	NURSING CARE AND CONSIDERATIONS
Surgical drains or GI drainage catheter (e.g., Penrose, Jackson–Pratt/Davol, etc.)	Placed near surgical site to remove excess fluid, drain abscess or monitor for postoperative complications (e.g., leak or abscess), or collect normal drainage (fluid, blood, pus). Prevents accumulation of drainage in the body The type and location of the drain inserted is based on surgical needs (e.g., type of surgery, drainage expected) and surgeon preference.	Blockage Dislodgement Periwound skin excoriation, denuded (MASD) Infection	Based on surgeon's orders, drains may be hooked to wall suction or a portable suction device or they may be left to use gravity to drain. Ensure accurate recording of the volume of drainage and appearance. Caregivers should know the location and purpose of drains; they should not manipulate surgical drains without input from the surgeon who placed them.
Large-bore nasogastric tube (sump tubes)	Placed for gastric decompression (e.g., with bowel obstruction).	Blockage (clogging, kinking) Dislodgement Pressure injury Gastric injury if not functioning correctly	Monitor and document output from NG tube. Ongoing assessment of the tube to ensure it doesn't become dislodged and is functioning properly is essential. If sump tube is in use, it is important to assure it is functioning and air is moving through the vent port' to avoid getting stuck on gastric mucosa.
PEG/JT catheter jejunostomy	Typically placed for long-term enteral nutrition needs or following extensive bowel surgery to aid in meeting nutritional needs.	Blockage (clogging, kinking) Dislodgement Pressure injury Periwound skin excoriation, denuded (MASD) Infection	Assess proper functioning, insertion site, and monitor the drainage.
Small-bore feeding tubes (gastric, duodenal, or jejunal)	Used for delivery of enteral nutrition. Can be used for gastric feeding or small bowel feeding.	Blockage (clogging, kinking) Dislodgement	Assess proper functioning; routinely flush with warm water to ensure patency.

GI, gastrointestinal; JT, jejunostomy tube; MASD, moisture associated skin damage; NG, nasogastric; PEG, percutaneous endoscopic gastrostomy.

REVIEW QUESTIONS

1. What test is used to diagnose an upper gastrointestinal (G) I bleed?
   A. Angiography of the abdomen
   B. Hemoglobin
   C. Colonoscopy
   D. O_2 saturation

2. Your patient presents to the unit and upon exam you identify that they are a candidate for nutrition support; oral intake has not been sufficient to meet daily caloric requirements and therefore a small-bore feeding tube was placed blindly at the bedside. What is your next course of action?
   A. Begin trickle feeding with standard solution
   B. Obtain radiographic confirmation of proper tube placement
   C. Wait 24 hours and then begin enteral nutrition
   D. Start enteral solution at goal rate

3. Which of the following factors contributes to a diagnosis of nonalcoholic steatohepatitis (NASH) cirrhosis?
   A. Female, seizure history, BMI
   B. Female, hypertension history, BMI, and diabetes
   C. BMI, low albumin, hypertension, and diabetes
   D. Male, elevated bilirubin, and BMI

ANSWERS

1. **Correct answer: A. Rationale:** Angiography of the abdomen. A colonoscopy will not be diagnostic; a low hemoglobin can be from other sources and O_2 saturation can be low from other causes.

2. **Correct answer: B. Rationale:** A variety of bedside tests are used to determine tube placement with varying degrees of accuracy. The gold standard for confirming correct placement of a blindly inserted tube is a radiograph that visualizes the entire course of the tube. You should not start any type of enteral nutrition until after placement is confirmed.

3. **Correct answer: C. Rationale:** Gender is not a risk factor for NASH. BMI, low albumin, hypertension, and diabetes are risk factors associated with metabolic syndrome and NAFLD.

REFERENCES

The complete reference and additional reading lists appear in the digital version of this chapter, at https://connect.springerpub.com/content/book/978-0-8261-7417-8/part/part01/chapter/ch10

Renal System

Clarissa Welbaum, Elizabeth Hudson-Weires, and Amy C. Shay

OVERVIEW OF THE RENAL SYSTEM

Renal system structures include the kidneys, ureters, bladder, and urethra. The renal system maintains homeostasis through the production and excretion of urine, detoxification of blood, production of red blood cells (erythropoiesis), and the regulation of fluid volume, electrolyte levels, and acid–base balance. The nephron is the functional unit of the kidney. Millions of nephrons filter blood as it flows through the glomerular capillary networks housed within the Bowman's capsule. Filtrate from the glomerulus flows through the proximal tubule, loop of Henle, and distal tubule. It is through this tubule system that alterations in filtrates and water, through absorption and reabsorption, occur. The filtrate then flows through the collecting ducts, where it eventually drains through the ureters and bladder and is subsequently eliminated as urine.

ACUTE KIDNEY INJURY

OVERVIEW

Definition

Acute kidney injury (AKI) is a newer and broader term that encompasses the previously used term, *acute renal failure*. AKI is a term that allows for inclusion of varying degrees of severity of kidney dysfunction throughout the disease continuum. *AKI* is defined as a sudden decrease in renal function that occurs over a few hours to days. This insult results in the inability to process nitrogenous waste and regulate fluid and electrolytes. AKI is potentially reversible.

Criteria for Diagnosis and Classification of Acute Kidney Injury

Diagnostic criteria have been developed by the Kidney Disease: Improving Global Outcomes (KDIGO) AKI Workgroup. The definition and staging of AKI were created through a compilation of studies, including the RIFLE criteria (risk, injury, failure, loss of kidney function, and end-stage kidney disease [ESKD]) and the Acute Kidney Injury Network (AKIN) criteria.

Kidney Disease: Improving Global Outcomes—Definition of *Acute Kidney Injury*

- Increased serum creatinine (SCr) of >0.3 mg/dL (>26.5 mcmol/L) within 48 hours, or
- SCr 1.5 times the baseline that is known or presumed to have occurred within the prior 7 days, or
- A urine volume of <0.5 mL/kg/hr for 6 hours.

Kidney Disease: Improving Global Outcomes—Staging of Severity

- *Stage 1*—SCr of 1.5 to 1.9 × baseline or an increase in SCr to >0.3 mg/dL (>26.5 mc/L); urine output <0.5 mL/kg/hr for 6 to 12 hours
- *Stage 2*—SCr of 2.0 to 2.9 × baseline; <0.5 mL/kg/hr for >12 hours
- *Stage 3*—SCr of 3.0 × baseline or increase in SCr to >4.0 mg/dL (>353.6 mcmol/L) or initiation of renal replacement therapy (RRT) or for patients <18 years, a decrease in estimated glomerular filtration rate (eGFR) to <35 mL/min/1.73 m^2, urine output <0.5 mL/kg/hr for >24 hours, or anuria for >12 hours (KDIGO, 2012a)

Risk Assessment

Identifying risk factors for AKI is key to prevention, early identification, prompt treatment, and reduction of morbidity and mortality. Risk factors include but are not limited to the following:

- Advanced age
- Black descent
- Hypertension
- Dehydration and operative hypoperfusion
- Nephrotoxic medications (e.g., nonsteroidal antiinflammatory drugs [NSAIDs], aminoglycosides, vancomycin, amphotericin B, chemotherapy medications)
- Preexisting chronic disease
- Radiocontrast agents
- Burns, trauma, and shock states
- Sepsis
- Chronic kidney disease (CKD) and anemia
- Diabetes mellitus (DM)
- Cancer

Etiology

The three categories of insult and etiology are as follows:

Prerenal—Due to a reduction in renal flow or hypoperfusion
- Causes
  - Hypotension and hypovolemia (blood loss, third spacing, dehydration, diuretics, diarrhea, vomiting)
  - Decreased blood circulation (sepsis, cardiac injury/failure, liver failure, shock states)
  - Medications (angiotensin-converting enzyme inhibitors [ACE], NSAIDs)
  - Renal artery involvement (stenosis, clot, occlusion, trauma, aneurysm)

The complete reference and additional reading lists appear in the digital version of this chapter, at https://connect.springerpub.com/content/book/978-0-8261-7417-8/part/part01/chapter/ch11

Intrarenal—Most often due to toxic insults, ischemia, or both
- Causes
  Glomerulonephritis—Wegener's granulomatosis; Goodpasture syndrome; Henoch–Schonlein purpura
  - Acute tubular necrosis (ATN)
    - Ischemia—Ineffective hypovolemia treatment
    - Nephrotoxic substances—Radiocontrast agents, nephrotoxic medications, environmental agents
  - Acute interstitial nephritis (AIN)
    - Autoimmune disease—Systemic lupus erythematosus (LSE), pyelonephritis, allergic reaction to medications, lymphomas and leukemias
  - Vascular diseases—Thrombotic thrombocytopenia purpura (TTP); hemolysis, elevated liver enzymes, and low platelets (HELLP); renal artery and vein involvement; Wilson's disease; sickle cell disease; DM; malignant hypertension

Postrenal—Occurs when urine flow from the kidneys is interrupted once it begins its path to the lower urinary tract (American Nephrology Nurses' Association, 2015)
- Causes of obstruction
  - Ureteral strictures
  - Benign prostatic hypertrophy
  - Kidney stones
  - Cervical cancer
  - Meatal stenosis
  - Retroperitoneal fibrosis
  - Neurogenic bladder
  - Pregnancy

Diagnosis
Early recognition of rising SCr and/or decreased urine output should prompt further investigation using the KDIGO classification and staging system criteria. Certain clinical situations can affect SCr levels and urine output, confounding the diagnosis of AKI:
- Medications (e.g., cimetidine, trimethoprim) can affect the secretion of creatinine.
- Liver failure can lead to a decrease in creatinine production.
- CKD can cause a gradual increase in SCr.
- Obesity: weight-based urine output calculations could lead to a misdiagnosis of AKI.
- Postoperative patients may have acute antidiuretic hormone release (ADH), which leads to oliguria secondary to fluid and electrolyte shifts.
- Fluid overload can have a dilutional effect on the SCr concentration.

Diagnostic Testing
Biomarker Sensitivity
- Interleukin-18 (IL-18)
- Kidney injury molecule-1 (KIM-1)
- Neutrophil gelatinase-associated lipocalin (NGAL), and cystatin C (KDIGO, 2012a)

Prevention and Treatment
Education
- *Education* of patients and families should include an understanding of the complexity of AKI, awareness of potential risk factors, and the need for close monitoring of kidney function (SCr and urine output) and early treatment interventions.

Preventive Measures
- *Fluid optimization:* Monitor through noninvasive (intake and output measurements) or invasive (central venous pressure, pulmonary artery pressure, etc.) means. Isotonic crystalloid solutions, such as 0.9% saline, are the fluid of choice for AKI volume expansion (Gilbert & Weiner, 2018). Albumin is considered a safe colloid for use in resuscitation of critically ill patents (The SAFE Study Investigators, 2004).
- *Vasoactive medication management:* Once fluid volume responsiveness is no longer occurring, vasoactive medications can be considered for management of cardiac output (Moore et al., 2018).
- *Polypharmacy:* Assess multiple medications and medication combinations for nephrotoxic risks.
- *Nutritional management:* Prevent protein-calorie malnutrition (KDIGO, 2012b). Enteral nutrition is the preferred route of feeding when feasible. Parenteral nutrition is utilized when the gastrointestinal (GI) tract cannot be utilized for feeding.
- *Renal replacement therapy (RRT):* The two forms of RRT are intermittent hemodialysis (IHD) and continuous renal replacement therapy (CRRT). RRT is initiated when medical management to correct metabolic acidosis, volume overload, hyperkalemia, and/or uremic symptoms has failed. Patients who are hemodynamically unstable may require CRRT. Factors such as severe hypotension, vascular access issues, and arrhythmias may delay the initiation of RRT.

CHRONIC KIDNEY DISEASE
OVERVIEW
The most common causes of CKD are diabetes and hypertension. It is important to note that CKD differs from ESKD, (also referred to as *end-stage renal disease [ESRD]*). ESKD is the complete, permanent failure of the kidneys with treatment options limited to kidney transplant or dialysis for life. ESKD is further described as CKD stage 5 (G5), where glomerular filtration rate (GFR) <15 mL/min/1.73 m² (Table 11.1).

Definition
CKD is defined as abnormalities of kidney structure or function, present for >3 months, with implications for health. CKD is further defined as an eGFR of <60 mL/min/m 1.73^2 for longer than 3 months and/or markers of kidney damage such as the following:
- Albuminuria >30 mg/d (a key marker in CKD)
- Electrolyte abnormalities and other abnormalities
- Urinary sediment abnormalities (i.e., urine casts, blood cells)
- Histological abnormalities
- Imaging abnormalities (i.e., hydronephrosis, polycystic kidney disease)
- Kidney transplant history (considered CKD without regard to other markers)

Treatment
The goal of CKD treatment is to slow the progression of the disease.
- *Blood pressure (BP) management:* A target BP of less than 140/90 mmHg is recommended for patients with CKD or DM.
- *Albuminuria reduction:* Risk factors for albuminuria are hyperlipidemia, obesity, hypertension, diabetes, smoking, high sodium intake, and chronic inflammation. Medications used to reduce the effect of proteinuria or that have renal protective properties are ACE inhibitors and angiotensin receptor blockers (ARBs).

TABLE 11.1 GLOMERULAR FILTRATION RATE CATEGORIES

| CKD | GFR CATEGORY | | | |
STAGE	CATEGORY	SEVERITY	GFR LEVELS (mL/min/m 1.73^2)	eGFR
Stage 1	G1	Normal or high	>90 and proteinuria	>60
Stage 2	G2	Mild decreased	60–89 and proteinuria	
Stage 3	G3a	Mild to moderately decreased	45–59	30–59
	G3b	Moderately to severely decreased	30–44	
Stage 4	G4	Severely decreased	15–29	<30
Stage 5	G5	Kidney failure (ESKD)	<15 requiring dialysis or transplant	

CKD, chronic kidney disease; eGFR, estimated glomerular filtration rate; ESKD, end-stage kidney disease; GFR, glomerular filtration rate.

- **Reduce cardiovascular risks:** Lifestyle modifications, treatment of diabetes and hypertension, and aspirin therapy. Statins have been found to reduce cardiovascular risk as well as slow the progression of CKD by decreasing proteinuria.
- **Dietary management:** Includes limited protein and sodium intake, blood glucose control, and weight management.
- **Diabetes management:** Can reduce the onset of albuminuria and the development of CKD.
- **Avoiding acute kidney injury:** Acute insults include drug toxicity and contrast media.
- **Managing related functions** (anemia, parathyroid hormone [PTH], calcium, phosphate)
  - *Anemia* (Table 11.2)
    - Complete blood count (CBC)
    - Serum transferrin saturation (TSAT)
    - Absolute reticulocyte count
    - Serum ferritin level
    - Serum vitamin B_{12} and folate level
      - Treatment: Recombinant erythropoietin and synthetic derivatives reduce the need for blood transfusions. Iron deficiency anemia can be treated with oral or intravenous (IV) iron.
    - *Mineral metabolism and bone disease* (hypocalcemia, hyperphosphatemia; Table 11.3)
      - Treatment: Dietary phosphorus restrictions; oral phosphorus-binding agents (with or without a calcium base) prescribed with meals. Maintain a serum phosphate level between 0.87 and 1.49 mmol/L.
    - *Hyperparathyroidism:* Vitamin D deficiency leads to hypocalcemia and hyperparathyroidism resulting in bone abnormalities. KDIGO recommends bone mineral density (BMD) testing for patients with CKD G3a to G5D.
      - Treatment: PTH, vitamin D, calcium, and phosphate levels determine type of treatment (Webster et al., 2017).

TABLE 11.2 MONITORING ANEMIA

CKD MONITORING HEMO-GLOBIN LEVEL FOR ANEMIA	MONITORING FREQUENCY AT LEAST
CKD 3	Annually
CKD 4–5 with HD	Two times a year
CKD 5 with HD and CKD 5 with PD	Every 3 months

CKD, chronic kidney disease; HD, hemodialysis; PD, peritoneal dialysis.

TABLE 11.3 MONITORING MINERAL METABOLISM

GFR GRADING LEVEL	SERUM BLOOD LEVELS FOR CALCIUM AND PHOSPHATE FREQUENCY	PTH MONITORING
CKD G3a–G3b	6–12 months	Monitoring based on baseline and CKD progression
CKD G4a	3–6 months	6–12 months
CKD G5 and G5D	1–3 months	3–6 months
G4–G5D*	Alkaline phosphatase monitoring every 12 months, or more when elevated PTH is present	

*CKD stage G4 or G5 and also receiving hemodialysis or peritoneal dialysis.

CKD, chronic kidney disease; GFR, glomerular filtration rate; PTH, parathyroid hormone.

CONTRAST-INDUCED NEPHROPATHY/ ACUTE KIDNEY INJURY

OVERVIEW

Definition and Epidemiology

Iodine-based contrast agents administered via vein or artery have been linked to the development of AKI (Contrast Materials, 2018; Newhouse & RoyChoudhury, 2013). *Contrast-induced nephropathy (CIN)* or *contrast-induced acute kidney injury (CI-AKI)* is defined by the KDIGO guidelines as meeting at least one of the following three conditions within at least 48 hours after the contrast agent has been given (Wichmann et al., 2015):

1. Absolute increase in SCr by >0.3 mg/dL from baseline
2. Relative increase in SCr levels by >50% from baseline
3. Urine output decreases to <0.5 mL/kg/hr for at least 6 hours
4. A 25% increase in SCr from baseline or a 0.5 mg/dL (44 mcmol/L) increase in absolute SCr value within 48 to 72 hours after IV contrast administration

The incidence of CIN is greater in those who have some degree of preexisting renal impairment. When AKI develops postcontrast procedure, there is a higher risk for further development of CKD.

Risk Factors

Patient-Related Risk Factors for CIN
- Preexisting renal impairment
- Advanced age
- Uncontrolled hypertension
- DM
- Hypotension
- Hypovolemia
- Congestive heart failure (CHF)
- Anemia—A decrease in oxygen delivery to the kidney leading to hypoperfusion that is exacerbated by CIN

Procedure-Related Risk Factors for CIN
- High volume and frequency of IV contrast exposure (i.e., percutaneous coronary intervention [PCI], CT, MRI)
- Nephrotoxic medication during contrast exposure (i.e., diuretics, NSAIDs)

Pathogenesis
Injected contrast agents cause cellular mitochondria to react by releasing unbound iron, which begins a cascade of events. This unbound iron then causes the production of hydroxyl (oxygen-free) radicals, which leads to the destruction of nephrons. Recovery from the insult at this point is impossible. Examples of other processes that cause a similar response in the kidneys are myoglobin release in rhabdomyolysis and heme exposure that occurs during cardiac surgery.

Management
Clinical signs of CIN include a rise in SCr, acidosis, hyperphosphatemia, and in rare situations oliguria. The patient may also develop a brown, gritty appearance to the urine due to epithelial cell casts and renal tubular cells (Rudnick, 2017). There may be only a slight change in GFR.

Prevention Strategies
- Avoid volume depletion and, if no contraindications are noted, consider isotonic saline prior to and several hours after contrast administration.
- Withhold NSAIDs due to their vasoconstriction effects on the renal vasculature, which can increase the risk of CIN.
- Administer the lowest volume of contrast possible to achieve optimal results.
- Utilize the least toxic contrast agent, especially for high-risk patents.
- Utilize a contrast media injection device that decreases the risk of overshooting the injection area.
- KDIGO guidelines recommend using either iso-osmolar or low-osmolar iodinated contrast media rather than a high-osmolar iodinated contrast media in patients who have a high risk of CI-AKI (Kidney International Supplements, 2012).

Pharmaceutical agents with potential renal protective effects are as follows: N-acetylcysteine, sodium bicarbonate, statins, ascorbic acid (vitamin C), dopamine, theophylline, beta 1 receptor antagonist, atrial natriuretic peptide (ANP), and prostaglandins.

There is no significant difference in renal outcome between IV administration of isotonic saline versus sodium bicarbonate to increase elimination of the contrast agent.

FLUID AND ELECTROLYTE IMBALANCES

OVERVIEW
Fluid and electrolytes regulate all cellular processes, and the kidneys contribute to the regulation of electrolyte and fluid balances. Imbalances create disorder in the system.

Assessment
- **History:** Injury, illness, medications, diet, fluid intake, and output
- **Physical exam:** Includes vital signs (VS), mucous membranes, tissue turgor, body weight, heart/lung auscultation, abdominal percussion/palpation
- **Serum laboratory values:** Serum osmolality, blood urea nitrogen (BUN)–creatinine ratio, electrolytes
- Urine electrolyte concentrations

Urine Evaluation
Urine electrolyte concentration: The concentration of an electrolyte indicates renal function of excreting or retaining the electrolyte.
Twenty-four-hour urine collection: Used to quantify daily electrolyte excretion. This is the gold standard.
Fractional Excretion (FE): Calculated from a spot urine sample and provides results quickly.

$$\text{FE electrolyte percentage} = \frac{\text{Urine electrolyte} \times \text{Serum Cr} \times 100}{\text{Urine Cr} \times \text{Serum electrolyte}}$$

Water, Sodium, and Chloride Homeostasis
Maintenance of body fluid homeostasis depends upon the following:
- **Kidneys:** Regulation of water and solutes
- **Hormones:** Aldosterone increases renal reabsorption of sodium
- **Antidiuretic hormone:** Stimulated by increased plasma osmolality or decreased blood volume (baroreceptors); water retention via renal reabsorbed into plasma
- **Renin–angiotensin system:** Decreased circulating volume → renin → angiotensin I converts to angiotensin II → aldosterone, which promotes sodium and water reabsorption
- **Atrial natriuretic peptide:** Released with increased atrial pressure (increased volume), which leads to renal elimination of sodium and water

Distribution of Body Water
- Intracellular fluid (ICF)
- Extracellular fluid (ECF)
  - Intravascular movement of fluid
    - The direction of fluid movement through capillary walls depends on the following:
      - Hydrostatic pressure: pressure exerted on the walls of blood vessels

- Osmotic pressure: pressure exerted by the protein in the plasma
- Interstitial movement of fluid
  - "Third spacing": loss of ECF into a space that does not contribute to equilibrium

WATER AND SOLUTE IMBALANCE

Water imbalance occurs due to changing osmotic gradients related to gain or loss of sodium chloride (salt). Water and solute alterations can be classified according to tonicity.

- Tonicity is the measure of the osmotic pressure gradient between two solutions.
- Osmolarity is the measure of solute concentration per unit volume of solvent.

Isotonic Alterations

Isotonic alterations refer to changes in water and electrolytes in equal proportion with no shrinking or swelling of cells.

- *Isotonic volume loss:* Isotonic loss of water and electrolytes
  - Causes: Hemorrhage; intestinal loss from vomiting, diarrhea, GI suctioning, excessive diaphoresis; decreased fluid intake
  - Manifestation: Symptoms of hypovolemia
- *Isotonic volume excess:* Isotonic gain of water and electrolytes
  - Causes: Excess infusion of IV saline, hypersecretion of aldosterone, steroid medications
  - Manifestation: Symptoms of hypervolemia

Hypertonic Alterations

Increased concentration of sodium or a deficit of water, ICF dehydration

- *Hypernatremia:* >147 mEq/L; deficit of total body water (TBW) relative to total body sodium content
  - Causes: Inappropriate administration of hypertonic saline, hyperaldosteronism, Cushing's disease (excessive secretion of adrenocorticotropic hormone [ACTH])
  - Manifestation: Thirst, hypotension, tachycardia, restlessness
  - Treatment: IV D_5W
- *Hypertonic volume loss:* Pure water deficit resulting in excess sodium: ICF dehydration. Pure water deficit is rare due to the thirst response and access to water.
  - Causes: Watery diarrhea; excessive diuresis; diabetes insipidus; excessive diaphoresis
  - Manifestation: Symptoms of dehydration and hypovolemia
  - Treatment: Water PO or IV D_5W

Hypotonic Alterations

Imbalance resulting in ECF concentration less than 0.9% salt solution

- *Hyponatremia:* <135 mEq/L, sodium loss or dilution, ICF edema
  - Causes: GI losses, burns, thiazide diuretics
  - Manifestation: Lethargy, headache, confusion, seizure, coma
  - Treatment: Replacement based on underlying disorder; water intake restriction for dilutional hyponatremia
- *Hypotonic volume excess:* Excessive pure water intake; ICF edema
  - Causes: Excessive hypotonic IV solutions, tap water enemas, syndrome of inappropriate antidiuretic hormone

(SIADH), decreased urine formation, psychogenic polydipsia, acute renal failure, liver failure; severe CHF conditions can precipitate water excess

- Manifestation: Confusion, convulsions
- Treatment: Withhold fluids for 24 hours; use balanced electrolyte IV solution such as Lactated Ringer's or normal saline; moderate to severe symptoms may call for hypertonic 3% normal saline or osmotic diuretic

Fluids

Fluids are an important medicinal treatment and must be used judiciously. First assess for fluid status and then plan the appropriate fluid, rate, and administration schedule to achieve treatment goals (Table 11.4). If the patient is taking adequate oral fluids, consider that IV fluids may not be necessary.

Sodium

Normal sodium: 135 to 145 mEq/L

- Most abundant cation in ECF
- Water balance and fluid shifts
- Enzyme activity and metabolism
- Muscle contraction
- Falls among older adults can often be attributed to hyponatremia

- *Hypernatremia:* >145 mEq/L
  - Cause: Inappropriate administration of hypertonic saline, hyperaldosteronism, Cushing's disease (excessive secretion of ACTH)
  - Symptoms: Confusion, thirst, restless, twitching, seizure
  - Treatment: IV D5W
- *Hyponatremia:* <135 mEq/L; excessive water relative to sodium
  - Cause: Excess sodium loss—GI losses, burns, renal loss from diuretics
  - Symptoms: Appear when <125 mEq/L: lethargy, headache, confusion, seizure, coma when <120 mEq/L
  - Treatment: Replacement based on underlying disorder; water intake restriction for dilutional hyponatremia

Potassium

Normal potassium: 3.5 to 5.0 mEq/L

- Major intracellular cation
- Most common electrolyte abnormality in hospitalized patients

TABLE 11.4 COMMON INTRAVENOUS FLUIDS AND THEIR CONTENTS

ELECTROLYTE	NORMAL SALINE 0.9%	LACTATED RINGER'S	D_5W
Na+, mEq/L	154	130	0
Cl, mEq/L	154	109	0
Ca, mEq/L	0	2.7	0
K, mEq/L	0	4	0
Lactate, mEq/L	0	28	0
pH range	4.5–7.0	6.0–7.5	3.2–6.5
Osmoles, mOsm/L	308	273	252
Dextrose, g/L	0	0	50

D5W, 5% dextrose in water.

- Vital to cardiac and neuromuscular function
- Acid–base balance (hydrogen ion exchange with potassium ions)

- *Hypokalemia:* <3.5 mEq/L
  - Cause: Diuretic loss in urine, GI loss (diarrhea), hyperaldosteronism
  - Symptoms: EKG (flattened or inverted T wave, U wave); cardiac dysrhythmias (premature atrial contractions [PACs], premature ventricular contractions [PVCs], paroxysmal atrial tachycardia [PAT], ventricular fibrillation [V-fib], ventricular tachycardia [V-tach]); increased risk of digoxin toxicity: confusion, lethargy, fatigue, muscle cramps, nausea, vomiting, ileus
  - Treatment: Oral or IV potassium replacement; potassium 40 to 60 mEq PO dose can raise the serum potassium level 1.5 mEq/L per dosage of PO replacement; maximum dose of diluted IV potassium chloride is 40 mEq/L infused at 10 mEq/hr; higher concentrations of IV potassium chloride must be infused via central line
- *Hyperkalemia:* >5 mEq/L
  - Cause: Renal insufficiency, medications (ACE, ARB, NSAIDs, potassium-sparing diuretics), metabolic acidosis, insulin deficiency, cell trauma
  - Symptoms: EKG (tall, peaked T wave; shortened QT, prolonged PR interval, wide QRS), bradyarrhythmias, cardiac arrest, muscle weakness, fatigue, nausea, abdominal cramping
  - Treatment: Underlying cause, oral or rectal sodium polystyrene (Kayexalate), insulin/glucose infusion, sodium bicarbonate, dialysis

Calcium

Normal calcium: 8.5 to 10.2 mg/dL
- Major role in muscle contraction and nerve conduction.
- 40% to 45% of calcium is bound to protein/albumin.
- Affected by albumin levels and nutritional status.
- Serum calcium levels fall about 0.8 mg/dL for every 1 g/dL drop in serum albumin.
- Hypoalbuminemia with critical illness or malnutrition can create normal serum calcium when the serum ionized calcium is high.
- Calcium and phosphorus move in opposite directions.
- Acute or chronic hypocalcemia may be mistaken for a neurologic disorder.
- *Hypocalcemia:* <8.5 mg/dL (<4.0 mg/dL ionized calcium)
  - Cause: Hypoparathyroidism, nutritional deficiency of calcium, vitamin D deficiency, excessive dietary phosphorus, blood transfusions (citrate in banked blood binds with calcium), neoplastic bone metastases (increased calcium bone deposits)
  - Symptoms: Paresthesia, spasms, tetany, seizures, bradycardia, prolonged QT interval, decreased cardiac output
  - Cardiac output
  - Signs:
    - Chvostek's sign—Tap the facial nerve anterior to the ear and watch for a facial muscle contraction
- Trousseau's sign—Carpal spasm after brachial artery occlusion
  - Treatment: Correction of acute symptomatic hypocalcemia: Correction of EAcute momatic Hypocalcemia
  - IV calcium with EKG monitoring

- Transition to PO calcium as values normalize
- Supplemental calcium: 1,500 to 2,000 mg/d in divided doses
- Elemental calcium: calcium carbonate or calcium citrate is given PO
- Calcium gluconate can be given IV at a rate of 1 to 2 g over 10 to 20 minutes
  - Identify root cause

Calculation for Corrected Calcium

Corrected calcium = (0.8 × 4[normal albumin] − patient's albumin) + serum Ca

Concurrent correction of magnesium levels is recommended.

- Low serum magnesium should be corrected.
- Magnesium level goal: 0.8 mEq/L

- *Hypercalcemia:* >10.5 mg/dL; more calcium enters the circulatory system than is eliminated by the kidneys or deposited in the bones.
  - Cause: The most common causes are hyperparathyroidism and malignancy (lung, breast, ovarian); mechanisms of malignancy are bone metastases with calcium resorption and PTH-secreting tumors; other causes are thyrotoxicosis, immobility, Paget's disease of the bone, and excessive vitamin D ingestion
  - Treatment: Correct the underlying cause with the goal of lowering serum calcium.
    - Use combination therapy with *normal saline hydration and bisphosphonates*, which inhibit calcium release and interfere with the bone resorption
    - Corticosteroids
    - IV fluids in combination with loop diuretic

Magnesium

Normal magnesium: 1.3 to 2.1 mEq/L
- Ensures sodium and potassium transport across cell membrane
- Significant role in nerve cell conduction

- *Hypermagnesemia:* Magnesium >2.1 mEq/L
  - Cause: Incidence is rare; aldosterone deficiency, excessive ingestion of Mg
  - Symptoms: Lethargy, impaired central nervous system (CNS) function, respiratory depression
  - Treatment: IV calcium gluconate, furosemide, HD in severe cases

- *Hypomagnesemia:* Mg <1.3 mEq/L
  - Cause: Alcoholism, severe malnutrition, malabsorption, diuretic therapy; often accompanied by hypocalcemia
  - Symptoms: Tremors, convulsions, arrhythmias, confusion
  - Treatment: For persistent levels <1.25 mg/dL. Begin with oral magnesium salts unless seizures or other severe symptoms, then 2 to 4 g of magnesium sulfate IV over 5 to 10 minutes

Phosphorus

Normal phosphorus: 2.5 to 4.5 mg/dL
- Energy (production of ATP)
- Neuromuscular function
- Acid–base balance (ECF buffer)

- *Hyperphosphatemia:* >4.5
  - Cause: Renal insufficiency, hyperthyroidism
  - Symptoms: Muscle cramping, calcifications in soft tissue
  - Treatment: Phosphate restriction, phosphate binders, saline diuresis or HD
- *Hypophosphatemia:* <2.5
  - Cause: TPN infusions, malnutrition, increased renal excretion
  - Symptoms: Slurred speech, dysrhythmias, anorexia, decreased level of consciousness (LOC), seizures
  - Treatment: Treat the underlying disorder; oral phosphate replacement with sodium phosphate or potassium phosphate; IV phosphate if <1 mg/dL or severe symptoms

Management of Fluid and Electrolyte Alterations

Urine osmolality can determine renal versus nonrenal water loss.

- *Low:* Acute renal insufficiency, glomerulonephritis, diabetes insipidus
- *High:* Dehydration, SIADH

Water deficit calculation:

Free water deficit = 0.6 × weight in kg × [(current serum Na/140) – 1]

Chronic hypernatremia does not usually produce neurologic symptoms.
Correction of hyponatremia should be done slowly to avoid cerebral edema. Correction should not exceed 12 mEq/L/d.

ACID–BASE IMBALANCES

OVERVIEW

Body fluid pH is maintained between 7.35 and 7.45 by the following mechanisms:

- *Buffers in extracellular fluid:* HCO_3, plasma proteins, hemoglobin, phosphates
- *Respiratory regulation:* Eliminating or retaining carbon dioxide
- *Renal regulation:* Excreting or conserving bicarbonate and hydrogen ions, slower response to changes in pH (minimum of 12 hours)

ARTERIAL BLOOD GAS ANALYSIS

- Assess for compensation:
  - Uncompensated: pH abnormal
  - Compensated: pH in normal range
  - Acid–base imbalances never overcompensate
    - pH in compensated acidosis: 7.35 to 7.40
    - pH in compensated alkalosis: 7.40 to 7.45

Categorize the pH: Acidosis or alkalosis
- Determine respiratory involvement (PCO_2 is abnormal)
- Determine metabolic involvement (HCO_3 is abnormal)
- Determine oxygenation
  - Is PaO_2 within normal range? What is the patient's baseline?
  - Is SaO_2 within normal range?

TABLE 11.5 NORMAL ARTERIAL BLOOD GAS

pH	7.35–7.45
$PaCO_2$	35–45 mmHg
HCO_3	22–26 mEq/L
BE	±2 mEq/L
PaO_2	80–100 mmHg
SaO_2	95%–100%
Hgb	13.5–17 g/dL, males 12–15 g/dL, females

BE, base excess; Hgb, hemoglobin.

  - Does the Hgb indicate adequate oxygen-carrying capacity (Table 11.5)?
- Clinical scenario
  - Does the patient have a chronic condition associated with long-term ABG alterations?

Anion gap calculation:

$$Anion\ gap = Na^+ - (Cl^- + HCO_3^-)$$

Normal gap range is 9 to 14.

- WAGMA (wide anion gap metabolic acidosis):
  - Lactic acidosis, ketoacidosis, renal failure
- Normal anion gap acidosis:
  - Diarrhea, pancreatic fistula, kidney failure to reabsorb HCO_3

Mixed Acid–Base Disorders

A mixed acid–base disorder is the simultaneous presence of more than one primary acid–base disturbance. A mixed disorder should be suspected when the ordinarily expected acid–base compensatory changes are inappropriate. Careful review of the medical history provides important clues to potential mixed disorders. Examples of mixed acid–base disorders are as follows:

- Patient with diabetic ketoacidosis (DKA) (metabolic acidosis) and pneumonia/respiratory failure (respiratory acidosis)
- Patient with chronic obstructive pulmonary disease (COPD) exacerbation (respiratory acidosis) and severe vomiting (metabolic alkalosis)
- Patient with prerenal failure (metabolic acidosis) and acute respiratory distress (respiratory alkalosis)

Estimating Compensation

HCO_3, $PaCO_2$, and pH have *normal compensatory relationships* that can be calculated. Analysis of these expected relationships can be conducted when a mixed acid–base disorder is suspected. If the actual ABG values and the predicted (calculated) values are not similar, then a mixed acid–base disorder is present. Normal acute compensatory relationships may be calculated as follows (Table 11.6):

- Compensation in metabolic acidosis
  - Predicted $PaCO_2 = 1.5 \times HCO_3 + 8$
- Compensation in respiratory acidosis
  - Predicted $HCO_3 = 24 + (PaCO_2 - 40) \times 0.1$
- Compensation in metabolic alkalosis
  - Predicted $PaCO_2 = 0.73 \times HCO_3 + 20$
- Compensation in respiratory alkalosis
  - Predicted $HCO_3 = 24 - (40 - PaCO_2) \times 0.2$

TABLE 11.6 COMMON ACID–BASE IMBALANCES

IMBALANCE	PRIMARY MECHANISM	PHYSIOLOGIC COMPENSATION	CAUSES
Metabolic acidosis HCO_3 <24	Endogenous acid accumulation or loss of HCO_3	Pulmonary compensation: Increased ventilation lowers $PaCO_2$	Hydrogen ion increase: DKA, renal failure, lactic acidosis HCO_3 decrease: diarrhea, hyperaldosteronism Elevated lactate: hypoxia, shock states Proper treatment involves determining which type of acidosis: Measure the anion gap
Respiratory acidosis $PaCO_2$ >45	Hypoventilation increases $PaCO_2$	Renal compensation: HCO_3 retention Hydrogen ion excretion	Oversedation, head trauma, drug overdose, anesthesia, COPD, OSA, neuromuscular disorders
Metabolic alkalosis HCO_3 >26	Excess plasma HCO_3	Pulmonary compensation: Hypoventilation raises PCO_2	Vomiting, NG suction, diuretics
Respiratory alkalosis $PaCO_2$ <35	Hyperventilation lowers $PaCO_2$	Renal compensation: HCO_3 excretion Hydrogen ion retention	Hypoxia, anxiety, fear, pain, fever

COPD, chronic obstructive pulmonary disease; DKA, diabetic ketoacidosis; NG, nasogastric; OSA, obstructive sleep apnea.

URINARY ELIMINATION ISSUES IN GERONTOLOGY

OVERVIEW

Physiologic changes in the urinary system occur during the normal aging process. However, it should not be assumed that incontinence is an inevitable consequence of aging. Caregiver misconceptions can negatively affect care.

AGE-RELATED CHANGES AFFECTING URINARY FUNCTION

- *Decreased thirst perception*—Increased risk of dehydration and increased bladder irritability
- *Bladder hypertrophy*—Limits expansion and comfortable urine storage to 200 to 300 mL
- *Relaxation of pelvic floor muscles*—Reduces sphincter tone
- *Cerebral cortex degeneration*—Delayed sensation of bladder fullness, decreased ability to fully empty the bladder
- *Estrogen*—Decrease is associated with urinary leakage and earlier onset of incontinence in women
- *Change in diurnal urine production*—More nocturia

Types of Urinary Incontinence

- *Stress*—Urine leakage from increased abdominal pressure (coughing, lifting, sneezing)
- *Urge*—Urine leakage due to inability to hold urine
- *Mixed*—Urine leakage and urgency
- *Overactive bladder (OAB)*—Urgency, nocturia, daytime frequency, with or without incontinence

Conditions With Increased Risk of Urinary Incontinence

- Pelvic floor dysfunction
- Benign prostatic hyperplasia (BPH)
- Urinary tract infection (UTI)
- Obesity
- Diabetes
- Neurologic disorders
- Acute illness/surgery that impairs mobility or mental status

Interventions to Promote Urinary Wellness and Function

- Initiate continence training programs—Voiding diary; schedule to increase time between voidings
- Pelvic floor muscle training—Improves urethral resistance; first-line treatment for stress and mixed incontinence in men and women
- Suggest environmental modifications—Remove obstacles, bathroom safety
- Use appropriate continence aids—Pessaries, external occlusive devices, and so forth
- Assess for medications that contribute to urinary incontinence (Table 11.7)
- Medications for urinary incontinence

TABLE 11.7 MEDICATIONS THAT CONTRIBUTE TO URINARY INCONTINENCE

DRUG CLASS	EFFECT ON URINARY FUNCTION
Diuretics	Frequency and polyuria
ACE inhibitors	Chronic cough exacerbates stress incontinence
Calcium channel blockers	Decreased bladder contractility, urinary retention
Alpha adrenergic agonists	Decreased bladder contractility, urinary retention
Alpha adrenergic blockers	Decreased sphincter tone
Anticholinergics	Decreased bladder contractility, urinary retention
Benzodiazepines	Sedation, cognitive impairment, loss of voluntary control

ACE, angiotensin-converting enzyme.
Source: Burcham, J. R., & Rosenthal, L. D. (2018). *Lehne's pharmacology for nursing care* (10th ed.). Elsevier.

URINARY TRACT INFECTIONS

CYSTITIS

Cystitis is an inflammation of the bladder, most often caused by bacterial contamination of urine via retrograde movement of Gram-negative bacteria (*Escherichia coli, Proteus mirabilis, Klebsiella pneumoniae*).

Risk Factors

■ Older age	■ Female gender
■ Diabetes	■ Poor hygiene
■ Indwelling catheters	■ Prostatitis
■ Pregnancy	■ Sexual activity
■ Neurogenic bladder	

Assessment

■ *Symptoms:* Reported symptoms include frequency, urgency, dysuria, and suprapubic pain. Older patients may be asymptomatic. Urine may be cloudy.

■ *Urinalysis results indicative of UTI:* Positive urinalysis should prompt urine culture and sensitivity.

■ Bacteria	5+ (rough equivalence to 100,000 CFU/mL)
■ Leukocyte esterase	Positive, indicates pyuria
■ WBC	>10, indicates pyuria
■ Nitrite	Positive, presence of bacteria that converts nitrate to nitrite (e.g., *E. coli*)
■ RBC	Hematuria, presence is common in infection
■ Epithelial cells	<5, indicates good urine sample; a high value indicates contaminated sample
■ pH	High pH may indicate presence of *P. mirabilis*

CFU, colony-forming units; RBC, red blood cell; WBC, white blood cell.

For first-line treatment of uncomplicated UTI, see Table 11.8.

PYELONEPHRITIS

Pyelonephritis is an acute infection of the kidney most commonly caused by Gram-negative bacteria. Complications include septicemia and renal failure.

Risk Factors

■ Urinary obstruction
■ Vesicoureteral reflux
■ Female gender

TABLE 11.8 FIRST-LINE TREATMENT FOR UNCOMPLICATED UTI

MEDICATION	DURATION
Trimethoprim–sulfamethoxazole 160/800 mg BID	3 days
Nitrofurantoin 100 mg BID	5 days
Fosfomycin 3 g once	1 day
Increase fluid intake	
If symptoms persist 48–72 hours after initiation of antibiotic, repeat urine culture. Rule out pyelonephritis.	

Source: Burcham, J. R., & Rosenthal, L. D. (2018). *Lehne's pharmacology for nursing care* (10th ed.). Elsevier.

Assessment

Symptoms: Acute-onset symptoms include fever, chills, flank pain, groin pain, frequency, dysuria, and costovertebral tenderness.

■ *Urinalysis results indicative of pyelonephritis:* Large amount of leukocytes, hematuria, WBC casts, protein
  ● Urine culture:100,000 CFU/mL of single organism
  ● Complete blood count: WBC >11,000; neutrophilia (<80%)
  ● Shift to left: Presence of immature neutrophils (bands) indicates serious infection.

For first-line treatment of uncomplicated pyelonephritis, see Table 11.9. Close follow-up is necessary. Mild to moderate infections can be treated at home. Severe pyelonephritis requires hospitalization and IV antibiotics.

Drug therapy recommendations should be based upon symptom scales score (International Prostate Symptom Score [IPSS]). IPSS guideline may be accessed from the Urological Sciences Research Foundation at: http://www.browardurologycenter.com/pdf//ipss.pdf

Table 11.10 lists medications used for overactive bladder. Table 11.11 lists medications used for BPH.

TABLE 11.9 FIRST-LINE TREATMENT FOR UNCOMPLICATED PYELONEPHRITIS

MEDICATION	DURATION
Trimethoprim–sulfamethoxazole 160/800 mg BID	14 days
Ciprofloxacin 250–500 mg BID	7–14 days
Levofloxacin 250 mg once daily	5–10 days

Source: Burcham, J. R., & Rosenthal, L. D. (2018). *Lehne's pharmacology for nursing care* (10th ed.). Elsevier.

TABLE 11.10 OVERACTIVE BLADDER MEDICATIONS

CLASS	ANTICHOLINERGIC/ANTIMUSCARINIC				
Mechanism	Inhibits detrusor muscle contractions				
GENERIC NAME (BRAND NAME)	INDICATIONS	CONTRAINDICATIONS	DOSAGE	COMMON ADVERSE EFFECTS	SAFETY AND PATIENT EDUCATION
Oxybutynin (Ditropan)	Overactive bladder	Urinary or gastric retention—uncontrolled narrow-angle glaucoma	5 mg PO BID to TID	Dry mouth Constipation Dizziness	Monitor for CNS anticholinergic effects such as hallucinations, agitation, confusion, and somnolence, particularly in the first few months of treatment
Tolterodine (Detrol)	Overactive bladder	Urinary or gastric retention—uncontrolled narrow-angle glaucoma	2 mg PO BID	Dry mouth, constipation, blurred vision (these decrease over time)	Limit dose in pts with renal/hepatic dysfunction—interacts with other medications metabolized by CYP3A4 inhibitors
CLASS	BETA 3 RECEPTOR AGONISTS				
Mechanism	Relaxes bladder smooth muscle				
GENERIC NAME (BRAND NAME)	INDICATIONS	CONTRAINDICATIONS	DOSAGE	COMMON ADVERSE EFFECTS	SAFETY AND PATIENT EDUCATION
Mirabegron (Myrbetriq)	For use in patients who are unable to tolerate increased antimuscarinic dose due to side effects or dose limits	None	25 mg PO once daily	Hypertension	Patients with severe or uncontrolled hypertension should not be prescribed mirabegron Contact provider immediately for dizziness, irregular heartbeat
CLASS	BOTULISM TOXINS				
Mechanism	Inhibition of the release of acetylcholine from the presynaptic nerve terminal, which prevents stimulation of the detrusor muscle				
GENERIC NAME (BRAND NAME)	INDICATIONS	CONTRAINDICATIONS	DOSAGE	COMMON ADVERSE EFFECTS	SAFETY AND PATIENT EDUCATION
Onabotulinumtoxin A (Botox)	Overactive bladder	Contraindicated in presence of UTI	100 U injection at intervals of every 6–9 months	Higher rates of transient urinary retention and UTI	Less likely to have dry mouth More complete resolution of incontinence

CNS, clinical nurse specialist; PTS, patients; UTI, urinary tract infection.

Source: Burcham, J. R., & Rosenthal, L. D. (2018). *Lehne's pharmacology for nursing care* (10th ed.). Elsevier.

TABLE 11.11 MEDICATIONS FOR BENIGN PROSTATIC HYPERPLASIA

CLASS	ALPHA ADRENERGIC ANTAGONISTS				
Mechanism	Relax smooth muscle tone at bladder neck and prostate				
GENERIC NAME (BRAND NAME)	INDICATIONS, CONTRAINDICATIONS	DOSAGE	COMMON ADVERSE EFFECTS	SAFETY AND PATIENT EDUCATION	
Terazosin (Hytrin)	Nonselective for BPH symptoms	1–10 mg PO at bedtime	May cause dizziness and hypotension	Do not stop medication suddenly; orthostatic hypotension	
Doxazosin (Cardura)				Orthostatic hypotension	
Tamsulosin (Flomax)	Uroselective: target bladder neck and prostate with fewer adverse cardiac side effects	0.4–0.8 mg PO once daily	Dizziness, nasal congestion, paranasal sinus congestion, rhinitis	Orthostatic hypotension Interaction with phosphodiesterase-5 inhibitors Ejaculatory dysfunction	
Alfuzosin (Uroxatral)					
CLASS	5-ALPHA REDUCTASE INHIBITORS				
Mechanism	Blocks 5-alpha reductase and inhibits conversion of testosterone to dihydrotestosterone. Results in 25% reduction in prostate volume over approximately 3 months.				
GENERIC NAME (BRAND NAME)	INDICATIONS, CONTRAINDICATIONS	DOSAGE	COMMON ADVERSE EFFECTS	SAFETY AND PATIENT EDUCATION	
Finasteride (Proscar)	Indicated for the treatment of symptomatic BPH in men and patients unable to tolerate alpha-1-adrenergics	5 mg PO daily	Ejaculatory disorder, erectile dysfunction, decreased libido, gynecomastia	Women should not handle crushed or broken Proscar tablets when they are pregnant or may potentially be pregnant because of the possibility of absorption of finasteride and the subsequent potential risk to a male fetus.	
Dutasteride (Avodart)		0.5 mg PO daily			

BPH, benign prostatic hyperplasia.

REVIEW QUESTIONS

1. Which of the following patients are at risk for acute kidney injury (AKI)?
   A. 55-year-old male with hypotension secondary to bleeding esophageal varices
   B. 23-year-old female receiving chemotherapy
   C. 69-year-old male with benign prostatic hypertrophy
   D. 87-year-old female taking vancomycin for a severe infection

2. A 43-year-old female with chronic kidney disease (CKD) comes to the primary care physician's office for her follow-up visit. During the interview, she states that she has been feeling tired for the past few months but just attributes it to being a busy working mother of three young kids. Upon examination, the patient exhibits pallor and has pale conjunctivae and slight pitting edema of her lower extremities. Lab values show the following:

Creatinine	0.75 mg/dL
Blood, urea nitrogen	32 mg/dL
Sodium	138 mEq/L
Potassium	4.0 mEq/L
Blood glucose	198 mg/dL
Hbg A1c	8.4%
Hemoglobin	9.7 g/dL
Estimated glomerular filtration rate	52 mL/min/1.73 m^2

The patient also has a past medical history of type 2 diabetes, hypertension, and diabetic nephropathy. For which of the following medications should the patient be evaluated?
   A. Epoetin and metformin
   B. Lasix and losartan
   C. Metformin and vitamin B_{12}
   D. Carvedilol and iron supplements

ANSWERS

1. **Correct answers: B and D. Rationale:** Both of these patients are at risk for intrarenal injury because of damage to the nephrons of the kidneys caused by nephrotoxic medication. Patient A has prerenal injury because there is a problem with perfusion to the kidneys secondary to bleeding from the esophageal varices. Patient C has postrenal injury because there is an obstruction that can cause backflow of urine into the kidneys, which leads to decrease kidney function.

2. **Correct answer: A. Rationale:** Epoetin is recommended because the patient is exhibiting signs and symptoms of anemia (been feeling tired for the past few months, has pallor, has pale conjunctivae, has slight crackles in the bases of her lungs and bilateral mild, pitting edema of her lower extremities) and is confirmed by laboratory results. Further lab testing (i.e., CBC, red blood cell [RBC] indices, reticulocyte count, serum ferritin concentration and transferrin saturation (TSAT) is warranted to assist with determining the best line of treatment for this patient. It's important to note that Metformin is contraindicated in patients with an eGFR below 30 mL/min/1.73 m^2. Metformin is used to treat the hyperglycemia and Hbg A1c, which determines the patient's average blood glucose control for the previous 3 months. Option B is incorrect because losartan (an angiotensin 2 receptor blocking agent) is not needed in this scenario for treatment. Although the patient does have symptoms of lower extremity pitting edema, it could be secondary to the combination of diabetes (hyperglycemia) and CKD. The Losartan medication would eliminate this as a choice. Although metformin would be appropriate in this situation, vitamin B_{12} is not necessary to prescribe at this time. Therefore, option C is incorrect. Option D is incorrect because carvedilol (a beta blocking agent) is not needed in this scenario for treatment. The need for iron supplements would need to be determined with further laboratory testing.

REFERENCES

The complete reference and additional reading lists appear in the digital version of the chapter, at https://connect.springerpub.com/content/book/978-0-8261-7417-8/part/part01/chapter/ch11

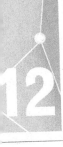

12 Integumentary System

Jan Powers, Katrina Hawkins, and Lynne Marie Kokoczka

OVERVIEW

The integumentary system is the largest system in the human body, and it is one of the fastest growing tissues in the body. It plays an important role in homeostasis.

Primary Functions

- Thermal regulation
- Barrier to external insults
- Prevents bacterial overgrowth (acidic pH 4.2–5.6)
- Provides sensory feedback
- Assists with regulation of fluid and electrolyte balance

The skin is composed of three layers (Figure 12.1).

- *Epidermis*—Outermost layer of the skin; provides a barrier
- *Dermis*—Contains tough connective tissue, hair follicles, and sweat glands
- *Subcutaneous tissue (hypodermis)*—Deepest layer made up of fat and connective tissue

Common problems related to the integumentary system include the following:

- Pressure-related injuries
- Wounds (neuropathic, vascular, surgical, burns)
- Allergic reactions/sensitivities

PRESSURE INJURIES

Pressure injuries are a primary area of focus for any clinical nurse specialist (CNS) regardless of practice area.

Definition

According to the National Pressure Ulcer Advisory Panel (NPUAP), a pressure ulcer is a localized injury to the skin and/ or underlying tissue, usually over a bony prominence, as a result of pressure, or pressure in combination with shear (National Pressure Ulcer Advisory Panel and European Advisory Panel [NPUAP], 2014).

Pathophysiology

Soft tissues can be compressed between bony prominences and contact surfaces causing microvascular occlusion, tissue ischemia, and hypoxia. The ability of pressure to cause tissue damage is related to the duration and intensity of pressure applied (NPUAP, 2014).

Etiology
Extrinsic Contributing Factors

- Pressure
- Shear
- Friction
- Moisture
- Temperature

Pressure over a bony prominence results in internal stresses that are highest in the soft tissue closest to the bony prominence. Pressure injury results when pressure blocks blood circulation, causing the skin and underlying tissues to die, leading to an open wound (Kuffler, 2015).

The greatest incidence of pressure injuries is on the sacrum, followed by the heels.

Moisture affects the skin by dissolving the collagen cross-linking, reducing the stiffness and strength of the skin up to 96%, which leads to erosion. Moisture increases the coefficient of friction, dilutes skin acidity, and with the pH shift promotes abrasion, slough, and ulceration.

Risk Factors

Risk factors for pressure injury should be evaluated using an approved risk assessment tool (NPUAP, 2014).

Risk factors for pressure injury include the following:

- Immobility
- Poor nutritional status
- Decreased perfusion and oxygenation
- Increased skin moisture (from incontinence, wound drainage, or diaphoresis)
- Increased body temperature
- Advanced age
- Increased temperature
- Decreased sensory perception

The presence of medical devices also places the patient at risk for medical device pressure-related injury. It is always important to select medical devices that have the least degree of ability to induce damage from pressure or shear (NPUAP, 2014).

Assessment

Head-to-toe skin pressure injury skin assessment

- Expose to assess all areas.
- Carefully assess skin folds and beneath hair.
- Examine posterior surface.
- Document any breakdown present on admission.

Pressure Ulcer Staging

The National Pressure Ulcer Advisory Panel redefined the definition of pressure injuries during the NPUAP 2016 Staging Consensus Conference held in 2016 (Table 12.1).

Prevention of Pressure Injuries
Comprehensive Pressure Injury Prevention Program

- Risk assessment
- Skin care–specific measures
- Pressure redistribution
- Friction and shear management

The complete reference and additional reading lists appear in the digital version of this chapter, at https://connect.springerpub.com/content/book/978-0-8261-7417-8/part/part01/chapter/ch12

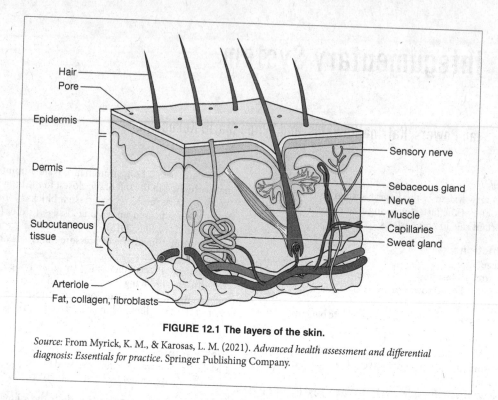

FIGURE 12.1 The layers of the skin.

Source: From Myrick, K. M., & Karosas, L. M. (2021). *Advanced health assessment and differential diagnosis: Essentials for practice.* Springer Publishing Company.

TABLE 12.1 PRESSURE INJURY STAGES

PRESSURE INJURY STAGES	DEFINITION	PRESENTATION
Stage 1	Nonblanchable erythema of intact skin	Presence of blanchable erythema or changes in sensation, temperature, or firmness may precede visual changes. May appear differently in darkly pigmented skin.
Stage 2	Partial-thickness skin loss with exposed dermis	The wound bed is viable, pink or red, and moist and may also present as an intact or ruptured serum-filled blister. These injuries commonly result from adverse microclimate and shear in the skin over the pelvis and shear in the heel. This stage should not be used to describe MASD, including IAD, MARSI, or traumatic wounds (skin tears, burns, abrasions).
Stage 3	Full-thickness skin loss	The depth of tissue damage varies by anatomical location; areas with significant adipose tissue can develop deep wounds. Undermining and tunneling may occur. Slough and/or eschar may be visible.
Stage 4	Full-thickness skin and tissue loss	Exposed or directly palpable fascia, muscle, tendon, ligament, cartilage, or bone in the ulcer. Slough and/or eschar may be visible. Undermining and/or tunneling often occur. Depth varies by anatomical location.
DTI	Persistent nonblanchable, deep red, maroon, or purple discoloration	Intact or nonintact skin with localized area of persistent nonblanchable deep red, maroon, purple discoloration or epidermal separation revealing a dark wound bed. Pain and temperature change often precede skin color changes. Discoloration may appear differently in darkly pigmented skin. This injury results from intense and/or prolonged pressure and shear forces at the bone–muscle interface. The wound may evolve rapidly to reveal the actual extent of tissue injury or may resolve without tissue loss.
Unstageable	Obscured full-thickness skin and tissue loss	Extent of tissue damage within the ulcer cannot be confirmed because it is obscured by slough or eschar. Stable eschar (i.e., dry, adherent, intact without erythema or fluctuance) on the heel or ischemic limb should not be softened or removed.

(continued)

TABLE 12.1 PRESSURE INJURY STAGES (*continued*)

OTHER SKIN CONDITIONS	DEFINITION	PRESENTATION
Medical device–related pressure injury	Any medical device that results in pressure injury	The resultant pressure injury generally conforms to the pattern or shape of the device. The injury should be staged using the staging system.
MASD (IAD)	General term for inflammation or skin erosion caused by prolonged exposure to a source of moisture, such as urine, stool, sweat, wound drainage, saliva, or mucus	Most common form is IAD.

DTI, deep tissue injury; IAD, incontinence associated dermatitis; MARSI, medical adhesive–related skin injury; MASD, moisture-associated skin damage.
Source: From National Pressure Ulcer Advisory Panel. (2016). *NPUAP Staging Consensus Conference.* http://www.npuap.org/wp-content/uploads/2014/08/Quick-Reference-Guide-DIGITAL-NPUAP-EPUAP-PPPIA-Jan2016.pdf

- Incontinence/moisture care
- Nutritional assessment and interventions
- Education of clinical staff and patients

Key measures for the prevention of pressure injuries include the following:
- Reposition frequently (at least every 2 hours) to relieve areas of pressure. Assure effective turn (typically 30°) to off-load sacral pressure. If the patient is bed bound or unable to move feed independently, elevate the heels off bed.
- Keep the skin clean and dry using a pH-balanced skin cleanser.
- Do not massage skin that is reddened or at risk for pressure injury as this may cause mild tissue destruction or provoke inflammatory reactions.
- Develop and implement an individualized continence management plan.
- Protect the skin from exposure to excessive moisture with a barrier product in order to reduce the risk of pressure damage.
- Consider using a skin moisturizer to hydrate dry skin in order to reduce risk of skin damage.
- Ensure that medical devices are correctly sized and fit appropriately to avoid excessive pressure.
- Ensure nutritional assessment and appropriate interventions.

Other considerations for prevention of pressure injuries include the following:
Prophylactic dressings—Apply a polyurethane foam dressing to bony prominences (e.g., heels, sacrum) to prevent pressure ulcers in anatomical areas frequently subjected to friction and shear. They may also be beneficial for reducing pressure ulcer incidence associated with medical devices (Clark et al., 2014).

Treatment of Pressure Injuries
Interventions
Implement appropriate treatment measures to facilitate wound healing and prevent new pressure injuries. Some standard treatment measures include providing pressure relief for pressure injuries; this includes avoiding positioning patients directly on their pressure injury, elevating heels off surface, and using pressure-reducing/relieving support surfaces.

Treat factors that may affect healing; maintain a clean wound bed; cleanse with wound cleanser, saline, or sterile water; deride wounds as needed; and treat infection if present and/or prevent infection.

Wound Treatment: Key Principles
- Cleanse the pressure ulcer at the time of each dressing change.
  - Consider using cleansing solutions with surfactants and/or antimicrobials to clean pressure ulcers with debris, confirmed infection, suspected infection, or suspected high levels of bacterial colonization.
- Debride nonviable or necrotic tissue within the wound bed or edge of pressure ulcers when appropriate.
  - Debridement should only be performed when there is adequate perfusion to the wound. Sharp debridement should only be performed by healthcare providers with appropriate training, credentialing, and competency.
  - The most common methods used for debriding pressure ulcers are
    - Surgical/sharp,
    - Autolytic,
    - Enzymatic:
      - Use mechanical, autolytic, enzymatic, and/or biologic methods of debridement when there is no urgent clinical need for drainage or removal of devitalized tissue.
      - Surgical/sharp debridement is recommended in the presence of extensive necrosis, advancing cellulitis, crepitus, fluctuance, and/or sepsis secondary to ulcer-related infection and must be performed by specially trained, competent, qualified, and licensed health professionals.
- Observe for local and/or systemic signs of acute infection, such as
  - Erythema extending from the ulcer edge,
  - Induration,
  - New or increasing pain or warmth,
  - Purulent drainage,
  - Increase in size,

- Crepitus, fluctuance, or discoloration in the surrounding skin,
- Fever, malaise, and lymph node enlargement, or
- Confusion/delirium and anorexia (particularly in older adults).
- Bacterial bioburden of the pressure injury is determined by tissue biopsy or quantitative swab technique.

■ Apply appropriate wound dressing based on individual needs of the wound. *Wound dressing selection* is based on the
  - Ability to keep the wound bed moist,
  - Need to address infection,
  - Nature and volume of the wound exudate,
  - Need for debridement,
  - Condition of the tissue in the ulcer bed,
  - Condition of peri-ulcer skin,
  - Ulcer size, depth, and location, and
  - Presence of tunneling and/or undermining.
■ Dressings should promote moist wound healing.
■ Dressing should also be selected to maintain absorption of drainage if present. Protect surrounding area for excess drainage/moisture.
■ Protect from friction, shear, pressure, moisture (including incontinence). Manage pain and nutrition as indicated (Molnar et al., 2016).
■ It is difficult to recommend one dressing or treatment over another with certainty. The clinician should decide which treatment to use based on wound symptoms, clinical experience, patient preference, and cost (Westby et al., 2017; Tables 12.2–12.4).

Nutritional Considerations

■ Optimizing nutrition should be considered an essential element in the prevention and healing of pressure ulcers. Understanding malnutrition in patients, the effect of nutrition on wound healing, and the application of evidence-based nutritional guidelines are important aspects for patients at high risk for pressure ulcers.
■ Appropriate screenings for nutritional status and risk for pressure ulcers, early collaboration with a registered dietician, and administration of appropriate feeding formulations and micronutrient and macronutrient supplementation to promote wound healing are practical solutions to improve the nutritional status of critical care patients (Cox & Rasmussen, 2014).

Nutrition Assessment and Plan

■ Screen nutritional status for each individual at risk for or with a pressure ulcer at admission to healthcare settings and with any significant change of clinical condition.
■ Use a valid and reliable nutrition-screening tool to determine nutritional risk.
■ Develop an individualized nutrition care plan for individuals with or at risk for a pressure ulcer. Collaborate with a registered dietitian; in consultation with the interprofessional team, develop and document an individualized nutrition intervention plan based on the individual's nutritional needs, feeding route, and goals of care, as determined by the nutrition assessment.
■ Provide 30 to 35 kcal/kg body weight for adults at risk for or with a pressure injury who are assessed as being at risk for malnutrition.

- Use of nutritional management and enteral feeding protocols may provide vital elements to augment nutrition and ultimately result in improved clinical outcomes (Cox & Rasmussen, 2014).

Barriers to wound healing include infection, necrotic material, perfusion, oxygenation, and poor nutrition. *Risk factors* that contribute to chronic wounds are venous disease, infection, diabetes, and metabolic deficiencies of older adults.

Clinical Practice Guidelines
Refer to NPUAP for detailed guidelines for prevention and management of pressure injuries (NPUAP.org).

SURGICAL WOUNDS

OVERVIEW
The Centers for Disease Control and Prevention (CDC) established and supports the surgical site infection (SSI) events reported to the National Healthcare Safety Network (NHSN), including the following classifications (Class I–Class IV). These are documented at the end of a case as a means of ranking the risk for developing an infection. They also impact the antibiotic selection.

A surgical wound is an incision made by cutting through skin or mucous membrane. Wounds are divided into four classifications:

Class I: Clean > no infection or inflammation; the respiratory, alimentary, genital, or urinary tracts are not entered; no breaks in aseptic technique; closed primarily; examples: mastectomy, vascular, hernia.

Class II: Clean-contaminated > no infection or inflammation; the respiratory, alimentary, genital, or urinary tracts are entered under controlled conditions; minor break in aseptic technique; examples: hysterectomy, cholecystectomy, colon surgery.

Class III: Contaminated > open, fresh accidental wounds, major break in aseptic technique, uncontrolled spillage from viscus; examples: penetrating wounds, ruptured appendix, bile spillage in cholecystectomy.

Class IV: Dirty or infected > purulent inflammation, old traumatic wounds, necrotic tissue, gross spillage from gastrointestinal tract; examples: peritonitis, wound debridement, perforated bowel.

SURGICAL SITE INFECTIONS
Infections that occur after surgery in the surgical incision, tissue, organ, or organ space are called *surgical site infections* (SSI; Anderson et al., 2014). The Centers for Medicare & Medicaid Services (CMS) includes the following SSI as hospital-acquired conditions (HAC): mediastinitis following coronary artery bypass graft surgery, SSI following bariatric surgery for obesity, SSI following certain orthopedic procedures (spine, neck, shoulder, and elbow), and SSI following placement of cardiac implantable electronic devices (CMS, 2018).

Etiology and Pathophysiology
The integumentary system acts as natural barrier to infection. Any break in this barrier, such as through a surgical incision, causes an increased risk of infection (Mangram et al., 1999). The four classifications of surgical wounds are clean,

TABLE 12.2 WOUND DRESSING INDICATIONS

DRESSING	INDICATION	SPECIAL CONSIDERATIONS
Hydrocolloid	Clean stage 2 in body areas where they will not roll or melt. Noninfected, shallow stage 3 pressure ulcers.	Avoid use with infected wounds.
Transparent film	Use for autolytic debridement when the individual is not immunocompromised. Use as secondary dressing for pressure ulcers treated with alginates or other wound fillers that will likely remain in the ulcer bed for an extended period of time.	Do not use with moderately to heavily exuding ulcers. Avoid use with fragile skin.
Hydrogel	Use for shallow, minimally exuding PIs that are not clinically infected and are granulating.	Can be used for treatment of dry ulcer beds.
Alginate	Use for treatment of moderately and heavily exuding pressure ulcers.	Caution with use in tunneling areas.
Foam	Use on exuding stage 2 and shallow stage 3 PIs.	
Silver-impregnated dressings	Use for PI that are clinically infected or at high risk for infection.	Avoid prolonged use of silver-impregnated dressings. Discontinue silver dressings when wound infection is controlled.
Medical-grade honey	Use for treatment of stages 2 and 3 PI.	
Cadexomer iodine dressings	Use for moderately to highly exuding PI.	Iodine products should be avoided in individuals with impaired renal failure, history of thyroid disorders, or known iodine sensitivity. Not recommended if taking lithium or for pregnant or breast-feeding women. Iodine toxicity has been reported in a few case studies, especially with large wounds. The risk of systemic absorption increases when iodine products are used on larger, deeper wounds or for prolonged periods.
Gauze	May be used on most wounds with exudate. Use to cover dressing to reduce evaporation when the tissue interface layer is moist. Consider using impregnated forms of gauze to prevent evaporation of moisture from continuously moist gauze dressings.	Avoid using gauze dressings for open pressure ulcers that have been cleansed and debrided because they are labor intensive, cause pain when removed if dry, and harm viable tissue if they dry. Avoid use of wet-to-dry gauze dressings. When other forms of moisture-retentive dressing are not available, continually moist gauze is preferable to dry gauze. Loosely fill (rather than tightly pack) ulcers with large tissue defects and dead space with saline moistened gauze when other forms of moisture-retentive dressing are not available, to avoid creating pressure on the wound bed.
Silicone foam	Use as a wound contact layer to promote atraumatic dressing changes.	Consider use to prevent peri-wound tissue injury when tissue is fragile or friable.

PI, pressure injury.

Sources: From Qaseem, A., Humphrey, L. L., Forciea, M. A., Starkey, M., Denberg, T. D., & Clinical Guidelines Committee of the American College of Physicians. (2015). Treatment of pressure ulcers: A clinical practice guideline from the American College of Physicians. *Annals of Internal Medicine, 162*(5), 370–379; National Pressure Ulcer Advisory Panel and European Advisory Panel. (2014). *Prevention and treatment of pressure ulcers: Clinical practice guideline.* National Pressure Ulcer Advisory Panel. http://www.npuap.org/resources/educational-and-clinical-resources/npuap-pressure-injury-stages

TABLE 12.3 KEY ASPECTS OF PRESSURE INJURY TREATMENT

STAGE	TREATMENT	GOALS
Stage 1	Relieve pressure from affected area.	Prevent wound progression.
Stage 2	Maintain moist wound bed; absorb exudate.	Promote reepithelialization.
Stage 3	Maintain moist wound bed; absorb exudate; debride any devitalized tissue.	Promote healing; prevent infection.
Stage 4	Maintain moist wound bed; fill any tunneling areas to prevent abscess; absorb exudate; debride any devitalized tissue. If bone is exposed, evaluate for presence of osteomyelitis.	Promote healing; prevent or treat infection.
DTI	Relieve pressure from affected area.	Prevent further damage.
Unable to stage	Debride as appropriate. Eschar on heels should not be removed; allow autolytic debridement.	Remove devitalized tissue.

DTI, deep tissue injury.

TABLE 12.4 PHASES OF WOUND HEALING

PHASE	DESCRIPTION	TIME FRAME
Hemostasis	Blood vessels constrict to restrict the blood flow. Platelets stick together in order to seal the break in the wall of the blood vessel. Finally, coagulation occurs and reinforces the platelet plug with threads of fibrin, which are like a molecular binding agent.	Starts immediately and lasts 5–10 minutes.
Inflammatory	Inflammation controls bleeding and prevents infection. The fluid engorgement allows healing and repair cells to move to the site of the wound; damaged cells, pathogens, and bacteria are removed from the wound area. These white blood cells, growth factors, nutrients, and enzymes create the swelling, heat, pain, and redness commonly seen during this stage of wound healing.	Begins right after injury and lasts 4–6 days.
Proliferation	Wound is rebuilt with new tissue made up of collagen and extracellular matrix. Wound contracts as new tissues are built. Granulation tissue is pink or red and uneven in texture.	Lasts 6–21 days.
Maturation or remodeling	Collagen is remodeled and the wound fully closes. Collagen laid down during the proliferative phase is disorganized and the wound is thick. During the maturation phase, collagen is aligned along tension lines and water is reabsorbed so the collagen fibers can lie closer together and cross-link, reducing scar thickness and also making the skin stronger.	Begins about 21 days after injury and can continue up to 1 year or more.

clean-contaminated, contaminated, and dirty/infected. The rate of infection for the different classifications increases with the amount of contamination (Mangram et al., 1999). The patient characteristics, type of surgery and the tissues, organs, and organ spaces involved determine the bacterial load and the subsequent risk of SSI (Table 12.5).

Patient

Nonmodifiable risk factors (Anderson et al., 2014):

- Age
- History of radiation
- History of previous SSI

Modifiable risk factors:

- Elevated blood glucose (Mangram et al., 1999)
- High body mass index (BMI; Anderson et al., 2014)
- Nicotine use (Mangram et al., 1999)
- Medications that cause immunosuppression (Mangram et al., 1999)

- Hypoalbuminemia (Anderson et al., 2014)
- Colonization of *Staphylococcus aureus* in the nares (Mangram et al., 1999)
- Preoperative infection (Anderson et al., 2014)

Procedure

- Inadequate skin preparation for patient and surgical team (Mangram et al., 1999)
- Inadequate or omitted antibiotic prophylaxis (Mangram et al., 1999)
- Poor surgical and/or aseptic technique (Mangram et al., 1999)
- Increased operative time and/or intraoperative complications (Anderson et al., 2014)

Environment

- Substandard operating room air ventilation exchanges (Mangram et al., 1999)

TABLE 12.5 TYPE OF SURGICAL SITE INFECTIONS

TYPE OF SSI	ASSESSMENT FINDINGS
Superficial incisional infection	Infections that involve only the skin and/or subcutaneous tissue of the incision and include one or more of the following: purulent drainage from the superficial incision; positive organism growth from wound culture; the superficial wound is intentionally opened by the practitioner; wound culture is not obtained, *and* the patient has one or more of the following symptoms at the surgical site: pain/tenderness, swelling, erythema, warmth; diagnosis by the practitioner.
Deep incisional infection	Infections that involve the deep soft tissues (fascia and/or muscle layers) and include one of the following: purulent drainage from the deep incision site; infection is assessed upon physical or microscopic exam or during imaging; the deep incisional wound is intentionally opened by the practitioner or spontaneously dehisces, *and* organism(s) are identified from a wound culture, *and* the patient has one or more of the following symptoms at the surgical site: temperature greater than 38 °C, pain/tenderness at the surgical site.
Organ/space infection	Infections that involve any part of the body that was surgically opened and/or manipulated during the operation and one or more of the following: does not include skin, subcutaneous tissue, fascia, and muscle *and* the organ/space wound has one or more of the following: Purulent drainage occurs from a drain in the organ/space; organism(s) are identified from fluid or tissue; infection is assessed upon physical or microscopic exam or during imaging.

SSI, surgical site infection.
Source: Centers for Disease Control and Prevention. (2019). *Centers for Disease Control and Prevention: Surgical site infection criteria*. https://www.cdc.gov/nhsn/pdfs/pscmanual/9pscssicurrent.pdf

TABLE 12.6 SURGICAL CARE IMPROVEMENT PROJECT: PERFORMANCE MEASURES

SCIP MEASURE	DEFINITION
Antibiotic timing	Administration of intravenous prophylactic antibiotics within 1 hour of surgical incision (within 2 hours of surgical incision for vancomycin and fluoroquinolones).
Antibiotic choice	Chosen prophylactic antibiotics must be consistent with the type of procedure in accordance with practice guidelines.
Antibiotic cessation after surgery	Prophylactic antibiotics discontinued within 24 hours of surgery (48 hours for cardiothoracic surgery).
Proper hair removal	Only remove hair if it will interfere with the operation; if removed, it should be with clippers outside of the operating room.
Glucose control for cardiac surgery patients	Maintain blood glucose of 180 mg/dL or less in the 18–24 hours after anesthesia end time.
Perioperative normothermia	Maintain temperature of 35.5 °C or more in the perioperative period for patients who receive 60 minutes or more of anesthesia.

SCIP, Surgical Care Improvement Project.
Source: From Anderson, D., Podgorny, K., Berríos-Torres, S., Bratzler, D., Dellinger, E., Greene, L., Nyquist, A.-C., Saiman, L., Yokoe, D. S., Maragakis, L. L., & Kaye, K. (2014). Strategies to prevent surgical site infections in acute care hospitals: 2014 update. *Infection Control & Hospital Epidemiology, 35*(S2), S66–S88. https://doi.org/10.1017/S0899823X00193869

- Traffic of personnel in and out of surgical rooms (Mangram et al., 1999)
- Inadequate sterilization of surgical equipment Bashaw & Keister, 2019; Mangram et al., 1999)
- Use of steam sterilization Bashaw & Keister, 2019; Mangram et al., 1999)

Prevention

Preventive measures focus on decreasing the bacterial load of the patient and adhering to strict aseptic technique (Anderson et al., 2014; Bashaw & Keister, 2019).

The Surgical Care Improvement Project (SCIP) focuses on the prevention of SSI by decreasing the bacterial load on the patient (Table 12.6).

Additional preventive methods include the following:
- Redose antibiotics during long procedures and those with excessive blood loss to maintain therapeutic levels (Anderson et al., 2014).
- Use weight-based antibiotic dosing for patients with a high BMI and those undergoing bariatric surgical procedures (Anderson et al., 2014).
- Treat *S. aureus* nasal colonization and other infections before surgery (Anderson et al., 2014).
- Maintain surgical asepsis and integrity of the sterile field (Anderson et al., 2014; Bashaw & Keister, 2019).
  - Perform surgical scrub for 2 to 5 minutes (Bashaw & Keister, 2019; Mangram et al., 1999).
  - Use double glove to identify glove perforation (Anderson et al., 2014).

- Prepare skin to decrease the bacterial load at the surgical site.
  - Use dual agents containing alcohol (Anderson et al., 2014).
- Use surgical technique that maintains tissue integrity of surrounding structures and removal of necrotic tissue (Mangram et al., 1999).
- Contaminated and dirty/infected surgical wounds should have delayed skin closure (Mangram et al., 1999).
- Minimize surgical and anesthesia time (Anderson et al., 2014).
- Administer oxygen during and immediately after procedures involving mechanical ventilation (Anderson et al., 2014).

Healthcare Organizations
- Use surgical safety checklists (Anderson et al., 2014).
- Maintain operating environment and sterilization per established guidelines (Anderson et al., 2014; Bashaw & Keister, 2019).

Clinical Practice Guidelines
- The Hospital Infection Control Practices Advisory Committee (1999): *Prevention of Surgical Site Infection.*
- The Society for Healthcare Epidemiology of America (2014): *Strategies to Prevent Surgical Site Infections in Acute Care Hospitals: 2014 Update.*

- American Society of Health-System Pharmacists (2013): *Clinical Practice Guidelines for Antimicrobial Prophylaxis in Surgery.*
- SCIP and the American Society of Health-System Pharmacists (2017): *Updated on Guidelines for Perioperative Antibiotic Selection and Administration.*

Foot Care
- Consider regular podiatric care to remove excessive callouses and monitor for potential foot ulcerations.
- Examine feet daily for any unusual changes in color or temperature and for the development of sores or callouses.
- Ensure that footwear is properly fitted to avoid points of rubbing or pressure and to allow adequate room for any deformities by consulting a podiatrist.
- Protect feet from injury, infection, and extreme temperatures.
- Never walk barefoot or wear open-toed shoes or sandals. Wear your shoes or at the very least slippers while in the house.
- *Avoid soaking feet:* Insensate feet can easily be scalded without the patient realizing it.

OTHER WOUND TYPES
There are many other various types of wounds. A short description of these with etiology and treatment is presented in Tables 12.7, 12.8, and 12.9.

TABLE 12.7 OTHER WOUND TYPES

WOUND	DESCRIPTION
Neuropathic	A result of peripheral neuropathy, these wounds typically occur in diabetic patients. Local paresthesia, or lack of sensation, over pressure points on the foot leads to extended microtrauma, breakdown of overlying tissue, and eventual ulceration.
Vascular	Vascular ulcers are chronic, or long-term, breaches in the skin caused by problems with the vascular system. Can be arterial or venous in origin. Vascular ulcers may not heal normally and can lead to an increased risk of infection.
Burns	A burn is a type of injury to skin, caused by heat, cold, electricity, chemicals, friction, or radiation. Burn wounds range from superficial to full thickness damage. Treatment varies based on type and etiology.

TABLE 12.8 WOUND DESCRIPTION, ETIOLOGY, AND TREATMENT

	DESCRIPTION	ETIOLOGY/CAUSES	TREATMENT/CARE
Neuropathic/diabetic	Typically appear on feet, balls of feet, outer surface or on great toe, or heel. Surrounding skin is often calloused. Small shallow crater, typically dry. Due to decreased sensation, patient may not be aware of wound.	Most common with diabetes. Caused by repeated stress on foot with diminished sensation.	Offload pressure around the wound Footwear considerations Keep wound bed clean with moist dressing, monitor signs of infection, avoid debridement Optimal glucose control Antibiotics if osteomyelitis or cellulitis present Podiatrist consult recommended Teach patient optimal foot care and prevention strategies
Venous ulcers	Wounds are typically on the lower extremities (ankles and calves). Lower extremity will be discolored. Highly exudating wounds. Increased edema of extremity. Pain increases when dependent.	Venous insufficiency Venous hypertension	Treat wound to control drainage, debride necrotic areas, keep wound bed moist. Using compression to treat venous hypertension is essential. Keep extremity elevated when seated.

(continued)

TABLE 12.8 WOUND DESCRIPTION, ETIOLOGY, AND TREATMENT (*continued*)

	DESCRIPTION	ETIOLOGY/CAUSES	TREATMENT/CARE
Arterial ulcers	Typically occur on toes, feet, heels, ankle. Well demarcated edges and a pale, nongranulating, often necrotic base. Surrounding skin may exhibit dusky erythema and may be cool to touch, hairless, thin, and brittle, with a shiny texture. Typically, little exudate and no edema. Ulcer is often very painful. Pain in the extremity increases with rest/elevation, alleviated by putting leg down.	Peripheral vascular disease, reduced circulation to extremity. Reduction in arterial blood supply results in tissue hypoxia and tissue damage.	Vascular surgery intervention may be indicated based on injury severity. Diagnostic testing required to assess vascular status. Treat wound topically, do not debride, monitor and prevent infection.
Dermatitis	Inflammation of the skin. Characterized by red, dry, and itchy skin. May have rash, crusty scales, painful cracks, or blisters that ooze fluid.	Contact dermatitis or allergic dermatitis is most common.	Identify causative agent and eliminate as possible. Treat with topical hydrocortisone and oral antihistamine agents. If no improvement is noted, steroid therapy may be indicated.
Shingles	Vesicular lesions follow dermatome pattern. Patient will complain of prodromal symptoms of intense burning, tingling, or muscular pain before breakout. After several days or a week, a rash of fluid-filled blisters, similar to chickenpox, appears in one area on one side of the body. Shingles pain can be mild or intense.	Herpes zoster virus, which remains dormant until resurfaces. A person with a shingles rash can pass the virus to someone, usually a child, who has never had chickenpox, but the child will develop chickenpox, not shingles. Shingles is a serious threat in immunosuppressed individuals.	Antiviral medications (e.g., Acyclovir) can shorten course but won't cure it. If healthy people receive treatment soon after the outbreak of blisters, the lesions heal, the pain subsides within 3–5 weeks, and the blisters often leave no scars. Treatments for postherpetic neuralgia include steroids, antidepressants, anticonvulsants (including pregabalin and gabapentin enacarbil), and topical agents. The varicella zoster virus vaccines Shingrix and Zostavax have been approved by the Food and Drug Administration for adults age 50 and older.
Skin cancer	Flat or slightly raised discolored patch that has irregular borders and is somewhat asymmetrical in form. Color varies.	Excessive exposure to the sun's UV radiation. Tanning beds are also a source of damaging UV rays.	Early stages of melanoma may be hard to detect, so it is important to check the skin regularly for signs of change. Avoiding overexposure to the sun and preventing sunburn can significantly lower the risk of skin cancer. Dermatology consult followed by oncology consult as indicated. Excision will be needed followed by treatments deemed necessary by oncologist.

Sources: From Boulton, A. J. M., Kirsner, R. S., & Vileikyte, L. (2004). Neuropathic diabetic foot ulcers. *New England Journal of Medicine, 351,* 48–55. https://doi.org/10.1056/NEJMcp032966; National Pressure Ulcer Advisory Panel and European Advisory Panel. (2014). *Prevention and treatment of pressure ulcers: Clinical practice guideline.* National Pressure Ulcer Advisory Panel. http://www.npuap.org/resources/educational-and-clinical-resources/npuap-pressure-injury-stages/; McGuire, J. (2010). Transitional off-loading: An evidence-based approach to pressure redistribution in the diabetic foot. *Advances Skin Wound Care, 23*(4), 175–178.

TABLE 12.9 DIFFERENCE BETWEEN VENOUS AND ARTERIAL ULCERS

	VENOUS	ARTERIAL
History	History of varicose veins, deep vein thrombosis, venous insufficiency, or venous incompetence	History suggestive of peripheral arterial disease, intermittent claudication, and/or rest pain
Classic site	Over the medial region of the lower leg	Usually over the toes, foot, and ankle

(*continued*)

TABLE 12.9 DIFFERENCE BETWEEN VENOUS AND ARTERIAL ULCERS (*continued*)

	VENOUS	ARTERIAL
Wound bed	Often covered with slough	Often covered with varying degrees of slough and necrotic tissue
Exudate level	Usually high	Usually low
Pain	Pain not severe unless associated with excessive edema or infection More pain when dependent	Pain, even without infection Increased pain with elevation
Edema	Usually associated with limb edema	Edema not common
Treatment	Compression is mainstay	Appropriate surgery for arterial insufficiency; drugs of limited value

Source: From Cleveland Clinic. (2019). Lower extremity (leg and foot) ulcers. *Cleveland Clinic*. http://my.clevelandclinic.org/heart/disorders/vascular/legfootulcer.aspx

BURNS
Assessment

- Many burn wounds have various burn depths.
- Burn extent is given as a percentage of the total body surface area (TBSA) burned.
- Two common methods of estimating the extent of a burn injury include the following:
  - Rule of nines
  - Lund and Browder methods
  - The rule of nines is commonly used in the prehospital setting because it is easy to remember and use
  - It divides the adult body into anatomical regions of 9% or a multiple of 9%
  - The patient's palm, including the fingers, represents approximately 1% of the patient's TBSA and can be used to estimate small scattered burns
- Location of the burn wound may cause additional complications initially or during the healing process.
  - Inhalation burns require endotracheal intubation.
  - Facial edema may prevent eyes from opening, impeding vision.
  - Circumferential limb or torso burns may lead to vascular compromise with subsequent edema and may require an escharotomy.
  - Burns to the perineum may cause urethral obstruction, necessitating an indwelling urinary catheter.
  - Burns over joints immediately affect the range of motion, which may be exacerbated later by hypertrophic scarring.

Treatment

- *Fluid resuscitation*
  - Critical burn patients require aggressive fluid resuscitation due to the loss of the natural barrier of the skin. A common equation used is the Parkland formula: (4 mL) × (body weight in kilograms) × (% body surface area [BSA] burned) = Total fluids for 24 hours. Half should be given in the first 8 hours.
- *Nutrition management*
  - Due to the hypermetabolism associated with burns, early aggressive nutrition is essential as the resting energy expenditure of burn patients is elevated 40 to 100 times normal (Clark, 2017).

- *Pain management*
  - Most burn wounds are painful. The most painful are superficial partial-thickness burns because the sensory nerve endings are intact and working but exposed because of the loss of the epidermis.
  - Burn pain is intense initially, during debridement and dressing changes, but usually moderates once dressings are applied, protecting the nerve endings.
  - Most patients require analgesics and will need opioid-based analgesics for wound care, physical therapy, and sleep.
- *Burn wound dressings/treatment*
  - Burned limbs should be elevated above the level of the patient's heart when not being actively exercised to decrease edema and pain.
  - Burned skin contracts so range of motion of any affected joints should begin with the first visit. This may necessitate referral to a physical therapist. Dressings applied over burned joints should facilitate range of motion, and fingers should be wrapped individually.
  - The burn wound dressing should keep the wound moist and clean, promote optimal function of affected joints, protect the wound from additional trauma, and provide for patient comfort. There are quite a variety of dressing types available to treat burn wounds on an outpatient basis, and there are several ways to accomplish the goals mentioned previously (Table 12.10).

SKIN CANCER

- People with certain types of skin are more prone to developing melanoma, and the following factors are associated with an increased incidence of skin cancer:
  - High freckle density or tendency to develop freckles after sun exposure
  - High number of moles (five or more atypical moles)
  - Presence of actinic lentigines (small gray-brown spots—also known as *liver spots, sun spots,* or *age spots*)
  - Giant congenital melanocytic nevus, brown skin marks that present at birth
  - Pale skin that does not tan easily and burns, plus light-colored eyes
  - Red or light-colored hair

TABLE 12.10 TYPE OF BURN WOUND AND DRESSING REQUIRED

TYPE/ DESCRIPTION	DRESSING	FREQUENCY/COMMENTS
Superficial burns (first degree) Involve the epidermis Red and very painful	Superficial burns are not open wounds and do not require dressings. Moisturizers for dry skin and comfort. Does not require antimicrobials. Cool compresses and analgesics are helpful. Assure use of sunblock.	Usually heal within 7–10 days
Superficial partial-thickness burns (second degree) Involve the epidermis and the superficial dermis. Red, moist, and very painful; here is blister formation.	Without adherent exudates or eschar can be treated with topical antimicrobial ointments such as bacitracin or vitamin A and D ointment. May require alginates, hydrofibers, or foam dressings for highly exudating burns; maintain a moist environment.	Apply bacitracin to fight against Gram-positive bacteria. Cover with nonadherent dressing and dry gauze and then secure with flexible elastic netting. Change one to two times per day depending on amount of drainage. Usually heal within 10–14 days.
Deep partial-thickness burns (third degree) Involve the epidermis and most of the dermis. Generally paler, dryer, and less painful than superficial second-degree burns.	Silver sulfadiazine 1% debrides devitalized tissue without harming healthy tissue and may speed healing, decrease the likelihood of a surgical procedure, or may be used when surgery is not an option. Broad spectrum of antimicrobial activity and better penetration of necrotic tissue. Can inhibit wound epithelialization and should be discontinued once exudates and eschar have separated from the wound, leaving a clean wound bed. Once the wound bed is clear of debris, another dressing may be used.	Change dressing one to two times per day depending on exudate. Do not use on patients with sulfa allergies. Typically take 2–4 weeks to heal and often with significant scarring.
Full-thickness burns (fourth degree) Involve epidermis and dermis. Can also include other structures (bones, tendons, etc.). Dry, leather-like texture due to destroyed collagen; variable in color depending on the causative agent; are insensate due to destruction of sensory nerve.	Silver sulfadiazine 1%. May require surgical debridement, escharotomy, and potential amputation. Surgeon will dictate care based on location and extent of wounds.	Varies based on surgical requirements.

- High sun exposure, particularly if it produces blistering sunburn, and especially if sun exposure is intermittent rather than regular
- Age, as cancer risk increases with age
- Family or personal history of melanoma

The **ABCDE examination** of skin moles is a simple way to identify and describe the characteristics for melanoma.

- *Asymmetric*: Normal moles are often round and symmetrical but one side of a cancerous mole is likely to look different from the other side—not round or symmetrical.
- *Border*: This is likely to be irregular rather than smooth—ragged, notched, or blurred.
- *Color*: Melanomas tend to contain uneven shades and colors, including varying black, brown, and tan, and even white or blue pigmentation.
- *Diameter*: A change in the size of the mole or a mole that is larger than a normal mole (more than 0.25 in. in diameter) can indicate skin cancer.
- *Evolving*: A change in a mole's appearance over a period of weeks or months can be a sign of skin cancer.

REVIEW QUESTIONS

1. A patient presents with a wound on the sacral area that is 4 cm × 3 cm in size and 1 cm deep with areas that are tunneling below the surface. What stage is this wound in?
   A. Stage 2
   B. Stage 3
   C. Stage 4
   D. Unstageable

2. Risk factors for the development of pressure injuries include all of the following except
   A. Adequate nutrition
   B. Immobility
   C. Moisture
   D. Advanced age

ANSWERS

1. **Correct answer: B. Rationale:** Tunneling is consistent with a stage 3 pressure ulcer. Wound depth is variable depending upon the location. There is no description of exposed muscle, tendon, ligament, or bone that would imply stage 4. Stage 2 only involves the dermis but does not have tunneling present. Unstageable ulcers are covered with eschar or slough, and one would be unable to determine the extent of the wound.

2. **Correct answer: A. Rationale:** Adequate nutrition does not increase risk for pressure injury. Malnutrition is a risk factor for pressure injury as well as immobility, moisture, and advanced age.

REFERENCES

The complete reference and additional reading lists appear in the digital version of this chapter, at https://connect.springerpub.com/content/book/978-0-8261-7417-8/part/part01/chapter/ch12

Musculoskeletal System

Judy Dusek and Amy C. Shay

OVERVIEW OF THE MUSCULOSKELETAL SYSTEM

The structures of the musculoskeletal system provide the framework for movement from place to place and for protection of internal organs. Musculoskeletal tissues may be bones, which make up the skeleton of the body, or they may be muscles, ligaments, tendons, cartilage, or joints.

OVERVIEW

Primary Functions
- Gives shape to the body.
- Protects internal organs and tissues.
- Stores minerals.
- Serves as site for hematopoiesis.
- Helps prevent injury to specific musculoskeletal structures or to other organs and tissues.

When the musculoskeletal tissues are unable to perform their usual functions, the affected tissue(s) influence a person's mobility, support, protection, and ability to carry on usual activities. Older adults are affected by rheumatic, inflammatory, and degenerative conditions of the musculoskeletal tissues (Mourad, 1991).

Physiology
- Bones are living structures that are continuously in the process of bone formation counterbalanced by bone resorption.
- Muscles are masses of tissues that cover bones and provide bulk to the body, help hold body parts together, and help move one or more parts from place to place.
- Ligaments are tough, relatively long bands of dense, connective tissues that hold bones to bones.
- Tendons are very strong, tough, long strands or cords of dense connective tissues that form at the ends of muscles.
- Cartilage is a semismooth layer of elastic, resilient supporting tissue found at the ends of bones.
- Collagen is the major supporting element in connective tissues, making up approximately half of the total body protein in adults.
- Synovium is a layer of cells that form a membrane to line the inner surfaces of synovial joints.
- Joints are articulations where bones are joined to one another or where two surfaces of bones come together.

COMMON PROBLEMS OF THE MUSCULOSKELETAL SYSTEM

IMMOBILITY
- Muscle strength decreases
- Joints become stiff
- Pain develops
- Loss of independence
- Pattern of disuse usually occurs after the person has experienced repeated falls

Key Points
- Physical activity and exercise are important to preventing disability from disorders in older adults.
- Loss of muscle means loss of strength and mobility, the two factors most associated with debilitation (McChance & Huether, 2018).

OSTEOARTHRITIS

Definition
Also known as *degenerative joint disease*, osteoarthritis is a noninflammatory disease of the joints. It is characterized by progressive articular cartilage deterioration with the formation of new bone in the joint space.

Pathophysiology
The articular cartilage thins and is lost, particularly in areas of increased stress. As the cartilage deteriorates, there is a proliferation of bone at the margins of the joints. When the joint cartilage is lost, the two bone surfaces come into contact with each other. This results in joint pain.

Joints Most Commonly Affected
- Distal interphalangeals
- Proximal interphalangeals
- Knees
- Hips
- Spine

Risk Factors
- Age
- Trauma
- Lifestyle
- Obesity
- Genetics

Etiology

The exact cause is not well understood.

Clinical Presentation

- Gradual onset of aching joint pain.
- Pain occurs with activity and is relieved with rest.
- Stiffness occurs after periods of inactivity.
- Crepitus, a grating sound and sensation, may be heard and felt with range of motion in affected joint.
- Affected joints have decreased range of motion.
- Degeneration of joint structure may result in muscle spasm, gait changes, and disuse of joint.
- Heberden's nodes may be seen on the distal interphalangeals.

Diagnosis

Diagnosis of the older adult patient with osteoarthritis (OA) includes the following:

- Pain related to inflammation and deterioration of the joint cartilage
- Impaired physical mobility related to lower extremity joint stiffness
- Self-care deficit related to limitations in joint movement and strength

Nonsurgical Interventions

- For those with mild pain, a gentle exercise program is recommended.
- Rest periods between activities are recommended.
- Heat or cold therapy applied to joints may be used to decrease joint pain.
- Warm bath or shower in the morning may help reduce early-morning stiffness.
- Nonsteroidal anti-inflammatory drugs (NSAIDs) may be used.
- Interventions for those with severe pain may include direct injections into the painful joint with steroids.

Surgical Interventions

When conservative measures for treating chronic arthritis pain fail and the patient becomes more disabled, surgical procedures may be considered. Main indications for surgery are severe pain and increasing disability.

- *Arthroplasty* is the surgical procedure to replace the involved joint.
- Arthroscopic joint fusion can be done to improve function and reduce pain.

Joint Replacement of the Knee and Hip

Postoperative goals are as follows:

- Prevent complications such as thromboembolism, joint and wound infection, blood loss, nerve injury, joint dislocation, and surgical pain.
- Relieve surgical pain.
- Assist patient in achieving a higher level of function and activity.

Precautions After Hip Surgery

- Sit with hips at a 90° or greater angle.
- Do not bend forward more than 90°.
- Do not lift the knee on the operated side higher than the hip.
- Do not cross legs at knees or ankles.
- Keep pillows between legs when lying on side or back.
- Do not bend to put on shoes; use a long shoehorn.
- Do not bend down to reach items on the floor.
- Do not sit in low chairs.

OSTEOPOROSIS

- Women lose an estimated 35% of cortical bone mass over the course of a lifetime.
- Occurs in approximately 30% of all women over age 45.
- Present in 70% of women over age 45 who experience bone fractures.
- Most common in postmenopausal women.
- Men develop osteoporosis at a ratio of 1:6 compared to women (men:women).
- Sedentary lifestyle is a contributing factor (McChance & Huether, 2018; Meiner & Lueckenotte, 2006).

Definition

A systemic condition of overall reduction in bone mass or density in which bone resorption is more extensive than bone deposition, upsetting the normal balance.

Pathophysiology

Osteoporosis stems from an imbalance of bone resorption and bone formation, resulting in decreased overall bone quality and bone density. The loss of bone density leads to frequent bone fractures. In bones with osteoporosis, trabecular (cancellous) bone is more porous and cortical bone is thinner.

Risk Factors

- Renal or hepatic failure
- Hyperthyroidism
- Hyperparathyroidism
- Heredity and genetic disposition
- Lifestyle factors: cigarette smoking, lack of exercise, consumption of alcohol, low intake of calcium
- Age

Etiology

- Decreased levels of estrogen and testosterone
- Reduced physical activity lessens muscle stress on bone
- Inadequate vitamins C and D
- Insufficient dietary magnesium and calcium
- Corticosteroid use
- Use of other medications, including phenytoin, phenobarbital, loop diuretics, methotrexate
- Prolonged immobility causing calcium excretion

Diagnosis

- Confirmed via bone densitometry with dual-energy x-ray absorptiometry (DEXA) of hips and lumbar spine.
- Criteria for diagnosis of osteoporosis have been established by the World Health Organization and are based on standard deviations from the norm.
- Laboratory blood studies are obtained to differentiate osteoporosis from other diseases that cause bone loss.
- Complete blood count (CBC), serum calcium, serum phosphorus, alkaline phosphatase, and urinary calcium are all normal in osteoporosis.

Interventions

- Calcium carbonate is the best supplement because it contains 40% elemental calcium.
- Exercise programs that include weight bearing and resistance help prevent bone loss.
- Exercise should be done three times a week for 30 to 60 minutes for best effect.

- Postmenopausal estrogen replacement therapy (ERT) will prevent or stabilize the process of osteoporosis.
- Estrogen has a direct role in regulating bone metabolism, attaching to receptor sites on osteoblasts and decreasing bone resorption.
- Estrogen has a positive effect on calcium absorption, promoting synthesis of calcitonin and increasing vitamin D receptors in osteoblasts.
- The benefits of ERT in decreasing hip fracture may outweigh other risks considered.
- Alendronate sodium (Fosamax) has been found to produce a reduction in bone resorption, and treatment has shown increased bone mass at lumbar spine and hip.
- Fosamax has been approved for treatment of postmenopausal osteoporosis and approved for prevention of osteoporosis in clients at risk.
- Another antiresorptive drug used for osteoporosis is calcitonin (Miacalcin) in either parenteral or nasal spray preparation.

RHEUMATOID ARTHRITIS

Definition
A chronic, systemic, inflammatory disease that causes joint destruction and deformity and results in disability.

Pathophysiology
In the initial phase of rheumatoid arthritis (RA), the synovial membrane becomes inflamed and thickens, with an increased production of synovial fluid. The change is called *pannus*. As the pannus tissue develops, it causes erosion and destruction of the joint capsule and subchondral bone. These processes result in decreased joint motion, deformity, and ankylosis or joint immobilization.

Etiology
The cause is unknown. The most widely accepted theory is that is it an autoimmune disease that causes inflammation, most often in the joints but sometimes in connective tissue.

Clinical Presentation
- Most often starts with the proximal interphalangeals, metacarpophalangeals, and wrists.
- In the later stages of the disease, knees and hips are affected.

Diagnosis
- Pain related to swollen, inflamed joint tissue
- Impaired physical mobility related to the joint deformities and inflammation
- Fatigue related to systemic disease process
- Potential for altered nutrition exists due to levels lower than body requirements related to loss of appetite
- Self-care deficits in activities of daily living (ADL) related to the loss of motion and strength in painful, swollen joints
- Body image disturbance related to the gradual onset of joint deformities

Interventions
- Application of heat and cold to the affected joints decreases cutaneous nerve stimulation.
- Ice packs should be applied to joints during periods of acute inflammation.
- Moist heat is useful in relaxing muscles and increasing joint mobility.
- Occupational therapy may be done to assist with the improvement of joint function and prevent disability.

- Splints may be used to protect joints, maintain joint function, and decrease pain.
- Physical therapy may be done for individualized exercise programs for strengthening and stretching exercises, range-of-motion exercises, and endurance training (McChance & Huether, 2018; Meiner & Lueckenotte, 2006).

OSTEOMYELITIS

Definition
A difficult-to-treat bone infection characterized by progressive and inflammatory destruction of the infected bone and new apposition of bone at the site of infection. It can be acute, subacute, or chronic in duration, although the differentiation between these designations is variable:
- *Acute*: 10 days' or 2 weeks' duration
- *Subacute*: Lasting less than 3 months but lacking acute symptoms
- *Chronic*: The development of bone necrosis, which is usually surrounded by sclerotic, hypovascular bone; thickened periosteum; and compromised surrounding soft tissues

The incidence of osteomyelitis has nearly tripled among older adults in past 30 years due to
- An increase in diabetes-related pedal osteomyelitis, and
- Posttraumatic osteomyelitis commonly due to open fractures.

Pathophysiology
Acute inflammation of marrow and cortex and impaired blood supply leads to necrosis. The pathogenic picture of bone infection is comparable to that in other body tissues. The invading pathogen provokes an inflammatory response that causes vascular engorgement, edema, leukocyte activity, and abscess formation. Once inflammation begins, the small terminal vessels thrombose and the exudate seals the bone's canaliculi. Inflammatory exudate extends into the metaphysis and the marrow cavity and through small metaphyseal openings into the cortex.

Etiology
The most common organisms causing bone and joint infections are *Staphylococcus aureus* and coagulase-negative staphylococci.

Clinical Presentation
Presentation varies with age of the affected individual, site of involvement, initiating event, infecting organism, and whether the infection is acute, subacute, or chronic.
- Acute: Abrupt onset of inflammation.
- Subacute: Signs and symptoms are vague.
- Chronic: RA is indolent or silent between exacerbations.
- Microorganisms persist in small abscesses or fragments of necrotic bone and produce occasional flare-ups.
- Patient has fever, pain, lymphadenopathy, necrotic bone as determined by radiographic imaging.

Diagnosis
- Laboratory data show an elevated white blood cell (WBC).
- Radiographic studies include radionuclide bone scanning, tomography, and MRI.

Interventions
- Administer antibiotics and drain inflammatory exudate.
- Tubes are placed into holes drilled into the bone cortex for continuous antibiotic irrigation and drainage.

- Chronic conditions may require surgical removal of inflammatory exudate followed by continuous wound irrigation with antibiotic solutions in addition to systemic treatment with antibiotics (Mandell et al., 2018).

GOUT

Definition

Gout is a metabolic disorder that disrupts the body's control of uric acid production or excretion. It is more prevalent in men than women.

Pathophysiology

Gout is closely linked to cellular metabolism of purines and kidney function. Uric acid is a breakdown product of purine nucleotides. Some individuals with gout have an accelerated rate of purine synthesis and other individuals break down purine nucleotides at an accelerated rate. Both conditions result in an overproduction of uric acid. A deficiency of the enzyme hypoxanthine guanine phosphoribosyl transferase (HGPRT) leads to the increased production of uric acid.

Kidney function is involved because most uric acid is eliminated from the body through the kidneys. Urate undergoes both reabsorption and excretion within the renal tubules. Sluggish urate excretion by the kidney may be caused by decreased glomerular filtration of urate or an acceleration in urate reabsorption.

High levels of uric acid accumulate in the blood and in other body fluids, including synovial fluid. When the uric acid reaches a certain concentration in fluids, it crystallizes. The crystals are deposited in connective tissues throughout the body. When crystallization occurs in synovial fluid, painful inflammation of the joint develops.

Clinical Presentation

- May present as an acute or chronic condition.
- Onset is sudden.
- Manifested by acute attack of pain in one or more joints.
- Occurs abruptly in a peripheral joint.
- Initial attack occurs in the metatarsophalangeal joint of the great toe in 50% occur of patients.
- Other involved joints are the heel, ankle, instep of foot, knee, wrist, or elbow.
- Affected joint becomes hot, red, and tender.
- Pain can be severe and interfere with mobility, self-care, and functional abilities.
- Acute attacks usually subside in 7 days.
- In chronic gout, uric acid crystals cause bone destruction and deformity.
- Uric acid crystals can also be deposited in kidney and cause nephrolithiasis.

Interventions

- Antiinflammatory drugs
- Low-purine diet (Table 13.1)
- High fluid intake to increase urinary output
- Antihyperuricemic drugs to reduce serum urate concentrations (McChance & Huether, 2018; Meiner & Lueckenotte, 2006)

See Table 13.2 for pharmacological treatments.

TABLE 13.1 LOW-PURINE DIET

FOODS TO EAT	FOODS TO LIMIT
Purine-rich vegetables New research shows they do not increase risk of gout attacks. These vegetables include mushrooms, green peas, dried peas and beans, spinach, asparagus, lentils, cauliflower	**Organ meats, shellfish, yeast extracts** Sweetbreads, liver, kidneys, brains, meat extracts, herring, mackerel, scallops, mincemeat, mussels **Seafood** Anchovies, sardines, tuna
Protein Focus on lentils, soybeans, poultry **Low-fat dairy** Nonfat or low-fat milk, yogurt, and cheese Eggs	**Red meat** Beef, lamb, pork
Beverages Water—Hydrate well with water Coffee (if no other health-related contraindications present)	**Alcohol** Beer and distilled liquor Sugary juices, sodas
Consider vitamin C Fresh fruit Cherries have been shown to reduce risk of gout attacks	Sugar-sweetened foods High-fructose corn syrup

Sources: From Lockyer, S., & Stanner, S. (2016). Diet and gout: What is the role of purines? *Nutrition Bulletin, 41*(2), 155–166; Mayo Clinic. (2020). Mayo Clinic gout diet.https://www.mayoclinic.org/healthy-lifestyle/nutrition-and-healthy-eating/in-depth/gout-diet/art-20048524

NECROTIZING FASCIITIS

Definition

Also known as *necrotizing soft-tissue infection*, necrotizing fasciitis (NF) is a severe, devastating infection of subcutaneous tissue, fascia, and muscles, characterized by rapid progressive tissue necrosis.

Pathophysiology

When the offending aggressive organism invades the superficial fascia, subcutaneous fat, and deep fascia, the bacteria rapidly track subcutaneously, producing endo- and exotoxins, causing tissue ischemia, liquefactive necrosis, and systemic illness. Infection can spread as fast as 1 inch per hour with little overlying skin change. Toxins cause endothelial damage, resulting in increased tissue edema, impaired capillary blood flow, phagocytosis, and neutrophil infiltration at the site of the infection and activation of the coagulation cascade, thus leading to vascular thrombosis and worsened tissue ischemia. Necrosis of subcutaneous tissue and fat is thought to be the work of bacterial enzymes such as hyaluronidase and the lipases.

Predisposing Factors

- Trauma
- Burns
- Insect bite

- Chronic skin ulcers
- Postoperative wound infection
- RA
- Systemic lupus erythematosus (SLE)
- Diabetes mellitus, type 2
- Renal transplantation
- Chronic renal failure
- Injection intravenous (IV) drug use
- Immunosuppressive therapy

Etiology

The most common cause of NF is Gram-positive bacteria, such as *Escherichia coli* and *Klebsiella*. Other bacterial organisms include group A streptococcal infections, methicillin-resistant *S. aureus*, and methicillin-sensitive *S. aureus*; some cases are caused by fungal infection (Candida).

Clinical Presentation

- Will present with intense pain, erythema, edematous; warm to touch.
- Affected areas lack defined margins.
- Pain may be uncharacteristically intense, more than expected with initial assessment.
- Tenderness of skin or area surrounding wound may extend into borders of wound.
- May have fever and tachycardia followed by hypotension and tachypnea as tissue destruction progresses.
- Infection may start along the fascial plane and include erythematous, painful, and edematous skin lesions that can deteriorate to hemorrhagic blisters, anesthesia, and gangrenous necrosis over several days.
- Commonly, the trunk and lower extremities are affected.
- Fournier's gangrene, a form of NF gangrene, which occurs in the perineum, genital, or perianal region, is seen in men but can be seen in women and children as well.

Diagnosis

- Ultrasound, CT, or MRI scan can be done in suspicious cases.
- Surgical exploration can establish a diagnosis.
- Operative findings of grayish necrotic deep fascia, lack of resistance to blunt dissection, lack of bleeding of fascia, and presence of foul-smelling "dishwater" pus aids in confirmation of diagnosis.
- Laboratory Risk Indicator for Necrotizing Fasciitis (LRINEC) score >6 has a positive predictive value of 92% in high-risk patients.
- Laboratory factors scored are
  - C-reactive protein, WBC, hemoglobin (HgB), sodium, sreatinine, and glucose.

Interventions

- Prompt treatment with aggressive surgical debridement, wide, extensive debridement of all tissues that can be elevated off of the fascia, is associated with a more rapid clinical improvement.
- IV broad-spectrum empiric antibiotic therapy, including Gam-positive, Gram-negative, and anaerobic organisms.
- Clindamycin should be the first line of antimicrobial therapy because of its effective toxin inhibition and rapid infusion

time (Brennan & LeFavre, 2019; Foldel & Smith, 2014; Kessenich & Babl, 2004).

NEUROMUSCULAR DYSFUNCTION RELATED TO CRITICAL ILLNESS

INTENSIVE CARE UNIT–ACQUIRED WEAKNESS

ICU-acquired weakness (ICUAW) is an acute syndrome occurring frequently among the critically ill. ICUAW is associated with prolonged mechanical ventilation weaning, longer hospital stays, and increased healthcare costs. Higher one-year mortality rates and long-term functional deficits are also linked to ICUAW. Public health concerns related to ICUAW increase as the ICU patient survival-to-discharge rate increases.

Definition

ICUAW is a syndrome of generalized weakness in critically ill patients for whom noncritical illness—related causes have been excluded. Neuromuscular dysfunction seen in ICUAW patients may involve critical illness polyneuropathy (CIP), critical illness myopathy (CIM), or a combination of both.

Etiology

No single causative mechanism for CIP and CIM has been identified. It is theorized that CIP and CIM may result from the same processes associated with multiorgan dysfunction syndrome, which include microcirculatory, cellular, and metabolic disturbances.

- Critical illness polyneuropathy
  - Diffuse distal axonal sensory-motor neuropathy
  - Affects limb and respiratory muscles
- Critical illness myopathy
  - Decreased muscle protein synthesis and increased muscle catabolism
  - Loss of myosin and myosin-associated proteins

Risk Factors

- Female sex
- Multiple organ failure
- Severity of disease—APACHE II score (Acute Physiology and Chronic Health Evaluation score)
- Sepsis
- SIRS (systemic inflammatory response system)
- Neuromuscular blockade agents (NMBA)
- Aminoglycosides
- Norepinephrine
- Duration of mechanical ventilation
- Parenteral nutrition
- Hyperglycemia
- Electrolyte disturbances
- Hyperosmolarity
- Lactate level

Prevention

There is no known specific treatment for ICUAW. Knowledge of risk factors helps identify patients at greatest risk. Early-prevention measures initiated within the first 48 to 72 hours of the diagnosis of the disorder may be most effective:

- Early recognition and treatment of sepsis
- Early prevention and treatment for organ failure
- Blood glucose control (110–180 mg/dL)
- Lung-protective mechanical ventilation strategies
- Early enteral nutrition

- Appropriate dose and short-term use of NMBA
- Examination of risks and benefits of aminoglycosides and norepinephrine to limit exposure to these medications
- Maintain fluid, electrolyte, and acid–base balance (Parotto et al., 2018; Yang et al., 2018)

TABLE 13.2 MUSCULOSKELETAL PHARMACOLOGY

GENERIC NAME (BRAND NAME)	SAFETY AND PATIENT EDUCATION	CLASS	MECHANISM OF ACTION	INDICATIONS/ CONTRAINDICATIONS	DOSE	COMMON ADVERSE SIDE EFFECTS
Acetylsalicylic acid (Aspirin)	Report signs of bleeding; inform provider if surgical procedure is planned	Salicylates	Anti-inflammatory, analgesic, antipyretic	Treatment of OA and RA pain Contraindications: Asthma, rhinitis, and nasal polyps; use in children or teenagers for viral infections with or without fever; acute gout	3 g daily in divided doses	GI irritation, GI bleeding
Ibuprofen (Motrin)	Report signs of stomach bleeding, tarry stools, persistent stomach pain Stevens–Johnson's syndrome/toxic epidermal necrolysis like red, swollen, blistered, or peeling skin	NSAIDs	Anti-inflammatory, analgesic	Treatment of pain associated with OA, RA Contraindications: Perioperative pain in CABG	1,200–3,200 mg daily in divided doses	Increased risk of serious and potentially fatal thrombotic events; MI, stroke, adverse cardiovascular events
Naproxen (Aleve)	Report signs of stomach bleeding, tarry stools, persistent stomach pain Stevens–Johnson's syndrome/toxic epidermal necrolysis like red, swollen, blistered, or peeling skin	NSAIDs	Anti-inflammatory, analgesic	Treatment of pain associated with OA, RA, acute gout	OA, RA: Starting dose 250–500 mg BID up to total 1,500 mg/d Acute gout: Starting dose is 750 mg followed by 250 mg q8h until the attack has subsided	
Celecoxib (Celebrex)	Report signs of stomach bleeding, tarry stools, persistent stomach pain Be alert for symptoms of cardiovascular thrombotic events Stevens–Johnson's syndrome/toxic epidermal necrolysis like red, swollen, blistered, or peeling skin	COX-2 selective inhibitor	Anti-inflammatory, analgesic, antipyretic	OA, RA	OA: 200 mg daily RA: 100–200 mg BID	Increased risk of serious and potentially fatal thrombotic events; MI, stroke, adverse cardiovascular events Increased risk of atrial fibrillation

(continued)

TABLE 13.2 MUSCULOSKELETAL PHARMACOLOGY (*continued*)

GENERIC NAME (BRAND NAME)	SAFETY AND PATIENT EDUCATION	CLASS	MECHANISM OF ACTION	INDICATIONS/ CONTRAINDICA-TIONS	DOSE	COMMON ADVERSE SIDE EFFECTS
Allopurinol (Zyloprim)	Notify provider of skin rash, blood in urine, painful urination Stevens-Johnson's syndrome/toxic epidermal necrolysis like red, swollen, blistered, or peeling skin	Xanthine oxidase inhibitor	Reduces production of uric acid	Gout	100–800 mg daily	Drowsiness, nausea, diarrhea
Colchicine (Colcrys)	Notify provider fmuscle pain or weakness, tingling or numbness in fingers or toes	Antigout agent	Blocks neutrophil-mediated inflammatory responses induced by monosodium urate crystals in synovial fluid	Gout Contraindication: Concomitant use of colchicine and CYP3A4 or P-glycoprotein inhibitors in patients with renal or hepatic impairment may cause fatal colchicine toxicity	0.6 mg, 1–2 times daily	Diarrhea, nausea, vomiting, and abdominal pain
Alendronate (Fosamax)	Take Fosamax at least 30 minutes before the first food, beverage, or medication of the day with plain water only Do not lie down for at least 30 minutes and until after first food of the day	Biphosphonate	Inhibits osteoclast-mediated bone resorption	Indications: osteoporosis Contraindications: esophageal disorders; inability to stand or sit upright for at least 30 minutes; hypocalcemia	Treatment of osteoporosis: 10 mg daily or 70 mg weekly	Heartburn, upset stomach; stomach pain, nausea; diarrhea, constipation; or. bone pain, muscle, or joint pain

CABG, coronary artery bypass graft surgery; COX-2, cyclooxygenase-2; GI, gastrointestinal; MI, myocardial infarction; NSAIDs, nonsteroidal anti-inflammatory drugs; OA, osteoarthritis; RA, rheumatoid arthritis.

Source: From Edmunds, M., & Mayhew, M. (2013). *Pharmacology for the primary care provider* (4th ed.). Mosby.

REVIEW QUESTIONS

1. The primary mechanism of osteoporosis is
   A. Inadequate mineralization
   B. Impaired synthesis of bone organic matrix
   C. Inadequate estrogen levels
   D. Formation of sclerotic bone

2. A 64-year-old man has developed osteomyelitis secondary to a diabetic foot ulcer. He has been on intravenous (IV) antibiotics for 4 weeks. There is current evidence of subperiosteal collection. The next course of treatment will likely be
   A. Nerve stimulation
   B. Debridement
   C. Arthrodesis
   D. Physical therapy

ANSWERS

1. **Correct answer: B. Rationale**: Impaired synthesis of bone organic matrix is the primary mechanism of osteoporosis. Osteoporosis is due to an imbalance in bone resorption and formation. Normally, continuous new bone matrix synthesis is followed by formation of newly formed bone. Osteoporosis occurs when creation of new bone does not keep up with loss of old bone. Inadequate mineralization is not the main reason for osteoporosis. Inadequate estrogen levels contribute to, but is not the primary cause of, osteoporosis. Formation of sclerotic bone is caused by excessive calcium deposits leading to bone thickening.

2. **Correct answer: B. Rationale**: Subperiosteal collection indicates continued infection. Patients may require surgical debridement to remove all infected material and surrounding scar tissue and to restore adequate blood flow to the area. Osteomyelitis is inflammation of the bone due to infection. Nerve stimulation, arthrodesis, and physical therapy are not treatments for infection.

REFERENCES

The complete reference list appears in the digital version of this chapter, at https://connect.springerpub.com/content/book/978-0-8261-7417-8/part/part01/chapter/ch13

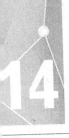

14

Nervous System

K. Denise Kerley, Debra A. Ferguson, JoEllen Rust, Theodore J. Walker, Jr., and Misti Tuppeny

HEAD AND BRAIN INJURY

OVERVIEW
Head and brain injury refers to any external structural damage or functional impairment of cranial content, including the scalp, skull, meninges, blood vessels, or brain (Cash & Glass, 2019).

Symptoms
Immediately following injury, symptoms may include any of the following (Table 14.1):
- Loss of consciousness or decreased awareness
- Memory loss particularly immediately pre- or postinjury
- Altered mental status
- Neurologic deficits involving motor strength, balance, vision, sensation, and speech

Common Complaints
- Headache (most common) may last days or weeks, can be constant, generalized or frontal, and occur usually within first 14 days of injury
- Amnesia surrounding impact
- Faintness
- Nausea/vomiting

TABLE 14.1 SIGNS AND SYMPTOMS OF HEAD INJURY

Physical	Reported or observed head injury Dizziness Fatigue Photophobia Sensitivity to noise Numbness/tingling Seizures, may be delayed post injury
Behavioral	Irritability Nervousness Depression
Cognitive	Difficulty concentrating Memory impairment such as short-term memory loss or repetition Confusion Slow response/difficulty processing Change in reaction time Disorientation Altered taste and smell
Sleep cycle disturbance	Feeling drowsy Difficulty falling asleep Sleeping more or less than normal

- Changes in vision, such as blurring
- Drowsiness
- Loss of consciousness
- Confusion

TYPES OF BRAIN INJURIES
Skull Fracture
A crack or break in one of the skull bones; if dented inward and pressed against the surface of the brain, it is a depressed skull fracture and may cause a bruise or contusion on the surface of the brain.

Mild Traumatic Brain Injury
- Symptoms are mild in nature, may go unrecognized, and medical attention is often not sought.
- Radiographic testing shows no anatomical abnormality.
- A Glasgow Coma Scale (GCS) score of 13 to 15 measured 30 minutes after the injury would be classified as a mild traumatic brain injury (mTBI).

Concussion
- Often used to describe mTBI:
- The American Academy of Neurology Guidelines for Grading Severity of Concussion
  - *Grade 1*—Transient confusion, no loss of consciousness, resolution of mental status changes in <15 minutes
  - *Grade 2*—Transient confusion, no loss of consciousness, symptoms of mental status changes with amnesia for >15 minutes
  - *Grade 3*—Loss of consciousness, with unresponsive period lasting seconds *or* unresponsive period lasting minutes

Postconcussion Syndrome
- *Dizziness*—Most common cause is vestibular system dysfunction
- *Cervical vertigo*—Related to whiplash causing musculoskeletal injury
- *Vision disturbances*—Frequently unrecognized

Intracranial Hemorrhage
Intracranial hemorrhage (ICH) refers to bleeding inside the brain or cranial vault. There are four types of ICH:
- *Epidural hematoma*—A collection of blood outside a blood vessel; occurs when blood accumulates between the skull and the outermost covering of the brain, usually accompanied by a skull fracture.
- *Subdural hematoma (SDH)*—A collection of blood on the surface of the brain; more common in older people and people with history of heavy alcohol use.

- *Acute SDH*—Most dangerous, typically caused by severe head injury, causes unconsciousness, 50% can be fatal.
- *Subacute SDH*—Symptoms may take days or weeks, and chronic symptoms may take weeks because of slow bleeding.
- **Subarachnoid hemorrhage (SAH)**—Bleeding into the subarachnoid space—the area between the arachnoid membrane and the pia mater (meninges) surrounding the brain; most common cause is trauma or rupture of a major blood vessel in the brain.
- **Intracerebral hemorrhage**—When blood suddenly bursts into cerebral or brain tissue, causing damage to the brain; most commonly occurs with stroke; also known as *intraparenchymal.*

Emergent treatment should be sought if the following conditions are noted:

- Focal neurologic deficit
- Decreasing level of consciousness (LOC)
- Persistent headache, nausea, and vomiting
- Seizures
- Any evidence of skull fracture
- Neuropsychologic dysfunction

Predisposing factors for traumatic brain injury (TBI) are as follows:

- Motor vehicle accidents
- Assaults
- Sports or recreation-related trauma
- Male gender
- Age of increased incidence: 0 to 4 years, 15 to 19 years, and 65 years and older
- Military occupation
- Falls are the number one risk factor for older adults; three times higher than other age groups

TBI pathogenesis: Two different types are found:

- *Primary injury*—Direct result of impact at time of injury
  - Mechanical in nature
  - May be focal (contusion or laceration or bone fragmentation)
  - May be diffuse [concussion or diffuse axonal injury (DAI)]
  - Usually does not require surgical intervention
- *Secondary injury*—Complication of primary injury, delayed onset (seconds, minutes, hours, or days)
  - Caused by a blood or cerebral spinal fluid–metabolism mismatch
  - Ischemic or hypoxic damage
  - Cerebral edema
  - ICH
  - Prolonged increased intracranial pressure (ICP)
  - Hydrocephalus
  - Infection

Diagnostic Tests

- Plain skull film does not typically provide significant information for treatment decisions.
- CT scan is preferred.
- Anteroposterior and lateral spine films if suspected soft tissue injury or vertebral fracture.
  - Patients with head injury should also be evaluated for concomitant spine injuries (especially cervical).

Patient Health History

- History of injury from patient or witness
- Identify cause: How did the injury occur and forcefulness of impact

- Confirm LOC at time of injury and after injury
- Any amnesia
- Obtain experienced symptoms or complaints, including description, location, severity, and onset
- Obtain medical history, any previous head injuries, learning disabilities, developmental disorders, depression, anxiety, sleep disorders, and mood disorders
- Review medications and drug and alcohol history

Physical Exam and Assessments

- Vital signs
- Inspect overall appearance; observe/palpate for facial fractures
- Periorbital ecchymosis ("raccoon eyes"), postauricular/mastoid ecchymosis (Battle's sign), or evidence of cerebral spinal fluid leak can indicate a basilar skull fracture
- Examine eyes for papilledema, proptosis, and periorbital edema
- Examine ears for signs of cerebrospinal fluid (CSF) or blood
- Examine for trauma to cervical spine (malalignment, abnormal curvature)
- Auscultation over globes of eyes and carotid arteries bilaterally
- Neurologic exam: Mental status and memory, orientation, behavior, mood and CNs, motor and sensory exam of all four extremities.

Treatment

- Admit for loss of consciousness, seizure activity, focal deficits, penetrating or depressed skull fracture, vomiting, serious facial injuries, and positive CT findings.
- Consider and manage any secondary injuries.
- Admission should be considered for patients who are homeless or have no home supervision.
- Patient should not be released if still under alcohol or substance use.
- Assess for suspected abuse privately with patient.
- Provide safety and accident prevention education.
- Assess driving ability of older adults (slower reflexes, visual problems, alcohol/substance use, medication effects).
- *Hyperosmolar therapy*
  Intravenous administration of hyperosmolar agents has become routine in the management of intracranial hypertension (IH) and herniation syndromes.
  - Mannitol and hypertonic saline are routinely employed hyperosmolar agents (Table 14.2).
  - Hypertonic saline administration may be hazardous for a hyponatremic patient.
  - Mannitol was previously thought to reduce ICP through simple brain dehydration; both mannitol and hypertonic saline work to reduce ICP, through reducing blood viscosity, leading to improved microcirculatory flow of blood, resulting in decreased cerebral blood volume and ICP.
- *Cerebrospinal fluid drainage*
  An external ventricular drainage (EVD) system zeroed at the midbrain with continuous drainage of CSF may be considered to lower ICP burden more effectively than intermittent use.
  - Use of CSF drainage to lower ICP in patients with an initial GCS <6 during the first hours after injury may be considered.
- *Ventilation therapies*
  - Normal ventilation is the goal for severe TBI in the absence of cerebral herniation and normal partial pressure of carbon dioxide in arterial blood ranges from 35 to 45 mmHg.

TABLE 14.2 MANNITOL

MEDICATION	CLASS	MECHANISM OF ACTION	INDICATIONS/ CONTRAINDI-CATIONS	DOSAGE	SIDE EFFECTS	SAFETY/ PATIENT EDUCATION
Mannitol (Osmitrol)	Osmotic diuretic agent	Filtered by the glomerulus, poorly reabsorbed from the renal tubule, causing an increase in osmolarity of the glomerular filtrate	Reduction of intracranial pressure and treatment of cerebral edema and intraocular pressure	1.5–2 g/kg IV infused over 30–60 minutes for reduction of intracranial pressure and treatment of cerebral edema and intraocular pressure	Fluid and electrolyte imbalance, pulmonary congestion	Monitor electrolytes and serum osmolality

IV, intravenous.
Source: Brain Trauma Foundation. (2018). *Guidelines for the management of severe traumatic brain injury* (4th ed.). American Association of Neurological Surgeons and the Congress of Neurological Surgeons.

- Prolonged prophylactic hyperventilation with partial pressure of carbon dioxide in arterial blood ($PaCO_2$) of 25 mmHg or less is not recommended.
- **Anesthetics, analgesics, and sedatives**
  - Propofol is recommended for the control of ICP; it is not recommended for improvement in mortality or 6-month outcomes. Caution is required as high-dose propofol can produce significant morbidity.
  - High-dose barbiturate administration is recommended to control elevated ICP refractory to maximum standard medical and surgical treatment. Hemodynamic stability is essential before and during barbiturate therapy.
- **Steroids**
  - The use of steroids is not recommended for improving outcome or reducing ICP. In patients with severe TBI, high-dose methylprednisolone was associated with increased mortality and is contraindicated.
- **Prophylactic hypothermia**
  - Early (within 2.5 hours), short-term (48 hours postinjury) prophylactic hypothermia is not recommended to improve outcomes in patients with diffuse injury.
  - Normothermia is helpful to reduce ICP.
- **Depressive craniectomy (DC)**—Surgical removal of a portion of the skull
  - Has been demonstrated to reduce ICP and to minimize days in the ICU.
- **Nutrition**
  - Feeding patients to attain basal caloric replacement at least by the fifth day and, at most, by the seventh day post injury is recommended to decrease mortality.
  - Postpyloric jejunal feeding is recommended to reduce the incidence of ventilator-associated pneumonia.
- **Infection prophylaxis**
  - Early tracheostomy is recommended to reduce mechanical ventilation days when the overall benefit is felt to outweigh the complications associated with such a procedure. However, there is no evidence that early tracheostomy reduces mortality or the rate of nosocomial pneumonia.
  - Antimicrobial-impregnated catheters may be considered to prevent catheter-related infections during EVD.
- **Deep vein thrombosis prophylaxis**
  - Low-molecular-weight heparin (LMWH) or low-dose unfractionated heparin may be used in combination with mechanical prophylaxis. However, there is an increased risk for expansion of ICH.
- **Seizure prophylaxis**
  - Prophylactic use of phenytoin or valproate is not recommended for preventing late post-traumatic seizures (PTS).

Monitoring

- **ICP monitoring** is recommended (see section Intracranial Hypertension).
  Management of patients with severe TBI using information from ICP monitoring is recommended to reduce in-hospital stay and 2-week post-injury mortality.
- **Cerebral perfusion pressure monitoring (CPP)**
  Management of patients with severe TBI using guidelines-based recommendations for CPP monitoring is recommended to decrease 2-week mortality.
- **Advanced cerebral monitoring**
  Jugular bulb monitoring of arteriovenous oxygen content difference ($AVDO_2$) as a source of information for management decision may be considered to reduce mortality and improve outcomes at 3 and 6 months post injury. See Table 14.3 for treatment thresholds.

TABLE 14.3 TREATMENT THRESHOLDS

Blood pressure	Maintaining SBP at ≥100 mmHg for patients 50–69 years old SBP ≥110 mmHg or above for patients 15–49 or over 70 years old may be considered to decrease mortality and improve outcomes
ICP	Treating ICP above 22 mmHg is recommended
CPP	Target CPP value for survival and favorable outcomes is between 60 and 70 mmHg Avoid aggressive attempts to maintain CPP >79 mmHg with fluids and vasopressors because of the risk of adult respiratory failure
Advanced monitoring	Jugular venous saturation of <50% may be a threshold to avoid in order to reduce mortality and improve outcomes

CPP, cerebral perfusion pressure; ICP, intracranial pressure; SBP, systolic blood pressure.

Outcomes

- Older adults have a higher mortality from TBI, increased frequency of intracerebral hematomas, and increased risk of cognitive deficits after TBI.
- Frailty rather than age can be predictive of earlier complaints and worsening outcomes.
- Older adults should be observed for falls, cognitive deficits, depression, and pain.
- Geriatric medication management should be based with attention to Beers criteria to avoid sedation and impact on attention, cognition, and motor performance.

INTRACRANIAL HYPERTENSION

OVERVIEW

Intracranial hypertention (IH) is the result of brain edema or an excessive amount of CSF within the skull. Under normal physiologic conditions, the body produces and absorbs circulating CSF in order to maintain pressure within the nonpliable cranial vault.

Pathophysiology

- The brain is housed and protected by bone within the non-flexible cranial vault. The brain is surrounded by blood and CSF that is tightly controlled through mechanisms of auto-regulation.
- The Monroe Kelli doctrine hypothesizes a constant balance among the brain, blood, and CSF, wherein if there is an increase in one component (e.g., brain edema), the other components should decrease (Dunn, 2002).

Alterations in Intracranial Pressure

- Normal ICP is <15 mmHg. ICP is auto-regulated by changes in the cerebral blood flow (CBF) and mean arterial blood pressure (MAP; Smith & Amin-Hanjani, 2019).
- Elevations >20 mmHg results in IH (Begley & Roberts, 2019; Smith & Amin-Hanjani, 2019).
- Untreated IH leads to cerebral herniation and brain death.
- Up to 40% of patients with severe TBI will develop elevated ICP that is refractory to standard forms of treatment (Seppelt, 2004)

Causes of Intracranial Hypertension

- **Acute IH** is the result of an acute event that is life threatening such as TBI, cerebral edema, obstructive hydrocephalus, lesions, and SAH.
- **Secondary IH** is chronic in nature and is traceable to a cause. Examples include head trauma, stroke, drug toxicity, infectious process, liver, and kidney failure (Intracranial Hypertension Foundation, 2019a).

Symptoms of Intracranial Hypertension

- **Universal symptoms** include headache caused by compression of cranial nerve (CN) V, change in LOC , and vomiting (Caceres & Goldstein, 2012; Smith & Amin-Hanjani, 2019).
- **Cushing's triad** is characterized by respiratory depression, bradycardia, and hypertension. The presence of Cushing's triad is considered a grave sign (Smith & Amin-Hanjani, 2019).
- **CN changes** V and VI are characterized by papilledema and periorbital swelling (Smith & Amin-Hanjani, 2019).

Treatment
Prehospital Setting

- Avoid hypoxemia and hypotension.
- Hyperventilation can be used as a temporizing measure in the presence of transtentorial herniation or acute neurologic deterioration.

Emergency Department

- Maintain adequate oxygenation and BP.
- Signs of transtentorial herniation or acute neurologic deterioration requires immediate head CT and neurosurgic intervention.
  - Hyperventilation may be used briefly for impending herniation but should be avoided as CBF is compromised and can lead to worsening cerebral edema.
  - Mannitol may be given prior to ICP monitoring.

Intensive Care Unit

- ICP monitoring
- Maintain optimal CPP
  - Maintain CPP >60 mmHg (CPP = MAP – ICP).
  - Drainage of CSF will decrease intracranial volume and may be as effective as mannitol.
- Administer osmotic diuretic (mannitol, hypertonic normal saline).
- Maintain adequate sedation and analgesia.
- Elevate head of bed at least 30° in euvolemic patients to promote cerebral venous drainage.
- Maintenance of normothermia is recommended. However, targeted temperature management (TTM) may be considered to reduce ICP but risks may outweigh benefits (i.e., risks of pneumonia, challenges with meeting target temperatures).
- High-dose barbiturate therapy is needed.
- Suppress cerebral metabolism.
- Continuous EEG monitoring or bispectral index monitoring needed to guide therapy.
- Decompressive craniectomy (Arifianto et al., 2016; Seppelt, 2004) may be needed.
  - Used as a last resort when all other treatment options have been exhausted.

Complications Associated With Intracranial Hypertension

- *Hyponatremia and hypernatremia* are caused by injury to the hypothalamus and the pituitary gland.
  - The pituitary gland and stalk work with the hypothalamus in controlling secretion of the antidiuretic hormone (ADH).
  - ADH is produced by the hypothalamus and stored in the posterior pituitary.
  - When injury occurs, osmoregulation is disrupted and results in the following:
    - Euvolemic hyponatremia due to excessive ADH release and water excretion (Sterns & Silver, 2016)
    - Hypovolemic hyponatremia due to renal sodium loss, more commonly seen in patients with neurological conditions or central nervous system surgical interventions (Rafiq, 2019; Sterns & Silver, 2016)
    - Hypervolemic hypernatremia due to lack of ADH production and ineffective ADH secretion (John & Day, 2012; Palmer, 2003; Table 14.4)

TABLE 14.4 FLUID IMBALANCES AS A RESULT OF INTRACRANIAL HYPERTENSION

HYPONATREMIA STATES			
CONDITION	ETIOLOGY	CLINICAL FEATURES	TREATMENT
SIADH	Volume expanded state related to increased ADH	Increased extracellular fluid volume Serum laboratory findings Normal hematocrit, albumin, potassium ↓ sodium, BUN/creatinine, uric acid, osmolality Urine laboratory findings ↑ osmolality, specific gravity ↓ urine output ↑ or normal urine sodium	Fluid restriction Slow sodium replacement (hypertonic saline): Approximately 4–8 mEq/day based on clinical condition and underlying cause Rapid increases in sodium may lead to osmotic pontine demyelination syndrome; desmopressin can be used to control rapid Na correction
CSW	Volume-depleted state. Kidneys cannot reabsorb sodium.	Decreased extracellular fluid volume Serum laboratory findings ↓sodium, osmolality ↑ BUN, hematocrit, albumin Normal or ↑plasma K+ Normal or ↓uric acid Urine laboratory findings ↑ osmolality, specific gravity, and sodium ↓ urine output	Normal saline
HYPERNATREMIC STATES			
Central diabetes insipidus	Reduce ADH secretion or ineffective renal response to ADH	Serum laboratory findings ↑ sodium, BUN/creatinine, osmolality Urine laboratory findings ↓ osmolality, specific gravity ↑ urine output ↓ or normal urine sodium	Fluid replacement Vasopressin Desmopressin (DDAVP)

ADH, antidiuretic hormone; BUN, blood urea nitrogen; CSW, cerebral salt wasting; DDAVP, D-amino D-arginine vasopressin; SIADH, syndrome of inappropriate antidiuretic hormone.
Sources: Data from John, C. C. A., & Day, M. W. (2012). Central neurogenic diabetes insipidus, syndrome of inappropriate secretion of antidiuretic hormone, and cerebral salt-wasting syndrome in traumatic brain injury. *Critical Care Nurse, 32*(2), e1–e7; Palmer, B. F. (2003). Hyponatremia in patients with central nervous system disease: SIADH versus CSW. *Trends in Endocrinology and Metabolism, 14*(4), 182–187; Sterns, R. H., & Silver, S. M. (2016). Complication and management of hyponatremia. *Current Opinion in Nephrology and Hypertension, 25*(2), 114–119.

INTRACRANIAL PRESSURE MONITORING, EXTERNAL VENTRICULAR DRAIN, AND LUMBAR DRAINS

OVERVIEW
Nursing care of the patient with an ICP monitor, external ventricular drain (EVD), or lumbar drainage device (LDD) is inherently complex. This complexity arises from the meticulous monitoring and multidimensional clinical decision-making required for provision of optimal care.

Intracranial Pressure Monitoring
ICP monitoring data are very useful to help predict outcomes and worsening intracranial pathology (cerebral edema, hemorrhage) and are useful for guiding therapy.
- ICP monitoring is an invasive monitoring tool used early in the course (Smith & Amin-Hanjani, 2019) for treating intracranial pathology at risk for elevated ICP.

- Goals of ICP monitoring are to assess and maintain cerebral perfusion and cerebral oxygenation and avoid secondary injury (Smith & Amin-Hanjani, 2019).
  - ICP monitor displays waveforms that provide a mean measure of ICP.
- ICP is used to calculate CPP (Slazinski et al., 2012):
  - CPP = MAP – ICP.
  - Based on the calculated CPP, clinical outcomes can be predicted, used to guide therapy, and identify worsening intracranial pathology (cerebral edema, hemorrhage).

Types of Intracranial Pressure Monitors
- **Intraventricular catheters** are considered the gold standard for measuring ICP.
  - Catheter is placed directly into the lateral ventricle via a burr hole in the skull and connected to an external pressure transducer (Slazinski et al., 2012; Smith & Amin-Hanjani, 2019).
  - Allows drainage of CSF fluid (Smith & Amin-Hanjani, 2019).

- **Intraparenchymal probe** is a fiberoptic device inserted directly into the brain tissue to monitor ICP.
  - The probe is inserted through a small opening in the skull. It is attached via a cable to a specially designed pressure monitor.
  - Does not facilitate drainage of CSF fluid.
  - Requires calibration, may result in miscalculation due to equipment failure or user error.
  - Smaller incidence of infections (Smith & Amin-Hanjani, 2019).
- **Subarachnoid catheter** or hollow open bolt placed through the skull and left in the subarachnoid space (rarely used)
- **External ventricular drain**
  - EVD has ICP monitoring capabilities but can assist with controlling increased ICP by allowing therapeutic CSF drainage.
  - The main disadvantage to an EVD is that it is the most invasive device that increases the risk of bacterial infection. Currently, antibiotic impregnated and coated ventricular catheters are commercially available (Table 14.5).

Lumbar Drainage

- LDDs are closed sterile systems that allow the drainage of CSF from the subarachnoid space in the spine. Placed at L2 to L3 level or below.

Potential Issues With All Types of Monitoring/Interventions

- Risk of infection
- Risk of overdrainage
  - CSF is produced by the highly vascular choroid plexus in the lateral ventricles at a rate of approximately 500 to 600 mL/d. At any one time, there is ~125 to 150 mL in the subarachnoid space. Drainage rates are specified per provider and can be continuous or intermittent.
    - Requires clamping of drainage system for any procedures or patient activities that cause an increase in intrathoracic pressure (movement of head above leveled drain, coughing, suctioning, movement for testing/daily activity).
    - Overdrainage can lead to a subdural hematoma due to rupture of bridging veins and brain shifts.
    - Supratentorial or transtentorial herniation may occur.
    - ICH related to placement or removal.

Diagnostic Tools

- Computerized axial tomography
- CT angiography
- MRI

TABLE 14.5 INDICATIONS FOR TYPES OF MONITORING OR MANAGEMENT

ICP	EVD	LDD
Traumatic brain injury with GCS <8		
		Adjuvant therapy in the management of traumatically brain-injured patients
Abnormal head CT with age >40, posturing, SBP <90		
		Treatment of patients with thoracoabdominal aortic aneurysms to improve spinal cord perfusion
Neurologic injury without clinical exam		
Obstructive hydrocephalus (communicating and noncommunicating)	Obstructive hydrocephalus (communicating and noncommunicating)	
		Medical therapy for the treatment of postoperative or traumatic dural fistulae, such as a CSF leak
SAH resulting in obstructive hydrocephalus	SAH resulting in acute hydrocephalus due to obstruction of arachnoid villi	
		Diagnostic evaluation of idiopathic normal pressure hydrocephalus
SAH Hunt Hess grade >3	SAH Hunt and Hess grade ≥3	
Cerebral edema	Cerebral edema	
Surgical mass lesions	Surgical mass lesions	
Infections (such as meningitis)	Infections (such as meningitis)	
Congenital abnormalities		
Chiari malformations	Chiari malformations	
Brain relaxation for the OR (with drainage)	Brain relaxation in the OR	
		Reduction ICP during a craniotomy
Benign intracranial hypertension	Shunt failure due to mechanical disruption or infection	Treatment of shunt infections
Craniosynostosis		
Traumatic subdural hemorrhage and intraventricular hemorrhage of the newborn		
Liver failure		

CSF, cerebrospinal fluid; EVD, external ventricular drain; GCS, Glasgow Coma Score; ICP, intracranial pressure; LDD, lumbar drainage device; OR, operating room; SAH, subarachnoid hemorrhage; SBP, systolic blood pressure.

BRAIN DEATH

OVERVIEW

Brain death is the irreversible loss of cerebral function secondary to a known cause that includes the loss of brain stem reflexes and spontaneous respiratory effort in the absence of confounding factors. This condition is secondary to inadequate cerebral perfusion.

Determination of Brain Death

- One neurologic examination is sufficient to pronounce brain death in most states in the United States. All providers making a determination of brain death require demonstration of competence with this complex examination.
- The determination of brain death consists of four steps.
  - Clinical evaluation
  - Neurologic assessment
  - Apnea test
  - Determination

Clinical Evaluation

- Establish irreversible and proximate cause of coma through history, drug screen, neuroimaging, and laboratory tests.
- Normal or near-normal temperature (>36 °C or 96.8 °F) is preferred during the apnea test.
- Systolic blood pressure (SBP) should be >100 mmHg.

Neurologic Assessment

- Coma, which is a lack all evidence of responsiveness
- Absence of brainstem reflexes (bilateral pupillary response, any ocular movements, corneal, pharyngeal, and tracheal)
- Any facial muscle movements to noxious stimulus

Apnea Test

- Prerequisites: Normotension, normothermia, euvolemia, eucapnia, absence of hypoxia, and no prior evidence of CO_2 retention
- Absence of a breathing drive, which is tested by a CO_2 challenge
- Documentation of an increase in $PaCO_2$ from baseline of eucapnea ($PaCO_2$ 35–45 mmHg)

Determination

- Absence of respiratory movements.
- Arterial CO_2 >60 mmHg or 20 mmHg over baseline.
- Positive apnea test.
- If test is inconclusive but the patient is hemodynamically stable, test may be repeated for a longer period of time (10–15 minutes) after patient is adequately oxygenated.
- Ancillary testing (EEG, cerebral angiography, nuclear scan, and transcranial Doppler) may also be completed if there are inconclusive results.
- Brain death determination is documented in the medical record (American Academy of Neurology, 2011).

ORGAN DONATION

OVERVIEW

Organ donation is a life-saving measure for individuals awaiting transplantation.

Organ Procurement Organization

- Federal regulations require that all hospitals notify the organ procurement organization (OPO) of every near death or actual patient death.

- For any suitable candidate, a representative from OPO travels immediately to the hospital.
- The representative will obtain information regarding donor registration and authorization from family.
  - A medical evaluation takes place after this process has been completed.
- After evaluation, the OPO contacts the organ procurement and transplantation network (OPTN).
  - Confirmation of brain death made.
  - OPTN enters donor information into a national database and a computer generates a list of best-matched patients
  - The transplant surgeon determines whether the organ is medically suitable.
    - Most organs go to patients in the vicinity where the organs were recovered.

Care of Potential Donors
Recovering and Transporting Organs

- The deceased donor organs are maintained on artificial support with management of any changes in physiologic status.

A transplant surgical team replaces the medical team for the recovery of the organs and tissues.

- Organs remain viable for only a short period of time.
  - The OPO representative arranges for transportation of the organs to the intended recipient.

Transplanting Organs

- The transplant operation takes place after the transport team arrives at the accepting hospital.

HYPOXIC/ISCHEMIC ENCEPHALOPATHY

OVERVIEW

Hypoxic/ischemic encephalopathy is the result of reduced oxygenated blood supply to cerebral tissues leading to permanent or temporary damage to affected parts of the brain.

Pathophysiology

- Loss of adenosine triphosphate (ATP) along with ATP synthesis leads to cerebral edema and atrophy and leads to cell death.
- Loss of oxygenated blood causes free radicals, which reprogram cells to destroy brain tissue (apoptosis).
- Influx of intracellular calcium causes damage to mitochondrial death.
- Damaged nitric oxide pathways cause vasoconstriction reducing blood flow.
- Neurotransmitters are excited, leading to glutamine release, cell death, and apoptosis (Heinz & Rollnik, 2015; McCance & Grey, 2010; Sekhon et al., 2017).

Contributing Risk Factors and Etiologies

- Sudden cardiac arrest
- Stroke
- Strangulation
- Carbon monoxide poisoning
- Near drowning
- Cerebral vasospasms
- Obstruction
- Living in high altitudes
- Traumatic brain injuries (Heinz & Rollnik, 2015; Sirvastava, 2017)

Assessment

Patient assessment is focused on obtaining a history and circumstances leading to the hypoxic event. This assessment includes patient's health and neurologic status prior to the event, preceding symptoms, acute episodes such as cardiac arrest, and current neurologic status (Weinhouse & Young, 2015).

Treatment

Goal: Preserve brain tissue and function by reducing demand and use of CBF.

Treatment Modalities

- TTM at onset of injury (Guanci & Mathiesen, 2016; Sekhon et al., 2017)
  - Core body temperature lowered to 32 °C to 36 °C to reduce cerebral metabolism.
    - Each degree lowered results in 5% to 10% reduction in CBF.
    - Hypothermia is maintained for 12 to 24 hours.
    - Body is gradually rewarmed.
  - Duration of TTM is determined by injury.
  - Adjunctive treatment includes use of sedatives, antipyretics, shivering control with neuromuscular blockage agents, and monitoring of electrolytes.

Ongoing and Postacute Management

- Evaluate and control seizures through continuous or intermittent EEG monitoring and use of antiepileptic medications (Arciniegas, 2012; Weinhouse & Young, 2015).
- Reduce disability and functional decline through neurologic evaluation and rehabilitation (Arciniegas, 2012).
  - Reduce cognitive decline by reducing delirium, speech therapy, social interaction, and medication therapies as indicated (Arciniegas, 2012).

MANAGEMENT OF THE PATIENT UNDERGOING TARGETED TEMPERATURE MANAGEMENT

OVERVIEW

TTM is achieved through surface or internal cooling mechanisms. The goal of TTM is to preserve brain function caused by reduced CBF after cardiac arrest and hypoxic and ischemic events (Dietrich & Bramlett, 2017; Herrero & Varon, 2019; Khan et al., 2018). Cooling is achieved by lowering the body's core temperature to a target temperature followed by a period of gradual rewarming.

- TTM is widely used after cardiac arrest; it may also be used to control ICP in TBI and for temperature control.
- Coordination and communication of the healthcare team is required to ensure smooth and timely implementation and monitoring of the patient receiving TTM (Mathiesen et al., 2015).

Benefits of Targeted Temperature Management

- Reduces cerebral oxygen demand by 6% for every degree Celsius of temperature lowered (Herrero & Varon, 2019)
- Promotes oxygen supply to the brain, reduces ICP (Muengtaweepongsa & Srivilaithon, 2017)

- Decreases cerebral metabolic rate by decreasing oxygen consumption (Cariou et al., 2018)
- Decreased inflammatory response by reducing free radicals that cause programmed cells to destroy brain tissue (apoptosis) (Cariou et al., 2018; Herrero & Varon, 2019)
- Decreased cerebral edema by decreasing protecting the blood–brain barrier (Dietrich & Bramlett, 2017; Muengtaweepongsa & Srivilaithon, 2017)

Cooling Methods

Invasive Endovascular Methods

- Special catheter placed intravascularly to cool infused fluids.

Surface Cooling Methods

- Application of surface pads designed for use with manufacturer-specific hypothermia cooling devices
- Cooling blankets
- Ice packs make it difficult to regulate temperature (Herrero & Varon, 2019)

Phases of Targeted Temperature Management

- *Induction or cooling phase:* Temperature targets should be based on clinical condition. Cooling temperature targets range from 32 °C to 36 °C (Cariou et al., 2018).
- *Maintenance phase*: Targeted cooling temperature maintained for a prescribed duration. This phase usually lasts 24 hours but may last longer as clinically indicated.
- *Rewarming phase*: Gradual increase in body temperature at prescribed rate and duration.
  - Rewarming rate is usually 0.2 °C to 0.5 °C/hr.
  - Rapid rewarming increases risk for neural injury.

Nursing Considerations

Core Temperature Monitoring

- Esophageal probe is preferred and superior (Rittenberger & Callaway, 2018); bladder probe acceptable; rectal probe least accurate.
- Pulmonary artery (PA) catheter may not be compatible with commercial hypothermia machines.
- Continuously monitor and control patient temperature.
  - Prior to start of cooling and rewarming phases
  - After initiation of chilled fluids
  - Minimally hourly
  - Treat episodes of fever and monitor response
    - Antipyretics
    - Chilled fluids
  - Monitor temperatures of surface or internal mechanical cooling devices
  - **Assess and control shivering:** Shivering is caused by the body's response to thermoregulation by peripheral vasoconstriction. Shivering increases metabolic demand (Logan et al., 2011; Rittenberger & Callaway, 2018)
    - Utilize tools to assess shivering. Use of standardized assessments is warranted (Logan et al., 2011).
    - Maintain adequate sedation (Mathiesen et al., 2015; May et al., 2015; Rittenberger & Callaway, 2018).
    - Neuromuscular blockade agents (NMBA) may help control shivering, but should be used with caution as they may also suppress seizure activity (Mathiesen et al., 2015; Rittenberger & Callaway, 2018).
      - Use only in well-sedated patient.

- Perform shivering countermeasures.
  - Cover distal extremities with socks (hands, feet); cover head.
  - Consider use of air-directed warming blanket.

Monitor and Treat Side Effects of Hypothermia

- Cardiac arrhythmias and hypotension: Treat based on clinical picture
- Bleeding tendencies
  - ↓Platelets, ↑INR
- Hyperglycemia caused by reduced insulin production (Polderman, 2009)
- Intracellular fluid shifts due to cold diuresis (Polderman, 2009)
  - ↓Potassium, ↓magnesium, ↓phosphate.
  - Use caution when replacing electrolytes as there will be electrolyte shifts when rewarming patient
- Infection risk increases with maintenance phase >24 hours (Cariou et al., 2018; (Rittenberger & Callaway, 2018))

MANAGEMENT OF THE PATIENT RECEIVING NEUROMUSCULAR BLOCKADE

OVERVIEW

- Neuromuscular blockades (NMBAs) are a select group of drugs used with sedation and mechanical ventilation to cause reversible muscular paralysis.
  - NMBAs do not have sedating or analgesic effects and therefore require sedating and antianxiety agents to a level of deep sedation (Murray et al., 2016).
  - NMBA agents should be short term to prevent complications associated with long-term use (Blauvelt et al., 2019).
- Use of NMBA should be used as adjunctive therapy in medical conditions not responsive to sedation alone (deBacker et al., 2017).
- Close patient monitoring during NMBA is required to ensure the least amount of drug provides the desired therapeutic effect and that the patient's level of sedation level is adequate.
- Monitoring post NMBA is required to determine return of muscular function.

Indications

- NMBAs used in procedures such as rapid sequence intubation, management of ventilator asynchrony, management of increased ICP (Bittner, 2017; Blauvelt et al., 2019; deBacker et al., 2017; Murray et al., 2016).
- Control shivering during TTM (Berlin et al., 2016; Bittner, 2017; Guanci & Mathiesen, 2016) with the use of a specific protocol (Murray et al., 2016).
- Aid in management of increased ICP refractory to other treatments.
- Facilitate ventilation in severe acute respiratory distress syndrome (ARDS) or other respiratory disorders requiring mechanical ventilation.
- Therapy goals should be individualized. Decision points should clinically controlling motor movement versus complete paralysis (Bittner, 2017).

NMBA is contraindicated in individuals with neuromuscular disorders (Bitters et al., 2016).

Caution should also be used with concomitant use of steroids.

Mechanisms of Action

NMBAs block nerve impulses through the effect of acetylcholine at the pre- or postneuromuscular junction motor endplate (Murray et al., 2016; Stawicki & Gessner, 2018; Table 14.6). NMBA mechanism of action is as follows:

> NMBA → Targets neuromuscular junction → Blocks nerve acetylcholine impulses → Relaxes skeletal muscles

- *Depolarizing NMBA work postjunction* results in prolonged depolarization by desensitizing the acetylcholine receptors
  - Inactivates voltage-gated sodium channels at the neuromuscular junction → Increases potassium permeability of the cell membrane → Stops action potential generation and causes muscular blockade.
- *Nondepolarizing agents work prejunctional* affecting the receptors at motor nerve endings. This prevents acetylcholine release (Bittner, 2017).
- Knowledge of each drug's mechanism of action, side effects, and interactions are necessary to adequately monitor patient receiving NMBA (Bittner, 2017).

Nursing Assessment

- Use ideal or adjusted body weight versus actual body weight in obese patients for dose calculations.
- *Sedation and anxiety*
  - Sedate patient prior to use of NMB (Blauvelt et al., 2019; Murray et al., 2016).
  - Sedation level should be deep sedation (Murray et al., 2016).
  - Measure sedation with use of Bispectral index sensor (BIS). BIS level should be 40 to 60 (Berlin et al., 2016; Blauvelt et al., 2019).
  - Monitor and control level of sedation and anxiety to reduce recall, awareness, pain, and discomfort.
  - Use sedation scales such as the Richmond Sedation Agitation Scale (RASS) or Riker Sedation–Agitation Scale (SAS).
- Determine level of NMB (Berlin et al., 2016; Blauvelt et al., 2019; Murray et al., 2016).

Peripheral Nerve Stimulator and Train of Four

- Peripheral nerve stimulator (PNS) with train of four (TOF) should be used as an adjunct to patient clinical assessment and not as a sole determinant for level of NMB (Murray et al., 2016).
- Patient conditions (i.e., edema, placement of electrodes) and variation in practice (i.e., staff assessment skill, PNS equipment models, lack of equipment) may create inconsistency in this method of monitoring.
- PNS determines level of NMB by delivering a transcutaneous electrical stimulus to specific peripheral nerves via leads and a PNS device.
  - Locations for monitoring level of NMB are described in Table 14.7. (Note all leads are placed on the same side.)

Determine level of supramaximal stimulation:

- Obtain baseline twitch prior to initiating NMB.
- Start at 20 mA; increase by 10 mA increments until twitch is seen.
- Observe for twitch; record baseline and subsequent responses.
- Use baseline mA to perform subsequent testing.
  - Increases by 25% mA may be needed once NMB is in progress.

TABLE 14.6 COMMON NEUROMUSCULAR BLOCKING AGENTS AND KEY POINTS

DEPOLARIZING AGENTS BIND TO POSTSYNAPTIC CHOLINERGIC RECEPTORS			
DRUG NAME/ METABOLIZED/ ELIMINATION	**PEAK ONSET (MIN)**	**DURATION (MIN)**	**KEY POINTS/PRECAUTIONS**
Succinylcholine	1	7–12	Causes hyperkalemia; caution in renal patient. May increase ICP; not recommended for prolonged use.

NONDEPOLARIZING AGENTS BIND TO PRESYNAPTIC CHOLINERGIC RECEPTORS			
AMINO STEROIDS			
DRUG NAME METABOLIZED/ ELIMINATION	**PEAK ONSET (MIN)**	**DURATION (MIN)**	**KEY POINTS/PRECAUTIONS**
Pancuronium *Renal/hepatic and biliary*	3–5	60–90	Limit use in neurologic injuries; caution in renal and hepatic impairment; vagolytic effect may increase HR.
Vecuronium *Hepatic/biliary*	3–5	20–35	CBF not affected with use; contains mannitol; may cause prolonged paralysis in liver disease.
Rocuronium *Biliary/hepatic*	1–2	20–35	Delayed recovery in liver disease; may reduce HR; vagolytic effect may cause tachycardia.
BENZYLISOQUINOLINIUMS			
Atracurium *Hoffman elimination*	3–5	20–35	Contains metabolites that may increase seizures. Preferred for hepatic and renal impairments.
Cisatrcurium *Hoffman elimination*	3–5	20–35	Does not increase ICP; may increase HR with bolus doses. Acidosis may prolong paralysis. Preferred for hepatic and renal impairments.
Mivacurium *Hoffman elimination*	2–3	12–20	3× more potent than atracurium; prolonged effect in renal and liver disease; facial, neck, and chest flushing common.

CBF, cerebral blood flow; HR, heart rate; ICP, intracranial pressure.
Sources: Data from Bitters, L., Love, J., & Perlstrom, K. (2016). Perioperative surgical consideration. In M. K. Bader, L. R. Littlejohns, & D. M. Olson (Eds.), *AANN core curriculum for neuroscience nursing* (6th ed., pp. 121–133). American Association of Neuroscience Nursing; deBacker, J., Hart, N., & Fan, E. (2017). Neuromuscular blockade in the 21st century management of the critically ill patient. *Chest, 151*(3), 697–706; Smetana, K. S., Roe, N., Doepker, B. A., & Jones, G. M. (2017). Review of continuous infusion neuromuscular blocking agents in the adult intensive care unit. *Critical Care Nursing Quarterly, 40*(4), 323–343.

TABLE 14.7 PERIPHERAL NERVE STIMULATOR LEAD PLACEMENT

NERVE ASSESSED	NEGATIVE LEAD PLACEMENT (BLACK)	POSITIVE LEAD PLACEMENT (RED)	PATIENT POSITION	TWITCH RESPONSE
Facial (Consider this location if peripheral edema is present)	Tragus of ear	Outer canthus eye same side negative lead		Facial twitch above eye—same side of leads
Ulnar	Base of fifth finger	3–5 cm above from lead 1	Arm relaxed in extension Keep palm up	Thumb twitch
Posterior tibia	2 cm behind medial malleolus next to Achilles tendon	2 cm above negative lead	Leg extended, toes facing up	Plantar flexion great toe

Note: Negative and positive leads are ipsilateral. .

- Increase or reduce NMB as prescribed, based on response to PNS.
  - Retest within 15 minutes after dose change.

Test for train of four: TOF delivery of four electrical impulses over 2 seconds. The response determines the degree of NMB.

- Four twitches = 0% to 75% of the receptors are blocked.
- Three twitches = approximately 75% of the receptors are blocked.
- Two twitches = 75% to 80% of the receptors are blocked.
- One twitch = 90% of the receptors are blocked.
  - When no twitches are seen, 100% of receptors are blocked.

Concomitant Patient Monitoring

- Monitor for hypotension, tachycardia, and bradycardia (Blauvelt et al., 2019; deBacker et al., 2017).
  - Monitor temperature and observe for signs of malignant hyperthermia when using depolarizing NMBA.
  - Monitor ICP—Depolarizing agents may increase ICP in patients with severe TBI.
  - Observe for ventilator synchrony.
    - Triggered respirations may be a sign of inadequate NMB.
- Reduce corneal injury.
  - Apply eye gels or drops to lubricate the eyes.
  - Manually close eyelids.
- Continue mobility strategies to prevent deep vein thrombosis and muscle atrophy.
  - Patient positioning
  - Range of motion
  - Adaptive devices as indicated

Discontinuing Neuromuscular Blocking Agents

- Avoid prolonged use of NMB to reduce the incidence of neuromuscular weakness.
- Include periods of no NMB to evaluate patient response and readiness for discontinuation (Bittner, 2017). Patient monitoring includes sedation adjustment movement and PNS testing prior to extubation (Blauvelt et al., 2019).
- Reversal agents may be used in the event of prolonged residual effects.

SPINAL CORD INJURY

OVERVIEW

A spinal cord injury (SCI) involves damage to the nerves within the bony protection of the spinal canal. The nerves can be severed, bruised, stretched, or crushed. The most common cause is trauma from vehicular accidents, falls, diving, violence, and sports injuries. SCI results in the loss of the ability to send and receive messages from the brain to the body's system that controls sensory, motor, and autonomic function (Maddox, 2017b).

Functioning after SCI depends on type and level of injury (Table 14.8).

Level of Injury: American Spinal Injury Association Scale

A = no motor control, no sensation
B = no motor control, some sensation
C = some motor function
D = motor function incomplete with more function below lesion area
E = normal

Complications Related to Spinal Cord Injury

- *Spinal shock* mechanism of injury is usually traumatic, occurs immediately, but can progress for several hours. Involves temporary loss of reflexes associated with level of injury as well as hypotension. Usually considered over when bulbocavernous reflex returns.
- *Neurogenic shock*—A serious life-threatening condition that can result from SCI, as a result of loss of sympathetic tone, it causes a severe hypotension and bradycardia resulting from widespread dilation of blood vessels. Usually occurs in SCI above T6 (see Chapter 16).
- *Autonomic dysreflexia*—Overactivity of autonomic nervous system (Maddox, 2017b; Previn 2019a).
  - Nerve impulses from the stimulus below the level of injury travel up the spinal cord and are blocked at the level of injury. A reflex is activated increasing the sympathetic portion of the autonomic nervous system. This causes narrowing of blood vessels, increasing BP. Nerve receptors in heart and blood vessels detect this rise in

TABLE 14.8 LEVEL OF INJURY OUTCOMES

LEVEL OF INJURY	MOTOR FUNCTION
C1–C3	Limited movement of head and neck.
C3–C4	Typically will have head and neck control. Patients at C4 level may shrug their shoulders.
C5	Has head and neck control,; can shrug shoulder and has shoulder control. Some upper extremity movement such as bending elbows and turn palms face up.
C6	Movement in head, neck, shoulders, arms, and wrists. Can shrug shoulders, bend elbows, turn palms up and down, and extend wrists.
C7	Similar movements to C6 along with ability to straighten elbows.
T1	Strength and precision of fingers that result in limited or natural hand function.
T2–T6	Normal motor function in head, neck, shoulders, arms, hands, and fingers. Increased trunk control with use of rib and chest muscles.
T7–T12	Added motor function from increased abdominal control.
L1–L5	Return of motor movement in the knees and hips.
S1–S5	Various degrees of return of voluntary bowel, bladder, and sexual functions depending on level of injury.

Source: Data from Sci Info Pages. (n.d.). *Spinal cord injury functional goals*. www.sci-info-pages.com/spinal-cord-injury-functional-goals

BP, sending message to brain, which results in heart rate slowing and the blood vessels above injury dilate; body is unable to regulate BP.

- *Life-threatening emergency* that occurs at injuries T6 and above, caused by irritant below level of injury. Patient or caregivers should know baseline BP, triggers, and symptoms.
- Symptoms vary by individual but include the following:
  - High BP
  - Pounding headache
  - Flushed face
  - Sweating above level of injury
  - Goose bumps below level of injury
  - Nasal stuffiness
  - Nausea
  - Slow pulse (<60/min)

Treatment

- Most important to remove offending trigger (bowel, bladder, skin issue, tight clothing)
  - Actions to take are as follows:
  - Sit or raise head to 90°.
  - Lower legs.
  - Loosen tight or restrictive clothing.
  - Check BP every 5 minutes (usually will be 20–40 mmHg above baseline in adults).
  - Check for full bladder (intake and output [I&O] catheterization).
    - Check for stool in rectal vault. Be aware this may exacerbate the dysreflexia, but it will most likely not resolve until stimulus removed. Stool will need evacuation.
- *Medications*: Only if stimulus cannot be identified and removed or if it continues after stimulus is removed.
  - *Prevention*
  - *Adhere to bowel and bladder schedules*
  - *Meticulous skin care*
    - *Proper size clothing*

Bladder Management

- SCI at any level can affect bladder control due to lower motor neuron (LMN) damage.
- Nerves controlling bladder are at levels S2 to S4.
- Primary complications are urinary tract infection, urinary reflux, and autonomic dysreflexia.

Treatment

- Intermittent catheterization program is the principal method for emptying bladder.
  - Typical schedule is every 4 to 6 hours a day.

Other Methods of Bladder Management

- Suprapubic catheter
- Continuous indwelling catheters: More prone to urinary tract infection, typical in acute SCI
- External condom catheters
- Monti or Mitrofanoff procedure—Create passage for catheterization via stoma on abdomen
  - Bladder augmentation—Enlarging the bladder with intestinal tissue to expand bladder capacity to reduce leaking and frequent catheterization

Neurogenic bladder: Both types of functional incontinence are common.

- *Spastic (reflex) bladder*: Usually occurs above T12
  - Bladder fills with urine; reflex triggers it to empty; may or may not empty; cannot control timing.
- *Flaccid (nonreflex) bladder*
  - Bladder fills with urine; bladder muscles are sluggish or absent.
  - Bladder becomes stretched or overly distended.
  - May not completely empty.

Bowel Management

There are two main types of neurogenic bowel, depending on the level of injury.

- *Upper motor neuron (UMN)*—An injury above the conus medullaris at L1, hyper-reflexic bowel; the sphincter remains tight, which causes stool retention and promotes constipation; connections between the spinal cord and colon remain intact, maintaining reflex coordination and stool propulsion; this allows a suppository or digital stimulation to initiate reflex activity; patient can schedule the bowel program at socially appropriate times.
- *Lower motor neuron*—Injury below L1; flaccid bowel results in loss of stool movement and slow stool propulsion causing constipation and higher risk of incontinence due to lack of a functional anal sphincter. Stool softeners minimize hemorrhoids; minimize straining and physical trauma during stimulation.

Bowel Program

- Follow a schedule to train the bowel.
- May be done at time that fits patient's schedule.
- Begins with insertion of suppository or mini-enema.
- Wait 15 to 20 minutes to allow stimulant to work.
- Perform digital stimulation every 10 to 15 minutes until the rectum is empty of stool (usually up to three times)
- Can be done on commode or in side-lying position.
- Entire program can typically be completed within 30 to 60 minutes. Sitting tolerance for 2 hours is usually sufficient.
  - Use side lying if skin breakdown is a concern.

Sexuality

- Men are affected both physically and psychologically. Women are less affected than males as it does not change their libido, their need to express themselves sexually, or their ability to conceive a child.
- It is physically easier for a woman to adapt; sexual intercourse is more passive and positioning may require accommodation.
- Partner communication is key for both sexes regarding changes, needs, and feelings.
- Major concerns for men are erection and ejaculation. Ability depends on level and extent of paralysis.
- Spasticity can interfere with sexual activity. With genital stimulation, it can be increased during sexual activity resulting in autonomic dysreflexia. This requires temporary cessation of activity.
- Erection may not be hard enough or last long enough for sexual activity (i.e., erectile dysfunction; Maddox, 2017a).

Treatment

- Viagra, Cialis, and Levitra can significantly improve the quality of erections and sexual satisfaction for men with injuries between T6 and L5 but cannot be used if the man has low/high BP or vascular disease.

- *Other treatment options available include* penile injection therapy, medicated urethral system erection, vacuum pumps, or penile prosthesis.

STROKE: CEREBRAL VASCULAR ACCIDENT OR CEREBRAL INFARCT

OVERVIEW

Sudden impairment of cerebral circulation in one or more of the blood vessels supplying the brain.

- Interrupts or diminishes oxygen supply causing serious damage or necrosis to brain tissue.
- Risk of stroke advances with age at 65 years or older; more prominent at ≤80 years of age; incidence doubles in octogenarians (Table 14.9; Cash & Glass, 2019).

TYPES OF STROKE

Transient Ischemic Attack

- Least severe type
- Temporary interruption of blood flow
- Common arteries are the carotid and vertebrobasilar arteries
- Clears within 12 to 24 hours
- Often referred to as mini-stroke or warning stroke

Signs and symptoms correlate with location of affected artery:

- Double vision
- Unilateral blindness
- Staggering or uncoordinated gait
- Unilateral weakness or numbness
- Falling from weakness in legs
- Dizziness
- Slurring or thickness of speech

Treatment

- Patient fully recovers; treatment is aimed at preventing a stroke.

Acute Ischemic Stroke

- *Cerebral thrombosis*—Most common cause in middle-aged and older patients; obstruction occurs in the extra cerebral blood vessels or can occur in intracerebral vessels.
- *Cerebral embolism*—Occlusion of a blood vessel due to a fragmented clot, tumor, fat, bacteria, or air. Develops rapidly

in 10 to 20 seconds and without warning. Most common vessel is left-middle cerebral artery. Causes necrosis and edema and if septic the infection can extend beyond the vessel leading to encephalitis.

Hemorrhagic Stroke

Intracerebral hemorrhage (ICH) or SAH involves a sudden rupture of a cerebral artery caused by chronic hypertension or aneurysm; diminishes blood supply to area served by the artery and blood accumulates deep within brain tissue, causing damage (13% of strokes).

Etiology

Vascular

- *Aneurysm*—Rupture of blood vessel
- *Arteriovenous malformation (AVM)*—Abnormal connection between arteries and veins that bypasses the capillaries; common location is the central nervous system; rupture of vessels within AVM creates hemorrhage.

Symptoms

- Dependent on the affected vessel and surrounding brain tissue
- Right-sided stroke affects the left side of body
- Left-sided stroke affects the right side of body
- Stroke involving the CNs creates deficits on the same side as the damage.
- Partial or total loss of consciousness
- Headache (often described as worst ever experienced)
- Limb weakness or numbness
- Contralateral hemiparesis
- Facial weakness/drooping
- Speech difficulty
- Dysphagia
- Visual changes
- Ataxia
- Other—Cognitive changes, behavioral changes, nausea and vomiting, fatigue, seizures

Long-Term Changes

- Hemiparesis
- Hemiplegia
- Spasticity

TABLE 14.9 RISK FACTORS FOR STROKE

CARDIAC	MODIFIABLE	NONMODIFIABLE	OTHER
Atrial fibrillation (5× greater risk for stroke) **Mitral and aortic valve disease** **Rheumatic heart disease** **Atrial and ventricular septal defects** **Carotid artery stenosis** **Thrombosis** **Embolism**	Hypertension—Major component of stroke prevention, effective for reduction across all ages and populations Smoking Diabetes Dyslipidemia Obesity Physical activity Sickle cell disease	Age: increases with age 65 and older; onset older in women, typically after age 70, increased prominence after age 80 Gender: Women at great risk than men Race/ethnicity: Increase in Blacks and Hispanics/Latinx Family history/genetic predisposition like inherited coagulopathies	Iatrogenic anticoagulation Illicit drug use Postsurgical complications Cerebral amyloidosis—Proteins called amyloids build up on the walls of the arteries in the brain. TIA Migraine with aura

TIA, transient ischemic attack.
Source: Data from Cash, J. C., & Glass, C. A. (2019). Seizures. In J. C. Cash, C. A. Glass, C. K. Bartoo, & K. D. Mullen (Eds.), *Adult-gerontology practice guidelines* (2nd ed., pp. 703–708). Springer Publishing Company.

- Contracture
- Emotional changes

Diagnostic Testing

- All patients admitted to hospital with suspected acute stroke should receive brain imaging evaluation on arrival to hospital.
  - Noncontrast CT (NCCT) will provide the necessary information to make decisions about acute management.
  - Should be performed within 20 minutes of arrival in the ED in at least 50% of patients, who may be candidates for IV alteplase and/or mechanical thrombectomy.
- Computed tomographic angiography (CTA) used to locate abnormalities and aneurysm.
- Magnetic resonance angiography (MRA) used to locate aneurysm.
- Cerebral angiography or cerebral arteriography used to determine size and location of blockages.
- Duplex Doppler studies.

Physical Examination

- Medical history: Symptoms before, during, and after event; timing; intensity; duration; any fluctuation
- Any pattern becoming more frequent or escalating; include witness or family members and emergency personnel regarding behavior, speech, gait, memory and movement, previous medical history; review medications, including use of illicit drugs and herbal supplements
- Overall appearance—Ability to interact, language, tremors, spasticity, walking
- Auscultation of heart, lungs, and carotid arteries (bruit)
- The use of a stroke severity rating scale, preferably the National Institutes of Health Stroke Scale (NIHSS) is recommended (Table 14.10)
- Neurological exam
  - Pupils
  - Fundoscopic exam—Optic disk
  - CN testing
  - Motor strength
  - Sensory testing
  - Gait and posture

Treatment

Refer to the *2018 Guidelines for the Early Management of Patients With Acute Ischemic Stroke: A Guideline for Healthcare Professionals* from the American Heart Association/American Stroke Association. An overview of the guidelines is provided but is not all inclusive.

- Patients with a positive stroke screen and/or a strong suspicion of stroke should be transported rapidly to the closest healthcare facilities that can capably administer IV alteplase (Table 14.11).
- IV alteplase should be administered to all eligible patients.
- Hypotension and hypovolemia should be corrected to maintain systemic perfusion levels necessary to support organ function.
  - Patients who have elevated BP and are otherwise eligible for treatment with IV alteplase should have their BP carefully lowered so that their systolic BP is <185 mmHg and their diastolic BP is <110 mmHg before IV fibrinolytic therapy is initiated.
- Antiplatelet treatment:
  - Administration of aspirin is recommended in patients with arterial ischemic stroke (AIS) within 24 to 48 hours after onset.
- Anticoagulants:
  - Urgent anticoagulation, with the goal of preventing early recurrent stroke, halting neurologic worsening, or improving outcomes after AIS, is not recommended for treatment of patients with AIS.
- Volume expansion/hemodilution, vasodilators, and hemodynamic augmentation:
  - Hemodilution by volume expansion is not recommended for treatment of patients with AIS.
- Neuroprotective agents:
  - At present, no pharmacologic or nonpharmacologic treatments with putative neuroprotective actions have demonstrated efficacy in improving outcomes after ischemic stroke and therefore other neuroprotective agents are not recommended (Table 14.12).
- Blood pressure:
  - In patients with AIS, early treatment of hypertension is indicated when required by comorbid conditions.

TABLE 14.10 NATIONAL INSTITUTES OF HEALTH STROKE SCALE

1a. Level of consciousness	0 = Alert; keenly responsive
	1 = Not alert, but arousable by minor
	2 = Not alert; requires repeated stimulation
	3 = Unresponsive or responds only with reflex
1b. Level of consciousness questions What is the month? What is your age?	0 = Answers two questions correctly
	1 = Answers one question correctly
	2 = Answers neither question correctly
1c. Level of consciousness commands Open and close your eyes. Grip and release your hand.	0 = Performs both tasks correctly
	1 = Performs one task correctly
	2 = Performs neither task correctly
2. Best gaze	0 = Normal
	1 = Partial gaze palsy
	2 = Forced deviation
3. Visual	0 = No visual loss
	1 = Partial hemianopia
	2 = Complete hemianopia
	3 = Bilateral hemianopia

(continued)

TABLE 14.10 NATIONAL INSTITUTES OF HEALTH STROKE SCALE (*continued*)

4. Facial palsy	0 = Normal symmetric movements 1 = Minor paralysis 2 = Partial paralysis 3 = Complete paralysis of one or both sides
5. Motor: Arm 　5a. Left arm 　5b. Right arm	0 = No drift 1 = Drift 2 = Some effort against gravity 3 = No effort against gravity; limb falls 4 = No movement
6. Motor: Leg 　6a. Left leg 　6b. Right leg	0 = No drift 1 = Drift 2 = Some effort against gravity 3 = No effort against gravity 4 = No movement
7. Limb ataxia	0 = Absent 1 = Present in one limb 2 = Present in two limbs
8. Sensory	0 = Normal; no sensory loss 1 = Mild-to-moderate sensory loss 2 = Severe to total sensory loss
9. Best language	0 = No aphasia; normal 1 = Mild-to-moderate aphasia 2 = Severe aphasia 3 = Mute, global aphasia
10. Dysarthria	0 = Normal 1 = Mild to moderate dysarthria 2 = Severe dysarthria
11. Extinction and inattention	0 = No abnormality 1 = Visual, tactile, auditory, spatial, or personal inattention 2 = Profound hemi-inattention or extinction

Total score = 0–42.

Score = 0 = No stroke
Score = 1–4 = Minor stroke
Score = 5–15 = Moderate stroke
Score = 15–20 = Moderate to severe stroke
Score = 21–42 = Severe stroke

Source: National Institutes of Health. www.stroke.nih.gov/documents/NIH_Stroke_Scale_508C.pdf

TABLE 14.11 ISCHEMIC STROKE PHARMACOLOGY—ACUTE TREATMENT

MEDICATION	CLASS	MECHANISM OF ACTION	INDICATIONS/ CONTRAINDI-CATIONS	DOSAGE	SIDE EFFECTS	SAFETY/PATIENT EDUCATION
Alteplase (Activase)	Thrombolytic agent	Binds to fibrin in thrombus and converts entrapped plasminogen to plasmin, initiates local fibrinolysis.	Management of acute ischemic stroke. Contraindicated in active internal bleeding, recent spinal or cerebral surgery/trauma.	Weight based, not to exceed 90 mg. Stroke—0.9 mg/kg over 1 hour. Administer.10% bolus over 1 minute.	Bleeding	Monitor for S&S bleeding, allergic reaction, angioedema, rash, and urticaria. Monitor BP frequently while administering, Notify provider of any S&S allergic reaction. Weigh benefits versus risk before administration.

BP, blood pressure, S&S, signs and symptoms.

TABLE 14.12 ISCHEMIC STROKE PHARMACOLOGY—SECONDARY STROKE PREVENTION

MEDICATION	CLASS	MECHANISM OF ACTION	INDICATIONS/ CONTRAINDICATIONS	DOSAGE	SIDE EFFECTS	SAFETY/PATIENT EDUCATION
ASA	Salicylate, nonsteroidal anti-inflammatory	Varies with dose. In stroke: inhibition of prostaglandin synthesis action to prevent the formation of platelet-aggregating substance thromboxane A_2.	To reduce risk of death and nonfatal stroke with previous stroke or TIA. NSAID allergy for those with pre-existing peptic ulcer disease, GI bleed, hemophiliacs.	81–325 mg PO daily	Fever, dysrhythmias, agitation, GI bleed, hearing loss	Care in patients with previous GI or other bleeding issues, true ASA allergy, increased risk of bleed with ETOH, may inhibit platelet function
Clopidogrel (Plavix)	Platelet aggregation inhibitor	Selectively inhibits the binding of ADP to its platelet receptor and subsequent ADP-mediated activation of glycoprotein GIIb/IIIa complex.	Reduce risk of stroke in patients with transient brain ischemia or complete thrombosis. Contraindicated in active pathologic bleeding.	75 mg daily in combination with ASA daily	Chest pain, influenza type symptoms, edema, HTN, headache	Check platelet counts before drug therapy, every 2 days in first week of treatment and weekly till therapeutic maintenance reached. Caution with other NSAIDs, warfarin.
Dipyridamole: ASA (Aggrenox)	Platelet aggregation inhibitor	Leads to increase in adenosine, which acts on platelet A_2 receptor to stimulate platelet adenylate cyclase and increase platelet cAMP levels.	For reduction of thrombotic-like events in those with recurrent stroke. Contraindicated in NSAID allergy, asthma, rhinitis, nasal polyps.	200/25-mg capsule, 1 BID	Headache, dyspepsia, abdominal pain, N&V.	Watch ETOH intake, due to increased risk of bleeding, contact provider for any S&S bleeding or allergic reactions; headaches are expected during initial treatment but if continues, may decrease dosage or pretreat with NSAID. Do not chew or crush.
Pradaxa (Dabigatran etexilate)	Direct thrombin inhibitor	Competitive direct inhibition of thrombin (factor IIa), including thrombin-mediated platelet activation and aggregation.	Prevention of stroke/systemic embolism associated with nonvalvular atrial fibrillation. Contraindications: Severe renal impairment, hemodialysis, hypersensitivity, mechanical heart valves **Black-box warning:** Premature discontinuation of medication increases risk of thrombotic events. If receiving neuraxial anesthesia, epidural/spinal hematomas can occur.	If CrCl>30mL/min = 50 mg PO BID If CrCl 15–30mL/min = 75 mg PO BID If CrCl <5 mL/min = no data available	Bleeding, gastritis, angioedema, neutropenia	Monitor for any signs of bleeding, inform provider if an invasive or elective surgical procedure to be performed. See reversal information.

(continued)

| Eliquis (Apixaban) | Direct factor Xa inhibitors | Prevents factor Xa-mediated conversion of prothrombin to thrombin. | Prevention of stroke or blood clots associated with nonvalvular atrial fibrillation. Contraindications: Active pathological bleeding. See reversal information. Avoid abrupt discontinuation in absence if adequate alternative anticoagulation. **Black-box warning:** Premature discontinuation of medication increases risk of thrombotic events. If receiving neuraxial anesthesia, epidural/spinal hematomas can occur | 5 mg PO QD= nonvalvular atrial fibrillation Reduce dosage to 2.5 mg PO BID if Cr > .5 mg/dL, body weight < 60 kg or > 80 years of age | Nausea, easy bleeding, unusual bruising | Monitor for any signs of unusual bleeding, concomitant use of medications that affect hemostasis should be avoided. Medication should be discontinued 48 hours before any elective surgical procedure/invasive procedure. |
| Warfarin (Coumadin) | Vitamin K–dependent coagulation factor inhibitor | Interferes with clotting factor synthesis by inhibition of the C1 subunit of the Vitamin K epoxide enzyme complex. | Prophylaxis and treatment of thromboembolic disorders associated with Afib. Contraindicated in hemorrhagic tendencies, central nervous system surgery or traumatic surgeries. | Adjust dosage based on INR. Initial 2–5 mg daily, may increase to 10 mg. | Fever, rash, abd. Pain, hepatic disorders, tissue/organ hemorrhage. | Maintain strict adherence to dose regimen; notify provider of all OTC medications. Do not stop medication without consulting provider, carry ID card stating drug is being taken; avoid cranberry juice and large amounts of green leafy vegetables. |

ADP, adenosine diphosphate; Afib, atrial fibrillation; aPTT, activated partial thromboplastin time; ASA, acetylsalicylic acid; cAMP, cyclic adenosine monophosphate; ETOH, ethanol; GI, gastrointestinal; HTN, hypertension; ID, identification; INR, international normalized ratio; NSAIDs, nonsteroidal anti-inflammatory drugs; N&V, nausea and vomiting; OTC, over-the-counter; S&S, signs and symptoms; TIA, transient ischemic attack; TTP, thrombotic thrombocytopenia purpura.

- Hypotension and hypovolemia should be corrected to maintain systemic perfusion levels necessary to support organ function.
  - Temperature:
    - Sources of hyperthermia (temperature >38 °C) should be identified and treated.
    - Antipyretic medications should be administered to lower temperature in hyperthermic patients with stroke.
  - Glucose:
    - Hyperglycemia during the first 24 hour after AIS is associated with worse outcomes than normoglycemia and should be treated to achieve blood glucose levels in a range of 140 to 180 mg/dL and to closely monitor to prevent hypoglycemia.
    - Hypoglycemia (blood glucose <60 mg/dL) should be treated in patients with AIS.
  - Dysphagia screening:
    - Should be performed before oral intake.
    - Speech therapist involvement required for dysphagia screening and treatment.
  - Nutrition:
    - Enteral diet should be started within 7 days of admission after an acute stroke.
    - For patients with dysphagia, use nasogastric tubes for feeding in the early phase of stroke and place percutaneous gastrostomy tubes in patients with longer anticipated persistent inability to swallow safely (>2–3 weeks).
    - Nutritional supplements are reasonable to consider for patients who are malnourished or at risk of malnourishment.
    - Implementing oral hygiene protocols to reduce the risk of pneumonia after stroke may be reasonable.
  - Deep vein thrombosis prophylaxis:
    - In immobile stroke patients without contraindications, intermittent pneumatic compression (IPC) in addition to routine care (aspirin and hydration) is recommended.
    - In ischemic stroke, elastic compression stockings should not be used.
  - Depression screening:
    - Administration of a structure depression inventory is recommended to routinely screen for poststroke depression, but the optimal timing of screening is uncertain.
    - Patients diagnosed with poststroke depression should be treated with antidepressants in the absence of contraindications and closely monitored to verify effectiveness.
  - Rehabilitation:
    - It is recommended that early rehabilitation for hospitalized patients with stroke be provided in environments with organized, interprofessional stroke care.
    - A functional assessment by a clinician with expertise in rehabilitation is recommended for the patient with an acute stroke with residual functional deficits.
  - Seizures:
    - Recurrent seizures after stroke should be treated; antiseizure drugs should be selected based upon specific patient characteristics.
    - Prophylactic use of antiseizure drugs is not recommended.

Surgical Intervention
- Mechanical thrombectomy
- Carotid endarterectomy (CAE)
- Carotid angioplasty and stenting (CAS)
- Extracranial–intracranial (EC–IC) bypass
- Endovascular stenting
- Open vertebral artery endarterectomy and vertebral artery transposition (Table 14.13)

Therapeutic Lifestyle Changes
- Physical activity
- Diet management (Mediterranean type, low sodium, low-fat/low cholesterol)
- Weight reduction
- Smoking cessation
- Alcohol consumption (1/d for women, 2/d for men)

Complications
- Pneumonia
- Swallowing difficulty: aspiration
- Bowel and bladder problems
- Clinical depression
- Pressure injury
- Limb contractures or spasticity
- Deep vein thrombosis

Prognosis
- Leading cause of disability in the United States.
- Nearly half have residual deficits, including weakness or cognitive dysfunction 6 months after stroke.
- Stroke mortality varies by geographic location: Southeastern and Pacific Northwest highest.
- One out of four people will have another stroke within 5 years.

Characteristic Impairments of Right Hemisphere Syndrome
- *Perception and attention deficits, including the following:*
  - Left visual field neglect, impulsivity, distractibility, poor attention to tasks, excessive attention to irrelevant information, anosognosia: denial of deficits
- *Affective deficits*
  - Difficulty expressing emotion or recognizing emotions of others, depression, apparent lack of motivation
- *Communication deficits*
  - Word retrieval, impaired auditory comprehension, reading and writing problems, impaired prosodic features of speech (rhythm, tone, stress, intonation), dysarthria
- *Cognitive deficits*
  - Disorientation, decreased attention span, poor integration of information, problems with logic, reasoning, planning and problem solving, comprehension of inferred meanings

MOVEMENT/DEGENERATIVE DISEASE

AMYOTROPHIC LATERAL SCLEROSIS
Amyotrophic lateral sclerosis (ALS) is a progressive neurologic disease in which gradual deterioration and death of the neurons responsible for controlling voluntary muscle movement occur.

Symptoms
- Early symptoms of ALS usually include muscle weakness or stiffness that progresses to gradual loss of voluntary muscle control and strength along with loss ability to speak, eat, move, and even breath.

Treatment
- There is no cure for ALS, nor effective treatment to halt, or reverse, the progression of the disease (Table 14.14).

TABLE 14.13 HEMORRHAGIC STROKE REVERSAL AGENTS

ANTITHROMBOTIC	MECHANISM OF ACTION	REVERSAL AGENT	
Vitamin K antagonists (Warfarin)	Inhibits vitamin K–dependent γ carboxylation of coagulation factors II, VII, IX, and X, reducing activity of clotting factors.	If INF >1.4: vtamin K 10 mg IV, plus 3 or 4 factor PCC IV (dosing based on weight, INR, and PCC type) or FFP 10–15 mL/kg IV if PCC not available.	
Direct factor Xa inhibitors (Edoxaban)	Prevents factor Xa-mediated conversion of prothrombin to thrombin.	Activated charcoal (50 g) within 2 hours ingestion, activated PCC (FEIBA) 50 mcg/kg or 4 factor PCC 50 mcg/kg IV.	
Direct factor Xa inhibitors (Apixaban)	Prevents factor Xa-mediated conversion of prothrombin to thrombin.	**Last apixaban dose: >5 mg or unknown**	
		<8 HOURS PRIOR TO EVENT OR UNKNOWN	**≥8 HOURS PRIOR TO EVENT**
		High dose of andexanet alpha: Initial IV bolus: 800 mg at a target rate of 30 mg/min. Follow on IV infusion: 8 mg/min for up to 120 minutes.	**Low dose of andexanet alpha:** Initial IV bolus: 400 mg at a target rate of 30 mg/min. Follow on IV infusion: 4 mg/min for up to 120 minutes.
		Last dose of apixaban ≤5 mg **Low dose of andexanet alpha** Initial IV bolus: 400 mg at a target rate of 30 mg/min. Follow on IV infusion 4 mg/min for up to 120 minutes.	
Direct factor Xa inhibitors (Rivaroxaban)	Prevents factor Xa-mediated conversion of prothrombin to thrombin.	**10 mg rivaroxaban or unknown**	
		<8 HOURS PRIOR TO EVENT OR UNKNOWN	**≥8 HOURS PRIOR TO EVENT**
		High dose of andexanet alpha: Initial IV bolus: 800 mg at a target rate of 30 mg/min. Follow on IV infusion: 8 mg/min for up to 120 minutes.	**Low dose of andexanet alpha:** Initial IV bolus: 400 mg at a target rate of 30 mg/min. Follow on IV infusion: 4 mg/min for up to 120 minutes.
		≤10 mg rivaroxaban **Low dose of andexanet alpha:** Initial IV bolus: 400 mg at a target rate of 30 mg/min. Follow on IV infusion 4 mg/min for up to 120 minutes.	
Direct thrombin inhibitors (Dabigatran)	Competitive direct inhibition of thrombin (factor IIa), including thrombin-mediated platelet activation and aggregation.	If available: 5 g idarucizumab (Praxbind) and activate charcoal for known recent ingestion within 2–4 hours. Consider hemodialysis or idarucizumab (Praxbind) redosing for refractory bleeding after initial administration.	
Direct thrombin inhibitors (Argatroban, Bivalirudin)	Reversible direct inhibition of thrombin (factor IIa), including thrombin-mediated platelet activation and aggregation.	Activated PCC (FEIBA) 50 mcg/kg IV of 4 factor PCC 50 mcg/kg IV.	
Direct thrombin inhibitors (Desirudin, Lepirudin)	Irreversible direct inhibition of thrombin (factor IIa), including thrombin-mediated platelet activation and aggregation.	Activated PCC (FEIBA) 50 mcg/kg IV of 4 factor PCC 50 u/kg IV.	
Unfractionated heparin (heparin)	Binds and activates antithrombin (blocks coagulation factors Xa and IIa).	Protamine 1 mg IV for every 100 units of heparin administered within the previous 2–3 hours (up to 50 mg in a single dose).	
Low-molecular-weight heparin (Enoxaparin)	Binds and activates antithrombin (blocks coagulation factors Xa and IIa).	Dosed within 8 hours: protamine 1 mg IV per 1 mg enoxaparin (up to 50 mg in a single dose) Dosed within 8–12 hours: protamine 0.5 mg IV per 1 mg Enoxaparin (up to 50 mg in a single dose) Minimal reversal in >12 hours from dosing.	

(continued)

TABLE 14.13 HEMORRHAGIC STROKE REVERSAL AGENTS (continued)

ANTITHROMBOTIC	MECHANISM OF ACTION	REVERSAL AGENT
Heparinoids (Dalteparin, Nadroparin, Tinzaparin)	Binds and activates antithrombin (blocks coagulation factors Xa and IIa)	Dosed with 3–5 half-lives of LMWH: Protamine 1 mg IV per 100 anti-Xa units of LMWH (up to 50 mg in a single dose) or rFVII 90 mcg/kg IV if protamine is contraindicated
Danaparoid	Binds and activates antithrombin thereby blocking factors Xa and IIb).	rFVII 90 mcg/kg IV
Pentasaccharides (Fondaparinux)	Binds with antithrombin and potentiates inhibition of free factor Xa, prevents formation of prothrombinase complex.	Activated PCC(FEIBA) 20 mcg/kg IV of rFVII 90 mcg/kg IV
Thrombolytic agents (Alteplase, Reteplase, Tenecteplase)	Catalyzes conversion of fibrin-bound plasminogen to plasmin. Plasmin exerts further proteolytic effects, including dividing of platelet GPIIIa and GP1B causing platelet function inhibition.	Cryoprecipitate 10 units IV or antifibrinolytics (tranexamic acid 0–15 mg/kg IV over 20 minutes or ε-aminocaproic acid 4–5 g IV) if cryoprecipitate is contraindicated
Antiplatelets		
Aspirin	Irreversible cyclooxygenase-1 and -2 enzyme inhibitor	Desmopressin 0.4 mcg/kg IV × 1. If neurosurgical intervention: Platelet transfusion (one pheresis unit)
Ibuprofen, naproxen	Reversible COX-1 and -2 enzyme inhibitor	Desmopressin 0.4 mcg/kg IV × 1. If neurosurgical intervention: Platelet transfusion (one pheresis unit)
Dipyridamole	Reversible adenosine reuptake inhibitor	Desmopressin 0.4 mcg/kg IV × 1. If neurosurgical intervention: Platelet transfusion (one pheresis unit)
Clopidogrel, prasugrel, ticlopidine	Irreversible inhibition of P2Y12 ADP receptor	Desmopressin 0.4 mcg/kg IV × 1. If neurosurgical intervention: Platelet transfusion (one pheresis unit)
Ticagrelor	Reverse inhibition of P2Y12 ADP receptor	Desmopressin 0.4 mcg/kg IV × 1. If neurosurgical intervention: Platelet transfusion (one pheresis unit)
Cilostazol	Reversible phosphodiesterase III inhibitor increases cAMP, induces platelet aggregation, causing vasodilation	Desmopressin 0.4 mcg/kg IV × 1. If neurosurgical intervention: Platelet transfusion (one pheresis unit)
Anagrelide	Reversible phosphodiesterase III inhibitor inhibits megakaryocyte formation	Desmopressin 0.4 mcg/kg IV × 1. If neurosurgical intervention: Platelet transfusion (one pheresis unit)
Abciximab	Irreversible glycoprotein IIB/IIIA antagonist	Desmopressin 0.4 mcg/kg IV × 1. If neurosurgical intervention: Platelet transfusion (one pheresis unit)
Eptifibatide, tirofiban,	Reversible glycoprotein IIB/IIIA antagonist	Desmopressin 0.4 mcg/kg IV × 1. If neurosurgical intervention: Platelet transfusion (one pheresis unit)
Vorapaxar	Reversible protease-activated receptor -1 thrombin receptor antagonist	Desmopressin 0.4 mcg/kg IV × 1. If neurosurgical intervention: Platelet transfusion (one pheresis unit)

ADP, adenosine diphosphate; cAMP, cyclic adenosine monophosphate; COX, cyclooxygenase isoenzyme; FFP, fresh frozen plasma; HR, heart rate; INF, intrinsic factor; IV, intravenous; LMWH, low-molecular-weight heparin; PCC, prothrombin complex concentrate.

TABLE 14.14 AMYOTROPHIC LATERAL SCLEROSIS: PHARMACOLOGIC TREATMENT

MEDICATION	CLASS	MECHANISM OF ACTION	INDICATIONS/ CONTRAINDICATIONS	DOSAGE	SIDE EFFECTS	SAFETY/ PATIENT EDUCATION
Riluzole (Rilutek)	Glutamate antagonist, benzothiozole	Unknown, thought to inhibit glutamate release.	Does not cure disease or improve symptoms but may prolong survival by 3 months; slows progression. Contraindicated in patients with known hypersensitivity to Riluzole or any of its components, known elevation of liver enzymes.	50–100 mg PO BID	H/a, nausea, drowsiness, asthesia, hypertension, pancreatitis	Call provider for any sign of febrile illness, assess for renal impairment, perform baseline LFTs.

H/a, headache; LFT, liver function test; PO, per os.

- Supportive care provided by multidisciplinary healthcare professionals can design individualized treatment plans and provide special equipment aimed at keeping people as mobile, comfortable, and independent as possible.
- The U.S. Food and Drug Administration (FDA)–approved medications are aimed to reduce damage to motor neurons by decreasing levels of glutamate.

Prognosis

- Death due to respiratory failure occurs within 3 to 5 years from onset of symptoms.
- Ten percent of people with ALS survive for 10 or more years (National Institute of Neurological Disorders and Stroke, 2019).

GUILLAIN-BARRÉ SYNDROME

Guillain-Barré syndrome (GBS) is an immune-activated demyelination disorder that affects the peripheral nervous system.

Incidence

- One in 100,000 individuals will be affected each year.
- Affects more men than women and can strike at any age (although it is more frequent in adults and older people).
- Rate of recovery is high (75%–85%); 10% will have residual effects, and 5% will die from this condition.
- More than 80% will be unable to ambulate during the illness (Cash & Glass, 2019).

Symptoms

- Onset is 2 weeks following a respiratory or gastrointestinal (GI) viral infection. Symptoms range from very mild brief weakness to devastating paralysis, with dependence on mechanical ventilation.
- Symptoms begin with unexplained sensations such tingling in hands and feet. Weakness increases, most often in an ascending manner.
  - Facial muscle weakness affecting vision and eye muscles, swallowing, speaking, or chewing.
  - Motor difficulty affecting coordination and balance, painful sensations in hands and feet (especially at night).
  - Autonomic changes affecting heart rate or BP, digestion, and/or bladder control.

Diagnosis

Recent illness with onset of symptoms ~2 weeks, abnormal sensations, absent or diminished deep tendon reflexes, elevated CSF proteins, abnormal nerve conduction velocity.

Treatment

There is no cure for GBS, only supportive therapies such as plasma exchange (plasmapheresis) and high-dose intravenous immunoglobulin therapy (IVIg; Yuki & Hartung, 2012). However, GBS is reversible, and 70% to 80% make a full recovery.

MULTIPLE SCLEROSIS

Multiple sclerosis (MS) is the most common immune-mediated inflammatory demyelinating disease of the central nervous system—the brain, spinal cord, and optic nerves—and is a leading cause of disability in young adults.

- Immune-mediated responses due to infection or genetic or environmental factors trigger inflammation that damages myelin—the fatty substance that surrounds and insulates the nerve fibers—as well as the nerve fibers themselves and the specialized cells that make myelin.
- Damaged or destroyed myelin or nerve fibers alter or stop messages within the central nervous system.
- Damaged areas develop scar tissue giving the disease its name—multiple areas of scarring, or MS.

Etiology

- The etiology of MS is unknown but is believed to be multifactorial; it results in abnormal immune response to some infectious or environmental trigger in a genetically susceptible individual. Each of these factors—immunologic, environmental, infectious, and genetic—is the subject of intensive ongoing research.
- Progression to disability over the first decade may be influenced by several factors.
  - *Gender:* MS affects more women than men (3:1). Men are more likely to have a progressive or malignant clinical course (Zaffaroni & Ghezzi, 2000).
  - *Race:* African Americans have a more rapidly progressive disease course (Kister et al., 2010).
  - *Pregnancy:* MS relapse rates decrease by ~70% in the third trimester of pregnancy. The risk of exacerbation increases following delivery of the baby. These observations suggest hormonal factors figure prominently in the mechanisms of immune modulation and the ultimate expression of MS.
- Ten years after diagnosis, 50% require ambulatory aids, and 15% require a wheelchair.
  - Approximately half of patients convert to the secondary progressive phase of the disease, where there is acceleration of disability and a paucity of effective therapy (Zaffaroni & Ghezzi, 2000).

Prognosis

Several factors affect prognosis of MS (Table 14.15).

Types of Multiple Sclerosis

- There are four disease courses (types of MS) with at least a dozen treatments to help modify the MS disease process.
  - *Clinical isolated syndrome (CIS)*: Criteria include first episode of neurologic symptoms lasting at least 24 hours with symptoms characteristic of MS but not yet meeting the criteria for a diagnosis of MS.

TABLE 14.15 FACTORS AFFECTING PROGNOSIS AND OUTCOMES OF MULTIPLE SCLEROSIS

FACTOR	FAVORABLE PROGNOSIS	UNFAVORABLE PROGNOSIS
Gender	Female	Male
Annual relapse rate	Low rate	High
Recovery after first attack	Complete	Incomplete
Symptom source	Afferent/sensory	Efferent/motor
Age of onset	Younger	Older
Disability at 2–5 years	Low	Significant
Onset of cerebellar involvement	Later	Early
Number of involved	One	More than one

Source: Adapted from Mowry, E. M. (2011). Natural history of multiple sclerosis: Early prognostic factors. *Neurologic Clinics, 29*(2), 279–292.

TABLE 14.16 FIRST- AND SECOND-LINE MEDICATION TREATMENT OF MULTIPLE SCLEROSIS

DRUG FORM	FIRST-LINE THERAPY	SECOND-LINE THERAPY
Injectable	*Interferon beta-1a* (Avonex, Betaseron, Extavia, Rebif) *Glatiramer acetate* (Copaxone) *Perinterferon beta-1a* (Plegridy)	*Alemtuzumab* (Lemtrada) *Mitoxantrone* (Novantrone) *Rituximab* (Rituxan): off label *Natalizumab* (Tysabri) Short-term steroid use: 3–5 days course of methylprednisolone or dexamethasone
Oral	*Teriflunomide* (Aubagio), *Dimethyl fumarate* (Tecfidera)	*Fingolimod* (Gilenya)

Source: Adapted from Cash, J. C., & Waltrip, K. D. (2019). Multiple sclerosis. In J. C. Cash & C. A. Glass (Eds.), *Adult-gerontology clinical practice guidelines* (pp. 689–693). Springer Publishing Company.

- *Relapse remitting (RRMS)* is found in 85% of all MS patients and is characterized by clearly defined attacks of new or increasing neurologic symptoms.
- *Secondary progressive (SPMS):* SPMS follows an initial relapsing–remitting course.
- *Primary progressive (PPMS)*: PPMS is characterized by worsening neurologic function (accumulation of disability) from the onset of symptoms, without early relapses or remissions.
- *Progressive relapsing*: steady decline since onset with superimposed attacks (National Multiple Sclerosis Society, n.d.).

Treatment

- MS is not a curable disease. Effective strategies can help modify or slow the disease course, treat relapses, manage symptoms, improve function and safety, and address emotional health.
- The U.S. FDA has approved disease-modifying medications to treat different forms of MS (Table 14.16).
  - These medications reduce the frequency and severity of relapses (also called attacks or exacerbations), reduce the accumulation of lesions in the brain and spinal cord as seen on MRI, and may slow the accumulation of disability for many people with MS (Capriotti et al., 2018; Cash & Waltrip, 2019).
  - Medications are prescribed specifically for the types of MS and may include a combination of therapies (Tables 14.17 to 14.19).

PARKINSON'S DISEASE

- Parkinson's disease (PD) is a progressive, neurodegenerative disorder affecting movement, muscle control, and balance as well as numerous other functions.
- PD is the most common movement disorder and the second most common neurodegenerative disorder, next to Alzheimer's disease.

- PD can significantly impair quality of life, not only for the patients but for their families and especially for the primary caregivers.

Pathophysiology and Associated Symptoms

- The hallmark symptoms of PD are asymmetric tremors at rest, rigidity, and bradykinesia (slowness in movement).
  - Clinical motor features may not present until approximately 50% to 80% of dopaminergic neurons are lost, making diagnosis challenging.
  - Motor symptoms are attributed to the loss of striatal dopaminergic neurons.
  - The presence of nonmotor symptoms supports neuronal loss in nondopaminergic areas.

Contributing Factors

- Contributing factors include hereditary traits, Lewy bodies, trauma, arteriosclerosis, toxins, and medications such as phenothiazine (Cash, 2019, p. 699).

Types of Parkinson's Disease

There are three types of PD grouped by age of onset (Table 14.20).

Prognosis

- There is no cure for PD; it is always chronic and progressive.
  - The rate of progression varies and symptom intensity varies from person to person.
  - PD is not a fatal disease; the mortality of PD patients is usually due to secondary complications, such as pneumonia or fall-related injuries.

Treatment

- Patients are always comanaged with a primary physician and a neurologist.

Medications

Polypharmacy is the hallmark of PD rather than the exception. Lowering dosage of multiple medications is a goal rather than using high doses of a single medication, thus minimizing side effects. Tapering of drug doses is imperative (Cash, 2019; Tables 14.21–14.25).

- First-line therapy: Levodopa
  - Second-line therapy
  - Dopamine agonists (Mirapex, Requip)
  - Ergot derivatives in combination with Levodopa (Parlodel, Permax)
    - Nonergot preferred due to fewer side effects (Mirapex)

SEIZURE DISORDERS/EPILEPSY

EPILEPSY

Epilepsy is a functional disorder of the brain in which neurons signal abnormally; unfortunately, in most clients the exact cause is unknown. It is the fourth most common neurologic disease and affects all ages. Seniors are the most rapid population developing this comorbidity (Table 14.26; Cash & Glass, 2019).

Diagnosis

Epilepsy is defined as at least two unprovoked (or reflex) seizures occurring more than 24 hours apart, or one unprovoked or reflex seizure. There is a probability of further seizures after two unprovoked seizures.

TABLE 14.17 MULTIPLE SCLEROSIS—INJECTABLE MEDICATIONS

MEDICATION	CLASS	MECHANISM OF ACTION	INDICATIONS/CONTRAINDICATIONS	DOSAGE	SIDE EFFECTS	SAFETY/PATIENT EDUCATION
Beta interferons (Avonex, Rebif, Betaseron/Extavia Plegridy)	Interferons	Enhances suppressor T cells, decreases release of metalloproteinases and proinflammatory enzymes	Indicated for relapsing form of MS. Contraindicated in patients with known hypersensitivity to albumin.	Avonex: 30 mcg IM every week. Rebif: Initials: 20% of prescribed dose SQ 3×/week. Titrate: Increase over a 4-week period to either 22 mcg or 44 mcg SQ 3 × week. Betaseron/Extavia: .25 mcg SQ QOD, Titrate over 6 weeks. Plegridy: Start treatment with 63 micrograms on day 1. On day 15 increase dose to 94 micrograms, on day 29 increase to full dose of 125 micrograms; continue with the full dose (125 micrograms) every 14 days thereafter	Injections site inflammation, flu-like symptoms, fatigue, depression/suicide.	Psychiatric disorders, injection site reaction, influenza-like symptoms, depression. Monitor LFTs, CBC, thyroid function, report any adverse reactions to MD.
Glatiramer acetate (Copaxone)	Immuno-modulatory agent	Synthetic polypeptides bind to MHC as a decoy for myelin proteins causing shifting immune response.	Indicated for relapsing–remitting forms of MS. Contraindicated in hypersensitivity to mannitol.	20 mg SQ daily and new 40-mg SQ dosing 3 ×/week.	Injections site inflammation, flu-like symptoms, fatigue, depression/suicide	Educate on self-injection techniques, rotate sites weekly.

CBC, complete blood count; IM; LFT, liver function test; MHC; MS, multiple sclerosis; SQ, subcutaneous.

TABLE 14.18 MULTIPLE SCLEROSIS—ORAL MEDICATIONS

MEDICATION	CLASS	MECHANISM OF ACTION	INDICATIONS/CONTRAINDICATIONS	DOSAGE	SIDE EFFECTS	SAFETY/PATIENT EDUCATION
DMF, Tecfidera	Anti-inflammatory, induces nuclear 1 factor	Unclear, neuroprotective properties, immunomodulating	Indicated for relapsing MS Contraindicated in immunocompromised patients, caution with hepatic patients	120 mg PO BID, increase to 240 PO BID after 7 days	Flushing, diarrhea, nausea, upset stomach	Drug may increase lymphocyte counts. Obtain CBC prior to induction of therapy, observe for worsening signs of neurologic status as PML can occur.
Fingolimod (Gilenya)	Sphingosine 1- phosphate receptor modulator	Fingolimod-phosphate blocks the capacity of lymphocytes to egress from lymph nodes, reducing the number of lymphocytes in peripheral blood	Indicated for relapsing MS and reduces frequency of exacerbations Contraindicated in those with heart blocks, alcoholism, angina, CAD, heart failure, QT prolongation. Patients with acute active or chronic infections should wait till clear before starting medication	0.5 mg PO daily.	Headache, diarrhea, elevated LFTs, fatigue, cough, HTN, bradyarrhythmia, AV blocks	Before starting, check CBC, LFT, EKG; perform eye exam and again in 4 months.

(continued)

TABLE 14.18 MULTIPLE SCLEROSIS—ORAL MEDICATIONS (continued)

MEDICATION	CLASS	MECHANISM OF ACTION	INDICATIONS/CONTRAINDICATIONS	DOSAGE	SIDE EFFECTS	SAFETY/PATIENT EDUCATION
Teriflunomide (Aubagio)	Pyrimidine synthesis inhibitors	Inhibits the de novo pyrimidine synthesis need for proliferation of lymphocytes	Indicated for those with relapsing forms of MS Contraindicated in those with severe hepatic disease	7–14 mg daily.	Diarrhea, nausea, hair thinning, renal failure, elevated ALT. May cause immunosuppression	Category X drug (contraceptive requirements for male and females), peripheral neuropathy may occur, risk of hypersensitivity or anaphylaxis.

ALT, alanine aminotransferase; AV, atrioventricular; CAD, coronary artery disease; CBC, complete blood count; DMF, dimethyl fumarate; HTN, hypertension; LFT, liver function test; MS, multiple sclerosis; PML, progressive multifocal leukoencephalopathy.

TABLE 14.19 MULTIPLE SCLEROSIS—INFUSION MEDICATIONS

MEDICATION	CLASS	MECHANISM OF ACTION	INDICATIONS/CONTRAINDICATIONS	DOSAGE	SIDE EFFECTS	SAFETY/PATIENT EDUCATION
Natalizumab (Tysabri)	Monoclonal IgG4k antibody	Prevents inflammatory events by inhibiting a4-integrin	Treatment of relapsing MS Contraindicated in pregnancy, patients who have or have had PML	300-mg infusion every 4 weeks	Increases risk of PML, hepatotoxicity, immunosuppression, h/a, fatigue, and muscle pain.	**Increased risk of infections, including herpes, PML,** infusion reactions, fatigue Check MRI every 6 months for PML surveillance. Patients must enter registry program while on medication.
Alemtuzumab (Lemtrada)	Humanized monoclonal antibody	Rapidly depletes the B&T lymphocytes	Treatment of relapsing MS **Restricted distribution is** contraindicated in patients with immunosuppression, autoimmune disease, ITP, leukopenia. Severe opportunistic infections may occur on treatment	Baseline monitoring before infusion, premedicate with high-dose steroids before infusion. 12 mg/d × 5 consecutive days (60 mg dose). Second treatment course 12 mg/d × 3 consecutive days (36 mg dose 12 months after first treatment course).	ITP, increased risk of malignancies, stroke, anti-glomerular basement membrane disease, infusion reactions, rash, h/a, fever.	Monthly monitoring program and continues 4 years after treatment. Monitor CBC, BUN/creatinine, and UA. Monitor patient in a setting with appropriate equipment to manage anaphylactic reaction and monitor 2 hours after infusion completion. Monitor for S&S of stroke during infusion.

BUN, blood urea nitrogen; CBC, complete blood count; h/a, headache; ITP, immune thrombocytopenia; MS, multiple sclerosis; PML, progressive multifocal leukoencephalopathy; S&S, signs and symptoms; UA, urinalysis.

TABLE 14.20 AGE OF ONSET OF PARKINSON'S DISEASE BY TYPE

TYPE	ADULT ONSET	YOUNG ONSET	JUVENILE ONSET
Age of onset	Average 60 years	21–40 years	Prior to age 21 years

Signs and Symptoms

- Aura, typically epigastric discomfort, fear, or unpleasant smells
- Automatic movements such as swallowing, chewing, fumbling, picking clothes, or lip smacking
- Stiffening, followed by jerking of limbs
- Staring, may or may not include repetitive movements

TABLE 14.21 PARKINSON'S DISEASE: PHARMACOLOGIC TREATMENT—DOPAMINERGICS

MEDICATION	CLASS	MECHANISM OF ACTION	INDICATIONS/ CONTRAINDICATIONS	DOSAGE	SIDE EFFECTS	SAFETY/PATIENT EDUCATION
Levodopa: Carbidopa (Sinemet)	Dopaminergic	Levodopa: Rapidly decarboxylated to dopamine in extra cerebral tissue. Carbidopa: Allows greater concentration of levodopa to reach brain.	Treatment of symptoms related to Parkinsons Contraindicated in patients with use of MAOIs within 14 days of use, narrow angle glaucoma, history of melanoma.	Initial: 100 mg levodopa/25 mg carbidopa TID. Increase by 1 tablet q24–48h. Maximum: 200/2,000 mg/d.	Dyskinesias, nausea, cardiac irregularities, hypotension, confusion, agitation.	Monitor LFTs, discoloration of body fluids may occur, do not chew or crush medicine. Monitor amount of protein consumed as it affects absorption.

LFT, liver function test; MAOI, monoamine oxidase inhibitor.

TABLE 14.22 PARKINSON'S DISEASE: PHARMACOLOGIC TREATMENT—DOPAMINE AGONISTS

MEDICATION	CLASS	MECHANISM OF ACTION	INDICATIONS/ CONTRAINDICATIONS	DOSAGE	SIDE EFFECTS	SAFETY/PATIENT EDUCATION
Bromocriptine (Parlodel)	Dopamine agonists	Activates postsynaptic dopamine receptors and modulates	Treatment of symptoms related to Parkinson's Contraindicated in uncontrolled HTN, postpartum with CVD	1.25–2.5 mg PO daily. May increase by 2.5–5 mg on alternate days. Maintenance: 2.5–100 mg PO daily in divided doses. Not to exceed 300 mg/d.	H/a, dizziness, GI effects, orthostatic hypotension, fatigue, arrhythmias	Monitor for somnolence, sudden sleep onset, confusion, seizures; *monitor BP*, prolactin, and LFTs.
Pergolide (Permax)	Dopamine agonists	Directly stimulates dopamine receptor cells in corpus striatum	Treatment of symptoms related to Parkinson's Can be used as a monotherapy/adjunct Use cautiously in patients with CVD	0.05 mg PO daily initially. May increase by 0.01–0.5 PO every third day over 2 weeks. Then increase by 0.25 mg every third day until response obtained. Total dosage 3 mg/24 hours in divided doses.	Nausea, hallucinations, dyskinesia, sedation and postural hypotension.	*Monitor BP*; sudden withdrawal may cause confusion, paranoid thinking, and severe hallucinations.
Ropinirole (Requip)	Dopamine agonists (nonergoline)	Stimulates the postsynaptic D$_2$-type receptors within caudate:putamen.	Treatment of symptoms related to Parkinson's	0.25 PO TID, increase weekly to 1 mg TID.	Neuralgia, increased BUN, hallucinations, somnolence, h/a, vomiting syncope.	Perform dermatologic screening periodically. Monitor eye exams, impulse control. *Monitor BP*, LFT, and renal functions. Use extreme caution while performing tasks, for example, driving.
Pramipexole (Mirapex)	Dopamine agonists (nonergot)	Stimulates dopamine receptors on the striatum.	Treatment of symptoms related to Parkinson's Contraindicated in pregnancy and acute history of PID	0.125 mg TID. Increase weekly by 0.5 mg TID.	Nausea, dizziness, somnolence, insomnia, constipation, visual abnormalities.	*Monitor BP*, renal functions, counsel on impulse control.

BP, blood pressure; BUN, blood urea nitrogen ; CVD, cardiovascular disease; GI, gastrointestinal; h/a, headache; HTN, hypertension; LFT, liver function test; PID, pelvic inflammatory disease.

TABLE 14.23 PARKINSON'S DISEASE: PHARMACOLOGIC TREATMENT—ANTICHOLINERGICS

MEDICATION	CLASS	MECHANISM OF ACTION	INDICATIONS/CONTRAINDICATIONS	DOSAGE	SIDE EFFECTS	SAFETY/PATIENT EDUCATION
Benztropine (Cogentin)	Anticholinergics	Selective inhibition of dopamine transporters, also has affinity for muscarine and histamine receptors.	Adjunct of all forms of parkinsonism Contraindicated in patients with hypersensitivity, acute glaucoma, chronic lung disease, acute/chronic kidney, cardia, liver disease.	1–2 mg PO daily. Range: 0.5–6 mg daily	Drowsiness, confusion, dizziness, loss of appetite, vision changes, dry mouth	Call for any signs of allergic reaction, tachycardia, Limited use in those >70 years of age. Can have additive/antagonistic effects with other Parkinson's drugs and anticholinergics.
Trihexyphenidyl (Artane)	Antispasmodic, anticholinergic	Blocks cholinergic activity in the central nervous system and increases availability of dopamine.	All forms of Parkinsonism Contraindicated in patients with hypersensitivity, acute glaucoma, chronic lung disease, acute/chronic kidney, cardia, liver disease.	1–2 mg on first day. Increase by 2 mg every 3–5 days. Maintenance: 5–15 mg PO daily in divided doses.	H/a, nervousness, dizziness, weakness, tachycardia, dry mouth.	May cause urinary retention in men with BPH.

BPH, benign prostatic hyperplasia; h/a, headache.

TABLE 14.24 PARKINSON'S DISEASE: PHARMACOLOGIC TREATMENT—MONOAMINE OXIDASE B INHIBITORS

MEDICATION	CLASS	MECHANISM OF ACTION	INDICATIONS/CONTRAINDICATIONS	DOSAGE	SIDE EFFECTS	SAFETY/PATIENT EDUCATION
Selegiline (Eldepryl)	MAOI inhibitor (type B)	Increases dopaminergic activity by blocking the breakdown of dopamine.	Adjunct to levodopa/carbidopa for management of Parkinson's. Concomitant use of Meperidine or other opioids.	5 mg BID. maximum: 0 mg daily. May reduce levodopa/carbidopa by 10%–30% after 2–3 days of therapy.	Nausea, dizziness, fainting, abdominal pain, confusion	Monitor for hypersensitivity reactions, myoclonic jerks, assess BP/HR. Avoid tyramine-containing foods and beverages.
Rasagiline (Agilect, Zelapar)	MAOI inhibitor (type B)	Blocks catabolism of dopamine and increases net amount of dopamine available.	Monotherapy in primary treatment of Parkinson's, adjunct to levodopa/carbidopa in later stages of Parkinson's. Concomitant use of meperidine or other opioids/MAOIs.	1.25 mg daily × 6 weeks. Titrate after 6 weeks. Maximum: 2.5 mg/d.	Nausea, dizziness, fainting, abdominal pain, confusion as a monotherapy. When used with levodopa—dyskinesias, GI symptoms, h/a, weight loss, orthostasis.	May have hypertensive crisis if tyramine foods ingested. Monitor for behavioral/mental status changes.

BP, blood pressure; GI, gastrointestinal; h/a, headache; HR, heart rate; MAOI, monoamine oxidase inhibitors.

TABLE 14.25 PARKINSON'S DISEASE: PHARMACOLOGIC TREATMENT—CATECHOL-O-METHYLTRANSFERASE INHIBITORS

MEDICATION	CLASS	MECHANISM OF ACTION	INDICATIONS/ CONTRAINDICATIONS	DOSAGE	SIDE EFFECTS	SAFETY/ PATIENT EDUCATION
Entacapone (Comtan)	COMT inhibitor	Selectively and reversibly inhibits COMT, increasing levodopa levels.	Adjunct to levodopa/carbidopa for Parkinson's specific to "wearing off" phenomenon.	200 mg with each levodopa/carbidopa dose. Maximum: 1,600 mg daily. Withdraw slowly for DC.	Sweating, back pain, dyskinesia, hyperkinesia, nausea, diarrhea, urine discoloration.	Monitor BP, LFTs, renal function. Monitor BP and assess for dyskinesias, hypotension.
Tolcapone (Tasmar)	COMT inhibitor	Alters plasma pharmacokinetics of levodopa, leading to more sustained levels of drug in system.	Adjunct to levodopa/carbidopa for Parkinson's. Patient must have significant fluctuations of symptoms unresponsive to other therapies. Contraindicated in patients with known liver disease.	Initial: 100 mg PO TID. Use 200 mg TID only if clinical benefit. May need to decrease levodopa dose.	Dyskinesia, nausea, dystonia, sweating, fatigue, urine discoloration, orthostatic complaints.	**Risk of fatal/acute/fulminant liver failure.** Monitor LFTs, renal functions tests, avoid ETOH, OTC agents, and central nervous system depressants.

BP, blood pressure; COMT, catechol-o-methyl transferase; DC, discontinue; ETOH, ethanol; LFT, liver function test; OTC, over-the-counter.

TABLE 14.26 PREDISPOSING FACTORS AND RISK FACTORS FOR EPILEPSY

Predisposing factors	Tumors, alcohol or drug use, stroke, hypoglycemia, Alzheimer's disease, head trauma, surgery, pregnancy (eclampsia), febrile illness, photosensitivity, hormone fluctuation, stress, obstructive sleep apnea, sleep deprivation
Risk factors for reoccurrence	Brain disease, mental retardation, abnormal neurologic exam/EEG, seizure onset after 10 years of age, multiple seizure types, family history, missed or poor response to AEDs, chronic alcoholism

AEDs, antiepileptic drugs.

- Eclampsia
- Does not remember seizure, impaired consciousness
- *Postictal (after seizure)*: Confusion, amnesia, fatigue, headaches, loss of bladder or bowel control

Diagnostic Testing
- Patient history, witness accounts/neurologic examination.
- *Labs*: Glucose, drug/alcohol screen, anticonvulsant levels, lumbar puncture if indicated for signs of infection (Mayo Clinic, 2019).
- *EEG*: The most common test used to diagnose epilepsy. With epilepsy, it is common to have changes in normal brain wave patterns, even when there is not a seizure (Mayo Clinic, 2019).
- *vEEG (video EEG)*: Video monitoring with continuous EEG recording, both awake and asleep.

- *MRI*: The gold standard for neuroimaging; more accurate than CT.

Key criteria for seizure classification include the following:
- Which brain structure triggered the onset of the seizure
- Person's level of awareness during seizure
- Symptoms accompanying the seizure
  - The most noticeable feature at the onset of the seizure should be used to determine seizure type and subtype.
  - Individuals may have symptoms that start as one subtype and then progress to another type.

Unknown-onset seizures are events that are motor or non-motor but cannot be clearly classified as focal or generalized types because the originating brain structure is not known. After careful history and diagnostic testing to clarify onset, the seizure type is changed to the appropriate classification.

Focal-onset seizures occur in one area of the brain (Table 14.27).

Generalized seizures occur in both sides of the brain at the onset of the event. This seizure type differs from those that progress from focal onset. Most generalized seizures include a degree of unawareness (Table 14.28).

STATUS EPILEPTICUS
Status epilepticus (SE) is a medical emergency occurring when a generalized motor or focal-onset seizure lasts longer than a set period and/or when there is no recovery of consciousness between two or more consecutive seizures. The time is defined in two intervals. Time (t1) indicates the time treatment should be initialized after seizure onset, and time (t2) indicates the duration of continuous seizure activity that may result in unfavorable neurologic outcomes (Table 14.29). Prolonged seizure activity without initial treatment may rapidly lead to adverse neurologic outcomes and may result in permanent damage to neurons.

TABLE 14.27 TYPES OF FOCAL-ONSET SEIZURES

SEIZURE CLASSIFICATION	CLASSIFICATION SUBTYPE	LOC/MOTOR SYMPTOMS
Focal-onset seizure	*FAS—* Previously known as *simple partial*	**LOC:** Awareness intact, able to interact, may not be able to speak; may include blank stare. Aura may be present. Last <2 minutes. **Motor:** May be unable to move.
	*FIAS—*Previously known as *complex partial*	**LOC:** Aura may be present. Impaired awareness during seizure; can have appearance of daydreaming; may have some or no recall post seizure. May have repetitive speech or exhibit emotional behavioral outburst. Seizures may occur at night while asleep. **Motor:** May include automatism (picking at clothes, air); abrupt movements. Can lead to generalized seizure.
	FMS	**LOC:** Includes focal impaired symptoms with motor. **Motor:** Jerking (clonic), tense or rigid (tonic), limp or weak (atonic), brief muscle twitching (myoclonus), may have automatisms rubbing hands, lip smacking, chewing or running; or repeated automatic movements such as clapping.
	FNMS	**LOC:** Changes in emotions, sensations, or feelings. *Cognitive seizure:* Delusions, hallucination, or distorted perception; May be aphasic or unable to recognize individuals. May include aggression. *Emotional seizures:* Anxious, fearful, tearful, joyful; emotions inconsistent with setting when individual would normally react appropriately. **Motor:** No movements involved; however, may experience changes in autonomic functions such as heartburn, surge of heat or cold, heart rate racing.
	Focal to bilateral tonic clonic seizure	**LOC/other:** Starts as focal aware or focal impaired. May be confused, crying, groaning. There is loss of consciousness/impaired breathing; loss of bowel or bladder function (clonic phases). **Motor:** Collapses or falls to floor; bilateral stiffening tonic jerking movements or face, arms, legs, repetitive flexing and relaxing (tonic phase).

FAS, focal awareness seizure; FIAS, focal impaired or unknown awareness seizure; FMS, focal motor seizure; FNMS, focal nonmotor seizure; LOC, level of consciousness.

TABLE 14.28 TYPES OF GENERALIZED SEIZURES

SEIZURE CLASSIFICATION	CLASSIFICATION SUBTYPE	SYMPTOMS
Generalized	Motor	**Tonic** clonic: Stiffening followed by jerking movement **Clonic:** Repeated jerking movements (contraction followed by relaxation) without the ability to stop if restrained **Tonic:** Stiffening Myoclonic Myoclonic–tonic–clonic Myoclonic–atonic **Atonic:** Sudden loss of muscular tone Epileptic spasms
	Nonmotor	Typical Atypical Myoclonic Eyelid myoclonia

TABLE 14.29 STATUS EPILEPTICUS TREATMENT

SEIZURE TYPE IN SE	TREATMENT INITIATION (T1)	TIME RISK OF UNFAVORABLE OUTCOMES (T2)
Tonic clonic	5 minutes	30 minutes
Focal impaired	10 minutes	>60 minutes
Absence	10–15 minutes	Time unknown

SE, status epilepticus.

SE requires prompt recognition with immediate and emergent medical treatment with appropriate benzodiazepines (Table 14.30). Antiepileptic drugs or medications that provide anesthesia may be necessary to cause cessation of SE. Admission to the ICU for continued monitoring, workup, and care is essential. As with all seizures, determine underlying causes for SE and correct treatable conditions.

SEIZURE TYPES AND PHARMACEUTICAL TREATMENT

PHARMACOLOGICAL TREATMENT

See Tables 14.31 and 14.32 for information on antiepileptic medications.

Other Treatments
- Vagus nerve stimulation (VNS)
- Responsiveness neurostimulation (RNS)
- External trigeminal nerve stimulation (eTNS)
- Ketogenic diet (Fisher et al., 2017)

Other Nervous System Pharmacologic Agents
For other nervous system pharmacologic agents, see Tables 14.33–14.37.

TABLE 14.30 PHARMACEUTICAL TREATMENT

SEIZURE TYPE	FIRST LINE	ADJUNCTIVE
Generalized tonic–clonic	Carbamazepine (Carbatrol), Lamotrigine (Lamictal): **Requires monitoring for Steven-Johnson syndrome** Oxcarbazepine Sodium valproate*	Clobazam (Onfi) Lamotrigine (Lamictal): **Requires monitoring for Steven-Johnson syndrome** Levetiracetam (Keppra, Spritam) Sodium valproate Topiramate (Topamax. Quedxy XR)
Tonic or atonic	Sodium valproate*	Lamotrigine (Lamictal): **Requires monitoring for Steven-Johnson syndrome**
Absence	Ethosuximide (Zarontin), Lamotrigine (Lamictal): **Requires monitoring for Steven-Johnson syndrome** Gabapentin (Neurontin, Gralise), Lacosamide (Vimpat), Sodium valproate	Clonazepam (Klonopin) Clobazam (Onfi) Clorazepate (Tranxene-T) Sodium valproate Levetiracetam (Keppra, Spritam), Phenytoin (Dilantin, Phenytek), Pregabalin (Lyrica), Tiagabine Vigabatrin
Myoclonic	Levetiracetam (Keppra, Spritam) Sodium valproate* Topiramate (Topamax. Qudexy XR)	Levetiracetam (Keppra, Spritam) Sodium valproate Topiramate (Topamax, Quedxy XR), Clobazam (Onfi) Gabapentin (Neurontin, Gralise)
Focal	Oxcarbazepine (Trileptal, Oxtellar XR), Carbamazepine (Carbatrol), Lamotrigine (Lamictal): **Requires monitoring for Steven-Johnson syndrome** Levetiracetam (Keppra, Spritam) Sodium valproate*	Carbamazepine (Carbatrol), Clobazam (Onfi) Gabapentin (Neurontin, Gralise), Lamotrigine (Lamictal): **Requires monitoring for Steven-Johnson syndrome,** Levetiracetam (Keppra, Spritam), Oxcarbazepine, Sodium valproate Topiramate (Topamax. Quedxy XR)
Prolonged and convulsive status epilepticus	IV diazepam (Valium, Diastat rectally) Buccal midazolam IV lorazepam (Ativan)	IV midazolam Propofol Thiopental

*Sodium valproate treatment must not be used in pregnant women.

IV, intravenous.

Sources: Healthline. *Epilepsy and seizure medication list*. www.healthline.com/health/epilepsy/medications-list; The National Institute for Health and Care Excellence. (2017). *Epilepsies: diagnosis and management. Pharmacological treatment. Guidance*. https://www.healthline.com/health/epilepsy/medications-list

TABLE 14.31 ORAL ANTIEPILEPTIC MEDICATIONS

MEDICATION	CLASS	MECHANISM OF ACTION	INDICATIONS/ CONTRAINDICATIONS	DOSAGE	SIDE EFFECTS	SAFETY/ PATIENT EDUCATION
Carbamazepine (Tegretol)	Carboxamide	Reduces postsynaptic response and blocks post tetanic potentiation	Treatment of partial seizures with complex symptomatology, GTC, and mixed seizure patterns Contraindicated in history of bone marrow depression, MAOI use within 14 days, hypersensitive to TCA	200 mg BID, increase by 200 mg/d every 7 days till therapeutic level reached. Not to exceed 1.2 g/d	Dizziness, drowsiness, N&V, unsteadiness, bone marrow depression, toxic epidermal necrolysis.	Counsel on S&S hematologic/ dermatologic complications, easy bruising, avoid ETOH and abrupt discontinuation.
Clobazam (Onfi)	Benzodiazepine	Not established, thought to enhance GABA-Anergic neurotransmission	Adjunctive treatment of seizures associated with Lennox Gastaut Watch with concomitant use of opioids or other depressants, may increase suicidal ideation	5 mg QHS, increase by 5 mg every week	Somnolence, sedation, agitation, urinary retention, skin reactions	Watch concomitant use with opioids and ETOH, is a weak CYP3A4 inducer, can be abused, strict care when withdrawing from patients.
Clonazepam (Klonopin)	Benzodiazepine	Not established, thought to enhance GABA activity	Adjunct/monotherapy in Lennox:Gastaut, akinetic/myoclonic/absence seizures Contraindicated in significant liver disease, acute narrow angle glaucoma, and untreated open angle glaucoma.	Initial dose not to exceed 0.5 mg PO TID. Increase by 0.5–1 mg every third day, not to exceed 20 mg daily	Somnolence, depression, ataxia, central nervous system depression, fatigue	May cause central nervous system depression, avoid abrupt withdrawal with use of machinery, ETOH, risk of pregnancy. Monitor blood counts with prolonged therapy, monitor for worsening seizures.
Diazepam (Valium)	Benzodiazepine	Enhances GABA type A receptors.	Adjunct therapy in convulsive disorders. Contraindicated in acute narrow angle glaucoma, untreated open angle glaucoma.	2–10 mg BID –QID, decrease dose in older adults. IV dose: load 10–20 mg (2 mg/min) can repeat in 15 minutes. Maintenance: 0.4 mg/kg/hr.	Drowsiness, fatigue, ataxia, paradoxical reactions.	Avoid ETOH/sedatives, caution while operating machinery, counsel on drug abuse/ dependence.
Ethosuximide (Zarontin)	Succinimide	Suppresses paroxysmal 3 cycles/ second spike wave activity	Absence (petit mal) seizures Extreme caution in liver/renal dysfunction, monitor blood counts, liver/renal function periodically, SLE; adjust dose slowly.	250 mg PO BID. Increase by 250 mg every 4–7 days PRN up to 1.5 g/d in 2 divided doses.	Anorexia, N&V, abdominal pain, blood dyscrasias	Contact provider if any infection develops, do not abruptly stop, therapy may impair mental/ physical abilities.
Gabapentin (Neurontin)	GABA analog	Suspected to bind to hippocampus and neocortex.	Adjunct therapy for partial seizures with/out secondary generalization. Avoid abrupt withdrawal, possible tumorigenic potential, sudden unexplained deaths.	300 mg PO at HS on first day. 300 mg PO BID on second day, 300 mg PO TID on third day. Maintenance 900–1,800 mg/d in 3 divided doses.	Somnolence, dizziness, ataxia, nystagmus	Can be taken with or without food, caution when driving or using machinery, watch for central nervous system depression if taking Maalox, separate dosing by 2 hours.

(continued)

Drug	Class	Mechanism	Indication/Use	Dosing	Side Effects	Notes
Lacosamide (Vimpat)	Anticonvulsant (miscellaneous)	Not well known, thought selectively enhance activation of sodium channels.	For use in partial onset seizures.	50 mg BID IV load: 200 mg. Maintenance: 200–400, divided doses BID, start 12 hours after PO: IV load	Suicidal ideation, dizziness, ataxia, cardiac/conduction abnormalities, syncope.	Notify provider immediately for any increase in suicidal ideation or psychiatric issues, if patient becomes pregnant to notify provider.
Levetiracetam (Keppra)	Anticonvulsant (SV2A inhibitor)	Unknown	For use of partial onset seizures, adjunct in JME, and primary GTC	Initiate dose with 1,000 mg daily dosed BID in 500 mg doses. Increase dosage every 2 weeks by 1,000 mg to a daily dose of 3,000 mg. IV load: 20–30 mg/kg	Psychotic symptoms, suicidal ideation, somnolence, fatigue, nervousness, anaphylaxis and hematologic abnormalities.	Notify provider immediately for any increase in suicidal ideation or psychiatric issues, panic attacks, anxiety, insomnia. Do not abruptly stop taking medication. Watch patients with kidney disease.
Lamotrigine (Lamictal)	Phenyltriazine	Suspected to inhibit voltage sensitive sodium channels, stabilizing neuronal membrane.	Adjunct therapy	If on carbamazepine, phenytoin, phenobarbital: 50 mg daily as a single dose for 2 weeks, then 50 mg BID for next 2 weeks, increase by 100 mg/d weekly to maintenance dose of 300–500 mg/d in 2 divided doses. If on Valproic: 25 mg QOD, increase to 300–500 mg daily q12h	Serious rash, dizziness, ataxia, somnolence, diplopia, xerostomia.	Notify provider immediately if rash, S&S of hypersensitivity reaction, blood dyscrasias, multiorgan failure, and suicidal ideation. Monitor drug levels with concomitant medications or with dosage adjustments.
Oxacarbazepine (Trileptal)	Dibenzazepine	Suspected to exert antiseizure effects by blocking voltage-sensitive sodium channels, thereby stabilizing neuronal membrane.	Monotherapy Risk of hyponatremia, cross sensitivity with carbamazepine, avoid abrupt withdrawal. Adjust dose with renal impairment, report serious dermatologic reactions, rare angioedema.	300–600 mg PO daily. Slowly titrate to 900–2,400 mg/d in 2–3 divided doses.	Dizziness, somnolence, diplopia, asthenia, nystagmus	Report any S&S angioedema, notify provider if fever with any other organ system involvement, serious skin reactions. Additive effects with ETOH, Verapamil, Phenytoin, Valproic acid, Carbamazepine Counsel females on efficacy with oral contraceptives, avoid operating heavy, machinery, avoid ETOH.
Phenobarbital (Luminal)	Barbiturate	Nonselective central nervous system depressant.	Treatment of GTC and cortical focal seizures	60–200 mg as single dose or 2–3 divided doses. IV load: 20 mg/kg (maximum rate 1–2 mg/kg/min) Check level immediately after, rebolus I flow.	Drowsiness, residual sedation, vertigo, resp. depression	Inform patient of psychologic/physical dependence, do not increase dosage without telling provider, may impair mental/physical activities, use caution with hazardous tasks.
Perampanel (Fycompa)	Noncompetitive AMPA receptor antagonist	Blocks glutamate activity at postsynaptic AMPA receptors	Treatment of drug-resistant partial onset seizures Contraindicated in those with preaggressive behavior or psychosis.	12 mg PO daily	Drowsiness, sleepiness, fatigue, weight gain, joint and back pain. Behavioral changes, psychiatric events psychosis have been reported.	Contact provider for signs of allergic reaction, skin rash, muscle aches, changes in mood/behavior, balance/coordination.

(continued)

TABLE 14.31 ORAL ANTIEPILEPTIC MEDICATIONS (continued)

MEDICATION	CLASS	MECHANISM OF ACTION	INDICATIONS/ CONTRAINDICATIONS	DOSAGE	SIDE EFFECTS	SAFETY/ PATIENT EDUCATION
Pregabalin (Lyrica)	Anticonvulsant	Unknown, but increases neuronal GABA levels	Adjunctive treatment of partial onset seizures w/o secondary generalization Contraindicated in patients with known hypersensitivity to pregabilin, use with caution with renal impairment	50 mg TID daily initially or 75 mg BID to maximum 600 mg/d.	Dizziness, drowsiness, blurred vision, peripheral edema, weight gain, h/a	May increase risk of suicidal ideation or depression, notify provider immediately if this occurs.
Phenytoin (Dilantin)	Hydantoin	Possibly promotes sodium efflux from neurons.	Control of GTC and CPS, prevention and treatment of neurosurgically induced seizures	Start 100 mg BID, increase by 50 mg every 7–10-day intervals. Maintenance 300–400 mg daily. IV load: 20 mg/kg (maximum rate 50 mg/min). Wait 1 hour to check level, rebolus if low.	Nystagmus, ataxia, slurred speech, dizziness, rash, hypersensitivity reactions.	Possibly teratogenic to fetus, avoid ETOH, notify provider if skin rash develops, use good dental hygiene; do not abruptly DC medication.
Topiramate (Topamax)	Sulfamate-substituted antiepileptic	Suspected to block voltage-dependent sodium channels	Monotherapy in partial onset or GTC. Adjunct in primary GTC or seizures associated with Lennox-Gastaut	50 mg initially, increase 50–400 mg daily q12h.	Somnolence, fatigue, speech disorders, depression, anxiety, memory difficulty, abnormal vision	Monitor for acute S&S of acute myopia, secondary angle glaucoma, cognitive impairment, speech difficulty. Take with food, maintain hydration, and seek immediate help with any visual difficulty.
Valproic acid (Depakote)	Valproate compound	Increases GABA concentration in brain.	Management of simple/ complex absence seizures, CPS. Treatment of mania associated with bipolar and migraine prophylaxis.	Multidrug therapy: 15 mg/ kg daily. Monotherapy: 5–5 mg/kg/d PO at weekly intervals. Maintenance 30–60 mg/kg/d PO in 2–3 divided doses. IV load: 10–20 mg/kg (maximum rate 150 mg/min).	Diarrhea, N&V, somnolence, dyspepsia, nystagmus, thrombocytopenia.	Avoid ETOH/sedatives, monitor LFT and platelet counts, hypersensitivity reactions.
Zonisamide (Zonegran)	Sulfonamide	Blocks sodium channels and facilitates both dopaminergic and serotonergic neurotransmission.	Adjunctive therapy in partial seizures. Care with those with sulfa allergies, renal impairment, may increase body temperature, use contraception, may cause psychiatric events.	100 mg PO daily. After 2 weeks, increase dose to 200 mg/d for 2 weeks, then to 300 or 400 mg daily.	H/a, abdomen pain, anorexia, dizziness, memory issues, depression	Avoid ETOH, may decrease sweating and increase body temperature, hydrate properly, notify provider if muscle pain, easy bruising.

AMPA, alpha amino-3-hydroxy-5-methyl-4-isoxazolepropionic acid; CPS, complex partial seizures; CYP3A4, cytochrome P450 3A4; DC, depressive craniectomy; ETOH, ethanol; GABA, gamma-aminobutyric acid; GTC, generalized tonic clonic; h/a, headache; IV, intravenous; JME, juvenile myoclonic epilepsy; LFT, liver function test; MAOI, monoamine oxidase inhibitor; N&V, nausea and vomiting; SLE, systemic lupus erythematosus; S&S, signs and symptoms; TCA, tricyclic antidepressant.

TABLE 14.32 IINTRAVENOUS ANTIEPILEPTIC MEDICATIONS (ONLY ROUTE)

MEDICATION	CLASS	MECHANISM OF ACTION	INDICATIONS/ CONTRAINDICA-TIONS	DOSAGE	SIDE EFFECTS	SAFETY/ PATIENT EDUCATION
Fosphenytoin (Cerebyx)	Prodrug of phenytoin, acute treatment of status epilepticus	Block frequency-dependent, use-dependent and voltage-dependent neuronal sodium channels, and therefore limit repetitive firing of action potentials	Prevention of general tonic–clonic seizures. Short term (up to 5 days use) of parenteral administration when other routes unavailable. Contraindicated in sinus bradycardia.	IV/IM load: 20 mg PE, maximum rate 150 mg PE/min). If IV, wait 2 hours to check level. If IM, wait >4 hours for level. Rebolus if low.	Bradycardia, heart block, nystagmus, pruritus, nausea	Cardiac monitoring while administering drug, monitor LFTs

IM, intramuscular; IV, intravenous; LFT, liver function test; PE, phenytoin equivalent.

TABLE 14.33 MYASTHENIA GRAVIS MEDICATIONS—CHOLINESTERASE INHIBITORS

MEDICATION	CLASS	MECHANISM OF ACTION	INDICATIONS/ CONTRAINDI-CATIONS	DOSAGE	SIDE EFFECTS	SAFETY/PATIENT EDUCATION
Edrophonium (Enlon, Reversol, Tensilon)	Cholinesterase inhibitor	Competes with acetylcholine for its binding site on acetylcholinesterase and potentiates the action of acetylcholine on both the skeletal muscle (nicotinic receptor) and the GI tract (muscarinic receptor	Used in diagnosis confirmation and treatment of MG. Use cautiously in patients with PUD, asthma, epilepsy, cardiac disease, and hypothyroidism	2 mg initially, if no response give 8 mg. May repeat in 30 minutes	Bradycardia, tachycardia, hypotension, cardiac arrest, salivation, fasciculations, diarrhea, cramps	Patients may feel flushed, hypotensive Overdosage can cause cholinergic crisis
Neostigmine (Prostigmin)	Cholinesterase inhibitor	Competes with acetylcholine for its binding site on acetylcholinesterase and potentiates the action of acetylcholine on both the skeletal muscle (nicotinic receptor) and the GI tract (muscarinic receptor	Used in diagnosis confirmation and treatment of MG. Use cautiously in patients with PUD, asthma, epilepsy, cardiac disease, and hypothyroidism	15–30 mg PO initially in divided doses or 0.5–2 mg q1–3h IM/IV. Maintenance: 75–150 mg daily. May go as high as 375 g/d	Bradycardia, tachycardia, hypotension, cardiac arrest, salivation, fasciculations, diarrhea, cramps	Patients may feel flushed, hypotensive Overdosage can cause cholinergic crisis
Pyridostigimine (Mestinon, Regonol)	Cholinesterase inhibitor	Competes with acetylcholine for its binding site on acetylcholinesterase and potentiates the action of acetylcholine on both the skeletal muscle (nicotinic receptor) and the GI tract (muscarinic receptor).	Used as a first-line treatment for MG. Use cautiously in patients with PUD, asthma, epilepsy, cardiac disease, and hypothyroidism. For patients receiving nondepolarizing agents for anesthesia, use extreme care for reversal.	600 mg in 60–120 mg PO initially 6–8 times/d or 2 mg IM/IV. May repeat q2h	Bradycardia, tachycardia, hypotension, cardiac arrest, salivation, fasciculations, diarrhea, cramps	Patients may feel flushed, hypotensive Avoid ETOH, may cause drowsiness, if a dose missed, do not double the next dose, take as soon as you remember it. Do not abruptly stop medication. Teach patient S&S of myasthenic and cholinergic crisis.

ETOH, ethanol; GI, gastrointestinal; IM, intramuscular; IV, intravenous; MG, myasthenia gravis; PUD, peptic ulcer disease; S&S, signs and symptoms.

TABLE 14.34 CEREBRAL PALSY MEDICATIONS

MEDICATION	CLASS	MECHANISM OF ACTION	INDICATIONS/ CONTRAINDICA- TIONS	DOSAGE	SIDE EFFECTS	SAFETY/ PATIENT EDUCATION
Baclofen (Lioresal)	GABA analog (peripheral)	Acts as an inhibitory neurotransmitter at the spinal level.	Used for the management of spasticity resulting from cerebral palsy. No absolute contraindications other than hypersensitivity.	5 mg PO BID– TID initially. May increase by 5 mg/d every 3–7 days for desired response. Do not exceed 80 mg/d.	Transient drowsiness, vertigo, confusion weakness.	Dose may need to be reduced for those with renal impairment.
Botulinum toxin (Botox)	Skeletal muscle relaxant (peripheral)	Inhibits acetylcholine release from nerve endings.	Used for the management of spasticity resulting from cerebral palsy. Contraindicated in patients with a known hypersensitivity to the drug or albumin, in patients with a neuromuscular disease, heart disease or patients with inability to hold head upright.	1.25–2.5 units/site every 3 months. Maximum: 400 units in a 3-month interval. Do not administer more than 50 units per muscle site.	Dysphagia, ptosis, headache and neck pain.	Cost to patient; neuropsychiatric signs (euphoria, depression paresthesias) are rare and difficult to discern from underlying disease state.
Cyclobenzaprine (Flexeril)	Skeletal muscle relaxant (central)	Blocks nerve impulses that increase muscle tone and contraction.	Used for the management of spasticity resulting from cerebral palsy. Do not stop spasms but reduce severity.	10 mg PO TID daily PRN. Range: 20–40 mg in divided doses. Not to exceed 60 mg/d.	Has significant anticholinergic effect (dry mouth, urinary retention, blurred vision).	Do not use longer than 2–3 weeks. May not be effective in those with CP.
Dantrolene sodium (Dantrium)	Direct-acting skeletal muscle relaxant	Reduces muscle contractility by inhibiting calcium release.	Used for the management of spasticity resulting from cerebral palsy. Contraindicated in active hepatic disease, where spasticity is utilized to sustain upright posture and balance in locomotion and when spasticity is utilized to maintain increased function.	25 mg PO daily x 7 days. Titrate dose by increasing by 25 mg 2–4 times/d PRN. Not to exceed 400 mg/d.	Dizziness, headache, blurred vision, confusion, euphoria. Prolonged high dosage use can cause hepatitis and hepatic necrosis.	Discontinue medication after 45 days if no benefits are not seen. May cause idiosyncratic liver injury.
Diazepam (Valium)	Benzodiazepine	Enhances GABA type A receptors.	Adjunct therapy in cerebral palsy. Contraindicated in acute narrow angle glaucoma, untreated open angle glaucoma.	2–10 mg BID– QID, decrease dose in older adults	Drowsiness, fatigue, ataxia, paradoxical reactions	Avoid ETOH/ sedatives, use caution while operating machinery, counsel on drug abuse/ dependence.

CP, cerebral palsy; ETOH, ethanol; GABA, gamma-aminobutyric acid.

TABLE 14.35 HEADACHE/MIGRAINE MEDICATIONS—SEROTONIN AGONISTS

MEDICATION	CLASS	MECHANISM OF ACTION	INDICATIONS/ CONTRAINDICATIONS	DOSAGE	SIDE EFFECTS	SAFETY/PATIENT EDUCATION
Almotriptan malate (Axert)	5-HT agonist	Selective 5-HT agonist	Acute treatment of migraine without aura. Contraindicated in ischemic heart disease, coronary artery vasospasm, uncontrolled BP.	6.25–12.5 mg at onset of h/a, May repeat after 2 hours. Maximum: 2 doses in 24 hours. Watch with hepatic dysfunction	Nausea, somnolence, h/a, coronary artery vasospasm, MI	Administer first dose in provider's office to monitor for cardiac issues, monitor for cardiac events. Advise to not take with SSRI/SNRI's, caution during hazardous tasks. Notify provider if pregnant.
Eletriptan (Relpax)	5-HT agonist	Selective 5-HT agonist	Acute treatment of migraine without aura. Contraindicated in ischemic heart disease, coronary artery vasospasm, uncontrolled BP.	20–40 mg PO at onset of headache, may repeat after 2 hours. Maximum: 30 mg/dose or 80 mg/d Do not crush/break tablets	Asthenia, chest tightness, dizziness, dry mouth, h/a, N&V, vasospasm, MI	Administer first dose in provider's office to monitor for cardiac issues, monitor for cardiac events Advise to not take with SSRI/SNRIs, caution during hazardous tasks Ischemic heart disease, coronary artery vasospasm, uncontrolled BP. Notify provider if pregnant.
Frovatriptan (Frova)	5-HT agonist	Selective 5-HT agonist	Indicated for use in those with headache without aura. Contraindicated in ischemic heart disease, coronary artery vasospasm, uncontrolled BP.	2.5 mg with fluids. If headache recurs, may repeat after 2 hours. Maximum: 7.5 mg/d Do not crush/break tablets.	Chest pain, dizziness, fatigue, headache, flushing	Administer first dose in provider office to monitor for cardiac issues, monitor for cardiac events. Advise to not take with SSRI/SNRIs, caution during hazardous tasks. Notify provider if pregnant.
Naratriptan (Amerge)	5-HT agonist	Selective 5-HT agonist	Acute treatment of migraine without aura. Contraindicated in ischemic heart disease, coronary artery vasospasm, uncontrolled BP.	1–2.5 mg PO as a single dose, may repeat in 4 hours up to 5 mg/24 hours.	Paresthesias, nausea, chest pain, GI upset	Administer first dose in provider office to monitor for cardiac issues, monitor for cardiac events Advise to not take with SSRI/SNRIs, caution during hazardous tasks Notify provider if pregnant
Sumatriptan (Imitrex)	5-HT agonist	Selective 5-HT agonist	Acute treatment of migraine without aura. Acute treatment of cluster headaches. Contraindicated in ischemic heart disease, coronary artery vasospasm, uncontrolled BP.	6 mg SQ, may repeat after 1 hour. Maximum: 12 mg/24 hr Spray: 5–20 mg single dose, may repeat after 2 hours. Maximum: 40 mg/24 hr. Tab- 25–100 mg, may repeat after 2 hours. Maximum: 200 mg/24 hr.	Tingling, burning, flushing, injection site reaction, neck pain, stiffness	Injectable form should be reviewed with healthcare provider. Administer first dose in provider office to monitor for cardiac issues, monitor for cardiac events. Advise to not take with SSRI/SNRIs, caution during hazardous tasks. Notify provider if pregnant
Zolmitriptan (Zomig)	5-HT agonist	Selective 5-HT agonist	Acute treatment of migraine without aura. Contraindicated in ischemic heart disease, coronary artery vasospasm, uncontrolled BP.	1.25–2.5 mg PO as single dose, may repeat in 2 hours to maximum 0 mg/24 hr. Spray: 5 mg as single dose, may repeat in 2 hours.	Chest pain, ischemia, hypertension, pressure sensations, dry mouth	Administer first dose in provider's office to monitor for cardiac issues, monitor for cardiac events. Advise to not take with SSRI/SNRIs, caution during hazardous tasks. Notify provider if pregnant.

BP, blood pressure; GI, gastrointestinal; h/a, headache; 5-HT, 5-hydroxytryptamine; MI, myocardial infarction; N&V, nausea and vomiting; SNRI, selective norepinephrine reuptake inhibitor; SQ, subcuta-

TABLE 14.36 HEADACHE/MIGRAINE MEDICATIONS—ERGOT ALKALOIDS

MEDICATION	CLASS	MECHANISM OF ACTION	INDICATIONS/ CONTRAINDICATIONS	DOSAGE	SIDE EFFECTS	SAFETY/PATIENT EDUCATION
DHE, Migranal	Ergot alkaloid	Binds with high affinity to 5HT receptors on intracranial blood vessels, causing vasoconstriction	Acute treatment of migraine with/out aura. Contraindicated in ischemic heart disease, coronary artery vasospasm, uncontrolled BP. Concomitant use with a CYP3A4 inhibitor is contraindicated.	SQ 1 mg single dose, may repeat up to 3 mg/d or 6 mg/wk IV maximum 2 mg/d or 6 mg/wk Spray: 1 spray (0.5 mg) into each nostril, may repeat in 15 minutes to maximum 4 sprays/24 hr or 8 sprays/wk.	Rhinitis, altered taste, NV, pharyngitis	Perform periodic cardiac evaluations. Potentiates BP elevation. Once applicator prepared, discard after 8 hours. Notify provider if pregnant. Prolonged administration /excessive dosage may produce ergot toxicity.
Ergotamine (Cafergot)	Ergot alkaloid/ caffeine	Binds with high affinity to 5HT receptors on intracranial blood vessels, causing vasoconstriction. Caffeine further enhances the vasoconstrictive effect.	Acute treatment of migraine with/out aura. Contraindicated in ischemic heart disease, coronary artery vasospasm, uncontrolled BP. Coadministration with potent CYP 3A4 inhibitors.	2 mg PO at onset of headache, then 1–2 mg every 30 minutes PRN to maximum 6 mg/episode or mg/wk. SL: tablet at onset of headache, then 1 tablet every 30 minutes to maximum 3 tablets/d or 5 tabs/wk.	N&V, paresthesias, vasoconstrictive issues (ischemia, absence of pulse)	Perform periodic cardiac evaluations. Potentiates BP elevation. Notify provider if pregnant. Prolonged administration /excessive dosage may produce ergot toxicity.

BP, blood pressure; CYP3A4, cytochrome P450 3A4; DHE, dihydroergotamine; 5HT, 5-hydroxytryptamine; IV, intravenous; N&V, nausea and vomiting; SL, sublingual; SQ, subcutaneous.

TABLE 14.37 HEADACHE/MIGRAINE MEDICATIONS—MISCELLANEOUS

MEDICATION	CLASS	MECHANISM OF ACTION	INDICATIONS/ CONTRAINDICATIONS	DOSAGE	SIDE EFFECTS	SAFETY/PATIENT EDUCATION
Topamax (Topiramate)	Sulfamate-substituted monosaccharide	Suspected to block voltage-dependent sodium channels	Migraine prophylaxis in adults.	Titrate: Week 1: 25 mg QPM, week 2: 25 mg PO BID, week 3: 25 mg PO QAM and QPM, week 4: 50 mg BID.	Somnolence, fatigue, dizziness, ataxia, speech disorders, abnormal vision.	Monitor for S&S myopia, hyperthermia. Assess for renal impairment.

S&S, signs and symptoms.

HEAD, EYES, EARS, NOSE, AND THROAT

For information specific to the head, eyes, ears, nose, and throat, see Table 14.38.

TABLE 14.38 NURSING CONSIDERATIONS FOR HEAD, EYES, EARS, NOSE, AND THROAT

HEENT NURSING INTERVENTIONS	EARS	NOSE	UPPER RESPIRATORY TRACT, THROAT, AND MOUTH	ORAL CAVITY	EYES
Physical assessment	System-specific questioning related to the following: ■ Perceived hearing loss ■ Ringing in ears, dizziness ■ Perceived motion ■ For any lesions, note: appearance growth changes, etc.	System-specific questioning related to the following: ■ Length of upper respiratory illness or dermal lesion. History of the following: ■ Trauma ■ Previous infections, recent fever ■ Pain related to the affected area or systemic signs of infection ■ Bleeding/discharge	System-specific questioning related to the following: ■ Immediate airway issues must be assessed. History of the following: ■ Fever or systemic signs of infection ■ Present illness ■ Pain ■ Smoking or oral tobacco use. ■ Assess when was the last oral cancer screen, possibly at a dental visit.	System-specific questioning related to the following: ■ Time of onset History of the following: ■ Prior medication, including chemotherapy ■ Last oral cancer screening possibly at a dental visit ■ Smoking or oral tobacco use ■ Any concurrent disease	System-specific questioning related to the following: ■ Loss of vision ■ Loss of areas of vision ■ Describe any floaters field of vision History of the following: ■ Dry eyes ■ Excessive tearing ■ Ocular pain ■ Seasonal allergies ■ Lesions on or around the eye ■ Fever or systemic signs of infection
Diagnosis	■ Hearing loss ■ Vertigo ■ Tinnitus ■ Lesion of external auditory tissue	■ Nasal polyps ■ Sinusitis ■ Loss of smell ■ Dermal lesion of face other than eyes	■ Acute pharyngitis ■ Peritonsillar abscess ■ Dysphagia ■ Visible lesion: base of tongue or oral pharynx	■ Oral mucosal dysfunction ■ Dry mouth ■ Burning mouth syndrome ■ Taste dysfunction	■ Glaucoma ■ Cataracts ■ Dry eye ■ Corneal abrasion ■ Macular degeneration ■ Ectropion ■ Dermal lesion
Intervention other than referral	■ Visually inspect the ear canal utilizing otoscope: ■ Exam for external auditory disease ■ Visualize canal and tympanic membrane ■ Perform a gross hearing and balance exam	■ Visual inspection of lesion, nasal cavity, and facial/orbital area: ■ Assess size, shape, color, and symmetry of any lesion. ■ Examine for any form of periorbital cellulitis. ■ Palpate the maxillary and frontal sinuses for pain or discomfort. ■ Consider review of systems, age, exposure to toxic substances or irritants and possible medical imaging for loss of smell.	■ Refer to appropriate clinical assessment for potential airway compromise. ■ Are they adequately handling oral secretions? ■ Assess hydration and nutrition status. ■ Direct assessment of upper oral pharynx. ■ Are there visible lesions? ■ Describe any secretions. ■ Are there visible tonsils, size, shape, and proximity to each other? ■ Assess the neck for swelling or fluid pockets/retention. ■ If no signs of infection, consider dysphagia as a possible emergency.	■ Encourage appropriate oral care ■ Discuss oral care in the presence of denture or oral prosthetics ■ Visually inspect oral cavity ■ Palpate under the tongue ■ Palpate the neck and lymph nodes	■ Description of any dermal lesions: ■ Limited visual field exam ■ Gross visual acuity exam ■ Ophthalmic examination: ■ Opacities ■ Fluorescein stain uptake ■ Conjunctiva ■ Tear production

(continued)

TABLE 14.38 NURSING CONSIDERATIONS FOR HEAD EYES EARS NOSE AND THROAT *(continued)*

HEENT NURSING INTERVENTIONS	EARS	NOSE	UPPER RESPIRATORY TRACT, THROAT, AND MOUTH	ORAL CAVITY	EYES
Pharmacology	Potential medication: ■ Antibiotic treatment for external auditory infections ■ Evaluate for fungal infection treat with antifungal agent. ■ Antiemetics for symptoms of nausea and vomiting related to tinnitus and vertigo refer to specialist.	Potential medication: ■ Consider topical intranasal steroids for sinusitis and intranasal swelling. ■ If fever, cellulitis palpation pain, or tooth pain consider antibiotic therapy for sinusitis or sinus infection. ■ Antihistamines could also be considered concurrently or apart from sinus rinses.	Potential medication: ■ Consider oral antibiotics with referral for complicated upper respiratory infection. ■ Steroids may be considered. ■ Use of antipyretic for fever. ■ Rinsing with a mild saline solution is also a possibility.	Potential medication: ■ Prescription fluoride paste ■ Appropriate ADA-recommended dentifrice ■ Moisturizing mouth wash	Potential medication: ■ Artificial tears
Special considerations	Referral to HEENT specialist	Referral to HEENT specialist	Referral to HEENT specialist	Referral to HEENT specialist	Referral to HEENT specialist

HEENT, head, eyes, ears, nose, and throat.

REVIEW QUESTIONS

1. A 19-year-old male is brought to the neurology ICU for observation after falling forward face down from his bicycle. On arrival, the patient is alert and oriented to person, place, time, situation. The patient is talking and texting on his cell phone. Glasgow Coma Scale (GCS) is 15, confusion assessment method for the ICU (CAM–ICU) is negative, Richmond Agitation Sedation Scale (RASS) score is 0, and muscle strength is 5/5. Blood pressure (BP) is 130/70, heart rate (HR) is 80, respiration is 18, and oxygen saturation is 100% on room air. The patient is NPO.

   The nurse conducting a routine neuro assessment 4 hours later notices the patient to be less active and slightly confused. The patient has not had any analgesia in the past 4 hours. The patient opens eyes to voice. When awakened the patient is sleepy and irritable. He is able to follow commands, state date, but thinks he is at home. Patient complains of a frontal headache. GCS is 13. BP is 170/95, HR 56, and respiration is 12. Oxygen saturation is 90% on room air.

   The nurse asks the adult-gerontology clinical nurse specialist (AG-CNS) who is rounding on another patient on the unit to consult. The AG-CNS's first course of action would be to do which of the following:

   A. Advise the nurse to give the patient Tylenol for headache and allow the patient to rest.
   B. Advise the nurse to administer 2 L O_2 to reduce cerebral O_2 demand and lower the head 0–15° to decrease CBF.
   C. Advise the nurse to contact the neurosurgeon stat and order a stat head CT.
   D. Raise the head of bed to 30°, administer oxygen to keep O_2 saturation about 94%, contact the neurosurgeon, and obtain an order for a stat head CT.

2. Intracranial hypertension (IH) can be managed through multiple methods, including the diversion of cerebrospinal fluid (CSF) by external ventricular drainage (EVD). In the techniques used for CSF diversion listed in the following, which would be the safest process used especially in a very busy neuroscience critical care unit?
   A. Continuous open drainage with ICP high range programmed in the monitor to alarm
   B. Closed drainage with opening only when the ICP is >20 mmHg (or ordered upper limit by provider)
   C. Closed drainage with opening only at the frequency and volume as ordered by provider
   D. Closed drainage with opening every 2 hours with neurochecks

ANSWERS

1. **Correct answer: D. Rationale**: The patient is having signs of increased ICP and Cushing's triad. The first course of action would be to maintain cerebral perfusion and reduce cerebral venous drainage by administering O_2 and raising the head of bed. Evaluation for cerebral edema and herniation through CT with neurosurgeon availability is imperative. Lowering the head of bed would increase CBF. Tylenol will have no effect for ICP and is not indicated. Contacting the neurosurgeon and ordering a stat head CT is indicated. However, raising the head of the bed to 30° and administering oxygen to keep O_2 saturation about 94% are comprehensive noninvasive measures to reduce ICP.

2. **Correct answer: B. Rationale**: Although inclusion of the high pressure range on the monitoring system is important, using a closed system with the inclusion of pressure ranges is ideal to avoid the risk of overdrainage with increased ICP as alarms only can have a delayed response time due to the high number of alarms in this environment and alarm fatigue.

REFERENCES
The complete reference and additional reading lists appear in the digital version of this chapter, at https://connect.springerpub.com/content/book/978-0-8261-7417-8/part/part01/chapter/ch14

Psychobehavioral Disorders

Nina M. Flanagan

ANXIETY DISORDERS

OVERVIEW
Etiology
- Not well understood
- Lifetime prevalence in older adults: 7.7% in women and 4.6% in men for generalized anxiety disorder (GAD)
- May be attributed to persistent activation of areas in the brain associated with mental activity and introspective thinking following worry-inducing stimuli

Risk Factors
- Chronic physical illness
- Female sex
- Presence of life stressors
- Onset—median age of 30

ANXIETY DISORDERS
Generalized Anxiety Disorder
Definition
- Excessive anxiety/worry
- Difficulty controlling the worry
- Anxiety associated with muscle tension, irritability, and difficulty concentrating

Assessment
- Fatigue
- Difficulty sleeping
- Trembling, feeling twitchy
- Sweating
- Irritability
- Restlessness

Differential Diagnosis
- Rule out organic causes such as thyroid disorders, anemias, infections
- Prior psychiatric disorders
- Medication review—decongestants, albuterol, levothyroxine
- Use of substances such as caffeine and energy drinks
- Exacerbation of chronic illness—chronic obstructive pulmonary disease (COPD), epilepsy

Screening for Generalized Anxiety Disorder
The Generalized Anxiety Disorder Scale (GAD-7) is a 7-item self-reported questionnaire for screening and measuring GAD: See www.mdcalc.com/gad-7-general-anxiety-disorder-7

Treatment
Nonpharmacologic:
- Cognitive behavioral therapy
- Desentization therapy

Pharmacologic:
- Selective serotonin reuptake inhibitors (SSRIs)
- Serotonin–norepinephrine reuptake inhibitors (SNRIs)
- Benzodiazepines not recommended due to risk of delirium or falls (American Geriatrics Society Beers Criteria® Update Expert Panel, 2019)

Panic Attacks
Definition
- Rapid/abrupt onset of intense fear (typically peaking in 10 minutes)
- Occur with a clear trigger

Etiology
- Familial predisposition in 48% of the population
- Abnormalities in the "fear network" (amygdala, hippocampus, thalamus, midbrain, and cerebellum)

Symptoms of Panic Attack
- Palpitations, pounding heart
- Sweating, trembling, shaking
- Feelings of choking
- Sensations of shortness of breath or smothering
- Chest pain or discomfort
- Fear of dying

Assessment
Differential Diagnosis
- Rule out organic causes such as thyroid disorders, anemias, infections, cardiac problems (myocardial infarction [MI], angina)
- Prior psychiatric disorders: depression, anxiety
- Medication review—decongestants, albuterol, levothyroxine
- Use of substances such as caffeine, energy drinks, alcohol, nicotine
- Exacerbation of chronic illness—COPD, epilepsy

Treatment
- Cognitive behavioral therapy—Recognize triggers
- Exposure therapy
- Relaxation techniques
- Stress management
- Improving sleep and physical activity

The complete reference and additional reading lists appear in the digital version of this chapter, at https://connect.springerpub.com/content/book/978-0-8261-7417-8/part/part01/chapter/ch15

TABLE 15.1 SELECTIVE SEROTONIN REUPTAKE INHIBITORS

CLASS	SSRIs			
Mechanism	Selectively inhibit the reuptake of the neurotransmitter serotonin into presynaptic terminals to enhance serotonergic neurotransmission			
GENERIC NAME (BRAND NAME)	**INDICATIONS, CONTRAINDICATIONS**	**DOSAGE**	**COMMON ADVERSE EFFECTS**	**SAFETY AND PATIENT EDUCATION**
Citalopram (Celexa)	Major depression Anxiety Phobia	10–20 mg daily Half-life 52 hours	Nausea, diarrhea, and appetite loss Impaired orgasm, ejaculation, and arousal Age > 60, risk of QT prolongation	GI side effects will usually decrease after 1 week. May take several weeks for full effect of medication. Do not abruptly stop the medication.
Escitalopram (Lexapro)	Major depression Anxiety	5–20 mg daily Half-life 45 hours	Nausea and appetite loss Impaired orgasm, ejaculation, and arousal Age > 60, risk of QT prolongation	May take several weeks for full effect of medication. Do not abruptly stop the medication.
Fluoxetine (Prozac)	Major depression Anxiety Most anticholinergic of SSRIs CYP2D6-2C9-3A4 inhibitor	5–60 mg daily Half-life 85 hours	Nausea and appetite loss Impaired orgasm, ejaculation, and arousal Dry mouth	May take several weeks for full effect of medication. Do not abruptly stop the medication.
Sertraline (Zoloft)	Major depression Anxiety	12.5–150 mg Half-life 25 hours	Nausea and appetite loss Impaired orgasm, ejaculation, and arousal	May take several weeks for full effect of medication. Do not abruptly stop the medication.
Vilazodone (Viibryd)	Major depression Anxiety	10–40 mg daily Half-life 25 hours	Nausea and appetite loss Impaired orgasm, ejaculation, and arousal	May take several weeks for full effect of medication. Do not abruptly stop the medication.
Paroxetine (Paxil)	Major depression Anxiety Most anticholinergic of SSRIs CYP2D6 inhibitor	10–40 mg Starting dose 5 mg	Dry mouth Nausea and appetite loss Impaired orgasm, ejaculation, and arousal	May take several weeks for full effect of medication. Do not abruptly stop the medication.

GI, gastrointestinal; SSRIs, selective serotonin reuptake inhibitors.
Source: From Boyd, M. (2016). *Essentials of psychiatric nursing.* Wolters Kluwer.

- Usually used in conjunction with pharmacotherapy
- SSRIs (Table 15.1)
- SNRIs (Table 15.2)
- Benzodiazepines not recommended due to risk of delirium or falls (American Geriatrics Society Beers CriteriaUpdate Expert Panel, 2019)

Phobias

Social Phobia/Social Anxiety Disorder

- Hallmark feature is fear of humiliation or embarrassment in front of others.
- Involves fear that others will notice one's physical symptoms such as blushing, sweating, or shaking.

Agoraphobia

- Hallmark feature is disproportionate fear of public places, often perceiving such environments as too open, crowded, or dangerous.

Symptoms

- Similar to anxiety and panic attacks

Assessment

- Same as anxiety and panic attacks

Differential Diagnosis

This is the same as for anxiety and panic attacks.

Treatment and Plan

- Cognitive behavioral therapy—Recognizing triggers
- Exposure therapy
- Relaxation techniques
- Stress management
- Improving sleep and physical activity
- Usually used in conjunction with pharmacotherapy
- SSRIs
- SSNIs

TABLE 15.2 SEROTONIN–NOREPINEPHRINE REUPTAKE INHIBITORS

CLASS	SNRIs			
Mechanism	Inhibit reuptake of serotonin and norepinephrine in synaptic clefts			
GENERIC NAME (BRAND NAME)	INDICATIONS, CONTRAINDICATIONS	DOSAGE	COMMON ADVERSE EFFECTS	SAFETY AND PATIENT EDUCATION
Duloxetine (Cymbalta)	Major depression/neuro-pathic pain Contraindicated if CrCL < 30	20–60 mg	Dry mouth, constipation, diarrhea, urinary hesitancy	Do not abruptly stop.
Venlafaxine (Effexor)	Major depression Anxiety Panic disorder Social phobia	75–225 mg in divided doses	May increase blood pressure and QT interval Hyponatremia May cause extrapyramidal symptoms May increase liver enzymes	Do not abruptly discontinue as it will cause withdrawal symptoms Has minimal sedative effect.
Desvenlafaxine (Pristiq)	Major depression Anxiety Postmenopausal symptoms	50–400 mg	Active metabolite of venlafaxine	Same as venlafaxine

CrCl, creatinine clearance; SNRIs, serotonin–norepinephrine reuptake inhibitors.

- Benzodiazepines not recommended due to risk of delirium or falls (American Geriatrics Society Beers Criteria® Update Expert Panel, 2019)

OTHER DISORDERS
Posttraumatic Stress Disorder
- Exposure to a highly traumatic event as a victim or as a witness in which life or injury was threatened is the situational trigger for posttraumatic stress disorder (PTSD).

Etiology
- Possible biologic factors include neurobiology and genetics, interactions with environmental stimuli such as childhood experiences, and the severity and extent of the traumatic exposure.
- Neurotransmitters involved in regulating fear conditioning include norepinephrine, dopamine, and opiate- and corticotropin-releasing hormones.

Symptoms of Posttraumatic Stress Disorder
- Exposure to actual or threatened death, serious injury, or sexual violence
- Presence of intrusion symptoms, that is, distressing memories of the event, distressing dreams related to the event, dissociative reactions (flashbacks), physiologic reactions (internal or external cues) that resemble the event
- Persistent avoidance of stimuli associated with the event
- Dissociative amnesia
- Irritable behavior and angry outbursts
- Duration of disturbance greater than 1 month
- Clinically significant impairment of function

Assessment and Treatment
See Anxiety Disorders.

Obsessive-Compulsive Disorder
- Hallmark feature is the presence of obsessions and compulsions that are a trigger for anxiety.

Symptoms of OCD
- Obsessions are recurrent thoughts and unwanted, intrusive ideas, thoughts, impulses, or images. Common thoughts are contamination, sexual imagery, repeated doubts, and need for order.
- Compulsions are ritualistic behaviors or mental acts carried out in response to an obsession. Common examples are hand washing, counting, or checking locks.

Assessment and Treatment
See Anxiety Disorders.

MOOD/AFFECTIVE DISORDERS
Depression
- Occurs in 30% to 40% of those with chronic medical illness.
- Older adults may complain of lack of energy and other somatic symptoms.

Risk Factors
- Prior episodes of depression
- Family history of depressive disorder
- Lack of social support
- Lack of coping abilities
- Presence of life and environmental stressors
- Current substance use or abuse
- Medical and/or mental illness comorbidity

Symptoms of Major Depression
Five of the nine listed symptoms are present continuously for a 2-week period; symptoms one and two must be included.
Five or more of the following:
- Depressed mood
- Loss of interest of pleasurable activities
- Significant weight loss or gain
- Insomnia or hypersomnia
- Psychomotor retardation or agitation

- Decreased ability to concentrate or make decisions
- Fatigue or loss of energy
- Feelings of worthlessness or excessive guilt
- Recurrent thoughts of death or suicide

Dysthymia
This is chronic depression characterized by symptoms for 2 or more years.

Assessment
Differential Diagnosis
Rule out organic cause for mood change (complete metabolic profile, B_{12}, thyroid-stimulating hormone [TSH], urinalysis [UA]). Dementia can coexist in 50% of cases in older adults.
Patient Health Questionnaire Screen for Depression (PHQ-2):
- Over the past 2 weeks, have you often had little interest or pleasure in doing things?
- Over the past 2 weeks, have you often been bothered by feeling down, depressed, or hopeless?
Geriatric Depression Scale (GDS)
- Fifteen-item questionnaire
- Yes/no questions
- Does not address sleep or somatic complaints

Treatment
- Nonpharmacologic
- Electroconvulsive therapy may be helpful in moderate to severe depression
For mild to moderate depression:
- Cognitive-behavioral therapy
- Mindfulness therapy
- Problem-solving therapy
For moderate to severe depression:
- Nonpharmacologic with pharmacologic
- First line—SSRIs (Table 15.3)
- Second line—Consider mirtazapine or vilazodone.

Bipolar Disorder
- Classified by periods of mania or hypomania that alternate with depression
- *Elevated mood*—Expressed as euphoria or elation
- *Expansive mood*—Characterized by a lack of restraint in expressing feelings, an overvalued sense of importance, and a constant and indiscriminate enthusiasm for interpersonal, sexual, or occupational interactions

Etiology/Risk Factors
- Possible genetic predisposition and psychosocial stress such as abuse or trauma
- Family history of mood disorders
- Lack of social support
- Substance abuse

Symptoms of Bipolar Disorder
- Inflated self-esteem or grandiosity
- Pressured speech
- Decreased need for sleep
- Fight of ideas or racing thoughts
- Distractibility
- Psychomotor agitation
- Excessive involvement in activities that have high potential for painful consequences (unrestrained shopping sprees, sexual indiscretion, or foolish business investments)
- Mood disturbance is sufficiently severe to cause impairment in social or occupational functioning.
- Episode not attributable to physiologic effects of substance abuse, medication, or medical condition.

Assessment
Differential Diagnosis
- Rule out organic cause for mood change (complete metabolic profile, B_{12}, TSH, UA, drug toxicology)

TABLE 15.3 OTHER COMMON ANTIDEPRESSANTS (NOT AN EXHAUSTIVE LIST)

GENERIC NAME (BRAND NAME)	MECHANISM OF ACTION	INDICATIONS, CONTRAINDICATIONS	DOSAGE	SIDE EFFECTS	SAFETY/PATIENT EDUCATION
Bupropion (Wellbutrin)	Norepinephrine Dopamine reuptake inhibitor	Major depression Smoking cessation Contraindicated in persons with history of seizures	75–150 mg	Dry mouth, constipation Headache, nausea, Weight loss	Do not stop abruptly.
Mirtazapine (Remeron)	Nonadrenergic and specific serotonergic antidepressant	Major depression Anxiety Can aid in sleep May improve appetite Contraindicated with MAOIs	7.5–45 mg daily	Drowsiness, dry mouth, constipation, weight gain, strange dreams	Can increase sedation, best taken at bedtime.
Methylphenidate (Ritalin)	Increased uptake of norepinephrine and dopamine in prefrontal cortex	Major depression with apathy ADHD Narcolepsy Contraindicated: thyrotoxicosis, seizures	5–10 mg in the morning	Nervousness anxiety, loss of appetite, nausea, insomnia	Best if taken 30 minutes prior to a meal.

ADHD, attention deficit hyperactivity disorder; MAOIs, monoamine oxidase inhibitors.

- Depression
- Other psychiatric mental illnesses

Treatment
- Hallmark of treatment is mood stabilizers (Tables 15.4 and 15.5)
- Cognitive-behavioral therapy
- High risk for suicide in depressive phase: Suicide assessment.

Suicide
Prevalence
- Highest rate of suicide in America is among people aged 45 to 64 years.
- Older adults are most likely to die on their first attempt.
- Men aged 85 and older are at highest risk.

Risk Factors
- Depression
- Prior suicide attempts
- Physical pain
- Social dependency and isolation
- Family discord or loss
- History of emotional, physical, or sexual abuse
- Inflexible or rigid personality
- Access to lethal means
- Chronic physical illness/cancer

Warning Signs
- Threatening to hurt or kill oneself
- Looking for access to medications or firearms
- Talking or writing about death or suicide

Assessment/Screen
- The U.S. Preventive Task Force (USPTF) indicates there is insufficient evidence for need to screen for suicide in older adults.
- Screen for depression, substance abuse, and warning signs.

DEMENTIA
- This is a chronic acquired decline in one or more cognitive domains (learning and memory, complex attention, language, visual–spatial, executive) sufficient to affect daily life (Table 15.6).
- Alzheimer's disease (AD) accounts for 60% to 70% of the affected population (Table 15.7).
- Other progressive disorders: these occur in 15% to 20% of the affected population (vascular, Lewy body dementia [LBD], fronto-temporal dementia [FTD], including primary progressive aphasia [PPA]).
- Dementia due to drug toxicity, metabolic changes, thyroid disease, head trauma, normal pressure hydrocephalus is completely reversible: comprises 2% to 5% of the affected population.

Risks for Dementia
- Age
- Family history
- APOE 4 (apolipoprotein E4) allele
- Down syndrome

Other Possible Risk Factors
- Head trauma
- History of depression
- Fewer years of formal education
- Cardiovascular risk factors

TABLE 15.4 MOOD STABILIZERS

CLASS	MOOD STABILIZERS			
Mechanism	Exact mechanism unknown. Becomes widely distributed in the CNS and interacts with neurotransmitters and receptors, decreasing norepinephrine release and increasing serotonin synthesis.			
GENERIC NAME (BRAND NAME)	INDICATIONS CONTRAINDICATIONS	DOSAGE	COMMON ADVERSE EFFECTS	SAFETY AND PATIENT EDUCATION
Lithium (Eskalith, Lithobid)	Interactions with diuretics, calcium channel blockers, NSAIDs Monitor serum sodium and BP	300–900 mg daily in divided doses	Thirst, drowsiness, diarrhea Muscular weakness, increased urination, loss of appetite, dry mouth	Maintain hydration. Do not take with any other antidepressants without discussing with provider.
Carbamazepine (Tegretol)	Increase risk of SIADH, pancytopenia Monitor Na$^+$	800–1,200 mg in divided doses	Drowsiness, dizziness, nausea, vomiting	Watch for any bruising or bleeding. Call provider with any acute onset of abdominal pain, rash, or sore throat, which can be an allergic reaction.
Valproic acid (Depakote)	Monitor LFTs, CBC Contraindicated in liver disease	750 mg daily in divided doses	Weight gain, tremor, thrombocytopenia	Call provider if rash occurs.
Lamotrigine (Lamictal)		100–200 mg daily in divided doses	Headache, dizziness, drowsiness, tremor, loss of coordination, blurred or double vision	

BP, blood pressure; CBC, complete blood count; CNS, central nervous system; LFT, liver function test; NSAIDs, nonsteroidal anti-inflammatory drugs; SIADH, syndrome of inappropriate antidiuretic hormone.

TABLE 15.5 ANTIPSYCHOTICS (SECOND GENERATION)

CLASS	ANTIPSYCHOTICS (SECOND GENERATION)			
Mechanism	Postsynaptic blockade of dopamine (D_2) receptors			
GENERIC NAME (BRAND NAME)	INDICATIONS, CONTRAINDICATIONS	DOSAGE	COMMON ADVERSE EFFECTS	SAFETY AND PATIENT EDUCATION
Aripiprazole (Abilify)	Psychotic disorders	30 mg daily maximum	Weight gain Dizziness Blurred vision Drowsiness Nausea/vomiting Constipation EPS symptoms	Need to monitor blood sugars in patients with diabetes. Medications should not be stopped abruptly.
Clozapine (Clozaril)		25–150 mg daily		
Lurasidone (Latuda)		40–80 mg daily		
Olanzapine (Zyprexa)		2.5–10 mg daily		
Quetiapine (Seroquel)		25–800 mg		
Risperidone (Risperdal)*		0.25–1 mg daily		

*May cause EPS symptoms.

EPS, extrapyramidail side effects.

TABLE 15.6 TYPES OF DEMENTIA

TYPE	ETIOLOGY	ONSET	DEFICITS	DISEASE PROGRESSION
MCI	Unknown	Gradual	Memory	Unknown, 12% progress to AD
AD	Neurodegenerative process Amyloid plaques/tau proteins, neurofibrillary tangles	Gradual	Memory, visual spatial, language	Gradual, 8–10 years
LBD	Neurodegenerative process	Gradual	Parkinsonism, visual hallucinations	Gradual, but faster than AD
Vascular	Cardiovascular risk factors	Can be abrupt or stepwise	Correlates with ischemia	Gradual, can be stepwise
Fronto-temporal	Tau or ubiquitin proteins in fronto-temporal dementia	Gradual, <less than 60 years old	Executive, visual spatial, disinhibited, apathy	Gradual, but faster than AD

AD, Alzheimer's disease; LBD, Lewy body dementia; MCI, mild cognitive impairment.

Source: From McCarron, R. (2018). *Primary care psychiatry*. Wolters Kluwer.

TABLE 15.7 STAGES OF ALZHEIMER'S DISEASE

Stage 1	No deficit
Stage 2	Complains of forgetting location of objects, subjective work difficulties
Stage 3	Decreased job function evident to coworkers
Stage 4	Decreased ability to perform complex tasks (planning, finances)
Stage 5	Requires assistance with dressing
Stage 6	Decreased ability to dress, bathe, and toilet independently (five substages that progress to incontinence of bowel and bladder)
Stage 7	Loss of speech, locomotion, and consciousness (five substages that progress to being unable to hold head up and nonverbal)

Source: From Reisberg, B. (1988). Functional assessment staging (FAST). *Psychopharmacology Bulletin*, 24(4), 653–659.

Screening

- Value of screening is controversial.
- Screening is a requirement of the Medicare Annual Wellness Visit (Table 15.8).
- Rule out organic cause: Complete metabolic profile, thyroid function tests (TFTs), CBC, rapid plasma reagin (RPR), HIV CT, or MRI if neurologic symptoms are noted

Differential Diagnosis

- Delirium
- Depression
- Neurologic disorder

Treatment

- Pharmacologic; see Table 15.9 for pharmacological treatment of AD.
- Nonpharmacologic
- Community services

TABLE 15.8 COGNITIVE SCREENING INSTRUMENTS

INSTRUMENT	SCORING	WEBSITE
Mini-Mental Status Exam	19-item score = 30	www.minimental.com
Mini-Cog	3-item score = 5	http://geriatrics.uthscsa.edu/tools/MINICog.com
MOCA	12-item score = 30	www.mocatest.org
SLUMS	11-item score = 30	https://www.slu.edu/medicine/internal-medicine/geriatric-medicine/aging-successfully/assessment-tools/mental-status-exam.php

MOCA, Montreal Cognitive Assessment; SLUMS, St. Louis University Mental Status.

Source: From McCarron, R. (2018). *Primary care psychiatry.* Wolters Kluwer.

TABLE 15.9 MEDICATIONS FOR TREATMENT OF ALZHEIMER'S DISEASE

CLASS	CHOLINESTERASE INHIBITORS			
Mechanism	Increase cortical acetylcholine			
GENERIC NAME (BRAND NAME)	INDICATIONS, CONTRAINDICATIONS	DOSAGE	COMMON ADVERSE EFFECTS	SAFETY AND PATIENT EDUCATION
Donezepil (Aricept)	5–10 mg daily		GI bleeding, bradycardia, nausea, vomiting, diarrhea	Notify provider if dark tarry stools or rectal bleeding. Notify provider if dizziness occurs.
Galantamine (Razadyne)	4–8 mg daily BID	Dose requires renal adjustment	GI, weight loss, broncho-constriction	Take with food.
Rivastigmine (Exelon)	Oral: 1.5–6 mg daily BID for PO dose Patch: 4.6 mg daily Maximum 9.5 mg		Syncope Weight loss Restlessness Irritability	Oral dose must be tapered.
CLASS	NMDA RECEPTOR AGONIST			
Mechanism	Blocks N-methyl-D-aspartate receptors			
GENERIC NAME (BRAND NAME)	INDICATIONS, CONTRAINDICATIONS	DOSAGE	COMMON ADVERSE EFFECTS	SAFETY AND PATIENT EDUCATION
Memantine (Namenda)	5–10 mg daily ER 7 mg daily Max 28 mg daily	Dose requires renal adjustment	Weight gain Aggression Somnolence	Must be tapered for discontinuation.

ER, extended release; GI, gastrointestinal; NMDA, N-methyl-D-aspartate.

Source: From McCarron, R. (2018). *Primary care psychiatry.* Wolters Kluwer.

- Advanced care planning—Now reimbursable
- Advanced directives
- Depression common for patient and caregiver

DELIRIUM

- Acute confusion
- Acute brain failure: inability to manage stressors
- Acute mental status change
- It is not dementia (Table 15.10)

Etiology

- Usually more than one cause

Risks and Precipitating Factors

- Advanced age (65 years and older)
- Surgery
- Functional impairment
- Sensory deprivation

- History of damage to brain (stroke, dementia)
- Medical complexity (infection)
- ETOH (ethanol) abuse
- Sleep deprivation
- Certain medications (anticholinergics, sedatives, sleeping pills, narcotics)
- Dehydration
- Malnutrition
- Use of restraints
- Extreme emotional stress (Badii, 2018; Khan & Boustani, 2014)

Screen/Assessment

- The confusion assessment method is most researched and widely used.
- Administration of the instrument requires education and training, which can be found at hospitalelderlifeprogram.org

TABLE 15.10 DIFFERENCES BETWEEN DELIRIUM AND DEMENTIA

DEMENTIA	DELIRIUM
■ Affects memory. ■ Level of consciousness is unaffected except in late stage. ■ Caused by anatomic, lasting changes in the brain. ■ Gradual onset (months to years). ■ Cognitive changes are permanent.	■ Affects attention. ■ Level of consciousness can fluctuate daily. ■ Can be caused by acute illness (infection, stroke, dehydration) or medications. ■ Onset is sudden: hours to days. ■ Can be reversible.

Source: From McCarron, R. (2018). *Primary care psychiatry*. Wolters Kluwer.

TABLE 15.11 SKILLS/PROCEDURES FOR MANAGEMENT OF AGITATION/AGGRESSION

De-escalation techniques for aggression	Use nonthreatening body language.
	Respect the person's personal space and boundaries.
	Speak softly and clearly.
	Have immediate access to a door in case you need to leave the room.
	Choose to leave a door open while talking with the person.
	Know where your colleagues are and make sure they know where you are.
Alternatives to restraints	Comfort rooms—Areas where the person can be provided with soothing music and alternative activities.
	Use of the comfort room is voluntary.
Management of restraints	Least restrictive
	Must use all nonrestraint alternatives with clear documentation
	Must be released every hour and skin checked and documented

Treatment

- Assume reversibility unless proven otherwise.
- Identify and correct underlying cause.
- Do a thorough review of medications and alcohol usage.
- Avoid anticholinergic medications.
- Avoid use of benzodiazepines and antipsychotics.
- Prevention and an interdisciplinary approach are the best interventions to minimizing the chance of the development of delirium (Khan & Boustani, 2014).

If delirium is not recognized and treated, it can lead to increased mortality, a decline in functional status, an increase in hospital-acquired complications, an increase in length of stay, and higher healthcare costs (Khan & Boustani, 2014, p. 197).

Capacity for Decision-Making

The capacity to make decisions for treatment/care can be determined by the following questions:

- Can the person comprehend risks and benefits?
- Does the person comprehend the implications?
- Does the person give reasons for the alternatives selected?
- Are supporting reasons rational?

If yes to all, the person has the capacity to make decisions. If no, the person should have shared decision-making with the healthcare proxy and healthcare team.

If no, person should be part of shared decision making with health care proxy and health care team

Agitation

- Unable to sit still or attend to others, accompanied by heightened emotion and tension.

Aggression

- May have behaviors or attitudes that reflect rage, hostility, and the potential for physical or verbal destructiveness (Table 15.11).

POST-ICU SYNDROME

- *Post-ICU syndrome* is defined as post-traumatic stress symptoms, anxiety, and depression after an ICU stay
- Prevalence: 19% to 48% of persons
- Affects recovery process, reduces quality of life, and increases burden on families
- Post-ICU clinics to address cognitive and psychologic issues, assess function, and determine at-home needs

MEDICAL NONCOMPLIANCE

Refers to deliberate or intentional refusal by the patient to take prescribed interventions.

MEDICAL NONADHERENCE

Adherence is defined as the extent to which patients take the medications or treatments prescribed by a healthcare provider. Nonadherence may be related to lack of understanding of medication, treatment, and unintended.

- Methods of measuring adherence are as follows:
- Direct observation
- Checking blood levels of medications
- Number of medication refills
- Pill counts

Consequences of Nonadherence

- Lack of progress toward goals and recovery
- Increased hospitalizations and ER usage
- Can increase polypharmacy

Important Communication Factors
- Trusting, caring patient–provider relationship
- Engagement in decision-making
- Positive expectancy/hope
- Person-centered approaches
- Clear explanation of disease process and medication
- simplify regimen if needed

REVIEW QUESTIONS

1. The hallmark signs of post-traumatic stress disorder (PTSD) are as follows:
   A. Intrusive thoughts, flashbacks, dissociative amnesia
   B. Hypersomnia, weight loss, irritability
   C. Feelings of helplessness, dissociative amnesia
   D. Psychomotor retardation, nightmares

2. As the clinical nurse specialist (CNS) assesses an older ICU patient, the CNS notes the patient seems confused. The CNS suspects delirium. What is the key sign that causes this suspicion?
   A. Acute change in mental status that affects attention
   B. Slow progressive change in mental status
   C. Difficulty with memory
   D. Weakness in both lower extremities

ANSWERS

1. **Correct answer: A. Rationale:** Intrusive thoughts, flashbacks, and dissociative amnesia are the hallmark symptoms of PTSD. Weight loss is not a hallmark symptom of PTSD. Although some patients with PTSD may feel helpless, it is not a hallmark symptom of PTSD. Psychomotor retardation is not associated with PTSD.

2. **Correct answer: A. Rationale:** Delirium is an acute change from baseline mental status. Dementia has a slow progression in change of mental status. Delirium is an acute change that occurs over hours to days, not a slow progressive change such as that associated with dementia. Delirium does not impair memory; this is more commonly associated with dementia. Delirium does not cause weakness; this symptom may be due to a neurologic event.

REFERENCES

The complete reference and additional reading lists appear in the digital version of the chapter, at https://connect.springerpub.com/content/book/978-0-8261-7417-8/part/part01/chapter/ch15

Multisystem Disorders

Lynne Marie Kokoczka, Joan Rembacz, Nicole Huntley, Marissa Diefenderfer, Eugena Bergvall, Margaret Skoog, and Ramona S. Irabor

SHOCK

OVERVIEW

Shock occurs when the body is unable to meet its oxygen and metabolic requirement to sustain normal body functions. The body initially compensates for the decrease in oxygen delivery but may progress to end-organ failure and death if compensatory measures fail. Treatment should be initiated even if the cause of the shock has not yet been determined. Once the underlying cause(s) are identified, additional treatment should be focused on the underlying cause(s) of the shock state (Puskarich & Jones, 2018; Tables 16.1 and 16.2).

CARDIOGENIC SHOCK

Cardiogenic shock is a state of end-organ hypoperfusion due to cardiac failure and the inability of the cardiovascular system to provide adequate blood flow to extremities and vital organs.

- In cardiogenic shock, myocardial dysfunction reduces stroke volume, cardiac output, and blood pressure, compromising myocardial perfusion, and exacerbates ischemia and further depresses the myocardial function, cardiac output, and systemic perfusion.
- Cardiogenic shock most commonly results from acute myocardial infarction.

ANAPHYLACTIC SHOCK

Anaphylaxis is a severe and life-threatening, systemic allergic reaction. It is a type of immediate hypersensitivity reaction. Anaphylaxis may lead to death by airway obstruction or vascular collapse. The most common symptoms are dermatologic and respiratory symptoms, occurring in 70% to 80% of episodes (Table 16.3).

Etiology and Pathophysiology

- Anaphylaxis can be due to either an immunoglobulin E- (IgE) mediated or a non–IgE-mediated allergic response (Grattan & Borzova, 2019).
- Almost any foreign substance can cause anaphylaxis, the most common cause is foods.
- Other causes of anaphylaxis are medications, blood and blood products, insect stings, and latex (Grattan & Borzova, 2019).

Assessment and Treatment

Immediate treatment of anaphylaxis includes administration of epinephrine at the first sign of respiratory or cardiovascular symptoms (Lieberman et al., 2015; (Table 16.4):

- Intramuscular (IM) route is the preferred route for initial administration in most settings (Lieberman et al., 2015).
- Intravenous (IV) route should only be given to patients with severe hypotension, who are unresponsive, or who are not responding to IM injections (Lieberman et al., 2015).
- Remove the allergen, if possible (Lieberman et al., 2015).
- Activate emergency response (Lieberman et al., 2015).
- Assess and treat airway obstruction (Lieberman et al., 2015).
- Optimize breathing and ventilation (Lieberman et al., 2015):
  - Administer oxygen at 8 to 10 L/min via face mask or use nonrebreather mask
  - Albuterol nebulizer or inhaler
- Maintain tissue perfusion (Lieberman et al., 2015):
  - Obtain IV access, if not previously established.
  - Treat hypotension with 0.9% sodium chloride or lactated ringers 1 to 2 L bolus.
  - Administer additional vasopressor if hypotension persists.
  - Initiate CPR if patient is pulseless.

Adjunctive treatment of anaphylaxis should not be used as the initial or the sole treatment for anaphylaxis (Lieberman et al., 2015). Medications used treat anaphylaxis include the following:

TABLE 16.1 SHOCK STATES: HEMODYNAMIC PARAMETERS

	PRELOAD (CENTRAL VENOUS PRESSURE)	PUMP FUNCTION (CARDIAC OUTPUT)	AFTERLOAD (SYSTEMIC VASCULAR RESISTANCE)
Cardiogenic	↑	↓	↓ ↔ ↓
Distributive	↓ or ↔	↑	↓
Hypovolemic	↓	↓	↑
Obstructive	↑	↓	↑

Source: Adapted from Franklin, C. M., & Darovic, G. O. (2002). Monitoring the patient in shock. In. G. O. Darvoic (Ed.), *Hemodynamic monitoring: Invasive and noninvasive clinical application* (3rd ed., pp. 361–401). W. B. Saunders.

The complete reference and additional reading lists appear in the digital version of this chapter, accessible at https://connect.springerpub.com/content/book/978-0-8261-7417-8/part/part01/chapter/ch16

TABLE 16.2 SHOCK STATES: ETIOLOGY AND TREATMENT

SHOCK STATES	ETIOLOGY	TREATMENT
Cardiogenic	Arrhythmias Myocardial infarction Valve insufficiency Aortic stenosis	Maintain oxygenation (PaO$_2$ > 60–70 mmHg) Maintain patent airway (endotracheal intubated as needed) Inotropic support Intra-aortic balloon pump Treatment of arrhythmias: cardioversion, pacing, medication Cardiac revascularization Valve replacement
Distributive	Anaphylactic shock Neurogenic shock Septic shock	Maintain oxygenation (PaO$_2$ > 60–70 mmHg) Maintain patent airway and adequate ventilation (endotracheal intubated as needed) Anaphylactic: epinephrine, identify allergen Neurogenic: spinal stabilization, vasopressors Septic: antibiotics, identify source and remove source (if able)
Hypovolemic	Hemorrhage Third spacing of fluids (burns, pancreatitis) Gastrointestinal losses Dehydration	Maintain oxygenation (PaO$_2$ > 60–70 mmHg) Maintain patent airway (endotracheal intubated as needed) Hemorrhagic: control bleeding, give blood and blood products, surgical consultation Treat electrolyte disturbances Treat underlying cause of fluid loss
Obstructive	Massive pulmonary embolism Tension pneumothorax Pericardial tamponade	Maintain oxygenation (PaO$_2$ > 60–70 mmHg) Maintain patent airway (endotracheal intubated as needed) Massive pulmonary embolism: thrombolysis Tension pneumothorax: needle decompression, chest tube insertion Pericardial tamponade: pericardiocentesis or pericardial window

Sources: Data from Leeper, B. (2014). Cardiovascular system. In S. M. Burns (Ed.), *AACN essentials of critical care nursing* (3rd ed., pp. 233–262). McGraw-Hill Education; Vincent, J.-L., & De Backer, D. (2013). Circulatory shock. *New England Journal of Medicine, 369,* 1726–1734. https://doi.org/10.1056/NEJMra1208943

TABLE 16.3 ANAPHYLAXIS SYMPTOMS

CATEGORY	SYMPTOMS
Cutaneous	Urticaria (hives) Angioedema Flushing Pruritus (itching)
Respiratory	Respiratory distress Laryngeal edema Bronchospasm Dyspnea Wheezing Persistent cough
Cardiovascular	Hypotension Tachycardia Cardiac dysrhythmias Chest pain Cardiopulmonary arrest
Other	Seizure Headache Abdominal pain Nausea/vomiting/diarrhea Anxiety, fear of impending doom

Source: Adapted from Grattan, C. E. H., & Borzova, E. (2019). Urticaria, angioedema, and *anaphylaxis*. In R. R. Rich, T. A. Fleisher, W. T. Shearer, H. W. Schroeder, A. J. Frew, & C. M. Weyand (Eds.), *Clinical immunology* (5th ed., pp. 506–521). Elsevier Saunders.

- Diphenhydramine 50 mg IV
- Methylprednisolone sodium succinate 125 mg IV
- Famotidine 40 mg IV or ranitidine 50 mg IV

Prevention
- Prevention of anaphylaxis includes identifying the allergen and limiting repeated exposure.
- Patients with a history of anaphylaxis should carry two units of auto-injector epinephrine (AIE) with them at all times and be taught how to avoid accidental exposures to the allergen.
- Patients with anaphylaxis should be referred to an allergist for further testing and management (Lieberman et al., 2015).
- To reduce reactions to IV radiocontrast media (RCM), premedication should be considered for patients with a previous allergic-like or unknown type of RCM reaction (American College of Radiology, 2020):
  - Elective premedication with oral medication is preferred (combinations of prednisone, diphenhydramine, methylprednisolone, dexamethasone, or hydrocortisone).

Clinical Practice Guidelines
- American College of Radiology's (ACR; 2020) *ACR Manual on Contrast Media*
- The American Academy of Allergy, Asthma and Immunology; the American College of Allergy, Asthma and Immunology; and the Joint Council of Allergy, Asthma and Immunology (2015)—*Anaphylaxis—A Practice Parameter Update*

TABLE 16.4 EPINEPHRINE ADMINISTRATION IN ANAPHYLAXIS

MEDICATION	MECHANISM OF ACTION	DOSAGE	SIDE EFFECTS	SAFETY/PATIENT EDUCATION
Epinephrine (alpha and beta agonists)	Stimulates alpha-1 adrenergic receptors (increases PVR causing vasoconstriction), decreases angioedema Stimulates beta-1 adrenergic receptors (increases contractility) Stimulates beta-2 receptors (bronchodilation) (Grattan & Borzova, 2019)	IM: 0.2–0.5 mg of 1:1,000 dilution IM to mid-outer thigh q5–15min up to 1 mg total (Lieberman et al., 2015) IV: 0.1 mg of 1:10,000 dilution IV repeated q1–2min as needed AIE (Patients greater than or equal to 30 kg): 0.3 mg of 1:1,000 dilution (Lieberman et al., 2015)	Anxiety, fear, headache, pallor, tremor, dizziness, palpation, decreased effects with beta blocker use, skin and soft tissue infections at injection site (Grattan & Borzova, 2019)	Recognition of signs and symptoms of anaphylaxis and when it is appropriate to use AIE Patient should always carry two units of AIE at all times in case a second dose is needed (Lieberman et al., 2015)

AIE, auto-injector epinephrine; IM, intramuscular; PVR, pulmonary vascular resistance.

SEPSIS/SEPTIC SHOCK AND MULTIPLE ORGAN DYSFUNCTION SYNDROME

OVERVIEW
- Sepsis is a life-threatening organ dysfunction caused by a dysregulated host response to infection.
- Sepsis is the leading cause of hospitalization and death from infection.
- Causes of sepsis can include community-acquired and healthcare-associated infections:
  - Pneumonia
  - Influenza
  - Urinary tract infections
  - Implanted port or indwelling catheter infections
  - Surgical-site infections
- *Septic shock* is defined as a subset of sepsis:
  - Clinical criteria representing this syndrome include the need for vasopressor therapy to maintain a mean arterial pressure (MAP) of 65 mmHg or greater and having a serum lactate level > 2 mmol/L despite adequate fluid resuscitation.
- Multiple organ dysfunction syndrome (MODS) is a progressive dysfunction of two or more major organs such that homeostasis cannot be maintained without medical intervention.

Pathophysiology
- Systemic inflammatory response syndrome (SIRS) is a clinical syndrome resulting from a dysregulated inflammatory response:
  - It can be infectious or noninfectious, for example, infection, ischemia, or trauma.
  - Infectious or noninfectious insult triggers cytokine production, causing inflammation.
  - Cytokines are released into circulation, causing growth factor stimulation, which recruits macrophages and platelets to attempt a return to homeostasis.
- Systemic reaction leads to activation of humoral cascades and activation of reticular endothelial system.
- Pro and antiinflammatory mechanisms are triggered by infection and are exaggerated in response:
  - These mechanisms are similar to SIRS stages.
  - Mechanisms are dysregulated and the antiinflammatory responses are overwhelmed by the proinflammatory responses, leading to systemic effects.
  - These mechanisms are initiated by endotoxin, perpetuating tumor necrosis factor (TNFα) release (a self-sustaining cascade), which causes further recruitment of leukocytes and macrophages.
- Damaged vascular endothelium leads to cell death.
- Altered coagulation leads to micro-thrombi formation and endothelial dysfunction, which impairs tissue oxygenation and can lead to disseminated intravascular coagulation (DIC).
- Tissue hypoperfusion is the effect of systemic vasodilation and hypotension and leads to MODS.

Identification
- Sepsis and potential sepsis screening is recommended at every shift or patient encounter (Tables 16.5 and 16.6).

Treatment
- Treatment is time sensitive and current evidence suggests completion of all of the following within 1 hour of actual or potential recognition of sepsis:
  - Check initial lactate level:
    - If >2 mmol/L but less than 4 mmol/L, without underlying organ dysfunction, the patient is likely in early sepsis.
    - If >4 mmol/L, without underlying organ dysfunction, the patient is likely in septic shock.
  - Obtain cultures (blood, sputum, urine, wound).
  - Administer broad-spectrum antibiotics.
  - Administer crystalloid fluid resuscitation:
    - Lactate ringers, normal saline, or plasmalyte are recommended.

TABLE 16.5 SEPSIS SCREENING

	SIRS	QSOFA	SOFA
Criteria	Temperature <36 °C or >38.3 °C Respiratory rate >20/min or $PaCO_2$ <30 mmHg Heart rate >90/min White blood cell count >12,000/mm³ or <4,000/mm³	Respiratory rate ≥22/min Altered mentation Systolic blood pressure ≤100 mmHg	See Table 16.6 (Vincent et al., 1996)
Screening	2/4 criteria is a positive screen	2/3 criteria is a positive screen	A score of 2 or more is associated with in-hospital mortality of >10%
Utility	Hospitals/facilities adhering to the CMS Core Measures are required to identify sepsis with SIRS criteria	ED and inpatient hospital units	Critical care trending of organ dysfunction to guide treatment

CMS, Centers for Medicare & Medicaid Services; QSOFA, quick sequential organ failure assessment; SIRS, systemic inflammatory response syndrome; SOFA, sepsis-related organ failure assessment.

TABLE 16.6 SEPSIS-RELATED ORGAN FAILURE ASSESSMENT SCORE

SOFA	SCORE				
SYSTEM	0	1	2	3	4
Respiratory: PaO_2 / FIO_2, mmHg (kPa)	≥400 (53.3)	<400 (53.3)	<300 (40)	<200 (26.7) with respiratory support	<100 (13.3) with respiratory support
Coagulation: Platelets, ×10³ mcL	≥150	<150	<100	<50	<20
Liver: Bilirubin, mg/dL (mcmol/L)	<1.2 (20)	1.2–1.9 (20–32)	2.0–5.9 (33–101)	6.0–11.9 (102–204)	>12 (204)
Cardiovascular	MAP ≥ 70 mmHg	MAP < 70 mmHg	Dopamine <5 or dobutamine (any does)	Dopamine 5.1–15 mcg/kg/min OR Epi nephrine ≤ 0.1 mcg/kg/min OR Norepi nephrine ≤ 0.1 mg/min	Dopamine > 15 mcg/kg/min OR Epi > 0.1 mcg/kg/min OR Norepi > 0.1 mcg/min
Central nervous system: Glasgow Coma Scale Score	15	13–14	10–12	6–9	<6
Renal: Creatinine mg/dL (mcmol/L)	<1.2 (110)	1.2–1.9 (110–170)	2.0–3.4 (171–299)	3.5–4.9 (300–440)	>5.0 (440)
Renal: Urine output, mL/d				<500	<200

Epi nephrine; MAP, mean arterial pressure; SOFA, sepsis-related organ failure assessment.
Source: From Vincent, J. L., Moreno, R., Takala, J., Willatts, S., De Mendoca, A., Bruining, H., Reinhart, C. K., Suter, P. M., & Thijs, L. G. (1996). The SOFA (sepsis-related organ failure assessment) score to describe organ dysfunction/failure. *Intensive Care Medicine, 22*, 707–710. https://doi.org/10.1007/BF01709751

- If the patient has a lactate >4 mmol/L or is hypotensive, 30 mL/kg resuscitation is recommended.
- Administer vasopressors as needed during or after fluid resuscitation to maintain MAP >65 mmHg.
- Continually reassess patient for perfusion effectiveness; for example:
  - Vital sign reviews
  - Cardiovascular and cardiopulmonary assessment
  - Skin assessment for mottling
  - Urine output
  - Peripheral pulse checks
  - Capillary refill
  - Recheck of lactate level until <2 mmol/L

Post-Sepsis Syndrome and Mortality

Similar to post-intensive care syndrome, post-sepsis syndrome can have major effects on a patient's quality of life and utilization of healthcare resources:

- Post-sepsis syndrome mortality has been shown to be anywhere from 7% to 46%.
- Post-sepsis utilization of healthcare resources increases markedly compared to nonsepsis utilization.
- Sepsis is an independent predictor of recurrent infections.
- Up to 50% of sepsis survivors can experience the following long-term effects:
  - Insomnia
  - Nightmares, hallucinations, and panic attacks

- Muscle and joint pains
- Extreme fatigue
- Poor concentration
- Decreased cognitive functioning
- Loss of self-esteem
- Significant and increased mortality has made this syndrome a regulatory performance metric.

Anti-Infective Medications
See Table 16.7 for a list of anti-infective medications.

Resources
Many guidelines are available as resources for recognition and treatment of sepsis.
- www.survivingsepsis.org/Pages/default.aspx
- www.sepsis.org
- www.cms.gov/medicare/quality-initiatives-patient-assessment-instruments/qualitymeasures/core-measures.html

---

ACID–BASE IMBALANCE

OVERVIEW OF ACID–BASE HOMEOSTASIS AND BUFFER SYSTEMS
Maintaining or restoring acid–base balance is necessary to ensure stable biologic processes, including the speed of cellular operations and permeability in cells and tissues (McCance & Huether, 2018).
- Assisted by buffer systems, acid–base homeostasis is regulated mainly by two body systems: the lungs (respiratory) and the kidneys (metabolic).
- The concentration of hydrogen ions (H+) represents pH: An acidic solution has a greater number of H+ ions, a basic solution has a lower number of H+ ions.
- An acid–base imbalance is caused by a change in H+ concentration (McCance & Huether, 2018).
- The following formula and its shift to the right or left represent the dynamic equilibrium reactions that occur to maintain acid–base balance (Hamilton et al., 2017).

$$CO_2 + H_2O \leftrightarrow H_2CO_3 \leftrightarrow HCO_3^- + H^+$$

Regulated by Lungs   Regulated by Kidneys

CO_2, carbon dioxide; H_2O, water; H_2CO_3, carbonic acid, HCO_3^-, bicarbonate.

- Acid–base imbalances or disorders are common among patients who are hospitalized and patients with chronic disorders.
- History and physical examination assists the clinician in determining if an acid–base imbalance exists and the cause of the acid–base imbalance.
- Lab diagnostics, specifically arterial blood gas (ABGs) and chemistries, play an important role in the assessment, diagnosis, and management of acid–base imbalances (Table 16.8).
- Treatment is determined by the underlying cause of the acid–base imbalance.

Classification of Acid–Base Imbalances
- Acidotic or alkalotic
- Metabolic, respiratory, or mixed acid–base disorders
- Acute or chronic (Foster & Prevost, 2012)

TYPES OF ACID–BASE DISORDERS
Anion Gap in Metabolic Acidosis
- This is used to help distinguish different causes of metabolic acidosis (Table 16.9).
- Anion gap is the difference between cations and anions in the plasma. It is calculated using the following formula: $(Na^+ + K^+) - (Cl^- + HCO_3^-)$. See Table 16.10.

COMPENSATION IN ACID–BASE IMBALANCES
The lungs, kidneys, and buffer systems attempt to correct an acid–base imbalance (Table 16.11):
- When the primary imbalance is metabolic, direct changes occur in bicarbonate levels, and compensation comes from the respiratory system via the respiratory rate within minutes to hours.
- When the primary imbalance is respiratory, direct changes occur in $PaCO_2$, and compensation comes from the kidneys by producing or excreting bicarbonate.

This process can take up to several hours or days (McCance & Huether, 2018).

Assessment
- Determining the cause or underlying disease process of an acid–base imbalance should be the clinicians' priority as this determines the best treatment for the imbalance.
- Signs and symptoms associated with acid–base disturbances vary depending on the underlying cause of the imbalance.

Diagnostics
- ABG and serum chemistry are the best diagnostic studies.
- Diagnostics that correlate with suspected differential diagnosis should be performed to determine the underlying cause.
- Other considerations of diagnostics include radiographs, EKG, CT, MRI, pulmonary function tests (PFTs), and blood tests such as chemistry, complete blood count (CBC), salicylate level, thyroid tests, beta human chorionic gonadotropin (hCG), urine anion gap, and ketone level.

Interpretation
Interpretation of the ABG and serum chemistry along with history and physical exam assists the clinician in diagnosing an acid–base imbalance. A simple step-by-step approach is shown in the following (Hamilton et al., 2017):

Steps in Interpretation
Step 1: Look at pH. Is acidemia or alkalemia present? Or is the pH normal? Note here that pH can be normal due to compensation and disorder might still be present.

Step 2: What are the bicarbonate levels? When bicarbonate levels are affected, we can suspect that a metabolic process is occurring. When the bicarbonate is reduced with acidemia, the condition is likely metabolic acidosis. When bicarbonate is elevated with alkalemia, the condition is likely metabolic alkalosis.

Step 3: What are the $PaCO_2$ levels? When there is a disturbance in $PaCO_2$, we can suspect that a respiratory process is occurring. If the value is increased when acidemia is present, the condition is likely respiratory acidosis. If the value is decreased when alkalemia is present, the condition is likely respiratory alkalosis. Remember that in respiratory disorders the primary markers move in opposite directions and in metabolic disorders the

TABLE 16.? ANTI-INFECTIVE MEDICATIONS

CLASS	1ST-/3RD-/4TH-GENERATION CEPHALOSPORIN				
Mechanism	Inhibition of bacterial cell wall synthesis				
Generic Name / Brand Name	**Indications and Contraindications**	**Dosage**	**Common Adverse Effects**	**Safety and Patient Education**	
Cefazolin sodium/ Ancef (1st generation)	INDICATIONS: ■ Genital infection ■ Infections of bone/joints ■ Infection of skin and/or subcutaneous tissues ■ Infective cholangitis ■ Infective endocarditis ■ Respiratory tract infection ■ Sepsis ■ Urinary tract infectious disease CONTRAINDICATIONS: ■ Hypersensitivity to cephalosporins	0.5–2 g IV q6–12h	■ Pruritus ■ Diarrhea/CDIFF ■ Drug induces eosinophilia ■ Stevens-Johnson syndrome ■ Leukopenia ■ Hypersensitivity or anaphylactic reactions ■ Encephalopathy ■ Seizure ■ Renal failure	■ Drug may cause diarrhea, nausea, vomiting, or thrombocytopenia ■ Severe diarrhea should be reported and healthcare professional consulted before taking antidiarrheal medication ■ Advise patient to maintain drug administration schedule	
Ceftriaxone sodium/ Rocephin (3rd generation)	INDICATIONS: ■ Sepsis ■ Bacteremia associated with intravascular line ■ Infections of the following: ● Skin ● Meninges ● Lower respiratory system ● Musculoskeletal system ● Abdomen ● Gonorrhea and pelvic inflammatory disease ● Urinary tract CONTRAINDICATIONS: ■ Hypersensitivity to cephalosporins ■ Monitor intravenous medication compatibility	1–2 g IV/IM q12h Maximum: 4 g/d	■ Induration at injection site ■ Stevens-Johnson syndrome ■ Diarrhea/CDIFF infection ■ Elevated eosinophil count ■ Hypersensitivity reaction ■ Renal failure ■ Lung injury	■ Longest cephalosporin half-life at 6.5 hours ■ Poor activity against pseudomonas ■ Educate patient about hypersensitivity symptoms ■ Educate patient to watch for signs of biliary obstruction/ hepatotoxicity	
Cefepime/ Maxipime (4th generation)	INDICATIONS: ■ Acute otitis media ■ Bacteremia associated with intravascular line ■ Endocarditis ■ Meningitis ■ Musculoskeletal infections ■ Chancroid ■ Epididymitis ■ Gonorrhea ■ Infections of the skin and subcutaneous tissues ■ Abdominal infections ■ Urinary tract infections CONTRAINDICATIONS: ■ Hypersensitivity to cephalosporins ■ Monitor intravenous medication compatibility	2 g IV q8–12h	■ Rash ■ Hypophosphatemia ■ Diarrhea ■ Positive direct Coombs test ■ Elevated liver enzymes ■ Stevens-Johnson syndrome ■ CDIFF infection ■ Anaphylaxis ■ Aphasia ■ Encephalopathy ■ Myoclonus ■ Neurotoxicity ■ Seizure	■ Educate patient to watch for hypersensitivity reactions and adverse reaction symptoms	

(continued)

CLASS	FLUOROQUINOLONE		
Mechanism	Inhibition of bacterial enzymes required for bacterial DNA synthesis		
Ciprofloxacin/ Cipro	INDICATIONS: ■ Prostatitis ■ Sinusitis ■ Acute exacerbation of chronic bronchitis ■ Campylobacteriosis ■ Febrile neutropenia ■ Gonorrhea ■ HIV infection ■ Hospital-acquired pneumonia ■ Infections of bone or joints ■ Infection of skin and/or subcutaneous tissues ■ Infectious diarrheal disease ■ Infectious disease of the abdomen ■ Inhalation anthrax ■ Lower respiratory tract infection ■ Otitis externa ■ Plague ■ Pyelonephritis typhoid fever ■ Urinary tract infectious disease CONTRAINDICATIONS: ■ Concomitant tizanidine administration ■ Hypersensitivity to Cipro or other quinolones	400–1,200 mg IV q8–12h	■ Rash ■ Diarrhea ■ Nausea ■ Vomiting ■ Headache ■ Irritability ■ Nasal discharge/pharyngitis ■ Aortic aneurysm or dissection ■ Cardiorespiratory arrest ■ MI ■ Torsades de pointes ■ Photosensitivity ■ Stevens-Johnson syndrome ■ Hypoglycemia ■ CDIFF ■ GI hemorrhage ■ Pancreatitis ■ Leukopenia ■ Pancytopenia ■ Thrombocytopenia ■ Hepatic necrosis ■ Hepatitis ■ Liver failure ■ Hypersensitivity reaction ■ Myasthenia gravis ■ Tendon rupture ■ Tendinitis ■ Disorientation ■ Guillain-Barré syndrome ■ Peripheral neuropathy ■ Increased ICP	■ Follow Beers Criteria for the older adult ■ Educate patient to watch for hypersensitivity reactions and adverse reaction symptoms ■ Avoid caffeine ■ Take drug 2 hours before or 6 hours after magnesium or aluminum-containing antacids or products containing calcium, iron, or zinc
Levofloxacin/ Levaquin	INDICATIONS: ■ Bronchiolitis ■ Prostatitis ■ Sinusitis ■ Community or hospital-acquired pneumonia ■ Plague ■ Pyelonephritis ■ Uncomplicated UTI and infections of the: ■ skin and subcutaneous tissues	250–750 mg IV/PO q24h	■ Seizure ■ Delirium ■ Depression ■ Paranoid disorder ■ Psychotic disorder ■ Suicidal behavior ■ Acute renal failure ■ Hemorrhagic cystitis ■ Diarrhea ■ Dizziness/headache ■ Aortic aneurysm or dissection	

(continued)

TABLE 16.7 ANTI-INFECTIVE MEDICATIONS (continued)

Generic Name / Brand Name	Indications and Contraindications	Dosage	Common Adverse Effects	Safety and Patient Education
CLASS	**FLUOROQUINOLONE**			
	CONTRAINDICATIONS: ■ Hypersensitivity reactions to quinolones		■ Cardiac arrest ■ Prolonged QT ■ Torsades de Pointes ■ V Tach ■ Stevens-Johnson Syndrome ■ Hypoglycemia ■ Anemia/pancytopenia ■ Liver failure ■ Hypersensitivity or anaphylactic reaction ■ Myasthenia gravis ■ Delirium ■ Guillain-Barré syndrome ■ Peripheral neuropathy ■ Retinal detachment ■ Renal failure	■ Educate patient to watch for hypersensitivity reactions and adverse reaction symptoms
CLASS	**EXTENDED SPECTRUM BETA LACTAMASE**			
Mechanism	Inhibition of cell wall synthesis by exerting bactericidal activity penetrating the cell wall to reach PBP targets			
Meropenem/ Merrem	INDICATIONS: ■ Bacteremia associated with intravascular line ■ Meningitis ■ Febrile neutropenia ■ Hospital-acquired pneumonia ■ Infection of skin and/or soft tissue ■ Infectious disease of the abdomen CONTRAINDICATIONS: ■ Hypersensitivity or anaphylaxis to beta lactams	500 mg–1 g IV q8h	■ Constipation ■ Diarrhea ■ Anemia ■ Headache ■ Pain ■ Cardiac arrest ■ Heart failure ■ Myocardial infarction ■ Shock ■ Syncope ■ Hemorrhage ■ Hypersensitivity or anaphylactic reaction ■ Cholestatic jaundice syndrome ■ Jaundice ■ Liver failure ■ Seizure ■ Renal failure ■ Hypoxia ■ Pleural effusion ■ Pulmonary edema ■ Pulmonary embolism ■ Angioedema ■ Sepsis	■ Educate patient to watch for hypersensitivity reactions and adverse reaction symptoms

(continued)

CLASS	COMBINATION BETA LACTAMASE AND CARBAPENEM			
Mechanism	■ Inhibition of cell wall synthesis by exerting bactericidal activity penetrating the cell wall to reach PBP targets ■ Exhibits a synergistic effect with imipenem by preventing renal enzymes from breaking down imipenem			
Imipenem and Cilastatin/ Primaxin	500 mg–1 g IV q6–8h	INDICATIONS: ■ Sepsis ■ Female genitalia infection ■ Bone/joint infections ■ Infection of the skin and/or subcutaneous tissues ■ Infectious disease of the abdomen ■ Infective endocarditis due to *Staphylococcus aureus* ■ Lower respiratory tract infection ■ Urinary tract infectious disease CONTRAINDICATIONS: ■ Hypersensitivity to beta lactamases	■ Phlebitis ■ Diarrhea ■ Nausea/vomiting ■ Thrombophlebitis ■ Stevens-Johnson syndrome ■ Toxic epidermal necrolysis ■ Hypersensitivity reaction ■ Seizure	■ Report severe diarrhea and consult healthcare professional before taking antidiarrheal medication ■ Educate patient to watch for hypersensitivity reactions and adverse reaction symptoms

CLASS	COMBINATION PENICILLIN AND BETA LACTAMASE INHIBITOR			
Mechanism	■ Inhibition of biosynthesis if cell wall mucopeptide ■ Inhibition of bacterial septum formation and cell wall synthesis ■ Inhibition of hydrolysis of ampicillin			
Ampicillin sodium and sulbactam sodium/Unasyn	1.5–3 g q6h	INDICATIONS: ■ Infection of skin and/or subcutaneous tissue ■ Infectious disease of the abdomen ■ Pelvic inflammatory disease CONTRAINDICATIONS: ■ History of jaundice/hepatic dysfunction associated with Unasyn ■ History of hypersensitivity reactions to medication classes	■ Injection site pain ■ Rash ■ Diarrhea/CDIFF ■ Hepatotoxicity	■ Development of rash to be reported ■ Diarrhea should be reported and healthcare professional consulted before taking antidiarrheal medication ■ Educate patient to watch for hypersensitivity reactions and adverse reaction symptoms
Piperacillin sodium and tazobactam sodium/Zosyn	3.375–4.5 g IV q6h	INDICATIONS: ■ Appendicitis, complicated by rupture or abscess ■ Community-acquired pneumonia ■ Hospital-acquired pneumonia ■ Infection of skin and/or subcutaneous tissue ■ Pelvic inflammatory disease ■ Peritonitis ■ Puerperal endometriosis CONTRAINDICATIONS: ■ Hypersensitivity reactions	■ Pruritus/rash ■ Constipation ■ Diarrhea/CDIFF ■ Nausea/vomiting ■ Headache ■ Insomnia ■ Fever ■ Stevens-Johnson syndrome ■ Agranulocytosis ■ Leukopenia ■ Pancytopenia ■ Thrombocytopenia ■ Hypersensitivity or anaphylaxis reactions ■ Seizure	■ Educate patient to report on the symptoms of bleeding ■ Diarrhea should be reported and healthcare professional consulted before taking antidiarrheal medication ■ Educate patient to watch for hypersensitivity reactions and adverse reaction symptoms ■ Educate patient with renal impairment to report symptoms of seizure ■ Educate patient with cystic fibrosis to report fevers or rash immediately

(continued)

ANTIINFECTIVE MEDICATIONS *(continued)*

Generic Name / Brand Name	Indications and Contraindications	Dosage	Common Adverse Effects	Safety and Patient Education
CLASS	**LINCOSAMIDE**			
Mechanism	Inhibition of bacterial protein synthesis			
Clindamycin phosphate/ Clindamycin	INDICATIONS: ■ Acne vulgaris ■ Bacterial infectious disease ■ Bacterial vaginosis ■ Endometritis ■ Infection of bone ■ Infection of skin and/or soft tissue ■ Infectious disease of the abdomen ■ Infectious disease of the joint ■ Lower respiratory tract infection ■ Pelvic inflammatory disease ■ Sepsis CONTRAINDICATIONS: ■ History of antibiotic-associated colitis ■ History of regional enteritis ■ History of ulcerative colitis ■ Hypersensitivity to lincosamides	600–2,700 mg IV q6–12h	■ Dry skin ■ Morbilliform eruption ■ Diarrhea ■ Nausea ■ Candida vaginitis ■ Vaginal pain ■ Stevens-Johnson syndrome ■ Epidermal necrolysis ■ CDIFF ■ Hemorrhagic diarrhea ■ Agranulocytosis ■ Increased liver function tests ■ Jaundice ■ Drug reaction with eosinophilia and systemic symptoms	■ See black-box warning about CDIFF infections ■ Educate patient to watch for hypersensitivity reactions and adverse reaction symptoms
CLASS	**GLYCOPEPTIDE**			
Mechanism	Inhibits bacterial cell wall synthesis, alters the permeability of membrane, and interferes with RNA synthesis			
Vancomycin hydrochloride/ Vancocin	INDICATIONS: ■ CDIFF ■ Infection of skin and/or subcutaneous tissue ■ Infective endocarditis ■ Lower respiratory tract infection ■ MRSA infection ■ Staphylococcal enterocolitis CONTRAINDICATIONS: ■ Allergy to corn or corn products ■ Hypersensitivity to vancomycin	**Varies:** For CDIFF: 125–500 mg PO q8h For MRSA: 30 mg/kg/d IV divided in 2 doses For endocarditis or lower respiratory tract infection: 2 g/d IV q6–12h	■ Hypokalemia ■ Abdominal pain ■ Nausea ■ Vomiting ■ Cardiac arrest ■ Hypotension ■ CDIFF ■ Agranulocytosis ■ Neutropenia ■ Thrombocytopenia ■ Anaphylaxis ■ Ototoxicity ■ Nephrotoxicity	■ Monitor drug peak and tough levels for best coverage ■ Educate patient to watch for hypersensitivity reactions and adverse reaction symptoms
Linezolid/Zyvox	INDICATIONS: ■ Community-acquired pneumonia ■ Hospital-acquired pneumonia ■ Complicated or uncomplicated infection of skin and/or subcutaneous tissue ■ MRSA infection ■ Vancomycin-resistant enterococcus faecium infection	400–600 mg IV q12h	■ Diarrhea ■ Nausea ■ Vomiting ■ Headache ■ Lactic acidosis ■ CDIFF ■ Myelosuppression	■ Report MAOI use prior to initiation of treatment ■ Avoid consumption of large quantities of food/beverages that contain tyramine (aged cheese, dried meats, alcohol, sauerkraut, soy sauce, yeast extract/supplements)

(continued)

CLASS	Mechanism	Drug	Dose	Indications / Contraindications	Adverse Effects	Patient Education
				CONTRAINDICATIONS: ■ Concomitant use of MAOIs (within 2 weeks of administration) ■ Hypersensitivity to linezolid	■ Injury of liver ■ Peripheral neuropathy ■ Seizure ■ Optic nerve disorder ■ Serotonin syndrome	Educate patient to watch for hypersensitivity reactions and adverse reaction symptoms, especially myelosuppression, lactic acidosis, and changes in vision
MACROLIDE	Interference with microbial protein synthesis	Azithromycin/ Zithromax	500–1,000 mg PO or IV daily	**INDICATIONS:** ■ Acute infective exacerbation of chronic COPD ■ Acute otitis media ■ Bacterial conjunctivitis ■ Bacterial sinusitis ■ Chancroid ■ Community-acquired pneumonia ■ Gonorrhea ■ Uncomplicated infection of skin and/or subcutaneous tissue ■ Nongonococcal cervicitis or urethritis ■ Pelvic inflammatory disease ■ Streptococcal pharyngitis or tonsillitis **CONTRAINDICATIONS:** ■ Cholestatic jaundice with prior azithromycin therapy ■ Hepatic dysfunction with prior azithromycin therapy ■ Hypersensitivity to azithromycin	■ Injection site reaction ■ Abdominal pain ■ Diarrhea/CDIFF ■ Nausea ■ Vomiting ■ Increased liver enzymes ■ Headache ■ Blurred vision ■ Prolonged QT interval ■ Torsades de pointes ■ Generalized exanthematous pustulosis ■ Stevens–Johnson syndrome ■ Hepatitis ■ Hepatic necrosis ■ Liver failure ■ Eaton–Lambert syndrome ■ Myasthenia gravis ■ Corneal erosion	■ Educate patient to watch for hypersensitivity reactions and adverse reaction symptoms—especially liver failure and CDIFF
AMEBICIDE	Inhibition of DNA synthesis and degradation	Metronidazole/ Flagyl	**Varies:** ■ CDIFF: 500 mg IV q8h *plus* vancomycin 500 mg PO/NGT QID	**INDICATIONS:** ■ Anaerobic abscess ■ Acute amebic dysentery ■ Amebic liver abscess ■ Bacterial meningitis ■ Infection due to anaerobic bacteria ■ Infection of bone/joint ■ Rosacea ■ Tichomoniasis **CONTRAINDICATIONS:** ■ Alcohol use during and for at least 3 days after administration ■ Concomitant use of disulfiram ■ Hypersensitivity to metronidazole or parabens	■ Abdominal discomfort ■ Diarrhea ■ Nausea ■ Jarisch–Herxheimer reaction ■ Dizziness ■ Headache ■ Vaginitis ■ Stevens–Johnson syndrome ■ Leukopenia ■ Hepatic failure/hepatotoxicity ■ Aseptic meningitis ■ Encephalopathy ■ Peripheral neuropathy ■ Seizure ■ Disorder of optic nerve ■ Ototoxicity ■ Hemolytic uremic syndrome	■ Educate patient to watch for hypersensitivity reactions and adverse reaction symptoms, especially aseptic meningitis, encephalopathy, or peripheral neuropathy ■ Avoid alcohol

CDIFF, *Clostridium difficile*; COPD, chronic obstructive pulmonary disease; GI, gastrointestinal; ICP, intracranial pressure; IM, intramuscular; IV, intravenous; MAOI, monoamine oxidase inhibitor; MI, myocardial infarction; MRSA, methicillin-resistant *Staphylococcus aureus*; NGT, nasgastric tube; PBP, penicillin binding protein; UTI, urinary tract infection.
Source: Drug Information. (2019). *Prescriber's digital reference, PDR.* www.pdr.net

TABLE 16.8 NORMAL RANGE OF COMMON LAB VALUES FOR ANALYSIS

pH	7.35–7.45 (7.40)
$PaCO_2$	35–45 mm/Hg
HCO_3^-	22–26 mEq/L
Anion gap	8–12 mEq/L

primary markers move in the same direction. However, the clinician must always consider the possibility of a mixed acid–base disorder.

Step 4: In cases of metabolic acidosis, calculate the anion gap, using the formula $(Na^+ + K^+) - (Cl^- + HCO_3^-)$. If the anion gap is above 12, the condition is high anion gap metabolic acidosis. If the anion gap is normal, the condition is normal anion gap metabolic acidosis. Again, this assists the clinician

TABLE 16.9 ACUTE STATES OF ACID–BASE DISORDERS AND THEIR CHARACTERISTICS

	METABOLIC ACIDOSIS	METABOLIC ALKALOSIS	RESPIRATORY ACIDOSIS	RESPIRATORY ALKALOSIS
pH	Decreased ↓	Increased ↑	Decreased ↓	Increased ↑
$PaCO_2$	Normal	Normal	**Increased ↑**	Increased ↑
HCO_3^-	**Decreased ↓**	**Increased ↑**	Normal	**Decreased ↓**
Pathophysiology	Caused by excess H^+ generated, a reduction in H^+ excretion, or a loss of HCO_3^- from the body	Caused by processes that increase HCO_3^-, usually from a loss of H^+ ions.	Occurs due to decreased ventilation, which results in increased $PaCO_2$.	Occurs due to increased ventilation, which results in decreased $PaCO_2$
Common causes	GI losses (loss of HCO_3^-), DKA and lactic acidosis (excess H^+ formation), renal failure (reduction in H^+ excretion), ingestions of salicylate, methanol or formaldehyde	GI losses from vomiting and suctioning, diuretic therapy, excessive bicarbonate intake, hyperaldosteronism, and decreased potassium (McCance & Huether, 2018).	Any condition or medication that can decrease respiratory drive, airway obstruction, and/or incorrect ventilation settings. Respiratory acidosis can be acute or chronic. Chronic causes of respiratory acidosis include COPD or neuromuscular disorders. (Hamilton et al., 2017).	Central nervous system stimulation, pain, fever, panic disorders, hyperventilation syndrome, trauma, hypoxemia, high altitudes and sepsis (Hamilton et al., 2017)
Signs and symptoms	Kussmaul respirations (deep/rapid), lethargy, confusion, diarrhea, headache, decreased appetite, and abdominal discomfort (McCance & Huether, 2018)	Weakness, cramps, hyperactive reflexes, tetany, seizures, and slow and shallow respirations; in severe alkalosis, confusion and convulsions can occur	Headache, anxiety, restlessness, increased respiratory rate initially that progresses to decreased respiratory rate, barrel chest, hyperresonance on percussion, and clubbing	Chest pain, tetany, dizziness, mental confusion, syncope, seizures anxiety, tachycardia, tachypnea, and cyanosis
Treatment	Bicarbonate can be used to treat acidosis. However, the underlying cause must be treated.	Volume status should be monitored. Antiemetics and H_2 blockers should be considered for patients vomiting or with GI suctioning. Diuretic medications may need to be adjusted (McCance & Huether, 2018). Sodium chloride and potassium should be given to stop HCO_3^- reabsorption/increase renal HCO_3^- loss to correct pH (Hamm et al., 2015).	Distinguish acute from chronic for treatment purposes. Treatment should focus on restoring alveolar ventilation and may include mechanical ventilation, opioid antagonists, corticosteroids, and bronchodilators. Oxygen should be given cautiously to prevent further respiratory depression (McCance & Huether, 2018).	Usually occurs in response to a stimulus; controlling the stimulus resolves the alkalosis. In mechanical ventilation, tidal volume or respiratory rate may need to be decreased. Pain control and sedation should be monitored to ensure it is adequate for the patient. Patients may need reassurance or benefit from breathing in a paper bag to increase $PaCO_2$ in the body (McCance & Huether, 2018).

Note: Bold type indicates the hallmark sign/direct change.

COPD, congestive obstructive pulmonary disease; DKA, diabetic ketoacidosis; GI, gastrointestinal.

Sources: Data from Hamilton, P., Morgan, N. A., Connolly, G. M., & Maxwell, P. (2017). Understanding acid-base disorders. *Ulster Medical Journal, 86*(3), 161–166; Hamm, L. L., Nakhoul, N., & Hering-Smith, K. S. (2015). Acid-base homeostasis. *Clinical Journal of the American Society of Nephrology, 10*(12), 2232–2242. http://doi.org/10.2215/CJN.07400715; McCance, K. L., & Huether, S. E. (Eds.). (2018). *Pathophysiology: The biologic basis for disease in adults and children.* Mosby Elsevier.

TABLE 16.10 SELECTED CAUSES OF METABOLIC ACIDOSIS CHARACTERIZED BY ANION GAP

	NORMAL ANION GAP (HYPERCHLOREMIC)	HIGH ANION GAP
Pathophysiology	Occurs due to bicarbonate loss with chloride retention (McCance & Huether, 2018).	Occurs when there is an accumulation of anions other than chloride (McCance & Huether, 2018).

Common causes	GI loss of bicarbonate/diarrhea
	Renal tubule acidosis
	Use of carbonic anhydrase inhibitors (acetazolamide)
	Urinary diversion/ureterosigmoidoscopy
	Excessive 0.9% saline administration
		Increased H^+
		  Ketoacidosis
		  Lactic acidosis
		  Ingestions = salicylate poisoning, glycol ingestion, methanol ingestion
		Decreased H^+ excretion
		  Uremia
		Distal renal tubule acidosis

Popular mnemonic	HARDUP	MUDPILES*

*See Table 16.17.

GI: gastrointestinal; HARDUP: hyperalimentation, acetazolamide, renal tubular acidosis, diarrhea, ureterosigmoid fistula, pancreatic fistula; MUD-PILES: methanol, uremia, diabetic ketoacidosis, paraldehyde, iron toxicity, lactate, ethylene glycol toxicity, salicylate toxicity.
Source: Data from Hamilton, P., Morgan, N. A., Connolly, G. M., & Maxwell, P. (2017). Understanding acid-base disorders. *The Ulster Medical Journal*, 86(3), 161–166; McCance, K. L., & Huether, S. E. (Eds.). (2018). *Pathophysiology: The biologic basis for disease in adults and children.* Mosby Elsevier; de Moya, M. A., Lee, J., & Yeh, D. D. (2017, November 29). *Acid-base balance.* https://www.facs.org/~/media/files/education/core%20curriculum/acid_base_balance.ashx

TABLE 16.11 COMPENSATION IN ACID–BASE IMBALANCES

	METABOLIC ACIDOSIS	METABOLIC ALKALOSIS	RESPIRATORY ACIDOSIS	RESPIRATORY ALKALOSIS
pH	Increasing to normal	Decreasing to normal	Increasing to normal	Decreasing to normal
$PaCO_2$	Decrease ↓	Increase ↑	Increase ↑	Decrease ↓
HCO_3^-	Decrease ↓	Increase ↑	Increase ↑	Decrease ↓
System	Lungs	Lungs	Kidneys	Kidneys
Process	Hyperventilation	Hypoventilation	Reabsorption of bicarbonate	Excretion of bicarbonate

in narrowing down the cause of the metabolic acidosis. Osmolar gap, the difference between measured and calculated osmolality, may also be used to assist in determining the diagnosis (Kitterer et al., 2015).

Clinical Nurse Specialist Competencies

Depending on cause and severity, the clinical nurse specialist (CNS) should be prepared to consult pulmonology, nephrology, and/or neurology. Other competencies required of the CNS in acid–base imbalance treatment include coaching the interprofessional team, initiating interprofessional meetings, and teaching patients and families about the diagnosis, causes, symptoms, and treatments.

TOXIC EXPOSURES, INGESTIONS, AND INHALATIONS

OVERVIEW

Poisoning is a significant public health concern that consumes healthcare resources and causes poison-related mortality and morbidity in the developing-world countries (Cline et al., 2016). Poisoned patients may not always appear acutely ill but should be treated as if they have a life-threatening intoxication. Regional poison control center consultation is highly recommended in all cases of suspected poisoning for expert advice on diagnosis and management:

- All healthcare providers and facilities should have the U.S. regional poison control center number: toll free 1-800-222-1222.
- Toxic exposures or poisoning occur most commonly by ingestion.
- Other routes include inhalation, insufflation, and cutaneous and mucous membrane exposure.

General Management

When treating a patient with suspected poisoning, the initial evaluation consists of a comprehensive assessment and an accurate history, when possible. A physical exam is essential to identify immediate threats to life, to evaluate the severity of the poisoning, and to assess for comorbid conditions. Initial management focuses on stabilization of the patient.

Initial Management and Evaluation

- Stabilization of the patient is the first priority in managing toxic ingestions.

Supportive Measures

Monitor airway, breathing, circulation, and vital signs.

- ***Obtain IV access:*** Consider IV thiamine, glucose, or naloxone for altered mental status (AMS; especially if presenting in a coma or with seizures).

Toxic Vital Signs

- Core temperature can be an indicator of numerous toxicities. Hyperthermia (core body temperature above 40.5 °C) can lead to irreversible neuron damage. Intoxicated patients can also be hypothermic, which can lead to AMS and cardiopulmonary dysfunction.

- Bedside capillary glucose should be obtained to identify hypoglycemia, a potentially fatal condition that can result from multiple medications and toxins.
- Supplemental oxygen, thiamine, glucose, and naloxone may be administered empirically to treat multiple toxicities that present as AMS (Cline et al., 2016).

Diagnosis

Clinical history and exam: History should include the five W's:

1. **Who:** Patient age, weight, relation to others present, and gender
2. **What:** Medication(s) name and dosage or substance of abuse, co-ingestants, and amount ingested; consideration of over-the-counter medications and local substance use patterns
3. **When:** The time and date of ingestion or exposure; whether single or chronic exposure
4. **Where:** The route of poisoning (ingestion, injection, nasal, rectal, etc.)
5. **Why:** Suicide attempt or therapeutic mistake (i.e., intentional or unintentional)

Physical Exams and Essential Laboratory Tests

Routine tests: The following tests are useful for providing clues to the diagnosis and management of poisoned patients.

- Serum glucose
- EKG
- Serum acetaminophen
- Electrolytes (anion gap, sodium, potassium, and bicarbonate)
- Ethanol level
- Serum osmolality and osmolality gap
- Complete blood count (CBC)
- Hepatic function tests (alanine aminotransferase [ALT], aspartate aminotransferase [AST])
- Blood urea nitrogen (BUN)
- Urinalysis and drug urine test
- Pregnancy (females of childbearing age)
- Creatine kinase to check for rhabdomyolysis

Decontamination

Following evaluation and stabilization of the poisoned patient, removal of the toxin from the patient is the next primary objective in treating the patient.

- **Dermal exposure:** Remove clothing and irrigate copiously with water, especially with chemical ocular exposure, preferably with an isotonic solution.
- **Gastrointestinal (GI) decontamination:** Gastric lavage and activated charcoal use remain controversial in the management of ingested poisons:
  - Gastric lavage or activated charcoal may not be beneficial if the ingestion had occurred more than 60 minutes prior (Olson et al., 2018).
  - Less toxic substances or rapidly absorbed drugs treated with either gastric lavage or activated charcoal have similar outcomes (Olson et al., 2018).
  - Highly toxic drugs that may require gastric decontamination include drugs that cannot be absorbed by charcoal,

massive amounts of a drug, enteric, and/or sustained release drugs.
  - When required, a preferred method in an awake patient with an intact airway is to give activated charcoal within 1 hour of ingestion, given as a ratio of 10:1 (charcoal: toxin).

Enhanced Elimination

This refers to the process of removing a toxin from the body after it has been absorbed.

Modalities include:

- **Multiple-dose activated charcoal (MDAC):** given over several hours in an attempt to increase the elimination of the toxin metabolites systematically absorbed.
- **Urinary manipulation:** The kidney is the contributor to total toxin clearance requiring forced diuresis. Urinary pH manipulation by forced diuresis increases the glomerular filtration rate and ion trapping. Forced diuresis may be used to produce urine volumes of up to 1 L/hr but needs to be used with caution due to the increase risk for fluid overload (Olson et al., 2018).
- **Hemodialysis:** Blood is pumped through an extracorporeal blood purification system; this allows for the concurrent correction of fluid and electrolyte abnormalities.
- **Gastric lavage** is rarely done but can occasionally be helpful within the first hour of ingestion:
  - Not used with acetaminophen overdose.
  - Removes 50% of pills at 1 hour.
  - Removes 15% of pills at 2 hours.

Antidote Treatment

After stabilization and assessment of the patient, antidote therapy should be assessed (Table 16.12). There are only a few antidotes that are indicated prior to initial stabilization:

- **Naloxone:** An emergency medication given for opiate toxicity
- **Cyanide antidotes:** Given for cyanide toxicity
- **Atropine:** Given for organophosphate poisoning
  See Table 16.13 for common toxic exposures.

COMMON MEDICATION OVERDOSES AND ENVIRONMENTAL FACTORS

Anticholinergic Toxicity

Pathophysiology

Anticholinergic drugs inhibit binding of the muscarinic acetylcholine receptors. Toxicity is primarily related to the antagonistic effects of the receptors at the peripheral and paraympathetic receptors.

- **Examples:** Atropine, scopolamine, diphenhydramine, promethazine, cyclobenzaprine, and phenothiazines

Presentation

- Blurred vision, dry mouth, fever, AMS, and flushed
- The phrase "blind as a bat, dry as a bone, hot as a hare, mad as a hatter, red as a beet" is often used to describe these patients' toxidrome

Management

- **Supportive measures:** IV hydration, external cooling
- Decontamination/elimination
- **Benzodiazepines:** Treat seizures or agitation

TABLE 16.12 COMMON ANTIDOTE TREATMENT

TOXIN	ANTIDOTE
Snake, black widow spider, brown recluse spider, scorpion	Antivenom
Clostridium botulinum	Botulinum antitoxin
Acetaminophen	NAC (mucomyst)
Cyclic antidepressants	Bicarbonate
Benzodiazepines	Flumazenil (Romazicon)
Opiates	Naloxone (Narcan)
Calcium channel blocker	Calcium
Digoxin	Digoxin immune Fab (Ovine; Digbind)
Beta blockers	Glucagon
Anticholinergic agents	Physostigmine salicylate (Antilirium)
Carbon monoxide	Oxygen/hyperbaric oxygen
Organphosphates	Atropine/pralidioxime (2-PAM)
Iron	Deferoxamine
Arsenic	Dimercaprol (BAL)
Lead and mercury	Succimer (DMSA)
Calcium channel antagonist	High-dose insulin
Heparin	Protamine sulfate
Local anesthetics	Lipid anesthetics
Methanol/ethylene glycol	Fomepizole
Coumadin	Vitamin K
Cyanide	Cyanide Kit (amyl nitrite, sodium nitrite, thiosulfate); cyanocobalamin

BAL, British anti-Lewisite; DMSA, dimercaptosuccinic acid; NAC, N-acetylcysteine; 2-PAM, 2-pyridine aldoxime methyl chloride.

- *Antidote:* Physostigmine (IV) reverses anticholinergic effect but is not considered for routine use because of increased risk for intractable seizures, atrioventricular (AV) heart block, or asystole

Acetaminophen Toxicity
Pathophysiology
Hepatic injury caused from cytochrome P450 (CYP) mixed-function oxidase enzymes is highly toxic; this reactive metabolite (N-acetyl-p-benzoquinone imine N-acetyl-p-benzoquinone imine [NAPQI]) is detoxified rapidly by glutathione in liver cells. Overdose increases production of NAPQI, which accumulates in the hepatocytes, causing hepatic injury.

Presentation
- *Four stages of poisoning*
  1. Asymptomatic: 0 to 24 hours
  2. Nausea and vomiting, abdominal pain (right upper quadrant): 24 to 72 hours
  3. Jaundice, fulminant hepatic failure, metabolic acidosis, encephalopathy: 3 to 5 days
  4. Recovery: 1 week after if patient survives stage 3 or goes into multisystem failure:
- Hypotension, hypothermia
- Encephalopathy (stage 3): AMS, stupor, delirium, coma, asterixis, (flapping tremor)

Management
- Acetaminophen levels should be checked after 4 hours after ingestion.
- Baseline liver function tests (LFTs), coagulations, and chemistry levels should be monitored every 24 hours.
- Activated charcoal may be administered within the first 4 hours of ingestion.
- Antidote: N-acetylcysteine (NAC) is a glutathione substitute.
- Acetylcysteine may be given via IV.

Key Points
- If patient has taken a toxic amount of acetaminophen (more than 8–10 g), then NAC should be given.
- Maximum dose of acetaminophen is up to 4 g every 24 hours.
- If overdose occurred more than 24 hours prior to presentation, there is no antidote.
- If the time of ingestion is unclear, the drug level should be checked.
- Charcoal can be given; it is not contraindicated with NAC.

Salicylates and Aspirin Toxicity
Pathophysiology
Aspirin metabolizes in the liver via glucuronidation, oxidation, and glycine conjugation. Excretion rate is variable on dose concentration; chronic use decreases the metabolic and

TABLE 16.13 COMMON TOXIC EXPOSURES

TOXIDROME	PATHOPHYSIOLOGY/ PHYSICAL EXAM	COMMON AGENTS	LABORATORY AND VITAL SIGN FINDINGS
Anticholinergic	Autonomic syndrome/altered mental status, agitation/delirium, mydriasis, dry skin, urinary retention, ↓ bowel sounds, hyperthermia, seizure, coma	Antihistamines, atropine and other anticholinergics, carbamazepine, glutethimide, tricyclic antidepressants	EKG findings of increased QRS interval > 0.10 second, sinus tachycardia, conduction abnormalities
Cholinergic	Autonomic syndrome/mixed effects occur when both muscarinic and nicotinic receptors are stimulated/miosis, diarrhea, vomiting, bronchorrhea, diaphoresis, urination, muscle fasciculation weakness, seizures, salivation, lacrimation, seizures	Organophosphate and carbonate insecticides, chemical warfare agents (Sarin)	EKG findings bradycardia, blood pressures can be labile
Ethanolic	Central nervous system depression/ataxia, dysarthria, odor of ethanol	Ethanol	Hypoglycemia, traced in urine for 7–12 hours
Sympatholytic	Autonomic syndrome, acting on alpha$_2$ agonist causing vasoconstriction/miosis (often pinpoint), ↓ peristalsis	Clonidine, opioids, valproic acid	Blood pressure and pulse rate decreased, elevated ammonia and hepatic panel
NMS	Increased metabolic rate/altered mental status, generalized muscle rigidity referred to as "lead pipe" rigidity	Antipsychotics	Hyperthermia >40 °C, metabolic acidosis, rhabdomyolysis, dehydration
Sympathomimetic	Agitation, hyperpyrexia, seizure, acute coronary syndrome, mydriasis, diaphoresis, chest pain, anxiety, euphoria	Amphetamines, cocaine, caffeine, hydrocodone, heroine	Tachycardia, hypertension, hyperthermia, positive for conditions caused by cocaine poisoning including myocardial infarction
Serotonin syndrome	Triad of features (mental status changes, autonomic hyperactivity, and neuromuscular abnormalities). Other findings may include clonus, diaphoresis, flushing, tremor, shivering, hypertension, tachycardia.	SSRI, MAOI, tricyclic antidepressants, amphetamines, St. John's wort, fentanyl	Hyperthermia, tachycardia, electrolyte imbalance, not likely to appear on a "drug of abuse" screen or other toxicology screen
Salicylates	Nausea, vomiting, hyperpnea, tinnitus, disorientation, lethargy, coma, seizure, diaphoresis, abdominal pain	Aspirin oil of wintergreen (methyl salicylate)	Hyperthermia, respiratory alkalosis with progressive anion-gap metabolic acidosis, hyperglycemia/hypoglycemia, hypernatremia/hyponatremia, hypokalemia
Sedative hypnotics	Central nervous system: depression, ataxia, dysarthria, stupor, coma, slurred speech	Benzodiazepines, barbiturates	Respiratory depression causing hypoxia, hypercarbia and respiratory acidosis; with severe overdose, hypothermia, bradycardia may be present
Opioid	Central nervous system: depression, sedation, slurred speech, miosis, decreased bowel sounds	Codeine, heroin, morphine	Respiratory depression, severe causing hypoxia, hypercarbia, respiratory acidosis, pulmonary edema, hypothermia, bradycardia

MAOI, monoamine oxidase inhibitors; NMS, neuromuscular malignant syndrome; SSRI, selective serotonin reuptake inhibitor.

excretion rates, leading to toxicity. The uncoupling effects of oxidative phosphorylation and interruption of glucose and fatty metabolism are the leading contributors to metabolic acidosis (Table 16.14).

Examples

- Acetylsalicylic acid (ASA), methyl salicylate, bismuth subsa-licylate (Pepto-Bismol, Kaopectate)
- Wintergreen food flavoring (1 teaspoon of oils contains 7 g of ASA)
- Methyl salicylate (BenGay, IcyHot muscle balm)

Management

- Ensure adequate ventilation to prevent respiratory acidosis.
- Treat metabolic acidosis with IV **sodium bicarbonate**; do *not* let the pH fall below 7.4.
  - Normal ABG pH: 7.38 to 7.42
- Decontamination: Whole-bowel irrigation is recommended to help remove the pills and charcoal through the intestinal tract.
- Enhanced elimination: Urine alkalization is effective to enhance urinary excretions but the goal is to continue to resuscitate and to maintain pH 7.5 or higher.
- **Hemodialysis** may be used to treat severe toxicity of acute ASA poisoning or chronic symptomatic toxicity.

Key Points

- The most common presenting symptom is respiratory alkalosis progressing to metabolic acidosis and increased anion gap.
- Aspirin causes multisystem toxicity, which leads to acute respiratory distress syndrome (ARDS), interferes with prothrombin production, and raises prothrombin time, which can lead to DIC.
- Aspirin also interferes with phosphorylation, which results in anaerobic glucose metabolism, which elevates lactate.
- Serial ASA levels should be monitored every 4 hours to ensure that levels do not rise due to bezoar formation secondary to enteric-coated pills, which delay metabolism.

Opioids and Opioids Toxicity

Pathophysiology

Opiate receptor agonist; usual peak effects occur within 2 to 3 hours, but absorption may be slowed by the pharmacologic effects of opioids on GI motility.

- *Opioid* refers to opiates and semisynthetic derivatives of naturally occurring opium (e.g., morphine, heroin, codeine, and hydrocodone).

- Total synthetic analogs (e.g., fentanyl, butorphanol, meperidine, and methadone) contain opioids in combination with either aspirin or acetaminophen.
- *Antidote:* naloxone IV is used to achieve normal levels of consciousness and ventilation (doses may be given every 2 to 3 minutes up to a maximum dose of 10 mg).

Key Points

- Caution should be applied when treating with additional opioids.
- Opioid withdrawal symptoms can develop more than 6 to 8 weeks with chronic daily use; signs and symptoms of withdrawal may be seen in up to 7 to 10 days (increased tremor, myoclonus, nausea, vomiting, and piloerection).

ALCOHOL AND ENVIRONMENTAL TOXICITIES

Alcohol

One of the most common toxicities is caused by alcohol. See Table 16.15 for common forms of toxicity, along with presentation and treatment.

Carbon Monoxide Poisoning

Pathophysiology

Toxicity occurs from cellular hypoxia and ischemia, because it has such a tight binding infinity to hemoglobin—of 250 times more than oxygen. This results in oxyhemoglobin saturation and decreases the oxygen-carrying capacity of the blood.

Examples of Sources

- Gas heaters, wood burning stoves
- Automobile exhaust, especially in a poorly ventilated environment

Presentation

- *Respiratory:* Short of breath, dyspnea
- *Central nervous system:* Headache, light-headedness, confusion, seizures, psychosis, paralysis
- *CV:* Chest pain, myocardial infarction (MI)
- *GI:* Nausea, vomiting, diarrhea

Lab/Diagnostic Findings

- Elevated carboxyhemoglobin level (10%–50%)
- Cardiac enzyme biomarkers indicating a MI
- *Cardiovascular:* Sinus tachycardia, premature ventricular contractions
- Metabolic acidosis

TABLE 16.14 PRESENTATION OF SALICYLATES AND ASPIRIN TOXICITY	
FIRST 8–12 HOURS	**WITHIN 24 HOURS**
<ul><li>Fever</li><li>Tinnitus</li><li>Hyperventilation leading to mixed respiratory alkalemia (respiratory alkalosis + metabolic acidosis), hyperpnoea, tachycardia, hypotension, diaphoresis, dysrhythmias</li><li>GI upset with epigastric pain, nausea, vomiting</li><li>Confusion</li></ul>	<ul><li>Death caused by central nervous system failure and CV collapse</li><li>Coma, cerebral edema, seizures</li><li>Noncardiogenic pulmonary edema</li><li>DIC</li></ul>

CV, cardiovascular; DIC, disseminated intravascular coagulation; GI, gastrointestinal.

TABLE 16.15 DIFFERENCES IN TOXICITY AMONG ALCOHOLS

ALCOHOL TYPE AND TOXICITY	ETHANOL	METHANOL	ETHYLENE GLYCOL	ISOPROPYL ALCOHOL
Common types of products	Commercial beer, wine, and liquor	Paint thinner, wood alcohol, cleaning solution	Antifreeze	Rubbing alcohol
Toxic metabolite	Acetaldehyde	Formic acid/ formaldehyde	Oxalic acid/oxalate	Acetone
Presentation	Central nervous system stupor	Ocular toxicity	Renal toxicity	Fruity breath
Initial diagnostic abnormality	↑ Serum ethanol level, hypoglycemia	Papilledema,	Hypoglycemia, envelope-shaped crystals in the urine	Falsely ↑ creatinine
Anion gap acidosis	No (except for ketoacidosis)	Yes	Yes	No
Management	Hemodialysis for severe toxicity Pretreat with thiamine, multivitamin, folic acids, fluids, and electrolytes as needed	Correct acidosis with fomepizole folate IV Dialysis for severe intoxications	IV fluids to increase renal clearance and to limit renal oxalates disposition **Fomepizole** (similar to methanol) Thiamine and pyridoxine **Beta hydroxybutyrate** levels are obtained to distinguish from alcoholic ketoacidosis	No antidote Enhanced elimination: hemodialysis for refractory hypotension Ethanol toxicity is often difficult to differentiate

IV, intravenous.

Management

- *Supportive measures:*
  - *Antidote:* Breathing 100% oxygen to help detach carbon monoxide from hemoglobin, which shortens the half-life of carboxyhemoglobin.
  - *Decontamination:* Remove from exposure.
- *Severe toxicity* requires hyperbaric oxygen, which shortens the half-life of carboxyhemoglobin even more.

Key Points

- Carbon monoxide is a colorless, odorless, tasteless, and non-irritating gas.
- Carbon monoxide is the most common cause of death in fires; high incidence of death after a fire is from carbon monoxide poisoning.
- Common exposures are from smoke inhalation, car exhaust fumes, and faulty or poorly ventilated charcoal, kerosene, or gas stoves.
- The oxyhemoglobin dissociation curve is displaced to the left, impairing oxygen delivery to the tissues.

Organophosphate (Insecticide) and Nerve Gas Poisoning

Pathophysiology

Both toxins cause a massive increase in the level of acetylcholine, inhibiting its metabolism. Clinical systems mostly are from the blockade of acetylcholinesterase (AChE).

Examples

- Pesticides, fungicides, herbicides, rodenticides
- *Medications:* pyridostigmine (used to treat myasthenia gravis)

Presentation

- *Muscarinic effects:* Bronchospasm, bronchorrhea, miosis, sweating, salivation, lacrimation, emotional lability, late peripheral neuropathy; usually bradycardia but muscarinic effects can cause tachycardia, abdominal pain, diarrhea, and polyuria (Table 16.16)

- *Nicotinic effects:* Tremors, slurred speech, seizures, and coma. Respiratory failure is the main cause of mortality from AChe inhibition.

Management

- *Supportive measures:*
  - *Decontamination:* Wash skin thoroughly to avoid self-contamination; wear gloves.
  - *Antidotes:* Antimuscarinic agent atropine and the enzyme reactivator pralidoxime (usually packaged together).

Key Points

- Resuscitators should take caution and wear protective measures to avoid contamination. They should wear neoprene or nitrile gloves.
- Organophosphate and nerve gas are identical in their effect except that nerve gas works faster and is more severe.
- Most organophosphate (OP) agents can be absorbed by any route: inhalation, ingestion, or absorption through the skin.
- *Atropine* will reverse its muscarinic but *not* its nicotinic effect.

TABLE 16.16 SYMPTOMS OF OP POISONING—DUMBBELSS

D	Diarrhea
U	Urination
M	Miosis
B	Bradycardia
B	Bronchoconstriction
E	Excitation (muscle, central nervous system nicotinic effects)
L	Lacrimation
S	Salivation
S	Sweating

Lead Poisoning
Pathophysiology
This is a multisystem toxicity that interferes with sulfhydryl-deprotonated enzymes mostly inhibiting heme synthesis to compete with essential cations like calcium, zinc, and iron.

Presentation
- Abdominal pain (lead colic), nausea, and vomiting
- Acute tubular necrosis (ATN): renal tubule toxicity
- Anemia (sideroblastic)
- Wrist drop from peripheral neuropathy
- *Central nervous system deficits*: memory loss, confusion, irritability
- Chronic toxicity: painful arthralgia, bluish "lead line" along gums

GENERAL MANAGEMENT: KEY POINTS
- If the offending ingested toxin is unclear, ask whether the overdose is acetaminophen or aspirin, the most common cause of death by unintentional overdose.
- **Herbal medications** do not require Food and Drug Administration (FDA) approval. Consumers often mistakenly believe that since these medications are "natural," this means they are safe. Ask for medical history, including use of herbal and alternative products, to assess for possible herb–disease interactions.
- *Osmolar gap* is the difference between the measured serum osmolality and the calculated osmolality. If calculated serum osmolality is 300 but the measured level is 350, alcohol toxicities such as methanol or ethylene glycol account for the extra osmoles. Ethanol alcohol can also increase the osmolar gap.

Serum osmolality = 2 times the sodium + BUN/2.8 + glucose/18

- Performing a physical assessment and examining all organ systems assist with the differential diagnosis.
- Evaluation of an unexplained metabolic acidosis oven includes ordering and then calculating the anion gap.
- Normal anion gap of 8 to 12 mEq/L accounts for unmeasured anions (e.g., phosphate, sulfate, and anionic proteins) in the plasma.
- The mnemonic **CAT MUDPILES** helps differentiate the common causes of an elevated anion gap (average normal 8–12 mEq/L; Table 16.17).

TABLE 16.17 MNEMONIC FOR CAUSES OF A WIDENED ANION GAP

C	Cyanide or carbon monoxide
A	Acetaminophen, aspirin, or alcoholic ketoacidosis
T	Toluene
M	Methanol, metformin: massive overdose
U	Uremia
D	Diabetic ketoacidosis
P	Paraldehyde or propylene glycol
I	Iron, isoniazid, or ibuprofen
L	Lactic acidosis
E	Ethylene glycol
S	Salicylates

Clinical Practice Guidelines
Refer to the following organizations for detailed updated guidelines for management for toxic exposures:
- American Academy of Clinical Toxicology: www.clintox.org
- American Association of Poison Control Centers: https://aapcc.org
- Agency for Toxic Substances and Disease Registry: www.atsdr.cdc.gov
- Centers for Disease Control and Prevention: www.cdc.gov
- Toxicology Net (TOXNET) databases: https://toxnet.nlm.nih.gov
  The U.S. Department of Health and Human Services Chemical Hazards Emergency Medical Management: https://chemm.nlm.nih.gov/index.html

MULTISYSTEM TRAUMA

OVERVIEW
This section is not meant to be a comprehensive discussion of trauma, but rather offers an overview of life-threatening and common traumatic injuries.

Resuscitation Considerations
- Resuscitation should be aggressive in all patients. Base deficit and lactic acid values should be immediately obtained during the initial trauma resuscitation. These values will help identify developing shock states (ACS TQIP, 2018).
- Age alone is not a predictor of morbidity or mortality.
- Traumatic injury in any patient requires prompt triage or direct transfer to an appropriate level of trauma center (Calland et al., 2016).

Resuscitation Assessment and Interventions
- An entire primary trauma survey (assessment of airway, breathing, circulation, neurologic disability) and then subsequent secondary assessment (including head-to-toe assessment) should be completed to identify possible injuries and treatments.
- No steps should be missed, and the assessment should be completed the same way every time to avoid missing injuries.
- Life-threatening injuries should be intervened upon when first identified, prior to moving on to other less critical injuries.

Basic Interventions for the Critically Injured Patient
- The airway should be assessed and secured.
- Breathing should be assessed and supported with the use of supplemental oxygen.
- Circulation should be assessed and supported. Any external uncontrolled bleeding should be controlled and volume resuscitation initiated with two large bore catheters.
- Neurologic status should be assessed: pupils and Glasgow Coma Score (GCS); or the Full Outline of Unresponsiveness (FOUR) Score should be used:
  - Impaired neurologic status may indicate reduced ability to maintain airway or a life-threatening head injury.
  - Head injury is poorly tolerated by the geriatric patient.
  - Assess for possible cervical spine injury, which may also impair airway and breathing status.
- Continuous cardiac monitoring, frequent vital signs monitoring, and possibly hemodynamic monitoring (central venous pressure, arterial line, pulmonary artery pressure

monitoring) should be completed based on patient status and severity of injury.

- Temperature should be measured frequently. Normothermia should be maintained.
- If the abdomen is distended or the patient is at risk for aspiration, a gastric tube should be inserted to decompress the stomach unless it is contraindicated.

THORACIC TRAUMA

Overview of Thoracic Trauma

- May be due to blunt or penetrating trauma.
- Most traumatic injuries to the chest can be cared for by pleural needle decompression or chest tube insertion.
- *Common exams, treatments, and goals:* Most examinations for traumatic injuries to the chest include chest x-ray, CT of the chest with or without radiographic contrast, or focused assessment with sonography for trauma (FAST).
- Injuries not remedied by simple interventions such as chest tube insertion and continue to destabilize or show signs of shock require interventional radiology or surgical treatment to control hemorrhage or repair structural damage to internal vasculature or organs.
- Intubation and mechanical ventilation may be needed to secure and maintain airway patency as well as to provide for adequate gas exchange, oxygenation, and ventilation.
- Goals are to increase gas exchange while minimizing the risk for additional pulmonary injury, reducing alveolar shear, and reducing work of breathing.
- Focusing on reexpansion of the lungs and preventing atelectasis, respiratory compromise, or infection should be accomplished by consistent and effective pulmonary hygiene measures to promote lung expansion:
  - Using inspirometers and encouraging deep breathing can reduce the risk for further pulmonary complications.
- Goals of all trauma resuscitation are to normalize respiratory and hemodynamic status, prevent or treat shock, maintain or restore cerebral and tissue perfusion, identify and treat all injuries, and restore the patient to optimal health post-trauma resuscitation (Tables 16.18–16.20).

Medication Considerations

- The use of antithrombotics, anticoagulants, direct or indirect oral anticoagulants, and antiplatelet agents increases the risk for life-threatening hemorrhage as well as the risk for intracranial hemorrhage; the risk needs be identified and treatment should be done quickly (ACS TQIP, 2018; Colwell, 2017).
- Coagulation profiles should be evaluated early in the resuscitation phase and treated if intracranial bleeding is present (Calland et al., 2016).
- Cardiac medications, such as beta blockers and angiotensin-converting enzyme (ACE) inhibitors, can impair the patient's normal physiologic response to decreased perfusion and shock states (ACS TQIP, 2018; Colwell, 2017).

ABDOMINAL TRAUMA

Overview

- Abdominal trauma can be divided into solid and hollow organ injury. Solid organ injury usually involves hemorrhage (Campbell, 2018; TNCC, 2015).
- Older patients do not tolerate blood loss, and it takes less blood loss to produce hypoperfusion. This is due to the loss in physiologic reserve and inability to compensate in hemorrhagic shock.

- Clinical presentation may be inconclusive. Assessments may not reveal a normal exam but also do not reveal an exam that is conclusive of serious intra-abdominal injury.
- Clinicians need to have a high index of suspicion for injury and a low threshold for performing FAST scans as well as ordering abdominal CT scans to identify abdominal trauma.
- Shock in the geriatric patient is more occult. This disguises significant blood loss into the abdomen from solid organ or vascular injury.

Diaphragmatic Trauma

Etiology

- This injury can occur in blunt or penetrating trauma.
- In penetrating trauma, an object penetrates both the thoracic and abdominal cavities by penetrating the diaphragm.
- In blunt trauma, the left diaphragm is more commonly injured due to the increased solid organ protection provided by the liver on the right.
- Although not life threatening acutely, this injury can significantly impact morbidity and mortality if not identified.
- Diaphragmatic trauma is usually associated with additional injuries of the chest or abdomen (ATLS, 2018; O'Connell, 2018; Simon & Burns, 2018; Williams, 2017).

Presentation

- Signs of chest or abdominal trauma
- Shortness of breath, orthopnea
- Difficulty swallowing
- Sharp epigastric pain or chest pain
- Abdominal and/or chest pain
- Kehr's sign (referred pain to the left shoulder with palpation)
- Bowel sounds heard in the chest
- Decreased breath sounds on the injured side (O'Connell, 2018; TNCC, 2015; Williams, 2017)

Diagnosis

- Chest x-ray demonstration of bowel in the chest cavity
- Abdominal/chest CT
- FAST scan
- Laparotomy/thoracoscopy

Immediate Treatment, Assessment, and Evaluation

- Stabilize the primary survey.
- Endotracheal intubation and mechanical ventilation may be needed for those presenting in acute respiratory distress or failure.
- Cover any open wounds with occlusive dressings and assess/monitor for development of tension pneumothorax and treat per protocol (O'Connell, 2018).
- Insert a gastric tube to decompress the stomach unless contraindicated.
- Assess the patient for additional potential injuries to the chest and abdomen (Table 16.21).
- Prepare the patient for laparoscopy, thoracoscopy, or other surgery to repair the diaphragm (ATLS, 2018; TNCC, 2015; Williams, 2017)

Trauma to the Small/Large Bowel

- Injury may be due to blunt or penetrating trauma.
- Small bowel may be compressed between the spine and abdominal wall, causing lap belt complex, which includes associated Chance fractures of the lumbar spine.
- Rapid deceleration mechanisms can also cause shearing injury of the small bowel and are usually related to motor vehicle crashes (Benjamin, 2018; Campbell, 2018).

TABLE 16.18 PULMONARY INJURIES

	DEFINITION	PRESENTATION	DIAGNOSIS	TREATMENT/INTERVENTION
Simple PTX	An abnormal collection of air in the pleural space due to injury to the lung that causes a reduction in negative intrapleural pressure (ATLS, 2018).	■ Dyspnea, tachypnea ■ Tachycardia ■ Diminished breath sounds on the affected side ■ Hyper-resonance on the affected side ■ Complaints of shortness of breath ■ Chest pain	Upright chest x-ray. Not identified well if the x-ray is taken with the patient flat due to movement of air to the anterior chest wall. CT of the chest is usually done for any patient presenting with significant chest wall injury.	Closely monitor the patient, including physical assessment, vital signs, pulse oximetry, and capnography for deterioration in respiratory status. Administer supplemental oxygen if warranted by clinical assessment findings, ABG, and/or pulse oximetry. If small, pneumothorax may be simply observed with repeat physical assessment, close monitoring of vital signs (including pulse oximetry and capnography), and repeat chest x-rays or CT of the chest. Administering high-flow oxygen can assist in reabsorbing small pneumothoraces (Daley, 2018). Larger pneumothoraces may be treated by chest tube insertion attached to a chest drainage device with suction to restore negative intrapleural pressure.
Open PTX	An abnormal collection of air in the pleural space due to an opening the chest wall from penetrating trauma.	■ Dyspnea ■ Tachypnea ■ Tachycardia ■ Decreased or absent breath sounds to the affected side ■ Shortness of breath and/or the inability to speak ■ Sucking noise heard on inhalation (size dependent) ■ Chest pain ■ Visible signs of chest trauma, penetrating wounds ■ Open wound(s) on the chest that bubbles with exhalation ■ Subcutaneous emphysema around the open chest wound may be present	Diagnosis is made by clinical findings of open bubbling or sucking chest wound(s) associated with hypoxia, respiratory distress or failure CT of the chest is performed to identify further thoracic injury due to penetrating trauma	*IMMEDIATE* Immediately cover the wound(s) with an occlusive dressing and tape securely on three sides. Alternatives include the use of chest seal dressings with one-way valves that allow air to escape from the chest. Administer supplemental oxygen as determined by clinical assessment findings, pulse oximetry/ABG results. Closely monitor the patient for signs of tension pneumothorax. If tension pneumothorax develops, remove the dressing to relieve the pressure that has developed in the chest and reevaluate the patient. Be sure to evaluate the patient's thorax for additional open wounds that may contribute to respiratory difficulty and treat as appropriate. *DEFINITIVE* Wounds need to be evaluated and closed. A chest tube may be inserted and attached to a chest drainage device with suction to reexpand the lung and restore negative intrapleural pressure. Frequently reevaluate the patient.

(continued)

TABLE 16.18 PULMONARY INJURIES (continued)

	DEFINITION	PRESENTATION	DIAGNOSIS	TREATMENT/INTERVENTION
Tension PTX	A tension pneumothorax is due to abnormal buildup of air in the pleural space that causes significant loss of negative intrapleural pressure, reduces venous return, and causes respiratory and hemodynamic compromise	■ Complaints of shortness of breath ■ Air hunger ■ Anxiety, restlessness ■ Severe respiratory compromise or distress ■ Diminished/absent breath sounds on the affected side ■ Signs of obstructive shock: Hypotension (not seen in a simple pneumothorax) Jugular venous distention that may include distention of the veins in the head, neck, and upper extremities (may or may not be present) Tracheal deviation away from the affected side (usually seen on chest x-ray on the portion of the trachea inside the chest cavity) Cyanosis (late sign)	Tension pneumothorax is not diagnosed by x-ray. It is a constellation of symptoms indicating a pneumothorax with obstructive shock due to air under pressure in the pleural space destabilizing the patient by impairing venous return and cardiac output. It is not diagnosed by size of the pneumothorax. Treatment should not be delayed to perform imaging to attempt to confirm the diagnosis.	*IMMEDIATE* Immediate pleural needle decompression with a large bore needle 6.5–8 cm in length (ATLS, 2018; Clemency et al., 2015). If related to an open pneumothorax, lift the dressing to allow air that has built up under pressure to escape. Administer high-flow oxygen if the patient continues in respiratory distress. Frequently reevaluate the patient. Chest tube may need to be inserted; if continued air leak is noted, work up for additional injuries (such as bronchial tear, esophageal tear) should be performed. *DEFINITIVE* Inset chest tube. Attach to chest drainage device with suction to reexpand the lung and restore negative intrapleural pressure.
Hemothorax	An abnormal collection of blood in the pleural space due to either blunt or penetrating trauma (ATLS, 2018).	■ Anxiety or restlessness ■ Complaints of shortness of breath ■ Dyspnea, tachypnea ■ Diminished lung sounds on the affected side ■ Dullness to percussion on the affected side chest wall ■ Hemoptysis ■ Flat neck veins	Upright chest x-ray should be performed to estimate volume loss (Mahoozi et al., 2016). Chest CT more accurately quantifies blood loss and may identify location of hemorrhage.	If hemothorax is identified on chest x-ray, insert a large bore chest tube to the 5th–6th intercostals space at the anterior axillary or midaxillary space to drain fluid and monitor output (ATLS, 2018). Suction may be used to help restore negative intrapleural pressures. If volume is estimated at less than 300 mL, the patient may be observed. Blood may subsequently reabsorb over the next several weeks. Monitor for ongoing blood loss. Embolization can also be used (Christmas & Jacobs, 2019).
Massive hemothorax	An abnormally large collection of blood in the pleural space due to blunt or penetrating trauma causing respiratory compromise and hemodynamic instability due to hemorrhagic shock.	■ Anxiety or restlessness ■ Complaints of shortness of breath ■ Dyspnea, tachypnea ■ Chest pain	Diagnosis may be made by clinical assessment of diminished or absent breath sounds on one side, flat neck veins, hypoxia, cyanosis and	*IMMEDIATE* Secure the patient's airway and administer high-flow oxygen via nonrebreather mask, bag mask device, or endotracheal tube as appropriate.

(continued)

	One third or more of the patient's blood volume accumulated in the chest (in adults >1,500 mL) or drainage of >200 mL/hr for 2–4 hours (ATLS, 2018; TNCC, 2015).	■ Signs of hypovolemic shock: tachycardia, hypotension, diaphoresis, thready pulses; ■ Diminished breath sounds on the affected side ■ Dullness to percussion of the affected side chest wall ■ Flat neck veins ■ Hemoptysis	signs of hypovolemic shock not attributable to other causes. Chest x-ray may not quantify blood loss if the patient is laid flat for the exam. FAST scan identifies blood in the pleural space but may not identify the location of hemorrhage.	Establish two large-bore IV catheters and volume resuscitate with warm isotonic crystalloid solution on blood tubing. Insert a large-bore chest tube at the fifth–sixth intercostals space at the anterior axillary or midaxillary line. Attach the chest tube to a chest drain device with suction. Provide immediate replacement of blood loss through massive transfusion protocols. Autotransfusion devices may be used to replace the patient's own blood from that lost into the chest. Fluid administration should be aggressive to provide euvolemic resuscitation (ATLS, 2018). Administer TXA according to local protocol. ***DEFINITIVE*** Prepare the patient for surgery, emergent thoracotomy, or other emergency procedures to control bleeding and repair vascular injury.
Pulmonary contusion	Lung tissue injury due to direct impact or rapid deceleration, causing blood to leak into the pulmonary capillaries, also causing edema and inflammation (Weiser, 2018). Concurrent injuries may include rib fractures or flail chest (ATLS, 2018; TNCC, 2015). Increased morbidity and mortality when accompanied by flail chest. Commonly associated with rib fractures and has the potential to become a lethal injury. Risk is increased in the older adult population (Weiser, 2018).	■ Sternal tenderness or pain ■ Shortness of breath, dyspnea ■ Crepitus on sternal palpation ■ Deformity/step-off may be present ■ Paradoxical chest wall motion may occur	Chest x-ray Chest CT	Administer supplemental oxygen. Continuously monitor respiratory status, physical assessment, pulse oximetry, and capnography. Provide adequate pain management. Encourage frequent cough and deep breathing to promote lung expansion. Older adults are at increased risk for atelectasis and respiratory complications. Perform intubation and mechanical ventilation if the pulmonary contusion is moderate to severe or if the patient develops hypoxia, hypercarbia, or respiratory distress (ATLS, 2018).

ABG, arterial blood gas; FAST, focused assessment with sonography for trauma; IV, intravenous; PTX, pneumothorax; TXA, tranexamic acid.

TABLE 16.19 INJURIES OF THE BONY CHEST

	ETIOLOGY	PRESENTATION	DIAGNOSIS	TREATMENT/INTERVENTION
Rib fractures	Caused by blunt trauma to the chest from motor vehicle crashes or falls. Rib fractures are common and increase morbidity and mortality among older adults(Colwell, 2017). Pulmonary complications increased in older adultsregardless of the number of ribs fractured (Colwell, 2017). Preexisting cardiopulmonary problems increase risk for mortality with rib fractures (Colwell, 2017).	■ Chest pain ■ Shortness of breath ■ Chest wall tenderness ■ Bony crepitus may be noted on palpation ■ Bruising, swelling, or evidence of trauma to the area	Chest x-ray Chest CT	Administer supplemental oxygen if needed, as determined by clinical assessment findings, pulse oximetry/ABG result. Provide appropriate pain management. Encourage frequent respiratory hygiene to promote lung expansion as older adults are at increased risk for atelectasis and respiratory complications.
Sternal fractures	Usually due to blunt anterior chest wall trauma from such mechanisms as motor vehicle crashes, sport injuries with direct chest wall trauma, falls (Felten, 2018). If trauma is severe, additional injuries of the thorax may occur, such as vascular disruption, cardiac, or pulmonary contusion. If sternal fracture is present have suspicion for additional thoracic or multisystem injury.	■ Sternal tenderness or pain ■ Shortness of breath, dyspnea ■ Crepitus on sternal palpation ■ Deformity/step off may be present ■ Paradoxical chest wall motion may occur	Chest x-ray (include lateral, sternal view; Felten, 2018) Chest CT to identify additional thoracic injury Laboratory tests and/or EKG if suspecting other injuries such as cardiac contusion	Administer supplemental oxygen. Admit for observation if unable to achieve adequate pain control. Cardiac monitoring. Provide adequate pain control. Pulmonary hygiene to promote lung expansion is critical as atelectasis and respiratory complications are more frequent in older adults.
Massive flail chest	Two or more adjacent ribs broken in two or more places or sternal fractures, causing a free floating segment disrupting chest wall continuity (ATLS, 2018; TNCC, 2015). Disruption of chest wall continuity does not determine prognosis. Energy absorbed by the lungs and underlying structures within the chest determine prognosis. Common underlying injury from massive flail chest is pulmonary contusion, which can be significant and lead to ARDS.	■ Dyspnea, tachypnea ■ Rapid shallow respirations ■ Paradoxical chest wall movement (may not be noticeable if the patient is able to splint) ■ Asymmetrical, uncoordinated movement of the chest with poor air entry ■ Respiratory failure ■ Palpable crepitus over bony fracture	Chest x-ray CT of the chest	*IMMEDIATE* Administer oxygen via the appropriate method based on clinical assessment, pulse oximetry, capnography, and ABG result. Provide adequate pain control as older adults are at increased risk for atelectasis and respiratory complications. Encourage frequent respiratory hygiene to promote lung expansion. Use continuous pulse oximetry and waveform capnography to monitor oxygenation and ventilation. Perform intubation and mechanical ventilation following ARDS protocols if deteriorating respiratory status occurs.

ABG, arterial blood gas; ARDS, acute respiratory distress syndrome.

TABLE 16.20 CARDIAC AND VASCULAR INJURIES OF THE CHEST

	ETIOLOGY	PRESENTATION	DIAGNOSIS	TREATMENT/INTERVENTION
Pericardial tamponade	This is a life-threatening injury Accumulation of blood in the pericardial sac Causes compression of the heart and equalization of atrial and ventricular chamber pressures This obstructs venous return, reduces stroke volume and impairs cardiac output	■ Beck's triad ■ Hypotension ■ Distended neck veins ■ Muffled heart tones ■ Chest pain ■ Tachycardia or pulseless electrical activity ■ Dyspnea ■ Cyanosis ■ Pulsus paradoxus greater than 10 mmHg ■ Electrical alternans	FAST scan reveals fluid in the pericardial sac. Acute traumatic pericardial tamponade does not usually present with cardiac silhouette enlargement and requires less fluid buildup in the sac to cause hemodynamic instability.	*IMMEDIATE* Rapid fluid boluses should be administered but pericardial tamponade is usually resistant to fluid therapy (ATLS, 2018). Immediate pericardiocentesis preferably guided by ultrasound or pericardial window should be performed as a life-saving measure. *DEFINITIVE* Thoracotomy should be done to further evaluate and repair the heart (ATLS, 2018; TNCC, 2015).
Aortic injury	Blunt or penetrating trauma	■ Fractures of the first/second ribs, sternum, scapula ■ Back or chest pain ■ Unequal pulses, blood pressure differences between upper and lower extremities ■ Hypotension, tachycardia and pale, diaphoretic and cyanotic skin ■ Paraplegia if spinal artery disruption occurs ■ Aortic changes noted on chest x-ray: ■ Widened mediastinum ■ Right-sided tracheal and/or esophageal deviation ■ Left hemothorax ■ Obliterated aortic knob ■ Elevated right mainstem bronchus ■ Obscured aortopulmonary window ■ Presence of a pleural or apical cap ■ Widened paratracheal stripe ■ Widened paratracheal interfaces (ACLS, 2018; Colwell, 2017; TNCC, 2015)	FAST scan Chest x-ray Helical chest CT with contrast Aortography	*IMMEDIATE* Continue to treat shock and fluid loss according to protocols, with use of massive transfusion protocol and TXA Emergency angiography Emergency thoracotomy to repair or dissect the injured area Endovascular repair (ACLS, 2018; TNCC, 2015)
Blunt cardiac injury	Injury due to blunt trauma to heart, usually to the anterior chest wall (Ottosen & Guo, 2012). Injuries can include but are not limited to cardiac contusions, myocardial rupture, and valve disruption (ATLS, 2018).	■ Chest pain or discomfort ■ EKG abnormalities such as premature ventricular contractions, atrial fibrillation, cardiac ischemic changes, S–T segment changes, AV conduction abnormalities such as right bundle branch block ■ Hypotension and signs of cardiac failure such as jugular venous distention or elevated central venous pressure ■ Wall motion abnormalities may be identified on cardiac ultrasound (ATLS, 2018; TNCC, 2015)	EKG Cardiac ultrasound Clinical presentation	Continuous observation with cardiac monitoring for 24 hours for patients who have abnormal EKGs due to increased risk for sudden dysrhythmias. Although troponin levels may be drawn, a positive or negative troponin is not indicative of blunt cardiac injury. Assess for signs of cardiac failure in those patients needing 24-hour-monitoring.

ABG, arterial blood gas; ARDS, acute respiratory distress syndrome; AV, atrioventricular; FAST, focused assessment with sonography for trauma; TXA, tranexamic acid.

TABLE 16.21 SOLID ORGAN TRAUMA IN THE ABDOMEN

	ETIOLOGY	PRESENTATION	DIAGNOSIS	TREATMENT/INTERVENTION
Spleen	Most common solid organ injured in blunt trauma Suspect with left abdomen or left lower chest trauma	Bruises, contusions, abrasions, lacerations noted to the left upper quadrant Left lower rib fractures Abdominal pain, tenderness, rigidity, and guarding to the left upper quadrant Left shoulder pain Signs of hypovolemic shock (ATLS 2018; Campbell, 2018; Coccolini et al., 2017)	FAST scan reveals free fluid in the abdomen indicative of splenic injury Abdominal CT demonstrates splenic injury, laceration, or vascular disruption Lab work indicative of blood loss and possible coagulopathy present	**Immediate** (ATLS, 2018; Campbell, 2018) Volume resuscitation as appropriate; use massive transfusion protocols and TXA to combat hemorrhagic shock; stabilize vital signs and replace blood loss Serial assessments and lab work to determine stability versus continued hemorrhage Observe whether patient is hemodynamically stable, without signs of continuing blood loss, and has minimal blood transfusion requirements Operative management if splenic blush or high-grade splenic injury is noted on CT scan, if hemodynamically unstable or has evidence of ongoing hemorrhage. Operative interventions include splenic salvage or splenectomy Angiography with embolization Provide analgesia and antibiotics to prevent infection if appropriate Pneumovax and hemophilus influenzae B vaccines should be given if splenectomy performed
Liver trauma	Most common solid organ injured in blunt and penetrating abdominal trauma combined Significant risk of massive hemorrhage with liver injuries (Campbell, 2018; Christmas & Jacobs, 2019) Suspect with any right abdomen or right lower chest trauma Additional injuries are commonly identified with liver trauma, most commonly chest and spleen (Christmas & Jacobs, 2019)	Signs of abdominal trauma to the right upper quadrant: bruises, abrasions, lacerations Right lower rib fractures Bruising around the umbilicus (Cullen's sign) Abdominal pain to the right upper quadrant: right upper quadrant tenderness, guarding, and rigidity Signs of hypovolemic shock (ATLS, 2018; Campbell 2018; Christmas & Jacobs, 2019; Mahoozi et al., 2016; TNCC, 2015)	Laboratory results indicative of ongoing blood loss and possible coagulopathy may be present Elevated liver enzymes Abdominal CT with contrast FAST scan indicating liver injury (not always identified on FAST scan)	Treat hemorrhagic shock with fluids, blood replacement, and possible massive transfusion protocol and TXA Observation may be appropriate for those who remain hemodynamically stable with low-grade liver injury and no sign of ongoing blood loss Angiography with embolization Prepare for operative intervention to control hemorrhage and/or repair injury (ATLS, 2018; Campbell, 2018; Christmas & Jacobs, 2019; Mahoozi et al., 2016; TNCC, 2015)

FAST, focused assessment with sonography for trauma; TXA, tranexamic acid.

- Large-bowel disruption causes intra-abdominal contamination with fecal contents and sepsis.
- With large bowel, blunt trauma more frequently injures transverse or sigmoid colon (Campbell, 2018; Table 16.22).

PELVIC AND FEMUR FRACTURES

Overview

- Falls are the most common etiology of orthopedic trauma for older patients (Peterson et al., 2015; Table 16.23).
- There are increased morbidity and mortality rates for this patient population due to lack of physiologic reserve and preexisting disease (Peterson et al., 2015).
- Because of this, geriatric patients are more likely to stay in ICU as opposed to a general medical or monitored unit (Peterson et al., 2015).
- Pelvic fractures are associated with increased morbidity and mortality regardless of type (Colwell, 2017).
- Fractures can be classified as stable or unstable. Stable fractures are minimally displaced and do not involve the pelvic ring. Unstable fractures are displaced and commonly disrupt the pelvic ring in two or more places (Washington State Department of Health, 2016).
- Mortality rates are high with presentation of systolic blood pressure less than 90 mmHg or with the presence of open fractures (Washington State Department of Health, 2016).

Femur Fracture

- There is increased risk for fractures in older adults due to weaker bones, balance or ambulation difficulties, medication side effects, and difficulty maneuvering (Table 16.24).
- Proximal femur fracture is the most common (Clement & Biant, 2014).
- Over 95% of hip fractures are due to falls, most commonly falling sideways (Yang et al., 2020)
- Concern for complications such as deep vein thrombosis should be addressed for all femur and pelvic fractures.

GERIATRIC TRAUMA CONSIDERATIONS

- Older patients are at increased risk for death and disability due to traumatic injury.
- Due to a loss of physiologic reserve, they have a diminished capacity to respond to extraordinary demands placed on the body due to trauma.
- Older adults do not tolerate blood loss, hypoperfusion (both cerebral and systemic), or hypoxia. Body systems altered by preexisting disease states may have already impaired vital systems within the body, causing older adults to be at increased risk for poorer outcomes.

Important Facts About Geriatric Trauma

- Older patients are usually under-triaged when presenting with trauma.
- Typical trauma scoring tools do not accurately take into account the special needs of the geriatric patient.
- The shock index scoring system, not the revised trauma score, is a more accurate predictor of acuity and mortality of geriatric trauma.
- Lower energy mechanisms can result in more severe injury.
- Older patients do not tolerate shock well and do not present with the same anticipated changes in vital signs or clinical status as compared to their younger counterparts.

- Manifestations of shock may be very subtle; it is often difficult to identify the severity and extent of traumatic injury and the physiologic impact on the geriatric patient (Calland et al., 2016; Llompart-Pou et al., 2017).
- Reviewing the patient's medical history may provide a framework regarding resuscitation priorities:
  - Life-threatening injuries should be intervened upon when first identified, prior to moving on to other less critical injuries.
  - Age alone is not a reason to withhold treatment as it is not a sole predictor of survivability posttrauma (Calland et al., 2016).

COMPARTMENT SYNDROME

OVERVIEW

Compartment syndrome occurs when there is an increase in the pressure of one or more muscle compartments. The syndrome can be acute, representing a surgical emergency, or be chronic (Stracciolini & Hammerberg, 2019).

Pathophysiology

Muscle groups are divided into compartments by fascia that does not easily stretch. When injury occurs to a muscle group causing muscle swelling or blood to build up within the compartment, the pressure increases. This pressure increase reduces arterial pressure and increases venous pressure, which in turn causes collapse of the capillary beds. When the capillary beds collapse, capillary permeability increases, causing more fluid to be released into the compartment. As the cycle continues, tissue death can occur from the lack of blood flow (Chung et al., 2019).

Etiology

- The most common cause of acute compartment syndrome is vascular injury, particularly arterial injury, leading to bleeding within a muscle compartment. It can be traumatic or non-traumatic (Stracciolini & Hammerberg, 2019; Table 16.25).
- It can occur in any muscle group. The lower leg is the most common site for compartment syndrome.

Risk Factors

- Male patients under 35 years of age (highest incidence)
- Traumatic injury
- Prolonged surgery
- Rhabdomyolysis
- Chronic or postoperative anticoagulant usage (Stracciolini & Hammerberg, 2019)

Presentation

- Pain (out of proportion to the injury, deep ache, burning)
- Paresthesias (onset within 30 minutes to 2 hours from injury)
- Rigidity of the compartment upon palpation
- Decreased distal sensation
- Muscle weakness (Stracciolini & Hammerberg, 2019)

Relevant Diagnostics/Imaging

The diagnosis of acute compartment syndrome is often made on the basis of history and physical assessment. The measurement of compartment pressures is not required to make a diagnosis. Measurement of compartment pressures can be painful and should only be performed by a practitioner trained in the technique (Stracciolini & Hammerberg, 2019).

TABLE 16.22 BOWEL INJURIES

	PRESENTATION	DIAGNOSIS	TREATMENT/INTERVENTION
Small bowel	Signs of abdominal trauma Abdominal pain, tenderness, rebound tenderness, distention, rigidity, guarding Tachycardia, hypotension Abnormal labs: elevated white blood cells, increased serum amylase Nausea, vomiting Peritonitis	Abdominal CT is the preferred test to identify bowel trauma and may reveal free fluid or air in the abdomen	Fluid volume resuscitation, including blood products for hemodynamic instability Abdominal CT performed on hemodynamically stable patients that may reveal free air or fluid in the abdominal cavity, mesenteric hematoma, or extravasation of CT contrast Diagnosis may be made during emergent surgery for those patients who present hemodynamically unstable and are taken for exploratory laparotomy to identify and stabilize injury Laparotomy/laparoscopy and/or surgical intervention if signs of deterioration, peritonitis, or hemodynamic instability (Benjamin, 2018; Campbell, 2018)
Colon	More frequently injured with penetrating trauma Abdominal tenderness, distention Signs of abdominal trauma Peritonitis Hypovolemic shock Bowel evisceration Gross blood on rectal exam may be present if rectal injury is present (Benjamin, 2018)	Abdominal CT performed on hemodynamically stable patients that may reveal free air or fluid in the abdominal cavity, mesenteric hematoma, or extravasation of CT contrast Diagnosis may be made during emergent surgery for those patients who present hemodynamically unstable and are taken for exploratory laparotomy to identify and stabilize injury (Benjamin, 2018)	Surgery for significant injuries to repair or resect damaged colon Fluid volume resuscitation and blood products for hemodynamic instability Observational management may occur if no signs of peritonitis or instability, but clinical condition must be closely monitored (Benjamin, 2018) Laparotomy/laparoscopy and/or surgical intervention if peritonitis or hemodynamic instability

TABLE 16.23 PELVIC INJURIES

	ETIOLOGY AND PRESENTATION	DIAGNOSIS	TREATMENT/INTERVENTION
Minor pelvic fractures	Involve low energy or repetitive stresses on more fragile bones Usually do not disrupt the stability of the pelvic ring Risk factors include osteoporosis, advanced age, glucocorticoid use, low body weight, smoking, excessive alcohol intake, and prior pelvic fracture (Fiechtl, 2017) **Common Sites** ■ Pubic rami ■ Sacrum ■ Iliac crest **Presentation** May present after a minor fall but may have no recall of traumatic injury May complain of hip, low back or groin pain, increased difficulty ambulating Abnormal leg positioning or shortening of a leg may be present There may be tenderness on palpation of the bony pelvis (Fiechtl, 2017)	Commonly made with pelvic x-rays May need CT or MRI (gold standard) to diagnose minor pelvic fractures (Fiechtl, 2017)	Management: Pain control, early mobilization. Only a small number of patients with minor fractures need to be nonweight bearing. Consider gait training and the use of crutches or walkers. Activity should be advanced as tolerated. If immobile, treatment for prevention of deep vein thrombosis. Have mortality rates of approximately 20%. Disruption of the pelvic ring integrity and can cause hemorrhagic shock. Require interventional radiology procedures or surgical intervention to tamponade hemorrhage and restore pelvic ring integrity (Fiechtl, 2017).

(continued)

TABLE 16.23 PELVIC INJURIES (continued)

	ETIOLOGY AND PRESENTATION	DIAGNOSIS	TREATMENT/INTERVENTION
Common major pelvic fractures	Anterior–posterior compression fracture (open book fracture) Lateral compression fracture Vertical shear fracture *Associated Injuries:* Life-threatening hemorrhage from arteries and veins in the pelvis that are unable to be controlled or from other internal injuries causing significant blood loss (Washington State Department of Health, 2016) Intra-abdominal and urinary system injury Nerve deficits from pelvic ring disruption or sacral fractures Disruption of thoracic aorta with massive hemorrhage (Clement & Biant, 2014; Washington State Department of Health, 2016)	CT of the pelvis: identify fractures, additional injuries, and hemorrhage (Fiechtl, 2018) X-ray of the pelvis can be used as well but will not be as specific regarding additional injury or blood loss as a pelvic CT scan (Washington State Department of Health, 2016)	Control hemorrhage that is a common priority in resuscitation of unstable pelvic fractures. Stabilize the pelvis with a commercial pelvic binder or wrapped sheet. Early consult with trauma and orthopedic surgery needed. Begin fluid resuscitation with warmed isotonic crystalloids and use of massive transfusion protocols and TXA if appropriate. FAST scan needed to identify surgical needs if hemodynamically unstable. Surgery needed for emergent pelvic stabilization with internal/external fixation. Caution if need to insert a urinary catheter as urethral trauma and bladder injury are more common with more severe pelvic fracture. (ATLS, 2018; Clement & Biant, 2014; Colwell, 2017; Fiechtl, 2018; Peterson et al., 2015; TNCC, 2015)

FAST, focused assessment with sonography for trauma; TXA, tranexamic acid.

TABLE 16.24 TYPES OF FEMUR FRACTURES

SITE	ETIOLOGY	PRESENTATION/DIAGNOSIS	TREATMENT
Femoral neck	About 50% are intracapsular, and about one third of those fractures are non displaced (Clement & Biant, 2014)	Hip pain Inability to walk or pain with ambulation May appear shortened and externally rotated Little bruising or external trauma may be noted with older patients	Refer to orthopedics for open reduction internal fixation or hemiarthroplasty/arthroplasty.
Intertrochanteric fracture	Is extracapsular and has an increased risk for displacement (Foster, 2019) May cause hypovolemia/hemorrhagic shock due to blood loss into the thigh	Hip pain, swelling, and bruising may be significant Injured leg may be shortened and externally rotated Tenderness over the trochanter Signs of blood loss Diagnosed by x-ray, MRI, or bone scan (Foster, 2019)	Arthroplasty or internal fixation Nonoperative management for selected populations
Trochanteric (greater or lesser trochanter)	May be due to direct trauma or pathologic fracture	Pain to the groin May also have knee or thigh pain, which increases with hip movement Anterior–posterior and lateral x-rays of the femur If pathologic trochanteric fracture is suspected and x-rays are not conclusive, MRI may be used to find evidence of fracture (Foster, 2019)	Usually nonoperative unless displacement indicates surgical management Surgical management is open reduction and internal fixation
Subtrochanteric	Occurs in the proximal femur If present in older adults, usually due more to low velocity energy (Medda & Pilson, 2019; Weatherford, 2018).	Hip or thigh pain Inability to ambulate, flex the hip, or abduct the affected leg Pain with movement	If displaced, reducing the fracture can assist in reducing blood loss as well as reducing pain and muscle spasm. Use of femoral traction devices is warranted in the ED as long as there is no evidence of open fracture

(continued)

TABLE 16.24 TYPES OF FEMUR FRACTURES (continued)

SITE	ETIOLOGY	PRESENTATION/DIAGNOSIS	TREATMENT
	Important to assess mechanism of injury in older patients to determine if low- or high-energy etiology (Medda & Pilson, 2019) Blood loss can be severe, as the long bone is involved in this fracture. The patient should be monitored for signs of hemorrhage/hemorrhagic shock	Swelling with tenderness to palpation of the proximal thigh Shortening and inward or outward rotation of the affected leg (depending on the fracture) (Lee, 2018; Weatherford, 2018)	Adequate pain control with observation if patient unable to tolerate a surgical procedure (Weatherford, 2018). This may also include use of skeletal traction (Lee, 2018) Nailing or plating of the bone, depending on fracture site and severity Aggressive and intensive physical therapy to rehabilitate the patient (Lee, 2018)

TABLE 16.25 CAUSES OF COMPARTMENT SYNDROME

TRAUMATIC CAUSES	NONTRAUMATIC CAUSES
Long bone fractures	Overly tight bandages
Crush injuries	Extravasation of IV fluids
Thermal injuries, particularly circumferential burns	Inadvertent arterial injection of medications or recreational drugs
Penetrating injuries	Prolonged limb compression due to surgery or following drug/alcohol intoxication
Envenomation	Coagulopathies leading to intramuscular hemorrhages

IV, intravenous.

Source: From Chung, K. C., Yoneda, H., & Modrall, J. G. (2019). Pathophysiology, classification and causes of acute extremity compartment syndrome. In K. A. Collins (Ed.), *UpToDate*. www.uptodate.com/home

Treatment

Early diagnosis and treatment of acute compartment syndrome are paramount to maintaining function of the extremity.

- Remove any external pressure to the extremity and keep the extremity in line with the heart.
- Provide analgesics for pain and supplementary oxygen to increase oxygen availability to the tissues.
- Treat hypotension with crystalloid solutions and vasoactive medications as systemic hypotension can further decrease tissue perfusion in the affected extremity.
- Fasciotomy is the definitive treatment for acute compartment syndrome (Stracciolini & Hammerberg, 2019).

RHABDOMYOLYSIS

OVERVIEW

Rhabdomyolysis is a condition caused by a breakdown of skeletal muscle tissue, leading to the release of large amounts of intracellular materials into the bloodstream. Rhabdomyolysis can range from an asymptomatic elevation of creatinine kinase (CK) to a life-threatening syndrome including an extreme derangement in electrolyte levels, elevation of CK, and acute kidney injury (Miller, 2019b).

Pathophysiology

Two mechanisms lead to the development of rhabdomyolysis: direct cellular injury or a depletion of adenosine triphosphate (ATP).

- Both mechanisms contribute to an intracellular influx of Na^+ and Ca^{2+}, causing disruptions to the intracellular space and cellular membrane. This disruption causes lysing of the cell and release of the intracellular contents, beginning a cycle of inflammation and apoptosis that can ultimately lead to necrosis of the muscle tissues (Miller, 2019b).

Etiology

The causes of rhabdomyolysis can be separated into three categories: traumatic, exertional, and nonexertional (Miller, 2019a; Table 16.26).

Presentation and Risk Factors

Patients with a personal or family history of malignant hyperthermia are at increased risk for developing rhabdomyolysis during an episode of malignant hyperthermia (Miller, 2019b). The classic triad occurs in <10% of patients:

- Myalgias
- Dark urine pigmentation
- Weakness

Systemic manifestations:

- Fever
- Malaise
- Nausea and vomiting
- Tachycardia (Miller, 2019b)

Relevant Diagnostics and Imaging

- Serum CK (can be elevated by as much as five times the upper limit)
- Urinalysis—Assess for myoglobinuria

TABLE 16.26 CAUSES OF RHABDOMYOLYSIS

TRAUMATIC (MOST COMMON)	EXERTIONAL	NONEXERTIONAL
Prolonged immobilization	Exertion during extreme temperatures	Myotoxic medications (i.e., statins, colchicine)
Crush injuries	Increase in exertion of an untrained individual	Carbon monoxide poisoning
Envenomation		Infectious agents

Source: Data from Miller, M. (2019a). Causes of rhabdomyolysis. In M. Ramirez Curtis (Ed.), *UpToDate*.www.uptodate.com/home

- Serum electrolyte panel, including kidney function tests
- Arterial or venous blood gas
- Complete blood count
- EKG (Miller, 2019b)

Treatment
- Aggressive rehydration with crystalloid solutions is the priority in the treatment of rhabdomyolysis, with the goal of maintaining a urine output of 2 to 3 mL/kg/hr or higher in adults.
- Acute kidney injury is a common complication that can be prevented through rehydration.
- Correction of electrolyte and metabolic abnormalities should occur as they arise (hyperkalemia, hypocalcemia, and metabolic acidosis are common).
- Hemodialysis may be initiated in patients whose kidney function is not improving with fluid resuscitation (Miller, 2019b).

MANAGING THE PATIENT WITH COMPLEX PAIN PROBLEMS

OVERVIEW
Chronic pain is pain that lasts longer than the normal healing time for acute injuries, typically longer than 6 months, and can be complex as well as difficult to manage when the cause is not readily identifiable. Complex pain problems interrupt daily life activities, lead to an increase in disabilities, and decrease quality of life. Managing complex pain can be exhausting, expensive, and time consuming as patients are referred to various providers, specialists, and therapists in search of a resolution to their pain (Barrie & Loughlin, 2014). Complex pain problems fall into several categories depending on the type and location of the pain (Czarnecki & Turner, 2018):
- Headaches
- Abdominal pain
- Low back pain
- Neuropathic pain
- Musculoskeletal pain
- Myofascial pain
- Pain related to chronic medical conditions (e.g., HIV)

Patients often report continued pain despite the use of prescribed medications and adverse side effects such as nausea, vomiting, respiratory depression, pruritus, dizziness, constipation, permanent debilitation, and addiction; even death may result.
- Many patients are treated with medications due to the healthcare provider's unfamiliarity with interventional pain procedures (Brooks & Udoji, 2016).
- Interventional options may not be offered in a location that is easily accessible to the patient.
- Interventional procedures provide the possibility to decrease or prevent unwanted adverse events and manage pain that has not responded to conservative treatment (Anitescu, 2014).

Also see Chapter 4 for a discussion of nonpharmacologic measures for pain management.

INTERVENTIONAL PROCEDURES TO MANAGE COMPLEX PAIN
Once it has been determined that pain and/or adverse effects can no longer be managed by traditional means, patients are generally referred to pain specialists or a pain clinic where interventional procedures are performed. A comprehensive pain assessment is recommended to determine the location and type of pain and the best treatment options to maximize functionality.
- A comprehensive pain assessment consists of the following:
  - Thorough history and physical and may include pain and/or depression questionnaires
  - Diagnostics such as labs
  - Imaging and scans to help determine a cause
- Most interventional procedures are elective and performed by a pain management specialist.
- Risks associated with interventional procedures include infection at the incision or insertion site, bleeding, nerve injury or nerve damage to the affected area, and continued or increased pain (Brooks & Udoji, 2016).

Injections
- Injection procedures block certain chemical substrates from nerves that cause pain (Tables 16.27 and 16.28).
- Injections can be performed in an office or clinic setting under fluoroscopy to provide temporary pain relief or to diagnose specific nerves that cause problems (Daftary & Karnik, 2015).
- The local anesthetic in the injection solution provides immediate relief, whereas it will take the steroid up to a week to be effective.

An alternate injection procedure called *dry needling* is a technique in which fine, sterile needles are used to pierce through the skin and stimulate specific tight, painful muscle bands to reduce pain and cramping. In this technique, no medication is injected. The goal of dry needling is to loosen the muscle and reduce pain (Espejo-Antúnez et al., 2017). It usually takes two to six treatments to notice effectiveness.

Nonsurgical Nerve Blocks
- Nonsurgical nerve blocks use local anesthetic to reduce pain by preventing pain signals from going to the brain from a group of nerves (Table 16.29).
- Nerve blocks are temporary, with effects lasting from a few hours up to 2 weeks.

TABLE 16.27 TYPES OF INJECTIONS

TYPE OF INJECTION	SOLUTION	INDICATION
Steroid	Steroid combined with a preservative-free local anesthetic	Administered adjacent to nerve roots or peripheral nerves responsible for pain propagation in order to reduce pain, inflammation, and swelling
Local anesthetic	Preservative-free anesthetic	Provides local temporary pain relief for quick procedures such as intravenous access or line placement. Also used in trigger point injections to reduce pain in well-localized areas
Botulinum	Botulinum toxins	FDA approved to cause muscle weakening and provide short-term pain relief in cervical dystonia (D'Arcy, 2011)

FDA, Food and Drug Administration.

TABLE 16.28 SITE-SPECIFIC INJECTIONS

INJECTION LOCATION	TREATMENT	INDICATION
Caudal	Steroid injection to decrease inflammation	Reduces muscle spasms to lower back and lower extremity pain.
Cervical	Steroid injection near herniated discs, spinal nerves, or area of stenosis	Deceases pain and inflammation to compressed nerves in the head, neck, or shoulders.
Facet joint	Local anesthetic or steroid injection	Lessens pain or inflammation to facet joints in neck and back.
Intracapsular (glenoid)	Local anesthetic injection	Reduces pain or inflammation to shoulders.
Lumbar epidural and lumbar transforaminal	Steroid injection near spinal nerves	Minimizes inflammation and swelling due to foraminal stenosis, spinal stenosis, and sciatica.
Sacroiliac	Steroid injection near the junction of the pelvis and spine	Diminishes inflammation pain and swelling resulting from arthritis to sacroiliac joints.
Trigger point	Local anesthetic injection to a specific area	Used to ease pain at specific pinpointed painful locations usually in taut muscle bands.

TABLE 16.29 NONSURGICAL NERVE BLOCKS

NERVE BLOCK	INDICATION
Occipital	One-sided occipital headaches
Celiac plexus	Blocks the anterior vertebrae at the T_{12}-L_1 level to cover nonmenstrual complex abdominal pain, mesenteric, and chronic pancreatic pain
Fascia iliaca	Used for refractory postsurgical hip, thigh, or knee pain
Sympathetic	Obstructs pain signals from sympathetically mediated pain (i.e., shingles, Raynaud's syndrome, phantom limb pain, excessive sweating, and CRPS

CRPS, complex regional pain syndrome.

- Risks include bleeding, infection, loss of sensation, and nerve injury or nerve damage to the area.
- Nerve blocks can be performed in pain clinics, surgery centers, and hospitals.

- The patient may experience pain for a few days after the procedure at the injection sites.
- It is possible for the pain to return after several months to years if the damaged nerve is able to repair itself or regenerate.

Surgical Nerve Blocks
- Surgical blocks reduce pain by preventing pain signals traveling from a group of nerves to the brain.
- Surgical blocks can be used to relieve terminal cancer or neuralgia-type pains and are more permanent in that the nerves are intentionally damaged or destroyed by physical destruction (e.g., cutting) or chemical destruction (e.g., instillation of a solution known to cause nerve damage).

Minimally Invasive Procedures
When optimal results are not achieved with medications, physical therapy, or minor interventional procedures such as nerve blocks, it may be necessary to perform more involved procedures to reduce pain, increase function, and improve quality of life (Giurazza et al., 2017). Most minimally invasive procedures are shorter in length, consist of smaller incisions, elicit less pain, and have a shorter recovery time (Table 16.30).

TABLE 16.30 PROCEDURES FOR BACK PAIN

PROCEDURE	INDICATIONS	TECHNIQUE	CONSIDERATIONS	RECOVERY
Discectomy	Herniated disc	A small tube is used to remove material pressing on nerve roots or spinal cord	If unrepaired can cause nerve damage to bladder, bowels, lower back, or legs	About 4 weeks
Percutaneous disc nucleoplasty	Bulging disc	A radiofrequency device is used to dissolve the glutinous center portion of a disc to cause contents to spread rather than bulge	Can cause nerve damage to bladder, bowels, lower back, or legs, new pain, or muscle spasms	Up to 6 weeks
IDET	Chronic low-back pain	A heated wire is inserted into a disc to expand collagen into minor tears and cracks	Infection, injury to nerve roots, disc herniation, epidural abscess, or spinal cord damage	Up to 4 months
Neurotomy	Neck, back, and sacroiliac joint pain	Radiofrequency waves are used to generate heat through needles to create a lesion on the nerve to relieve pain	Pain relief is temporary, may develop increased pain, infection, bleeding, or nerve damage	Patient specific
Vertebroplasty	Repair collapsed vertebrae	Uses imaging to inject cement into the vertebral column	Bleeding, infection, increased back pain, nerve damage, or cement leaking out of position	24 hours
Kyphoplasty	Repair vertebrae damaged from spinal fractures or cancer	Uses an orthopedic-type balloon to push vertebrae back into place; the cement is injected to maintain the position	Bleeding, infection, increased back pain, nerve damage, or cement leaking out of position	6 weeks

IDET, intradiscal electrothermal therapy.

Spinal-Cord Stimulation
- Spinal-cord stimulation is FDA approved for intractable neuropathic pain of the limbs and trunk
- It is currently used for failed back surgery, chronic regional pain syndrome (CRPS), diabetic neuropathy, ischemic limb pain, and other chronic pain.
- Leads are placed in the epidural space and connected to a generator to send electrical impulses into the nerves, interfering with pain signals sent to the brain (Ehrhardt et al., 2018).
- If effective in relieving the pain, then the spinal cord stimulator may be inserted permanently, which requires a surgical procedure. Risks include bleeding, infection, pain at the insertion site, and dural puncture.
- Recovery time for the percutaneous trial is typically 24 hours, whereas recovery time following the implantation procedure is about 6 to 8 weeks.

Intrathecal-Implanted Pump
An intrathecal pump is an option used to manage cancer pain, pancreatitis, and CRPS. It can also be used to manage spasticity from multiple sclerosis and cerebral palsy.
- The intrathecal pump is inserted in the intrathecal space of the spinal column and has a reservoir in which the medication is placed.
- The patient undergoes a trial and adjustment period for 24 hours up to 2 weeks to determine an appropriate medication dose that relieves the pain or spasm.
- After the trial period, the intrathecal pump is permanently inserted, typically implanted subcutaneously in the patient's lower abdomen, allowing for dose adjustment using an external device and refills through needle insertion into a port underneath the skin (D'Arcy, 2011).

- Risks of an intrathecal pump placement are infection, bleeding, meningitis, spinal headaches, and medication withdrawal with pump malfunction (D'Arcy, 2011).
- Recovery time is 4 to 6 weeks after permanent implant of the intrathecal pump.
- Only three medications are approved by the U.S. FDA for use in the intrathecal pump (D'Arcy, 2011):
  - *Preservative-free morphine*—An opioid to provide pain relief
  - *Ziconotide (Prialt)*—A nonopioid for pain relief medication
  - *Baclofen (Lioresal)*—An antispasmodic to manage spasms

Interventional options, such as simple injections, to more minimally invasive procedures and implanted devices can provide alternatives when pharmacologic and nonpharmacologic methods have proven ineffective.

REVIEW QUESTIONS

1. A trauma patient sustains possible head injury after being hit in the head with a shovel and is currently comatose. The patient is at immediate risk for what type of shock?
   A. Cardiogenic
   B. Distributive
   C. Hypovolemia
   D. Obstructive

2. You are caring for a patient and you suspect an acid–base imbalance. You order a simultaneous arterial blood gas (ABG) and serum chemistry. The results are as follows:
   pH: 7.50
   $PaCO_2$: 30
   HCO_3^-: 25

Based on these lab values, you suspect the patient is suffering from which of the following?

A. Metabolic acidosis
B. Metabolic alkalosis
C. Respiratory acidosis
D. Respiratory alkalosis

3. A patient presents with the following injuries. Which injury must be treated in the primary survey?

A. Closed femur fracture
B. Diaphragmatic tear
C. Splenic hematoma
D. Tension pneumothorax

ANSWERS

1. **Correct answer: B. Rationale**: Patients with head injuries are also at risk for spinal cord injuries, putting the patients at risk for neurogenic (distributive) shock. Based on the mechanism of injury (isolated head injury), the patient would not immediately be at risk for cardiogenic, hypovolemia, or obstructive shock.

2. **Correct answer: D. Rationale:** The pH is above the normal value, indicating an alkalemia, and the $PaCO_2$ is below the normal value, indicating a respiratory disorder. Metabolic alkalosis would also have a pH above normal but would have a HCO_3 below normal. Respiratory acidosis and metabolic acidosis would have a pH below normal.

3. **Correct answer: D. Rationale:** Tension pneumothorax is a life-threatening injury that would be identified and treated in the primary survey of airway, breathing, and circulation. Although closed femur fractures can cause hemorrhage, they are not an immediate threat to life. Diaphragmatic tears and cause respiratory difficult; it is not an immediate threat to life needing intervention in the primary survey. Splenic hematoma can cause hemorrhage; it is not an immediate threat to life.

REFERENCES

The complete reference and additional reading lists appear in the digital version of this chapter, at https://connect.springerpub.com/content/book/978-0-8261-7417-8/part/part01/chapter/ch016

17

Family Planning

Brittany Waggoner

OVERVIEW

The scope of contraception in relation to reproductive health is ever evolving. Knowledge of current recommendations is an important step toward providing the highest quality of care to patients (Gavin & Pazol, 2016).

Providing a range of family planning services, including contraception and counseling, is an essential element of patient-centered reproductive care. Care considerations include the patient's desired number and spacing of children, emphasizing client-centered counseling, and a full range of contraceptive methods for those seeking to prevent pregnancy (Gavan & Pazol, 2016).

Choosing a contraceptive method is complex. The clinical nurse specialist (CNS) plays an important role in providing information and supporting patient decision-making about contraceptive methods. Women should receive contraceptive counseling and identify conditions that may limit the range of available methods. Selection of the appropriate contraceptive method is accomplished through a shared decision-making process with the patient (Dehlendorf et al., 2019).

Types of Contraception
Contraceptive Methods
- Progestin-only
  - Oral contraceptives
  - Injections
- Combined estrogen and progestin
  - Oral contraception
  - Transdermal patches
  - Vaginal ring
- Long-acting reversible contraception (LARC)
  - Progestin intrauterine device (IUD)
  - Copper IUD
  - Implant
- Barrier method
  - Diaphragm
  - Sponge
  - Cervical cap
  - Condom
- Fertility awareness
- Sterilization
  - Male
  - Female
- Other
  - Withdrawal (American College of Obstetricians and Gynecologists [ACOG], 2019; Table 17.1)

Contraceptive outcomes can be measured as follows:
- Unintended pregnancy with the most effective contraceptive methods
- Unintended pregnancy with moderately effective contraceptive methods
- Unintended pregnancy with a LARC method

TABLE 17.1 TYPES OF CONTRACEPTION MEASURES

CONTRACEPTION OPTIONS	PREGNANCY RISK (%)	PLACEMENT TIMEFRAME	SIDE EFFECTS	OTHER CONSIDERATIONS
Female sterilization	0.005	Permanent	Pain, bleeding, infection	Permanent protection
Male sterilization	0.0015			
IUD	Progestin, 0.002	Lasts 3–12 years	Pain with placement	Estrogen free
	Copper, 0.008			Hormone free
Implant	0.0005	Lasts up to 3 years		Estrogen free
Injection	4	Every 3 months	Increase in appetite/weight gain	
Oral	8	Every day at same time	Nausea, breast tenderness	May improve acne and menstrual cramps Lowers risk of ovarian and uterine cancer

(continued)

The complete reference and additional reading lists appear in the digital version of this chapter, at https://connect.springerpub.com/content/book/978-0-8261-7417-8/part/part01/chapter/ch17

TABLE 17.1 TYPES OF CONTRACEPTION MEASURES (*continued*)

CONTRACEPTION OPTIONS	PREGNANCY RISK (%)	PLACEMENT TIMEFRAME	SIDE EFFECTS	OTHER CONSIDERATIONS
Patch	9	Each week		
Ring	9	Each month		
Diaphragm	12	Prior to sex	Irritation, allergic reaction	Hormone free
Male condom	13			Hormone free No prescription necessary
Female condom	21			
Withdrawal	20		None	Hormone free No cost associated
Sponge	12–24		Irritation, allergic reaction	Hormone free No prescription necessary
Fertility awareness	24	Daily	None	Hormone free Increase in awareness
Spermicides	28	Prior to sex	Irritation, allergic reaction	Hormone free No prescription necessary

IUD, intrauterine device.

- After a live birth with a most effective contraceptive method within 3 to 60 days postdelivery
- After live birth with a LARC method within 3 to 60 days postdelivery

REVIEW QUESTIONS

1. You and a patient are discussing pregnancy prevention options. She has three children and would like the best option for permanently preventing future pregnancies. While utilizing the patient-centered reproductive care planning model, you would counsel her to chose which method of contraception?
   A. A one-time intrauterine device (IUD) placement
   B. Female sterilization
   C. Oral contraception
   D. Fertility awareness

2. When counseling a patient to choose the highest quality of contraceptive care, the CNS should take into consideration which of the following measures?
   A. How many children she has
   B. Her access to contraception methods
   C. The effectiveness of the methods
   D. Both B & C

ANSWERS

1. **Correct answer: B. Rationale:** Female sterilization is a permanent option to prevent future pregnancies, this is the best option after counseling her to ensure she does not want any future pregnancies. IUD and oral contraception are temporary measures. Fertility awareness has no bearing on this decision.

2. **Correct answer: D. Rationale:** Effectiveness of the birth control method is the highest priority, but it is also important to ensure the client has access to the contraception method chosen. The number of children may help the client make the decision from a personal perspective, but does not affect the method the CNS should choose.

REFERENCES

The complete reference and additional reading lists appear in the digital version of this chapter, at https://connect.springerpub.com/content/book/978-0-8261-7417-8/part/part01/chapter/ch17

Section II
Nurses and Nursing Practice

Response to Illness

Jeanna Ford, Francesca C. Levitt, Valerie Pfander, and Amy C. Shay

PHYSIOLOGIC STRESS RESPONSE

OVERVIEW

The body adapts to potentially stressful challenges by activating response mechanisms in the autonomic nervous system. The autonomic nervous system regulates the rate of breathing, blood pressure, heart rate, body temperature, and digestive processes. The autonomic nervous system has two main divisions: sympathetic and parasympathetic. When a stressful or emergency situation is perceived, the body's sympathetic nervous system responds by triggering a release of hormones to prepare the body to react. The sympathetic nervous system stimulates the adrenal glands, which triggers a release of catecholamines including epinephrine and norepinephrine. The release of these hormones causes a physiologic reaction, often called the fight-or-flight response. This fight-or-flight response occurs when a harmful event or threat to survival is perceived. Physical changes that occur in the body during the fight-or-flight response include tachycardia, tachypnea, muscle tension, dilated pupils, and diaphoresis.

Pathophysiology of Stress

The stress response begins in the amygdala, an area of the brain that contributes to emotional processing. The amygdala interprets sounds and images; when danger is perceived, a distress signal is sent to the hypothalamus. The hypothalamus communicates the stress to the rest of the body through the autonomic nervous system. The fight-or-flight response is triggered, and the body responds with an epinephrine-induced burst of energy as a preparatory response to danger. As the initial surge of epinephrine subsides, the hypothalamus activates the second component of the stress response system called the hypothalamic–pituitary–adrenal axis. If the brain continues to perceive danger, the hypothalamus releases corticotropin-releasing hormone (CRH), which travels to the pituitary gland, triggering the release of adrenocorticotropic hormone (ACTH). This hormone travels to the adrenal glands, prompting them to release cortisol. The release of these hormones results in the body being energized and on high alert. When the threat passes, the stress response subsides (Table 18.1).

Impact of Early Life Stress on Adult Health

Emerging research is exploring the link between childhood stress and adult health. Stress occurring early in life may be associated with increased physical and emotional health issues throughout adulthood. Children who experience chronic stressors have an increased connection between peripheral inflammation and neural circuitries involved in threat-related, reward-related, and executive control–related processes. This connection can lead to chronic low-grade inflammation, which in turn can contribute to obesity, insulin resistance, and other predisease states. Chemical mediators of inflammation act on the cortico-amygdala threat and cortico-basal ganglia reward circuitries in a way that predisposes individuals to self-medicating behaviors like smoking, drug use, and consumption of high-fat diets. These behaviors combined with chronic inflammation can hasten emotional and physical health problems. Major childhood stressful events can be emotional, physical, sexual, or related to family dysfunction. Future research is needed to explore additional childhood stressors such as bullying, discrimination, and natural disasters to see if they lead to similar neuroimmune changes in the body.

Coping

Stress, health, and coping are interrelated. Stress can lower the body's resistance and disrupt the homeostasis that is essential for health and well-being. Bodily stress may arise from disease or illness. Patients with chronic illness will often have stress from both emotional and physical mechanisms. When emotional stress occurs, teaching relaxation and stress-reduction techniques to patients can improve their overall health and increase the likelihood of their living a disease-free life.

Effective coping mechanisms are an important predictor of well-being. Religion and acceptance are the most common coping strategies used by patients. Other methods used to cope with chronic illness include humor, emotional or social support, and positive reframing. There are several tools available for the clinical nurse specialist (CNS) to use to assess a patient's coping ability. One tool is the COPE inventory scale and another is the Temporal Satisfaction with Life Scale (TSWLS). The COPE inventory scale indicates how people respond when confronted with stressful events in their lives. The TSWLS assesses a patient's life satisfaction.

IMPACT OF COMORBIDITY

OVERVIEW

Aging is associated with the development of chronic comorbid conditions. Biologic changes of aging occur at the cellular structural level. As these cellular defects accumulate over time, age-related illness and disease develop. Multimorbidity is defined as the presence of two or more chronic conditions in a single patient. Multimorbidity is a significant problem among older adults, leading to increased healthcare utilization, hospitalizations, readmissions, and poorer outcomes in terms of

TABLE 18.1 STRESS-RESPONSE THEORIES

THEORY	THEORIST	KEY CONCEPT
GAS	Hans Selye	Three theoretical stages: ■ Alarm: The body experiences physiologic responses to a threat (fight or flight). ■ Resistance: Stress-activated responses continue; the body attempts to adapt to the stress. ■ Exhaustion: The body has depleted its reserves and can no longer maintain responses to the stressors.
Allostasis and allostatic load theories	Sterling and Eyer	This theory proposes that homeostasis is the body's ability to regulate balance, such as blood oxygen level, blood glucose, or blood pH. Failed adaptation to stress results in pathology and chronic illness. ■ Allostasis is the process by which the body responds to stressors in order to regain homeostasis. ■ Allostatic load is the "wear and tear" on the body that accumulates when an individual is exposed to repeated or long-term stress.
RAM	Sister Callista Roy	This theory places emphasis on the person's own coping abilities to achieve health. ■ Focal stimuli are the internal and external demands immediately confronting the organism (e.g., a need for cancer surgery). ■ Contextual stimuli are all other internal and external factors in the given situation (e.g., fear of dying). ■ Residual stimuli are factors that may be affecting current emotions and behaviors but whose effects are not clearly validated (e.g., having a mother who died from cancer).
PSM	J. Toth Midrange theory	■ Stressors (physiologic, psychologic, environmental, and sociocultural) ■ Psychophysiologic stress ■ Conditioning effects ■ Stressors cause increases in heart rate, blood pressure, and myocardial oxygen consumption, potentially leading to an increase in myocardial ischemia and the possibility of fatal dysrhythmias or infarction. ■ Assessing stress levels, particularly at hospital discharge, is important to determine who may be at risk for a cardiac event.
Stress appraisal and coping theory	Lazarus and Folkman	This theory states that stress is a product of a transaction between a person and their environment. ■ Primary appraisal involves determining whether the stressor poses a threat. ■ Secondary appraisal involves the individual's evaluation of the coping strategies available. ■ Coping involves the individual using the coping processes to attempt to change the stressor or think about the stressor in a different way.
Theory of emotion	James and Lange	■ Emotions do not immediately succeed the perception of the stressor or the stressful event; they become present after the body's response to the stress. ■ It is not possible for emotional behavior to occur unless it is connected to the brain.

GAS, general adaptation syndrome; PSM, psychophysiological stress model; RAM, Roy's Adaptation Model.

morbidity, mortality, and quality of life. Traditional chronic disease management is based on care of patients with a single chronic illness in the absence of other concurrent conditions. Care of multimorbid patients can be highly specialized, fragmented, and duplicative, which may lead to increased treatment burden and cost. Older adults experience diminished ability to adapt to the physiologic stress of illness. Stressors of acute illness may affect multiple organ systems, including those unrelated to the initial complaint. Patients with multimorbidity require a holistic, individualized, and coordinated management approach (Box 18.1).

Common Chronic Comorbidities

■ Heart disease	■ Diabetes
■ Neoplasm	■ COPD
■ Stroke	■ Chronic kidney disease

COPD, congestive obstructive pulmonary disease.

BOX 18.1. Multimorbidity Approach to Care Principles

Personalize assessment.	Reduce unplanned or uncoordinated care.
Individualize management plan.	Consider patient health and treatment priorities.
Reduce treatment burden.	Consider frailty assessment.
Consider nonpharmacologic alternatives.	Be alert for anxiety and depression.
Identify medicines with higher risk of adverse events.	Be alert to care transitions as periods of vulnerability lead to errors and follow-up confusion.

Additional Chronic Conditions Associated With Increased Surgical Risk

■ Alzheimer's disease	■ Chronic pain syndrome
■ Morbid obesity	■ Obstructive sleep apnea
■ Liver disease	■ Dementia

SYMPTOMATIC RESPONSE TO ILLNESS PAIN

OVERVIEW

A myriad of circumstances and coexisting factors leads to the experience of pain, including a symptomatic response to illness. Pain can manifest as a response to illness when accompanied by tissue damage, inflammation, ischemia, nerve irritation, concomitant anxiety, and a stress response. The CNS is in a perfect position as an advanced practice nurse to gain expertise in pain management, educate patients and families, and act as a role model to other clinicians to promote optimal patient outcomes through the development of patient-specific plans of care.

Nurses must consistently assess and reassess pain after an intervention and make a multimodal approach of pharmacologic and nonpharmacologic interventions the standard of care.

Definition

The International Association for the Study of Pain (IASP) describes *pain* as "an unpleasant sensory and emotional experience associated with actual or potential tissue damage, or described in terms of such damage" (https://www.iasp-pain.org/PublicationsNews/NewsDetail.aspx?ItemNumber=10475). Regardless of the definition of *pain*, it is clear that there is complexity in the experience that must be appreciated to individualize care.

Pathophysiology

In the peripheral nervous system (PNS), pain messaging involves nociceptive and primary afferent fibers that travel to the dorsal horn of the spinal cord. Free nerve endings are found in the muscle, fascia, blood vessels, knee joint, and dura. Nociceptors respond to potentially harmful thermal, chemical, or mechanical stimuli. Specific nociceptors are associated with afferent A (myelinated) and C (unmyelinated) fibers. A fibers (A delta and A beta) produce a sharp, pricking, or aching pain, whereas C fibers evoke a burning pain sensation.

- **Nociception** includes transduction, transmission, perception, and modulation. **Transduction** involves stimulation of afferent fibers by thermal, chemical, or mechanical stimuli. If there is tissue damage, neurochemical mediators (substance P, K^+, bradykinin, prostaglandin, histamine, and serotonin) are released, causing an exchange of ions and resultant action potential. **Transmission** occurs when the impulses are sent to the dorsal horn of the spinal cord and then to the brain via the spinothalamic tract.
- **Perception** occurs after the neurons continue to transmit nociceptive messages to the thalamus and midbrain. In the somatosensory cortex, parietal lobe, frontal lobe, and limbic system, the painful sensation is perceived.
- **Modulation** occurs in the dorsal horn during descending pathway activation and can work to decrease the amount of pain felt through the release of neurotransmitters serotonin and norepinephrine.

Other physiologic manifestations of the pain response include the body's response to pain via the sympathetic nervous system, neuroendocrine system, immune system, and limbic system, which impact the stress response, hormone regulation, response to infection, and emotional health.

In nursing, pain is categorized as acute pain (nociceptive), persistent or chronic pain, cancer pain, and neuropathic pain. The patient's description of pain will help determine the likely pain mechanism. Explaining the pain mechanism to patients in terms they can understand will help establish a therapeutic relationship and movement toward a mutual plan for the delivery of targeted interventions (Table 18.2).

Assessment

Pain assessment is more than determining a pain score on a numeric pain rating scale, yet many staff nurses focus exclusively on this component. Although no pain assessment tool is comprehensive, one approach to pain assessment includes the components listed in Box 18.2. A list of pain assessment tools is found in Table 18.3.

Factors Affecting Pain Presentation

Depending on the situation, culture, genetics, coping skills, medical history, and past experience, patients will communicate any discomfort they might be experiencing to care providers differently, as pain tolerance varies and a uniform pain threshold is nonexistent. Cultural competence and communication must be considered when discussing pain with patients. The clinician should be prepared to discuss goals and expectations while being sensitive to language, eye contact preferences, personal space, style of speech, nonverbal communication, spiritual or religious beliefs, health beliefs, and familial relationships.

Risk Factors

- Nonverbal and cognitively impaired patients: Such patients are at risk for undertreatment of pain secondary to their inability to adequately communicate discomfort to those providing care and treatment.
- *Delirium:* Pain may be a risk factor for delirium; therefore, regular pain and delirium assessments are necessary to more effectively manage both pain and delirium.
- *History of substance use disorder (SUD):* Patients with a SUD who experience pain are at risk for inadequate pain management. Bias, judgment, or inexperience on the part of the clinician can impact pain assessment, treatment, and evaluation of response. Patients in recovery may communicate

TABLE 18.2 PAIN TYPE, NATURE, AND TREATMENT

TYPE OF PAIN	SENSATIONS	LOCATION	TREATMENT
Somatic pain	Constant, dull, aching, throbbing, sharp	Skin, subcutaneous tissues, bone, muscle, blood vessels, connective tissue	Nonopioid analgesics Adjuvants (anticonvulsants, antidepressants) Opioids Nonpharmacologic modalities
Visceral pain	Cramping, splitting, squeezing, aching, pressure	Internal organs or body cavity linings	Nonopioid analgesics Adjuvants (anticonvulsants, antidepressants) Opioids Nonpharmacologic modalities
Neuropathic pain	Shooting, burning, electric shock like, tingling, itching, sharp, stabbing, numb, motor weakness	Peripheral nerves, spinal cord, brain	Nonopioid analgesics Adjuvants (anticonvulsants, antidepressants) Nonpharmacologic modalities

BOX 18.2. Pain Assessment Components

Location: Mark the location on a figure drawing or pointing to the body part(s).

Intensity: Use a 0 to 10 numeric pain scale with anchors of 0 = no pain and 10 = worst possible pain.

Comfort–function goal: Refers to an acceptable 0 to 10 pain level that does not interfere with functional activity.

Pain constancy: Ask whether the pain is constant or breakthrough pain.

Quality of pain: Identify the underlying pain mechanism (e.g., throbbing, shooting, sharp, cramping, aching, tender, pricking, burning, or pulling).

Onset, duration, variation, rhythm: Ask when the pain began, how long has the pain been present, is the pain better or worse at certain times?

Manner of expressing pain: Note hesitancy or embarrassment when discussing pain; ask whether the pain scale is acceptable.

What relieves the pain: Include pharmacologic and nonpharmacologic modalities.

What makes the pain worse: Note activity, positions, or other events.

Effects of pain: Ask how pain interferes with function, sleep, quality of life, and healing.

Comments: Solicit anything else the patient or family wishes to add.

the desire to avoid opioids while hospitalized, and it is the responsibility of the healthcare providers to develop a pain management plan in collaboration with the patient that utilizes nonopioids and nonpharmacologic modalities. Patients may also be in a medication assisted treatment (MAT) program with buprenorphine, methadone, or naltrexone. Medications for opioid use disorder (MOUD) is a more recent term that is more specific to opioid use disorders. Consulting with the MAT/MOUD prescriber to determine the best course of treatment during a healthcare episode supports

the patient's recovery. Depending on the reason for the hospitalization of treatment episode, if acute pain is present, a tailored pharmacologic treatment plan that might need to include opioids should be developed in conjunction with the provider and pharmacist.

- **Surgical patients:** These patients typically experience postoperative pain and are at risk for chronic opioid use. Considering the opioid epidemic, it is important to manage acute pain in the immediate postoperative phase and minimize opioid use by using a multimodal approach and limiting opioids to the first few postoperative days.
- **Opioid-induced respiratory depression:** This is a dangerous side effect that can lead to failure to rescue if monitoring is inadequate. When opioids are prescribed to opioid naive patients or those with obstructive sleep apnea or other obstructive conditions, end tidal CO_2 monitoring can detect breath-to-breath ventilation and periods of obstruction or apnea and alert the nurse.
  - The **Pasero Opioid Sedation Scale (POSS)** is used to assess unintended sedation that can occur with the administration of opioids. POSS with interventions includes adjusting the opioid dose for an increased level of sedation to reduce the risk of ventilatory compromise while maintaining adequate analgesia. For somnolent or unarousable patients, the nurse would administer naloxone per protocol and activate a rapid response team. To accurately evaluate the patient for signs of unintended sedation, the nurse observes the patient without stimulation.

Pathophysiological Consequences of Pain

- Poorly managed acute pain can lead to the **development of persistent pain,** thought to occur secondary to immune system involvement, stress response, and inflammatory processes.
- *Bowel function* always needs to be addressed when initiating opioids. A bowel regimen should be started when opioids are prescribed.
- Nonsteroidal antiinflammatory agents can cause **digestive irritation** and **impact renal function**. Assessing for symptoms and monitoring laboratory values can assist in dosing decisions.

TABLE 18.3 PAIN ASSESSMENT TOOLS

PAIN ASSESSMENT TOOL	INDICATIONS FOR USE	ADVANTAGES/DISADVANTAGES
BPI	Self-report of pain severity and interference with function	Valid, reliable tool in outpatient settings; available in many languages.
NRS	Self-report of pain intensity	Valid, reliable; more accurate when a copy of the tool is provided. Available in many languages. Must be anchored when providing an explanation; uses 0–10 scale.
FPS-R	Self-report of pain intensity	Valid, reliable. Provide a copy of the tool for the patient to select one of six faces that best describes the current pain or discomfort.
VDS	Self-report of pain intensity	Can assign numbers to the descriptor; consistency during the episode of care is essential.
PAINAD	Observation of pain behaviors	Valid and reliable; documented for use in advanced dementia patients. Scale ranges from 0 to 10.
CNPI	Observation of pain behaviors	Valid and reliable; a score ≥1 assumes pain is present; scale ranges from 0 to 12.
CPOT	Observation of pain behaviors	Valid, reliable tool for nonverbal, unable-to-self-report, critically ill patients. Scale ranges from 0 to 8.

BPI, Brief Pain Inventory; CNPI, Checklist for Non-Verbal Pain Indicators; CPOT, Critical Care Pain Observation Tool; FPS-R, Faces Pain Scale-Revised; NRS, Numeric Rating Scale; PAINAD, Pain Assessment in Advanced Dementia; VDS, Verbal Descriptor Scale.

- *Hepatotoxicity* can be a concern with acetaminophen (APAP). Doses should be limited to 3,000 to 4,000 mg/d since the medication is metabolized by the liver. The upper threshold on the maximum daily allowed dose of APAP has been the subject of controversy, and doses have been reset from 4,000 mg/d to either 3,000 mg/d or 3,250 mg/d for consumers taking the 500- or 325-mg tablet preparations, respectively. Prescription combination (opioid and acetaminophen) drug products now have 325 mg of APAP per dosage unit.
- *Sleep hygiene* should be assessed and managed, especially in patients experiencing persistent pain. Pain can interfere with sleep, and sleep disturbances can exacerbate pain.

Interventions

- The pain mechanism must be accurately identified to determine effective pharmacologic treatment and to avoid unnecessary and potentially dangerous opioid use. In light of the current opioid epidemic, responsible, evidence-based prescribing and treatment practices are essential.
- *Patient education* has been shown to improve movement, exercise ability, and thinking about pain differently.
- A *multimodal approach* that combines targeted pharmacologic (opioids and nonopioids) and nonpharmacologic interventions to manage acute and/or chronic pain states is an evidence-based strategy. Multimodal pharmacologic analgesia uses two or more medications that act by different mechanisms and may be administered via the same or different routes. The aim of multimodal analgesia is to improve pain relief and increase function, while reducing opioid requirements and opioid-related adverse effects.
- *Example of multimodal approach*: Treatment for a surgical patient undergoing a colectomy for diverticular disease could include preemptive analgesia with preoperative acetaminophen, a bilateral transverse abdominus plane block, low dose of an intraoperative opioid, and ketorolac in the postanesthesia care unit. Postoperatively, scheduled acetaminophen, ketorolac, and gabapentin would be prescribed. In addition, the patient may practice mindfulness and meditation and keep a gratitude journal. Social support from family and regular physical activity to increase blood flow also helps manage the postoperative discomfort.
- An *interdisciplinary pain management approach* is ideal and can lead to patient engagement and inclusion in decisions about care. Collaboration of interprofessional team members along with the patient and family allows for the development of a comprehensive, individualized plan of care.
- The *Empiric Analgesia Trial* is beneficial when pain is assessed and identified through appropriate tools for nonverbal adults with or without cognitive impairment. Using an analgesic trial or nonpharmacologic intervention with subsequent reassessment will more accurately determine if pain was present and the efficacy of the intervention (Box 18.3).
- Reasons to initiate an empiric analgesia trial include the following: Pathologic conditions are likely to cause pain. Scheduled procedures are likely to cause pain.
- Scores of an observational behavioral pain assessment tool.
- Pain behaviors continue after addressing the suspected cause of pain.
- Pain behaviors after basic needs are met and comfort measures administered.
  - Reports from surrogates or family that behaviors are indicative of pain.

Information should be shared during handoff to establish continuity of pain treatment and care. When caring for patients

BOX 18.3. Nonpharmacological Interventions

Aroma therapy
Activity
Acupuncture
Biofeedback
Cognitive behavioral therapy
Deep breathing
Distraction
Environmental modification
Guided imagery
Heat/cold
Healing touch
Gratitude journal
Immobilization
Light massage
Meditation
Mindfulness-based stress reduction
Movement
Music
Pain education
Pet therapy
Positioning/repositioning
Prayer/spiritual practices
Progressive muscle relaxation
Relaxation
Self-hypnosis
TENS
Yoga

TENS, transcutaneous electrical nerve stimulation.

who have difficulty communicating, family members should be included during the assessment process.

ANXIETY

OVERVIEW

Definition

Anxiety is a nonspecific feeling of dread or foreboding, particularly of the unknown, and is highly subjective. Anxiety is the psychologic response to a perceived threat that activates the body's physical stress response. The physiologic stress response is an adaptive function with the primary purpose of self-preservation. Anxiety levels can be labeled as debilitating when the stressor experienced by the individual overbears the ability to cope. Diagnosis of a serious illness can invoke feelings of anxiety or distress. However, some people have feelings of anxiety without the diagnosis of a serious or chronic illness (Ford, 2016).

Presentation

Anxiety can be considered a normal reaction to any stressor or stimulus. Most individuals need a small amount of anxiety to function and in mild forms, anxiety can be considered healthy, serving as a powerful motivator. However, disproportionate anxiety reactions to stressful situations are not considered therapeutic. Anxiety is considered a treatable condition with medication and psychotherapy. If left untreated, these symptoms can have a detrimental effect on a patient's quality of life and overall function (Ford, 2016). Anxiety disorders include generalized anxiety disorder (GAD), phobias, and panic disorders (Yohannes et al., 2018).

Assessment, Risk Factors, Interventions (See Chapter 15, "Psychobehavioral Disorders.")

SHORTNESS OF BREATH/DYSPNEA

OVERVIEW

Definition

Shortness of breath, or *dyspnea*, is defined by the American Thoracic Society as "a subjective experience of breathing discomfort that consists of qualitative distinct sensations that can vary in intensity" (Parshall et al., 2012, p. 436). The overall experience of shortness of breath or dyspnea originates from interactions of physiologic, psychologic, social, and environmental factors (Baldwin & Cox, 2016). Qualities of dyspnea can be derived from three categories: air hunger, work, and tightness. Each category may stem from different pathophysiologic processes, making accurate assessment critical.

Presentation

Dyspnea can affect multiple dimensions of life, reducing activity level and functional capacity and causing distress and discomfort. Signs and symptoms include tachypnea, pallor, cyanosis, nasal flaring, accessory muscle use, chest pain, coughing, and tachycardia. Dyspnea is a subjective experience and patients may describe feelings of dyspnea without physical symptoms. Symptoms may not correlate with disease severity. Emotional distress associated with dyspnea may worsen symptoms, creating a vicious cycle.

Assessment

A thorough assessment must include comprehensive history including timing, precipitating factors, associated symptoms, and overall quality. It may be difficult to distinguish dyspnea from pain, fatigue, loss of energy, or weakness. Presence and degree of dyspnea does not always correspond to level of hypoxia.. The clinical assessment of dyspnea initially should focus on eliciting the underlying pathology.

- *Risk factor assessment*—Includes smoking history, cancer treatments, comorbid conditions, medications, and history or patterns of dyspnea including exacerbating and relieving factors
- *Physical findings*—Pulse oximetry to identify hypoxia, percussion, auscultation, inspection of facial expression, and work of breathing
- *Laboratory tests*—Arterial blood gas (ABG), complete blood count (CBC), electrolytes
  Diagnostic tests—Chest x-ray, spirometry, pulmonary function test, EKG
- *Dyspnea assessment tools*—Examples are the Respiratory Distress Observation Scale (RDOS), Visual Analogue Scale (VAS), Chronic Respiratory Questionnaire (CRQ), and Cancer Dyspnea Scale (CDS).
- *Other conditions* associated with dyspnea include superior vena cava obstruction, cachexia, ascites, obesity, and anxiety/panic.

Etiology

- *Airflow obstruction and increased mechanical impedance*: Resistance to airflow can be related to obstruction and hyperinflation seen in patients with congestive obstructive pulmonary disease (COPD), pleural effusions, endobronchial lesions, or parenchymal infiltrates. Respiratory muscles that allow chest wall expansion and lung inflation may also not be able to match the input received from mechanical receptors, vagal receptors in the airways and lungs, or extra thoracic receptors in the central nervous system.

- *Increased ventilatory demand:* Causes increased minute ventilation, disruption of physiologic balance, and respiratory muscle dysfunction.
- *Anxiety:* May lead to or amplify dyspnea.
- *Environmental factors:* High altitude is a factor.

Interventions

The CNS must manage both the disease and the symptoms of dyspnea. There is no evidence to support the use of oxygen for feelings of dyspnea. However, if it provides psychologic comfort to the patient or their family, it will not cause harm. See Table 18.4 for management of dyspnea by some common etiologies.

FATIGUE

OVERVIEW

Definition

Fatigue is described as a distressing, persistent, subjective sense of tiredness or exhaustion that is not proportionate to recent activity and interferes with usual functioning including a decreased capacity for physical and mental work. Fatigue is highly subjective and is very much like pain in that it is what the patient says it is. Fatigue is multidimensional and has mental, physical, and emotional components.

Presentation

Fatigue is among the most prevalent and distressing symptoms reported by people living with chronic illness. Common signs and symptoms include feeling weary, sluggish, irritable, and forgetful, as well as having difficulty with concentration and communication. Mental and physical fatigue prevents the individual from participating in activities and relationships, increasing loneliness and isolation (Malik & Sadaf, 2018).

Assessment

Assessment of fatigue is a routine component of the clinical evaluation of patients with serious illness. Patient self-reports and information from family members should be solicited regarding day-to-day functioning and activities of daily living (ADL). A thorough health history, review of systems, and physical examination should be done. Laboratory tests can rule out underlying issues (See Table 18.5). The National Comprehensive Cancer Network (NCCN) Intensity Tool offers an easy and quick assessment of fatigue.

Risk Factors

- Lower socioeconomic status
- Cancer
- Congestive heart failure (CHF)
- COPD
- Renal disease and hemodialysis
- HIV/AIDS
- Multiple sclerosis

Etiology

Fatigue can be a side effect of treatment as well as a biologic effect of disease itself. The pathophysiology of fatigue varies by underlying clinical condition. Fatigue may be acute, chronic, or secondary in nature. Etiology and treatments differ accordingly.

TABLE 18.4 TREATMENT OF DYSPNEA BY SPECIFIC ETIOLOGY

ETIOLOGY	TREATMENT
Chronic obstructive pulmonary disease Asthma Pulmonary fibrosis	Bronchodilators Corticosteroids Opioids
Congestive heart failure with pulmonary edema	Diuretics opioids
Pneumonia	Antibiotics appropriate for pathogenic organism
Superior vena cava syndrome	High-dose corticosteroids Radiotherapy Chemotherapy
Pleural effusion	Thoracentesis
Pericardial effusion	Pericardiocentesis Pericardial window
Ascites	Paracentesis Diuretics Chemotherapy
Lymphangitic carcinomatosis	Corticosteroids Anxiolytics
Obstruction from primary tumor or related	Radiotherapy Stent placement Cryotherapy Laser therapy
Pulmonary embolism	Anticoagulant Oxygen Benzodiazepines
Anemia	Transfusion of packed red blood cells

TABLE 18.5 LABORATORY TESTS FOR DIFFERENTIAL DIAGNOSIS

TEST	RATIONALE
CBC and differential	Rule out anemia and underlying infection.
TSH and T4 levels	Evaluate thyroid function.
Electrolyte level	Evaluate nutritional status; rule out electrolyte imbalance.
BUN and creatinine	Evaluate renal function as a potential factor in fatigue.
LFTs (aspartate aminotransferase, alanine aminotransferase, alkaline phosphatases, and bilirubin)	Rule out liver dysfunction or metastatic disease as a potential cause of fatigue.
Bone scan, CT scan, or other diagnostic imaging tests	Rule out metastatic disease-causing pain that in turn causes fatigue.

BUN, blood urea nitrogen; CBC, complete blood count; LFT, liver function test; TSH, thyroid stimulating hormone.

- *Acute fatigue:* A protective state linked to a single cause in a usually healthy individual; rapid onset and short duration; viewed as normal in a healthy person. Acute fatigue can be alleviated by restorative techniques such as rest, diet, exercise, and stress management.
- *Chronic fatigue:* No known physiologic purpose and can occur without any relationship to exertion or activity; seen in severe deconditioning or limited mobility patients with chronic conditions. It is insidious in onset and persists generally longer than 6 months.
- *Secondary fatigue:* Results from the stress and pathology of chronic disease or cancer whereby body reserves are depleted. Occurs in the advanced stage of chronic disease with concurrent malnutrition, anemia, and cachexia. It is reported in 100% of patients undergoing radiation and in 95% receiving chemotherapy.

Interventions

The optimal intervention for fatigue is prevention. Treat or eliminate causes such as nutritional deficiencies, anemia, pain, emotional distress, and sleep disturbances, thus avoiding the concomitant impacts of these. Focus on eliminating stressors and increasing patient resistance to stressors. Therapy may include modification of drug regimens and correction of metabolic abnormalities. Symptomatic interventions may include exercise, activity and rest modification, cognitive therapies, and nutritional support. See Table 18.6 for pharmacologic therapies.

NAUSEA

OVERVIEW

Definition

Nausea is defined as an unpleasant sensory and emotional experience associated with the feeling of fullness in the epigastric and upper abdominal area with or without a need to vomit (Moorthy & Letizia, 2018). Nausea may be described as a feeling of queasiness, upset stomach, or sour stomach. Nausea has also been described as having a more negative impact on quality of life than vomiting or even pain (Lynch, 2016).

Presentation

Nausea is a very common and distressing symptom encountered by most people at some point in life. It is even more common in patients with advanced illness. Nausea can lead to further complications such as dehydration, electrolyte imbalance, malnutrition, aspiration, and esophageal tears. Persistent nausea can lead to feelings of hopelessness, depression, and social isolation (Lynch, 2016).

Assessment (Measurement Instruments Most Commonly Used)

A detailed health history and physical examination are essential in attempting to uncover the cause of nausea, which will then guide the management of symptoms (Moorthy & Letizia, 2018).

TABLE 18.6 PHARMACOLOGICAL THERAPIES FOR THE TREATMENT OF FATIGUE

CLASS OF DRUG	EXAMPLE	MECHANISM OF ACTION	COMMENTS
Corticosteroids	Dexamethasone 4–8 mg BID	Unclear: Low dosing recommended	Mitigate fatigue in advanced cancer. May mask the signs of acute infections. Effectiveness may be short lived.
Stimulants	Methylphenidate 5–20 mg daily or qam and at noon	Stimulates central nervous system and respiratory centers, increases appetite and energy levels, improves mood, reduces sedations	Treats fatigue related to depression, hypoactive delirium, drowsiness due to opioids. Titrate to effect. Rapid onset of action; fewer side effects than many antidepressants. May cause agitation; risk of toxicity increases with dosage.
Selective serotonin reuptake inhibitors	Paroxetine 20 mg daily	Inhibits serotonin reuptake	Give once daily in the morning, Some SSRIs have longer half-lives and should be used cautiously in the older adult.
Norepinephrine dopamine reuptake inhibitor	Bupropion 100 mg daily for 3 days; then 100 mg TID	Acts as stimulant	
Tricyclic antidepressants	Amitriptyline 10–25 mg PO QHS	Blocks reuptake of various membranes; can improve sleep	Amitriptyline contraindicated in patients with MAOIs or post-MI.
Cholinesterase inhibitors	Donepezil 5 mg PO QHS	Reversible acetylcholinesterase inhibitor	
Erythropoietin	150–300 units/kg SQ TID a week	Increases hemoglobin with effects on energy, activity, and overall quality of life while decreasing transfusion requirements	Monitor H&H. Safety concerns associated with higher mortality rates and not recommended in the treatment of cancer-related fatigue.

H&H, hemoglobin and hematocrit; MAOI, monoamine oxidase inhibitor; MI, myocardial infarction; SQ, subcutaneous; SSRIs, selective serotonin reuptake inhibitors.

Source: From Matzo, M., & Soltani, C. (2015). Fatigue. In M. Matzo, & D. Sherman (Eds.), *Palliative care nursing* (4th ed., pp. 589–625). Springer Publishing Company.

Characteristics of nausea that should be included in the assessment are frequency, duration, severity, and presence of vomiting. Weight change, abdominal distention with or without bowel sounds, tenderness, masses, or fecal impaction are other factors to be assessed.

Nausea assessment tools include patient-reported tools, such as the numeric 0 to 10 rating scales: the Edmonton Symptom Assessment Scale, Visual Analog Scale, Verbal Categorical Scale, or Adapted Symptom Distress Scale (Blush & Larsen, 2015). It is important to remember that nausea is a subjective symptom. Following are the risk factors:

- Female gender
- Younger age
- Anxiety
- Any cancer diagnosis but more prevalent in gynecologic, stomach, and esophageal tumor
- CHF
- COPD
- Upper GI disorders (erosive gastritis, ulcerative esophagitis, and duodenitis)
- AIDS
- Hepatic disease
- Renal disease

- Metabolic derangements (hypercalcemia or fluid and electrolyte imbalances)
- Patients on opioids, antidepressants, cholinesterase inhibitor
- Patients undergoing chemotherapy and/or radiation
- Central nervous system disorders
- End of life

Etiology

The pathology of nausea and vomiting is complex, and the etiology guides the treatment. Nausea is triggered in the vomiting center (VC) in the brainstem, which is responsible for triggering the vomiting reflex. This reflex receives input from four major neural pathways: the chemoreceptor trigger zone, the gastrointestinal system, the vestibular system, and the cerebral cortex. The pathways are activated by the receptor's histamine, acetylcholine, dopamine, and serotonin. Treatment depends upon which pathway and receptor is involved (Figure 18.1).

Interventions

Both pharmacologic and nonpharmacologic interventions should be utilized. The pharmacologic interventions are dependent on the origin of the nausea (see Table 18.7 for all

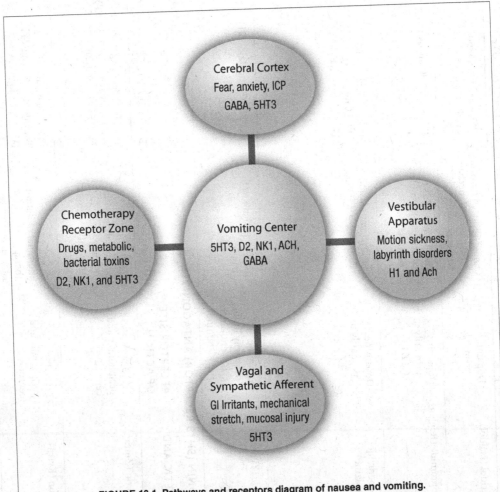

FIGURE 18.1 Pathways and receptors diagram of nausea and vomiting.

ACH, acetylcholine; GABA, gamma-aminobutyric acid; GI, gastrointestinal; 5HT3, 5-hydroxytryptamine; ICP, intracranial pressure; NK1, neurokinin.

TABLE 18.7 PHARMACOLOGIC INTERVENTION OF NAUSEA AND VOMITING BY PATHWAY

DOPAMINE ANTAGONISTS

ANTIEMETIC AND COST	RECEPTOR SITE OF ACTION	INDICATION	DOSAGE/ROUTE	SIDE EFFECTS	COMMENTS
Haloperidol (Haldol) $0.36	Dopamine primarily in the CTZ	Opioid-induced nausea, chemical and mechanical nausea	PO: 0.5–5 mg q4–6h IV: 0.5 mg q3–4h	■ Dystonia ■ Dyskinesia ■ Akathisia	Side effects are low at low doses.
Metoclopramide (Reglan) $0.91	Dopamine-primarily in the CTZ	Gastric stasis Ileus in absences of complete obstruction	PO, IV: 10–30 mg q4–6h	■ Dystonia ■ Akathisia ■ Esophageal spasm ■ Colic in GI tract obstruction	Has prolonged half-life in renal failure.
Prochlorperazine (Compazine) $5.52	Dopamine primarily in the CTZ	Low level nausea and vomiting	PO: 5–25 mg q4–6h PR: 25 mg q6–8h IV: 20–40 mg q4–6h	■ Allergic reaction ■ EPS ■ Headache ■ Dry mouth ■ Hypotension ■ Drowsiness ■ Irritation ■ Anxiety	May cause excessive drowsiness in older adults.
Olanzapine (Zyprexa) $17.47	Dopamine primarily in the CTZ serotonin and histamine	CNIV or patients with cancer	PO: 2.5–10 mg daily BID	■ Sedation ■ Hyperglycemia ■ Reduced seizure threshold ■ Increased serum lipids	Has other beneficial effects such as increased appetite and weight gain.

SEROTONIN (5HT3 RECEPTOR) ANTAGONISTS

ANTIEMETIC AND COST	RECEPTOR SITE OF ACTION	INDICATION	DOSAGE/ROUTE	SIDE EFFECTS
Ondansetron (Zofran) $7.74	5HT3 both peripherally and centrally	CINV Abdominal radiation therapy Postoperative nausea GI irritants	PO/ODT: 8–24 mg in divided doses depending on etiology IV: 0.15 mg/kg q12h	■ Constipation ■ Headache ■ Diarrhea ■ Mild sedation
Granisetron (Kytril) $37.70	5HT3 both peripherally and centrally	CINV Abdominal radiation therapy Postoperative nausea	PO: 1 mg q12h Transdermal: 3.1 mg/24 hr IV: 10 mcg/kg q12h	■ Constipation ■ Headache ■ Diarrhea ■ Mild sedation

(continued)

CLASS	ANTIEMETIC AND COST	RECEPTOR SITE OF ACTION	INDICATION	DOSAGE/ROUTE	SIDE EFFECTS	COMMENTS
Corticosteroid	Dexamethasone $0.64	Possibly reduces release of serotonin or activation of corticosteroid receptors in the central nervous system	■ Cerebral edema ■ Intracranial tumors ■ CINV ■ Bowel obstruction	PO: 2–4 mg q6h IV: 2–4 mg q6h	■ Insomnia ■ Anxiety ■ Euphoria ■ Perirectal burning with IV administration ■ GI upset	Taper to prevent withdrawal effects.
Substance P	Aprepitant (Emend) $154.42	NK1 receptor	■ Acute CINV ■ Delayed CINV	PO: 125 mg 1 hr prior to chemotherapy then 80 mg daily BID and TID		
Anticholinergic	Hyoscine Scopolamine $15.50	Acetylcholine	■ Intestinal obstruction ■ Peritoneal irritation ■ Increased intracranial pressure ■ Excess secretions ■ Motion sickness	Transdermal: 500–1,500 mg q72h	■ Dry mouth ■ Urinary retention ■ Blurred vision ■ Agitation	Useful when nausea and vomiting coexist with colic.
Antihistamine	Cyclizine (Meclizine) $0.69	Histamine	■ Motion sickness ■ ICP ■ Bowel obstruction	PO: 25–50 q8h	■ Sedation ■ Dry mouth ■ Blurred vision	Use is less sedating tthan antihistamines.
Antihistamine	Diphenhydramine (Benadryl) $0.56	Histamine	■ Motion sickness ■ ICP ■ Bowel obstruction	PO/IV: 12.5–50 mg q6–8h	■ Sedation ■ Dry mouth ■ Blurred vision	
Antisecretory	Octreotide (Sandostatin) 50 mg/mL, $110	Somastostatin receptors in brain, pituitary, GI tract	■ Bowel obstruction	SC: 100–150 mg TID	■ Pain at injection site ■ Worsening GI symptoms	Reduces peristalsis and intestinal secretions
Benzodiazepines	Lorazepam (Ativan) $0.33	GABA	■ Anxiety	0.5–1 mg daily TID	■ Sedation ■ Amnesia ■ Delirium ■ Depression	Not FDA approved as an antiemetic.

CINV, chemotherapy-induced nausea and vomiting; CTZ, chemoreceptor trigger zone; EPS, extrapyramidal side effects; FDA, Food and Drug Administration; GABA, gamma-aminobutyric acid; GI, gastrointestinal; ICP, intracranial pressure; NK1, neurokinin; ODT, orally disintegrating tablet; PO, per os; PR, prothrombin ratio.

pharmacologic interventions). Nonpharmacological therapy can be used for all forms of nausea. The most effective have shown to be distraction/relaxation, dietary modifications, and small/slow feedings. Environmental therapies such as strong cooking smells, fragrances, and unpleasant odors should be eliminated when possible. The use of a fan has been shown to be very effective for patients. Some patients have found relief with acupressure, acupuncture, transcutaneous electrical nerve stimulation, and guided imagery.

GRIEF

OVERVIEW

Definition

Grief can be defined as an emotional response to any loss and includes the emotional state and actions of those who experienced the loss. Grief reaction to major loss is often characterized by a period of sorrow, emotional numbness, and even guilt or anger. Grief is a healthy, normal response to perceived loss. There are various forms of grieving depending on loss, culture, and norms. Although grief is not an illness, it can have devastating effects on emotional, mental, and physical health.

- *Anticipatory grief:* Refers to the emotions and feelings before an anticipated loss. This is often exhibited by family members who have watched a loved one with a prolonged, terminal illness.
- *Disenfranchised grief:* Hidden and socially marginalized or unacceptable. This can be someone who has lost someone due to suicide or experienced the death of an ex-spouse or partner.

Presentation

Grief can be understood as the response to an actual or potential loss. Although most known grief is related to a loss of a relationship or the loss of a person, there are many other triggers of grieving. This can be from the loss of safety after going through a traumatic event, loss of an experience, loss of health, or the loss of identity for the future.

Although there is no normal way to grieve, grieving can become maladaptive when the painful emotions are so long-lasting and severe that the affected person is unable to resume their normal daily activities after a prolonged period of time (approximately 6 months). This is called complicated grief or pathologic grief. Signs and symptoms of complicated grieving include difficulty accepting the death, intense yearning for the deceased loved one, focusing on events of the death, feelings of numbness and detachment, withdrawal from social activities, or disproportionate irritability or agitation (Burke et al., 2015; Table 18.8).

Grief does not follow a linear progression but is a unique experience for each individual. Grief ebbs and flows, with periods of intensity remitting with eventual acceptance of the loss and integration. This can be impacted by the individual's culture and personal, historical, and social contexts (Bottomley et al., 2015).

Assessment

There are a variety of screening instruments to identify individuals who may need a higher level of service or a mental health referral. The Inventory of Complicated Grief (ICG) measures symptoms along four domains: separation, cognitive/emotional, social impairment, and duration; it differentiates complicated

TABLE 18.8 SYMPTOMS OF GRIEF

CATEGORY	SYMPTOMS
Feelings	<ul><li>Sadness</li><li>Anger</li><li>Guilt</li><li>Anxiety</li><li>Fatigue</li><li>Helplessness</li><li>Loneliness</li><li>Shock</li><li>Relief</li><li>Numbness</li><li>Irritability</li><li>Identity Issues</li><li>Jealousy</li><li>Idealization</li></ul>
Physical symptoms	<ul><li>Tightness in the chest</li><li>Tightness in the throat</li><li>Hollow stomach</li><li>Increased sensitivity to noise</li><li>Low energy</li><li>Dry mouth</li><li>Breathlessness</li><li>Sense of unreality</li><li>Muscular weakness</li><li>Malaise or persistent fatigue</li></ul>
Thoughts	<ul><li>Preoccupation with the loss</li><li>Disbelief</li><li>Confusion</li><li>Hallucinations (visual or auditory)</li></ul>
Behaviors	<ul><li>Sleep disturbance</li><li>Absentmindedness</li><li>Withdrawal</li><li>Changes in appetite</li><li>Restlessness</li><li>Crying</li></ul>

grief from normal grief. The Brief Grief Questionnaire assesses risk for complicated grief (Guldin, 2014).

Risk Factors

Certain populations are at higher risk for grief and complicated grief (Hurley & Archer-Nanda, 2016):

- Loss of a loved one from a complicated relationship
- Suffering multiple significant losses or unresolved past losses
- History of mood or anxiety disorders
- Losing someone to a violent death
- Losing someone to an unexpected death
- Losing someone to suicide
- Loss of a child
- Loss of significant other
- Missing person/absence of a body
- Notoriety/news coverage
- Shock of discovery
- Poor health
- Poor social support
- Lower socioeconomic status

Interventions

- Interdisciplinary death preparation
- Life review
- Bereavement support
- Referral to mental health services
- Counsel and support patients and families
- Establish a safe plan of care
- Education on what is to be expected
- Decrease caregiver stress
- Use of advance directives
- Referral to chaplain
- Referral to social worker
- Involve palliative care specialists
- Encourage self-care

REVIEW QUESTIONS

1. All of the following medications are recommended as standard pharmacologic therapy of nausea in patients with serious illnesses except:
   A. ABHR (lorazepam, diphenhydramine, haloperidol, metoclopramide) gel
   B. Prochlorperazine
   C. Haloperidol
   D. Lorazepam

2. Which of the following treatments represents a multimodal approach to acute pain?
   A. IV opioids initially and then transitioning to oral opioids.
   B. Opioids, nonopioid pain relievers, adjuvant medications including nerve blocks, and nonpharmacologic interventions.
   C. Nonopioid pain relievers and nonpharmacologic interventions.
   D. Physical therapy and self-hypnosis.

ANSWERS

1. **Correct answer: A**. **Rationale:** Prochlorperazine is often used as a first-line therapy for nausea and acts both at the chemoreceptor trigger zone (CTZ) and at the vomiting center (VC). Haloperidol is often used a second-line agent and works at the cerebral cortex and CTZ. Lorazepam primarily works at the level of cerebral cortex with the GABA receptor. Although ABHR gel is sometimes used at end of life, it is not a first or second line and should only be used when all other methods are exhausted.

2. **Correct answer: B**. **Rationale:** The multimodal approach is represented by the combination of opioid and nonopioid medications along with nerve blocks (addressing multiple pain pathways) used together with nonpharmacologic interventions. The multimodal approach to acute pain must address multiple pain pathways and include nonpharmacologic interventions.

REFERENCES

The complete reference and additional reading lists appear in the digital version of this chapter, at https://connect.springerpub.com/content/book/978-0-8261-7417-8/part/part02/chapter/ch18

Care of the Older Adult

Erica Newkirk, Monica D. Coles, Jessica Green, JoEllen Rust, K. Denise Kerley, Mary H. Fischer, and Amy C. Shay

ABUSE AND NEGLECT

OVERVIEW

One in 10 older adults suffers some form of abuse worldwide on a monthly basis (Beach et al., 2016; Center for Medicare and Medicaid Services [CMMS], 2013). The ratio of reported elder abuse is 1:24. Elder abuse is a form of mistreatment and can occur in any relationship where there is a purported element of trust (CMMS, 2013).

Elder abuse involves one of two concepts:

- Either an act was committed (abuse) or omitted (neglect) and can be classified as either intended or unintended, a single act or repetitive acts.
  Abuse of older adults is inclusive of psychological/emotional, physical and sexual abuse, neglect of basic needs (passive or self), and financial exploitation.
- Offenders who commit these acts of abuse can be children, other family members, and spouses, as well as nursing facility staff (Beach et al., 2016; CMMS, 2013).
- There is a 300% higher risk of death in older adults subjected to any form of abuse.

It is important for the clinical nurse specialist (CNS) to recognize elder abuse, neglect, and exploitation. The CNS must also understand the effects abuse has on older adults and be aware of what and where to report suspicions of abuse.

Theories

Multiple theories address vulnerability of elders and the reasons for elder abuse (Momtaz et al., 2013; Table 19.1).

Recognizing Abuse in Older Adults

Abuse can manifest in unexpected behavioral or obvious physical changes that would indicate to observers that something is not right (Beach et al., 2016).

Behaviors exhibited by someone subjected to abuse can include the following:

- Fear of one or many person(s)
- Irritability
- Depression and anxiety
- Lack of interest
- Change in sleep habits

TABLE 19.1 SUMMARY OF ELDER ABUSE THEORIES

THEORY NAME	KEY COMPONENT	DESCRIPTORS
Feminist theory	Man as head of household	Abuse is a product of a family whereby the male dominates as the head and the female has no authority.
Political economic theory	Dependency	Older adults may no longer work and independence has changed.
Psychopathology of the caregiver theory	Caregiver behaviors	Behavioral features of the abuser are contributing factors in the abuse.
Role accumulation theory	Environmental stressors	Domestic supporters are not able to distinguish their responsibilities and do not manage their stress effectively. Abuse may manifest as a coping mechanism.
Situational theory	Caregiver stressors	Caregivers who are overloaded often cannot cope with the demands of caring for others, which can foster an avenue for abuse.
Social exchange theory	Costs and rewards	Role reversal; the older adult and the caregiver have increased demands on each other.
Social learning theory	Learned behavior	Violence can pass through generations.
Stratification theory	Caregiver stressors	Caregivers who are not satisfied with their employment or who are poorly educated can become abusers.
Symbolic interactionism theory	Cultural beliefs	Behaviors deemed abusive by cultural tenets and beliefs.

Source: Adapted from Momtaz, Y. A., Hamid, T. A., & Ibrahim, R. (2013). Theories and measures of elder abuse. *Psychogeriatrics, 13*(3), 182–188. https://doi.org/10.1111/psyg.12009

The complete reference and additional reading lists appear in the digital version of this chapter, at https://connect.springerpub.com/content/book/978-0-8261-7417-8/part/part02/chapter/ch19

- Change in eating habits
- Suicidal ideations
- Panic attacks
- Crying outburst
- Rigidity
- Feelings of helplessness, hopelessness, or sadness
- Statements are contradictory in the absence of confusion
- Unwillingness to speak openly
- Avoids contact—Eye, physical, or other
- Allows others to answer for them

Risk Factors

Experienced advocates identify influences linked to abuse and that the presence of one or more of these influences puts a person in jeopardy of abuse incidents (Beach et al., 2016).

- Significant risk factors for abuse include caregiver stress, dependence, family conflict, seclusion, psychologic problems, and addictive mannerisms.

Caregiver Stress

When a person is frail or has disabilities, becoming a primary caregiver can be stressful. In numerous instances, other causative aspects are present and together can be the prompt for abuse (Beach et al., 2016; CMMS, 2013). Contributing factors for development of an abusive affiliation are as follows:

- Financial problems
- Lack of other sources of care or relief
- Poor support systems
- The cost, both physical and emotional, of caring for someone else
- Personal stress: "the sandwich effect"
- Ill prepared to assume the role of being a caregiver to an older parent/grandparent

Dependency

- A relationship that involves one being dependent on another for care puts an elder at risk for abuse (Beach et al., 2016; CMMS, 2013).
- Physical deficits such as frailty, disability, or cognitive impairments such as dementia can be contributing factors for abuse.
- These are also reasons that make it difficult for the abused to report abuse or leave abusive situations (Liu et al., 2017; Pillemer et al., 2016).
  - Offenders are often themselves dependent on the person for whom they care in order to meet their own physical, psychologic, social, emotional, or financial needs and might have feelings of confinement or helplessness and commit abuse out of distress or frustration.

Family Conflict

- Abuse can emerge from a domestic or family violence situation that has now manifested into a caregiver situation, that is, a child formerly abused may now be providing primary care and the cycle of abuse continues (Liu et al., 2017; Pillemer et al., 2016; Schmeidel et al., 2012).
- Violence enacted in some families is a normal stress reaction and may become generational. More than one generation cohabitating together adds to this risk and conflict presents.
- Cross-cultural situations also place dependent persons at risk for abuse.

Isolation

- The caregiver may be secluded and have nonexistent social interaction or support. In this instance, abuse may manifest in the following ways:
  - Misappropriation of funds, valuables, or property
  - Changes to wills or other legal documents are forced or obtained improperly from those without decision-making capacity
  - Denying one access to their personal finances while they remain capable of maintaining them
  - Forging of signatures
  - Abusing power of attorney
  - Keeping the change from shopping
  - Physical, social, and emotional isolation

Medical/Psychologic Conditions

- In the case of physical and psychologic abuse, compromised mental health of the perpetrator is the contributing element (CMMS, 2013; Liu et al., 2017).
- Abuse in these situations relates to mental illness, difficulty in controlling anger, and/or frustrations and low self-regard or feelings of low self-confidence.
- Older persons who suffer from cognitive decline may also be at risk especially in the presence of aggressive behaviors.

Addictive Behaviors

- Caregivers or family members who have a substance abuse dependency, both prescription and illicit, alcohol, or a gambling problem, are at risk for being abusers (Tables 19.2 and 19.3; Figures 19.1 and 19.2).

Prevention

Tips to share with older people to help them keep themselves safe (Pillemer et al., 2016) are the following:

- Remain active in the community and maintain a support network friends, neighbors, and family.
- Maintain contact with healthcare workers/medical practitioners.
- Query nonfamilial others when making any changes to your financial or living arrangements.
- Never make legal or financial decisions or sign documents until you have all the required information.
- Keep a list of important numbers by your bed.
- Seek assistance the first time abuse occurs.

Assistance

- Adult Protective Services (APS, n.d.; Ernst et al., 2013; National Adult Protective Services Association [NAPSA], 2012) is a social services program provided by state and local governments nationwide.
- This department provides assistance to seniors and adults with disabilities.
- APS workers frequently serve as first responders in cases of abuse, neglect, or exploitation and work closely with professionals such as physicians, nurses, paramedics, firefighters, and law enforcement officers.
- If one suspects that an older adult is in immediate, life-threatening danger, that person should call 911 and the local APS office. Most states have mandatory reporting statutes for elder abuse. Many professionals are required to report suspected mistreatment, and some states require that all citizens report suspected abuse. A call to APS is not made to get someone in trouble; it is to get someone help.
- Approximately 2 million adult Americans 65 years of age or older are victimized by some form of elder abuse annually (Acierno et al., 2010). Nearly 85% of cases go unreported to the APS.
  - Underreporting is likely though as it relates to the differences in guidelines that govern reporting as well as the definition of elder abuse being unclear.

TABLE 19.2 TYPES OF ELDER ABUSE

	PSYCHOLOGIC	PHYSICAL	SEXUAL	FINANCIAL	NEGLECT
Definition	Mental distress that originates from using actions that incite fear through violence, seclusion, or deprivation, as well as provoking feelings of shame, indignity, or powerlessness Verbal or nonverbal	Physical abuse is the infliction of physical pain or injury and could include coercion or physical/drug-induced restraint	Sexual abuse is any sexual contact that is nonconsensual with an older person	Financial abuse involves improperly and illegally misusing a person's finances or property without their permission	Failure to provide an older adult with life's necessities, including but not limited to food, clothing, shelter, medical care, therapeutic devices, or other physical assistance and exposing that person to the risk of physical, mental, or emotional harm Intentional or unintentional
Signs	Loss of interest in self or milieu Uncertainty toward family member or caregiver Apathetic Fear Fails to make eye contact with practitioner, caregiver, or others Nervousness around caregivers or others Reluctance to talk openly/deferral of questions to caregiver or abuser Helplessness Withdrawal Depression/anxiety Insomnia/sleep deprivation Paranoid behavior or confusion	Discrepancies between injury and history Facial swelling or missing teeth Burns Seen by different doctors or hospitals Unexplained accidents or injuries Bruising/abrasions/lacerations or fractures Conflicting stories between client and caregivers or family members Depression	Difficult to recognize as humiliation and indignity may prevent the victim from talking about it Bruising/abrasions, lacerations around the breasts, ano-genital, or abdominal areas, or inner thighs Unexplained venereal disease or genital infections, especially if the person resides in a nursing home Underclothing that is torn, stained, or bloody Presence of sperm in the vagina or anus Vaginal bleeding not associated with menses	Disinclination to make a will Unable to locate personal property or financial material Unmatched fund transfers Improperly obtained power of attorney Bills not paid when money entrusted to a third party Sudden inability to pay bills, rent, buy food, obtain medication, or participate in social activities Unexplained withdrawal from bank accounts Noncompliance with medication regimen Malnutrition and/or weight loss without a related medical condition	Live in squalor and may be hoarders May exhibit malnutrition, anorexia, weight loss, cachexia, and dehydration because of not having adequate food sources Isolation Physical needs, such as decaying teeth or overgrown nails, are unmet Clothing does not match the season or may be in ill repair The older person may be unclean and have a strong smell of urine or have lice Incontinence-associated dermatitis or pressure injury development is possible
Examples	Verbal bullying, shaming, and harassing through name calling, degrading in a public or private place, treating them like a child Threatening physical harm	Hitting, slapping, pushing, punching, kicking, beating, biting, scratching, shaking, grabbing forcefully, arm twisting, dragging, or burning	Touching, fondling, intercourse, sodomy, coerced nudity, and explicitly sexual photography Rape	Improper use of property, money, or valuables Forcing changes to wills or other legal documents, that is, obtaining a power of attorney from an older person who does not have decision-making capacity	Abandonment, improper/misuse of medication, that is, to induce sleep so that the caregiver can leave the older person alone; poor hygiene; or refusing to allow others to provide care

(continued)

TABLE 19.2 TYPES OF ELDER ABUSE (continued)

	PSYCHOLOGIC	PHYSICAL	SEXUAL	FINANCIAL	NEGLECT
	Threatening to institutionalize Withholding affection Denying access to grandchildren Elimination of decision-making powers	Physical restraint such as tying the person in a chair, putting them in a chair they cannot get out of, or locking the person in a room	Sexual harassment—improper remarks	Denying an older person the right to make financial decisions when they are capable of doing so Falsified signatures	Older person who refuses or fails to provide themselves with adequate food, water, clothing, shelter, personal hygiene, medication, and safety precautions

Sources: Acierno, R., Hernandez, M. A., Amstadter, A. B., Resnick, H. S., Steve, K., Muzzy, W., & Kilpatrick, D. G. (2010). Prevalence and correlates of emotional, physical, sexual, and financial abuse and potential neglect in the United States: The National Elder Mistreatment Study. *American Journal of Public Health, 100*(2), 292–297. https://doi.org/10.2105/AJPH.2009.163089; Centers for Disease Control and Prevention. (2015). *Elder abuse: Definitions.* CDC; Fulmer, T., Rodgers, R., & Pelger, A. (2014). Verbal mistreatment in the elderly. *Journal of Elder Abuse and Neglect, 26*(4), 351–364. https://doi-doi.org/10.1080/08946566.2013.801817; New York County District Attorney/NAPSA Elder Financial Exploitation Advisory Board. (2013). *Nationwide survey of mandatory reporting requirements for elderly and/or vulnerable persons.* http://www.napsa-now.org/wp-content/uploads/2012/04/Mandatory-Reporting-Chart.pdf; Liu, P.-J., Conrad, K. J., Beach, S. R., Iris, M., & Schiamberg, L. B. (2017). The importance of investigating abuser characteristics in elder emotional/psychological abuse: Results from adult protective services data. *Journals of Gerontology, Series B, Psychological Sciences and Social Sciences, 74*(5), 897–907. https://doi.org/10.1093/geronb/gbx064

TABLE 19.3 ELDER ABUSE SCREENING TOOLS

TOOL	DESCRIPTION
BASE	Assists practitioners to assess the probability of abuse.
EASI	Raises suspicion about elder abuse to a level that may mandate reporting.
H-S/EAST	Identifies those at high risk for the need for protective services.
Questions to Elicit Elder Abuse	Specific questions constructed to determine if abuse is occurring: Physical/sexual abuse: 1. Do you feel safe at home? 2. Has anyone hit, slapped, or kicked you? 3. Has anyone tied you down or locked you in a room? 4. Has anyone touched you in your private areas without your permission? Emotional abuse: 1. Do you ever feel alone? 2. Has anyone threatened you with punishment, deprivation, or institutionalization? 3. Have you received the "silent treatment"? 4. Has anyone ever fed you forcefully? 5. What happens when you and your caregiver disagree? Neglect: 1. Do you lack aids such as eyeglasses, hearing aids, mobility devices, or false teeth? 2. Have you been left alone for long periods of time? 3. If you need assistance, how do you obtain it? 4. How do you get help? 5. How many meals do you get each day? 6. How do you use the bathroom? Financial abuse: 1. Does your caregiver depend on you for shelter or financial support? 2. Has anyone stolen money from you? 3. Are you able to get your medication?

(continued)

TABLE 19.3 ELDER ABUSE SCREENING TOOLS (*continued*)

TOOL	DESCRIPTION
Screen for various types of abuse or neglect	General questions to screen an older person for various types of abuse or neglect: 1. Have you ever been hurt by anyone in your home? 2. Has anyone ever touched you without your consent? 3. Has anyone ever made you do things against your will? 4. Has anyone taken anything that was yours without asking? 5. Have you ever been scolded or threatened? 6. Have you ever signed any documents that you did not understand? 7. Are you afraid of anyone at home? 8. Are you alone a lot? 9. Has anyone ever failed to help you take care of yourself when you needed help?
Suspected Abuse Tool (Bass et al., 2001)	Assists with recognition of common signs or symptoms of abuse

BASE, Brief Abuse Screen for the Elderly; EASI, Elder Abuse Suspicion Index; H-S/EAST, Hwalek-Sengstock Elder Abuse Screening Test.

Note: Screening tools are available at https://medicine.uiowa.edu/familymedicine/research/research-projects/elder-mistreatment-elder-abuse/em-screening-instruments

Sources: Bass, D. M., Anetzberger, G. J., Ejaz, F. K., & Nagpaul, K. (2001). Screening tools and referral protocol for stopping abuse against older Ohioans: A guide for service providers. *Journal of Elder Abuse and Neglect, 13*(2), 23–38. https://doi.org/10.1300/J084v13n02_03; Centers for Disease Control and Prevention. (2015). *Elder abuse: Definitions.* CDC; Yaffe, M. J., Wolfson, C., Lithwick, M., & Weiss, D. (2008). Development and validation of a tool to improve physician identification of elder abuse: The Elder Abuse Suspicion Index (EASI). *Journal of Elder Abuse and Neglect, 20*(3), 276–300. https://doi.org/10.1080/08946560801973168

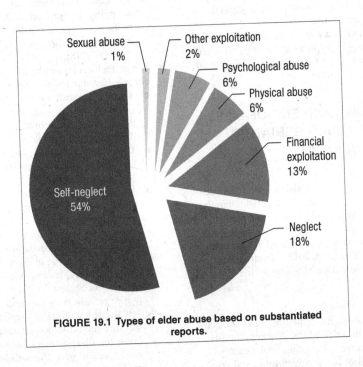

FIGURE 19.1 Types of elder abuse based on substantiated reports.

- Reasons that healthcare professionals are reluctant to report abuse even though they are mandated reporters include (Schmeidel et al., 2012) the following:
  - Worried about making the situation worse for the patient
  - Patient and/or family denies mistreatment
  - Lacks understanding of reporting procedure—who to call?
  - Lacks awareness of signs/symptoms of elder abuse
  - Patient and/or family loyalty
  - Patients may refuse what they feel is interference, thereby leaving the healthcare professional thinking that to report is useless
  - Fear of damaging relationship with patient and/or family

Tips for Reporting Elder Abuse

- Spend some time alone with your patient; this might be the only chance to discuss freely concerns/issues/fears about their current living arrangements, their safety, or their financial security.

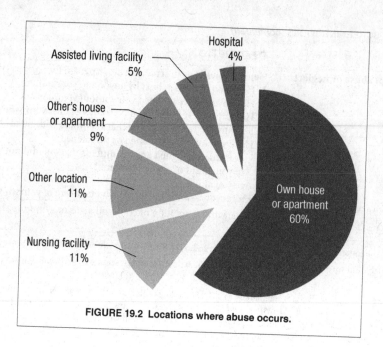

FIGURE 19.2 Locations where abuse occurs.

- Be alert to cultural differences, which could impede a patient's willingness to disclose issues about a caretaker's behaviors that might suggest abuse.
- Know the laws in your state that relate to reporting.
- Remember, it is not up to you to prove abuse. It is, however, up to you to protect your patient and report suspicions of elder abuse (Schmeidel et al., 2012).

HEALING, COMFORT, AND END-OF-LIFE CARE FOR THE ADULT–GERIATRIC POPULATION

OVERVIEW

The assessment and treatment of the geriatric patient is specialized and must be thorough, including the patient, family, and caregivers. When performing a geriatric assessment, it is very important to gather data not only from the patient and diagnostic tests but also from family and support systems connected to the patient (Ward & Reuben, 2018). Treatment goals should be directed toward the patient's quality of life (QOL) and wishes.

Geriatric Assessment

Geriatric conditions are common and frequently unrecognized or not addressed adequately in older adults. A comprehensive geriatric assessment identifies medical, psychosocial, functional, spiritual, financial, social, end-of-life and environmental components that influence an older adult's health.

- Patients over the age of 65 have a much higher risk of falling.
  - A fall can lead to losing independence.
  - Patients should have a fall risk assessment integrated into their history and physical examination (Hartford Institute for Geriatric Nursing [HIGN], n.d.).
- Functional status is the ability to perform activities necessarily for daily life.
  - The Katz' Activities of Daily Living Scale includes self-care tasks like bathing, dressing, toileting, maintaining continents, grooming, and feeding.

- The Lawton Instrumental Activities of Daily Living are shopping for groceries, driving, using the telephone, housework, home repairs, preparing meals, doing laundry, taking medications, and handling finances (Ward & Reuben, 2018).
- Dementia increases with age especially in those over 85 years old (see Chapter 15 for more information).
  - There are many tools used to evaluate cognitive function and if these tools raise suspicion for any cognitive impairment, additional evaluation is needed, such as neuro-psychologic testing, bloodwork, or imaging.
  - Tools used to evaluate cognitive function are the Clock Drawing Test, Mini-Mental Status Examination (MMSE), and the Mini-Cog.
  - All hospitalized geriatric patients have a high risk for delirium, especially if they have dementia.
- Geriatric patients should be screened for depression.
  - Depression is underdiagnosed and inadequately treated in the older adult population.
  - Examples of tools available to help with this screening are Patient Health Questionnaire-9 (PHQ-9) and The Geriatric Depression Scale (HIGN, n.d.; Ward & Reuben, 2018). Screen caregivers for depression or caregiver burnout.
- Review the older adult's medication list at each visit as many patients are subject to polypharmacy.
  - Look for discrepancies between what the medical record says and what the patient actually states when they are taking.
  - When possible, ask to see the medications.
  - Older adults are at risk for adverse drug reactions and side effects from medications they may be taking.
  - Check the BEERS Criteria for possible medication contraindications (American Geriatrics Society 2015 Beers Criteria Update Expert Panel [AGSBCUEP], 2015).
- It is important to discuss the goals of care with the geriatric patient. Discuss what outcomes are important for them and their families, advanced care preferences, decision-makers, durable power of attorney, and healthcare representatives (Ward & Reuben, 2018).

Age-Related Changes
- Age-related changes are more prominent after age 85 (Table 19.4).
- *Frail elderly* is a term used to identify older adults.

GERIATRIC SYNDROMES

OVERVIEW
Geriatric syndromes are common conditions that typically reflect the loss of the older adult's physiologic reserve and are brought on by the aging process and comorbidities (Khan & Boustani, 2014).
- The classification of geriatric syndromes includes three syndromes: delirium, dementia/cognitive decline, and gait/mobility issues (Health in Aging Foundation [HAF], 2017; Khan & Boustani, 2014; O'Hara, 2013).
- Some additional syndromes include urinary incontinence, frailty, sleep problems, and skin breakdown (HAF, 2017; O'Hara, 2013; Sloane et al., 2014).

DELIRIUM AND DEMENTIA
Dementia/Cognitive Impairment
Dementia is an umbrella term that reflects the various cognitive disorders such as Alzheimer's disease, vascular dementia, frontotemporal dementia, Lewy body dementia, and Parkinson's dementia (Khandelwal & Kaufer, 2014). For more information refer to Chapter 15.

Delirium
Delirium symptoms include acute change in consciousness, fluctuating course, attention and memory impairment, sleep disturbances, and psychomotor activity changes (Khan & Boustani, 2014):
- *Hyperactive:* Aggressive, restless, hallucinations
- *Hypoactive:* Lethargic, flat affect
- *Mixed:* Demonstrates varying behaviors throughout the day

If delirium is not recognized and treated, it can lead to increased mortality, a decline in functional status, an increase in hospital-acquired complications, an increase in length of stay, and higher healthcare costs (Khan & Boustani, 2014).
- Prevention and an interdisciplinary approach are the best interventions to minimize the chance of developing delirium (Khan & Boustani, 2014).

FALLS/GAIT INSTABILITY
Difficulty with ambulation and mobility are common complaints with the older adult population (Alexander, 2014). As impairments progress, debilitation and falls may occur.

TABLE 19.4 REVIEW OF SYSTEMS AND AGE-RELATED CHANGES

SYSTEM	OVERVIEW	AGE-RELATED CHANGES
Integumentary (Heitkemper, 2004)	As the body ages, there is a decrease in the water content and a loss of subcutaneous fat. The epidermis loses elasticity. This causes the first layer of skin to heal more slowly, increasing the risk for skin tears, bruising, and the skin to be a less effective barrier to microorganisms.	■ Sweat glands decrease ■ Cells turn over slower ■ Sebaceous gland activity decreased ■ Sensory receptors decreased
Immune (Heitkemper, 2004; HIGN, n.d.)	Immune function decreases and patients are more susceptible to infections. Signs and symptoms of infections manifest atypically in the older adult. Watch for subtle signs like mental status changes, incontinence, falls, and decreased appetite.	■ Malignancy incidence increases ■ Follow the CDC recommendations for vaccines
Musculoskeletal (Heitkemper, 2004; HIGN, n.d.)	As the adult ages, lean body mass is replaced with fat and there is reduced muscle strength and slowed motor skills. Sarcopenia is a decline in muscle mass and strength associated with aging.	■ Slowed cognitive processing ■ Intervertebral desk narrowed ■ Muscle fibers atrophy ■ Flexions of joints increase ■ Calcium deposits increase ■ Range of motion is limited ■ Osteoarthritis ■ Increased risk for fractures
Gastrointestinal (Heitkemper, 2004; HIGN, n.d.)	The older adult has a decrease in taste, thirst perception, gastric emptying, and mobility. There is a risk for decreased nutrition from chewing impairment from dental changes, malabsorption, and vitamin deficiencies.	■ Taste threshold for salt and sugar increases ■ Motility decreases ■ Lipase production decreases ■ Constipation increases
Respiratory (Heitkemper, 2004; HIGN, n.d.; Taffet, 2017)	The older adult has a stiffer chest wall and reduced pulmonary functional reserve. Ciliary and macrophage activity decrease, which can cause decreased cough and clearance of foreign substance in the lungs.	■ Increased likelihood of hypoxia ■ Respiratory muscles atrophy ■ Alveoli decreases ■ Elastic recoil decreases
Cardiovascular (Heitkemper, 2004; Taffet, 2017)	The older adult has an increased risk for hypertension and coronary artery disease.	■ Increased the risk for hypertension and coronary artery disease ■ Force of contraction decreased ■ Heart muscle decrease ■ Mitral valve stretching

(continued)

TABLE 19.4 REVIEW OF SYSTEMS AND AGE RELATED CHANGES (continued)

SYSTEM	OVERVIEW	AGE-RELATED CHANGES
Neurologic (Heitkemper, 2004)	Older adults will have a loss in neurons in the cerebellum and cerebral.	<ul><li>Increased risk for sleep disorders, delirium, and dementia</li><li>Loss of neurons in the brain and spinal cord</li><li>Brain size decreases</li><li>Major neurotransmitters decreased</li><li>Reaction time increases</li><li>Response times slow</li><li>Potential for altered balance</li><li>Syncope</li><li>Postural hypertension increases</li><li>Sensory input decreases</li></ul>
Genitourinary (Heitkemper, 2004; HIGN, n.d.; Taffet, 2017)	The genitourinary system increases the older person's risk for urinary incontinence, urinary tract infection, erectile dysfunction, and dyspareunia.	<ul><li>Globular filtration rate decreased</li><li>Sphincter control decreased</li><li>Reduced drug clearance</li><li>Reduced bladder elasticity and muscle tone</li><li>Males have an increased risk of prostate enlargement</li></ul>
Visual (Heitkemper, 2004)	The older adult has structural changes in the eye: atrophy, relaxed eyelids, and cornea sensitivity.	<ul><li>Dry eyes</li><li>Tear production decreases</li><li>Elasticity of eye muscles decreases</li><li>Presbyopia</li><li>Peripheral vision decreases</li><li>Incidence of cataracts increase</li></ul>
Auditory (Heitkemper, 2004)	The older adult will experience decrease in high-frequency hearing (presbycusis) and cerumen impaction.	<ul><li>Sensitivities to high tones decreases</li><li>Understanding of speech decreases</li><li>Equilibrium and balance deficits</li><li>Potential conductive hearing loss</li></ul>

CDC, Centers for Disease Control and Prevention.

- *Falls* are defined as any unplanned decent to the ground or any lower surface, which was not caused by loss of consciousness (Reuben et al., 2017).
- Falls can lead to substantial morbidity and mortality and continue to contribute to the gait instability issues, leading to immobility (Rubenstein & Dillard, 2014). As reported by Alexander (2014), some common causes leading to gait impairment and subsequent falls include the following:
  - Cardiopulmonary disease
  - Musculoskeletal disease
  - Impaired strength
  - Reduced vision
  - Impaired balance
  - Sedentary lifestyle
  - Previous falls and a fear of falling again
  - Medications
  - Cognitive impairment
  - Malnutrition

Assessment

- A thorough history, including performance-based assessment, should be obtained. A common performance-based assessment is the Timed Up and Go test (also known as the *Get Up and Go test*).
  - The test requires the adult to get up from a chair with armrests, walk 3 meters, turn around and walk back to the chair, and sit down.
  - A baseline score of 14 seconds or higher is the threshold for identifying an adult at risk for falls; new evidence has questioned that time, but the test's validity remains.

Other tests include the Performance-Oriented Mobility Assessment, the Short Physical Performance Battery, and the 6-minute walk (Alexander, 2014).

- Management of gait instability and falls varies based on the etiology. Alexander (2014) identifies some possible interventions to help minimize progression:
  - Treatmedication side effects
  - Replace vitamin deficiencies
  - Physical therapy, strength training
  - Walking
  - Behavioral and environmental modifications (improved lighting and removal of clutter)
  - Appropriate/well-fitting shoes, assistive devices (cane, walker)
  - Surgery (orthopedic replacements)

URINARY INCONTINENCE

Reuben et al. (2017) defines *urinary incontinence* as any involuntary leakage from the bladder, which is linked to multiple causes.

- Etiologies include lower urinary tract defect, inability to cognitively control voiding, comorbidities, and anatomical changes resulting in impairment.
- Three common types of urinary incontinence include
  - Stress (increased pressure),

- Urgency (sudden need to void), and
- Mixed (both urgency with an increased pressure) (Reuben et al., 2017).

FRAILTY

A basic definition of *frailty* includes an increased susceptibility to developing complications after exposure to a stressful event (Old & Woolley, 2014; Reuben et al., 2017).

- A frailty model has been developed to help guide in the defining process.
- Three or more of the identified symptoms must be present to formally classify as frailty. These symptoms include (Old & Woolley, 2014)
  - Unintentional weight loss,
  - Exhaustion,
  - Weakness or low physical activity,
  - Decreased walking speed,
  - Changes in cognition,
  - Changes in mood, and
  - The experience of pain.

FAILURE TO THRIVE

Not considered a geriatric syndrome, failure to thrive is a state of decline that is multifactorial and is caused by chronic conditions and functional impairments (Robertson & Montagnini, 2004).

- If frailty is identified and is exacerbated by other comorbidities and complications, failure to thrive should be something a CNS should consider.
- Common manifestations that present in failure to thrive present with frailty as well. Four prominent symptoms include (Robertson & Montagnini, 2004)
  - Weight loss,
  - Decreased appetite,
  - Poor nutrition, and
  - Inactivity.

SLEEP PROBLEMS

Older adults report more nighttime insomnia, daytime sleepiness, sleep apnea, and restless leg syndrome than the younger adult population (Martin & Alessi, 2014). Refer to Chapter 20 for a more in-depth review.

- Physiologic changes that cause sleep disturbances include (Martin & Alessi, 2014)
  - Changes in the circadian rhythm (shift to earlier),
  - Changes in upper airway (more fatty tissue and reduced muscle tone),
  - Musculoskeletal (arthritis, chronic pain),
  - Genitourinary (nocturia), and
  - Menopause.

SKIN BREAKDOWN/PRESSURE INJURY

- Changes to the older adults' skin make it more susceptible to skin breakdown.
- The skin in older adults is less tolerant to pressure or shear. It can also be adversely affected by microclimate, nutrition, repositioning and mobility, comorbidities, and the patients' baseline skin condition (National Pressure Ulcer Advisory Panel [NPUAP], 2016).
- Aggressive, 24/7, preventive efforts need to be implemented to reduce the development skin breakdown (Garcia & White-Chu, 2014). For more information see Chapter 12.

FUNCTIONAL ASSESSMENT OF OLDER ADULTS

OVERVIEW

Functional status refers to a person's ability to perform tasks that are required for living.

The **adult or geriatric functional assessment** begins with a review of the two key divisions of functional ability: activities of daily living (ADL) and instrumental activities of dailly living (IADL; Table 19.5).

- Assessment is made by simple observation of tasks performed and provides significant information on function. IADL are required to live independently. Functional status may be affected by impairment in speech and/or hearing, along with motor function.
- Assessment tools that are available to determine functional ability include the Katz Index of Independence in ADL, Lawton IADL Scale, and Cleveland Scale for Activities of Daily Living (CSADL; Miller, 2012).

NEUROLOGICALLY BASED COMMUNICATION DISORDERS

Speech
- **The left hemisphere** is known as the *hemisphere of language function* (phonology, syntax, and simple level semantics).
  - The **right hemisphere** is primarily responsible for complex linguistic processing and the nonverbal, emotional aspects of communication.
- **Speech disorders**
  - *Motor speech disorders*
    - *Dysarthria:* Motor speech disorder resulting from muscle impairment.
    - *Apraxia:* Motor speech disorder resulting from neurologic damage; normal muscle tone and coordination present but brain prevents completion of precise, purposeful muscle movement.
    - *Aphasia:* Loss of language function due to brain injury in the area associated with the comprehension and production of language, most often caused by a stroke or cerebral vascular accident (CVA).
      - *Expressive aphasia (Broca's aphasia)*—Can understand but unable to express or verbalize
      - *Receptive aphasia*—Difficulty understanding written and spoken communication

TABLE 19.5 DESCRIPTION OF FUNCTIONAL ABILITIES

FUNCTIONAL ABILITY	DESCRIPTION
ADL	Eating, dressing, bathing, ambulation, transfers, toileting, controlling bowel and bladder functions
IADL	Doing housework, preparing meals, medication administration, financial management, using a telephone

ADL, activities of daily living; IADL, instrumental activities of daily living.

- Characteristic behavior and communication deficits of aphasia:
  - Impaired auditory comprehension
  - Impaired verbal expression
  - Presence of paraphasias (words are jumbled; sentences are meaningless)
  - Perseveration
  - Grammatical errors
  - Nonfluent or nonmeaningful speech
  - Impaired prosodic features of speech (rhythmic aspects of speech such as intonation, tone, stress, and rhythm)
  - Difficulty repeating words, phrases, and sentence
  - *Anomia*—Problems naming or word finding
  - *Dyslexia or alexia*—Impaired reading ability
  - *Agraphia (or dysgraphia)*—Impaired writing ability; can be confounded by loss of use of dominant right hand with hemiparesis
  - If bilingual, unequal impairment between the two languages
  - Pragmatic deficits (i.e., response **hearing**; Shipley & McAfee, 2009b)

Classification of Hearing Loss

- *Conductive loss*: Transmission of sound is interrupted and occurs in the outer or most frequently the middle ear.
- *Sensorineural hearing loss*: Damage to the hair cells of the cochlea or the acoustic nerve. Loss of hearing occurs through bone conduction. It is considered a permanent impairment.
  - *Causes*
    - Ototoxicity (side effects of drugs)
    - Infection
    - Genetic factors
    - Anoxia or syphilis contracted through birth delivery
    - **Presbycusis**—Gradual loss of hearing that occurs as people age. One in three older adults over age 60 have hearing loss. Half of people over age 75 have hearing loss.
    - Ménière's disease
- *Mixed hearing loss*: A combination of conductive and sensorineural hearing loss
- *Auditory processing disorder (APD) or central auditory processing disorder (CAPD)*: Neurologic condition stemming from problems in the auditory center of the brain. The patient is unable to process auditory information normally and may have difficulty detecting or localizing sound or discriminating speech.
- *Retrocochlear pathology*: Damage to the nerve fibers along the ascending auditory pathways from the internal auditory meatus to the cortex, often the result of a tumor; patients often perform poorly on speech recognition tasks. Auditory brainstem response (ABR) tests and other auditory-evoked potentials identify presence of this pathology.

Diagnostic Tests

- Audiograms
- Tympanograms
- Speed audiometry
- ABR
- Auditory evoked potentials

Treatment Options

- Hearing aids (ITE—in the ear, BTE—behind the ear, canal aids, body aids)
- Cochlear Implant
- Vibrotactile aids

END-OF-LIFE AND PALLIATIVE CARE

OVERVIEW

Palliative care is a subspecialty of care for people living with serious illness with a focus on providing relief from the symptoms and stress of serious illness. The focus is to provide improvement in the quality of life (QOL) for both the patient and the family.

- Some illnesses that may be appropriate for palliative care would include cancer, congestive heart failure (CHF), liver failure, kidney failure, congestive obstructive pulmonary disease (COPD), stroke, and neurologically deteriorating conditions such as multiple sclerosis, amyotrophic lateral sclerosis, Parkinson's disease, and dementias.
- Palliative care combines a focus on symptom management with attention to patient autonomy and advanced directives.
- Symptom alleviation focuses on the physical, psychologic, and spiritual domains of patient suffering.
- APRNs address acute pain (and often acute on chronic pain), fatigue, anorexia, agitation, dyspnea, and nausea/vomiting, as well as symptom management in the care of patients who are having life-sustaining treatments withdrawn toward the goal of comfort care.

Palliative care differs from hospice care, in that palliative care can be provided along with active treatment for the disease process, whereas hospice care is provided for patients who have a life expectancy of 6 months or less and for whom curative treatment is no longer beneficial and so has been stopped.

Principles of Palliative Care

- Recognizes dying as a normal process
- Neither hastens nor postpones death
- Provides relief from pain and other distressing symptoms
- Integrates the psychologic and spiritual aspects of patient care
- Offers support for patients to live as fully as possible until death
- Offers support to help the family cope during the patient's illness and in their own grief

SYMPTOM MANAGEMENT

Suffering at the end of life prevents enjoying the remaining time that patients do have, causing depression, isolation, and an inability to fulfill the tasks of dying.

- Suffering (physical, emotional, spiritual) diminishes QOL and fulfills patients' worst fears of dying in misery.
- Symptoms that cause the most suffering at end of life include pain, dyspnea, nausea and vomiting (N/V), anorexia/cachexia, fatigue, and delirium. Suffering is the amount of distress associated with the symptom.

Pain

- More than 60% of patients reported moderate to severe pain at the end of life.
  - Twenty-five percent of patients with advanced illness rated their suffering as moderate to severe, which is most commonly associated with physical pain.
- Patients reported unrelieved pain as an important factor decreasing dignity at the end of life.

The assessment of pain may be evaluated on the PQRST mnemonic:

P—Provocative or palliative features: what makes the pain better or worse

Q—Quality of the pain such as burning or stabbing

R—Radiation or referral of pain

S—Severity, often measured by the numeric scale 0 to 10

T—Temporal factors such as onset, duration, daily fluctuations

Even if disease-modifying treatment is still being attempted (i.e., dialysis or chemotherapy), patients with moderate to severe pain often need help with adequate pain relief.

- Pharmacotherapy is the main approach to pain relief, and there are three main categories of drugs used to treat pain:
  - Nonsteroidal anti-inflammatory drugs (NSAIDs) and acetaminophen
  - Opioids
  - Adjuvant analgesics

The World Health Organization's (WHO's) analgesic ladder is a simple framework used for drug selection and titration of opioids, which can be used to provide effective pain management (Figure 19.3).

Step One: Mild Pain

- Nonopioid medications like acetaminophen or NSAIDs such as ibuprofen.
- PRN dosage may be sufficient.
- Next, try scheduled dosing.
- Alternate acetaminophen and ibuprofen on a schedule.
- Adjuvant medications may be used for targeted treatment of a specific sort of pain.
  - Adjuvant medications can be very useful for patients with cancer-related or neuropathic pain. Antidepressants control the way pain is perceived from the spinal cord to the brain.

- *Tricyclic antidepressants (TCAs)*—Amitriptyline
- *Selective serotonin reuptake inhibitors (SSRIs)*—Duloxetine
- Anticonvulsants prevent certain types of nerve transmission:
  - Gabapentin
  - Pregabalin
- Glucocorticoids inhibit prostaglandin synthesis and reduce vascular permeability to reduce tissue edema and can reduce spontaneous discharge in an injured nerve, which reduces neuropathic pain.
  - Dexamethasone
- Topical therapies
- Capsaicin for treatment of neuropathic pain and arthritic pain
- Topical lidocaine for focal musculoskeletal pains

Step Two: Moderate Pain

- Tramadol
- Hydrocodone
- Low starting dose of oxycodone or oral morphine
- Opioids combined with acetaminophen providing acetaminophen use is within limits
- Scheduled medication is most effective
- Continued use of adjuvant medications for appropriate types of pain

Step Three: Persistent or Severe Pain

- Morphine
- Oxycodone
- Oxymorphone
- Hydromorphone
- Methadone

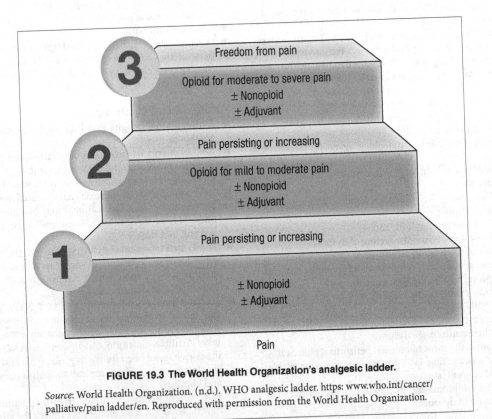

FIGURE 19.3 The World Health Organization's analgesic ladder.

Source: World Health Organization. (n.d.). WHO analgesic ladder. https: www.who.int/cancer/palliative/pain ladder/en. Reproduced with permission from the World Health Organization.

- Fentanyl
- Around-the-clock treatment with PRN short-acting medication for breakthrough pain. Routes of administration for breakthrough pain can be PO, IV, intravenous, SC, or sublingual.
- Long-acting medications are
  - Oral sustained release versions of morphine or oxycodone,
  - Transdermal versions of fentanyl, and
  - Continuous versions of a patient-controlled analgesia (PCA)-delivered medication, such as
    - Morphine,
    - Hydromorphone, and
    - Fentanyl.

Opioid treatment must include attention to bowels:
- Encouraging activity as tolerated.
- Fluids as tolerated.
- Encourage high-fiber foods.
- Take stool softener and/or stimulant daily.
- Take plyethylene glycol daily or PRN.
- Bowel protocols, for the appropriate patient population, can be valuable in providing stepwise treatment choices, starting with stool softeners all the way to enemas if needed.

Dyspnea

Dyspnea is a sensation of air hunger with increased work of breathing:
- Assessment of dyspnea is subjective.
- Work of breathing is directly correlated to survival rate.
- Tends to worsen as patients near death.

Treatment for dyspnea may rely on a combination of strategies. Nonpharmacologic approaches
- Instruct on decreasing energy and attention to comfortable positioning upright seated position.
- Improve air circulation with fans or open windows; adjustment of humidity.
- Consider triggers of anxiety that lead to breathlessness and teach relaxation and mindfulness techniques.
- Supplemental oxygen usually required to palliate dyspnea and improve symptoms and exercise tolerance.
- High-flow nasal cannula has recently allowed the administration of up to 40 L/min of oxygen; however, its availability in home care and hospice is currently limited.

Pharmacologic approaches
- Opioids are the first-line pharmacologic agents for managing dyspnea.
  - Morphine, oxycodone, and hydrocodone promote symptom relief; they
    - Decrease the chemoreceptor response to hypercapnia,
    - Promote vasodilation, and
  - Decrease anxiety and the feeling of dyspnea.
  - Routes of medication administration may include IV, subcutaneous, oral, sublingual, or nebulization, so morphine may be the better agent.
  - Scheduled or long-acting opioids may be considered in patients with persistent dyspnea.
- Anxiolytics prevent the cyclic effect of dyspnea, causing anxiety, which then causes more dyspnea.
  - Lorazepam is the most often used benzodiazepine as it is relatively quick acting, lasts 4 to 6 hours, and is available in an oral concentrate.
- Diuretics offer symptom relief as pulmonary edema can be a significant cause of dyspnea:

- Furosemide may be used palliatively.

Congestion and upper airway secretions, creating a loose noise often called the *death rattle*, can be very distressing to family at the bedside. Generally, patients are unresponsive, unaware, and unbothered by this.
- Anticholinergics may be used to dry up secretions.
  - These medications do not dry up the secretions already in the airway but dry up the mucosa to slow down further accumulation and are generally only used at the end of life for patients, as they can cause thickening of secretions and mucus plugging.
  - Scopolamine is available as a patch, so it is easy for home usage.
  - Atropine drops may be given sublingually to patients who are unresponsive.
  - Glycopyrrolate may be given PO, IV, or SC.

Nausea and Vomiting

Nausea and vomiting (N/V) are common and distressing symptoms in terminally ill patients, especially in patients with cancer (see Chapter 10 for more detailed information on N/V).
- Prevalence is 60% or higher in terminally ill patients.
- Can be as distressing as or more distressing than pain.
- Can lead to weight loss, dehydration, malnutrition, diminished QOL, and noncompliance with cancer therapy.

Appropriate treatment for N/V depends upon determining the source of the nausea, hopefully prior to the initiation of vomiting.
- Nonpharmacologic approaches
  - Remove foods with strong odors or tastes.
  - Offer frequent small sips of fluids.
  - *Teach relaxation and mindfulness techniques:* attention to any psychosocial or spiritual factors.
  - Aromatherapy, particularly ginger and peppermint, have shown some positive results.
- Pharmacotherapy
- Various causes such as increased intracranial pressure or anxiety, vertigo or vestibular/inner ear complications, medication side effects, or gastrointestinal (GI) tract complications
- Treatment varies based on etiology

Anorexia and Cachexia

- Unintentional weight loss leading to muscle atrophy and weakness
- Shift of energy use from carbohydrates to fat
- Increase in ketones and decrease in amino acid metabolism
- Decrease in urine volume and decrease need for water.
- Reversible causes of anorexia (pain, nausea, depression, cancer treatments and medications) may be addressed, but it is often part of the disease process and a natural part of life coming to a close.
- Food often represents nurturing and love; therefore, families often focus on a patient's eating or lack of eating. They may attempt to force food, which can lead to conflict, psychosocial distress, and impact on QOL.
- Patients should be allowed to choose favorite, easy-to-swallow foods. In the last few weeks or months of life, it may make sense to liberalize restrictions on sugar and salt intake. Artificial nutrition and hydration (ANH) in terminal illnesses has not been shown to prolong life and may actually shorten it as a result of aspiration, pulmonary congestion, and vomiting.
- With severe distress, a limited trial of appetite stimulant(s) may be tried but their efficacy is limited; the stimulants may

relieve anorexia to the extent that the patient may enjoy having meals with their family.

Fatigue

A persistent sense of tiredness that may be caused by an illness or its treatment.

- Almost always an indicator for worsening of the disease process
- Caused by changes in energy metabolism or inflammatory changes and cytokines
- The Edmonton Assessment Scale is a validated tool for assessment of fatigue
- Reversible causes include endocrine disorders, anemia, malnutrition, depression, and pain
- Educate in energy conservation strategies, including prioritization of activities so that the most important ones that promote QOL come first and less essential tasks are postponed

Delirium

- Common and distressing symptom in patients nearing end of life
- Many patients with life-limiting or end-of-life illnesses have limited cognitive reserves due dementia, pain, depression, sleep deprivation, auditory and/or visual impairment, or dehydration (see Chapter 23, "Quality Improvement and Safety," for more information).
- Delirium near end of life (often termed terminal restlessness) is characterized by skin mottling, respiratory pattern changes, calling out for deceased family members, mentioning plans for leaving, and periods of deepening somnolence. This constellation of symptoms indicates that death is imminent.

COMPLEMENTARY MODALITIES

When conventional therapies for any or all of these symptoms do not provide adequate symptom management or carry the burden of unpleasant side effects, patients and/or caregivers may choose to include complementary medicine techniques. Complementary therapies can be used with palliative care with the aim of optimizing QOL.

Complementary modalities include the following:

- Acupuncture
- Aromatherapy
- Art therapy
- Massage therapy
- Breathing methods
- Hypnotherapy, meditation
- Movement therapy
- Music therapy
- Pet therapy
- Reflexology
- Reiki
- Yoga

WHEN DEATH NEARS AND IS IMMINENT

- Helping the family understand the signs that death is nearing will help them be more prepared and understand what they are seeing.
- Each disease process has specific symptoms, but as death nears, there is a constellation of physical changes that occur that are fairly universal.
- Almost all families will ask for an estimated time of death. Based on the patient's condition at the present time and

experience with patients with similar condition, it's best to give a time frame in ranges of weeks to months, days to weeks, or hours to days.

Anticipatory grief occurs when families begin the grieving process well before the patient dies, typically when they learn of their loved one's diagnosis or terminal condition (Table 19.6).

- Allow family time to express their feelings. Sometimes, grief begins to significantly impair function; -this is known as *complicated grief.*
- Family members who have had a history of difficulty dealing with previous deaths, who are isolated, or who have inadequate coping skills can be most at risk for complicated grief.
- When patients are within hours to minutes of dying they exhibit the following (Table 19.6):
  - Large, fixed pupils
  - Motionless
  - Rapid thready pulse
  - Noisy breathing
  - Irregular breathing patterns
- Clinical signs of death
  - No response to external stimuli
  - No muscular movement
  - No reflexes
  - No breathing
  - No pulse

At the moment of death, just as throughout the whole process, family and caregivers need continued education and support. Multidisciplinary palliative care teams are attuned to needs of families as they grieve.

Withdrawal of Life-Sustaining Treatment

When making the decision to either withhold or withdraw life-sustaining treatment, a patient with the capacity to make their own healthcare decisions has the right to decline any medical procedure/intervention or ask for interventions to be stopped/withdrawn, whether they are terminally ill or not, even if refusal will lead to their death. When a patient lacks decision-making capacity, the patient's healthcare representative (HCR) may enact the patient's advanced directives to decline or stop life-prolonging therapies such as ANH, dialysis, and ventilatory support.

ANALGESIC MEDICATIONS

ANALGESICS

Analgesic medications relieve pain without loss of consciousness.

OPIOIDS

Opioids are natural or synthetic medications with actions similar to those of morphine.

- Metabolized by the liver
- Excreted by the kidneys
- **Pregnancy category C:** The fetal blood–brain barrier is readily crossed by opioids; use with caution in pregnant or breastfeeding women; prolonged use in pregnancy can cause neonatal withdrawal syndrome in the newborn.

Drug Enforcement Agency Classifications of Controlled Substances

Drug preparations are federally regulated to reduce the chance of drug diversion from legitimate sources to abusers by tracking purchases, dispensing, and transfers. The Drug Enforcement

TABLE 19.6 SIGNS OF IMPENDING DEATH

PHYSIOLOGIC CHANGES	SIGNS/SYMPTOMS	INTERVENTION
CARDIAC AND CIRCULATION CHANGES		
Decreased blood perfusion	Skin may become mottled and discolored. Mottling and cyanosis of the upper extremities appear to indicate impending death versus such changes in the lower extremities.	Provide good skin care. Turn patient q2–3h if this does not cause discomfort. Apply lotion to back and extremities. Support extremities with soft pillows.
Decreased cerebral perfusion	Decreased level of consciousness or terminal delirium. Drowsiness/disorientation.	Orient patient gently if tolerated and if this is not upsetting. Allow patient to rest.
Decrease in cardiac output and intravascular volume	Tachycardia. Hypotension. Central and peripheral cyanosis and peripheral cooling.	Comfort measures. Space out activities.
URINARY FUNCTION		
Decreased urinary output	Possible urinary incontinence. Concentrated urine.	Keep patient clean and dry. Place a Foley if skin starts to break down or if patient is large and difficult to change diapers or if caregiver is unable to provide diaper and linen changes.
FOOD AND FLUIDS		
Decreased interest in food and fluid	Weight loss/dehydration.	Do not force fluid or foods. Provide excellent mouth care.
Swallowing difficulties	Food pocketed in cheeks or mouth, choking with eating/coughing after eating.	Soft foods and thickened fluids (e.g., nectar) as tolerated. Stop feeding patient if choking or pocketing food.
SKIN		
Skin may become mottled or discolored.	Patches of purplish or dark pinkish color can be noted on back and posterior arms/legs.	Keep sheets clean and dry; avoid paper chux directly to skin. Apply lotion as tolerated.
Decubitus ulcers may develop from pressure of being bedbound, decreased nutritional status.	Red spots to bony prominences are first signs of stage I decubiti, and open sores may develop.	Relieve pressure to bony prominences or other areas of breakdown with turning and positioning q2h if tolerated. If patient has increased pain or discomfort with position changes, decrease the frequency. Special mattress as needed. Dressings for skin changes and pressure injuries. Promote comfort and prevent worsening rather than healing since healing most likely will not occur. Consider application of specialized products such as charcoal or metronidazole paste (compounded) if odors are present.
RESPIRATORY		
Retention of secretions in the pharynx and the upper respiratory tract	Noisy respirations—usually no cough or weak cough.	Head of bed up at 45°. Can fold small soft pillow or towel behind neck for extra support.
Dyspnea	Shortness of breath	Oxygen at 2–3 L may help for some patients and often helps families to feel better.

(continued)

TABLE 19.6 SIGNS OF IMPENDING DEATH (*continued*)

PHYSIOLOGIC CHANGES	SIGNS/SYMPTOMS	INTERVENTION
Cheyne–Stokes respirations	Notable changes in breathing.	A gentle fan blowing toward the patient may provide relief. Educate families that this is normal as the patient is dying.
GENERAL CHANGES		
Profound weakness and fatigue	Drowsy for extended periods. Sleeping more.	This is normal. Educate family.
Disoriented with respect to time and a severely limited attention span	More withdrawn and detached from surroundings. May appear to be in a comatose-like state.	This is normal. Educate family.
Patient may speak to persons who have already died or see places others cannot see.	Family may think these are hallucinations or a drug reaction.	

Source: Data from Palliative Care. (2019). *Symptom management at the end of life.* https://palliative.stanford.edu/transition-to-death/symptom-management-at-the-end-of-life

Agency (DEA) is responsible for handling of controlled substances and has categorized drugs according to their approved medical use and potential for dependence and abuse. There are five DEA categories or schedules.

- *Schedule I controlled substances:* The drug or other substance has a high potential for abuse and has no currently accepted medical use in treatment in the United States.
- *Schedule II controlled substances:* This class has the highest potential for abuse and dependence.
- *Schedule III controlled substances:* These substances are less potential for abuse less than schedules I and II
- *Schedule IV controlled substances:* Substances have low potential for abuse relative to the drugs or other substances in schedule III.
- *Schedule V:* These drugs have ow potential for abuse relative to the drugs or other substances in schedule IV.
  The majority of prescribed opioid analgesics are categorized as schedules I and II.

Class: Opioids
Mechanism: Primarily activate opioid receptor binding sites altering perception of pain
Indications: Moderate to severe pain
Contraindications: Patients with significant respiratory depression, paralytic ileus, severe asthma, hypercapnia in unmonitored settings
Common adverse reactions: Sedation, miosis, euphoria, constipation, urinary retention, cough suppression
Safety: Use with caution in older adults, pregnant women, and the opioid naive; see also Table 19.7.
Patient education: Avoid driving and other hazardous activities until effects of the medication are known; use gradual tapering when stopping treatment; discuss the potential for drug dependence; avoid alcohol (Tables 19.8–19.10)

Prescribing Management and Safety Concerns
Schedule opioids based on the duration of action. If pain control does not last for the drug's known duration, increase the **dose** rather than the frequency. Use opioids around the clock for persistent pain, with a rescue medication available for breakthrough pain. Begin with immediate release opioids at the lowest effective dose. Conduct frequent reassessment of effectiveness and side effects. Consider adjuvant or nonopioid analgesics. Always consult the package insert for dosing instructions

TABLE 19.7 OPIOID–DRUG INTERACTIONS

OPIOID ADVERSE DRUG REACTIONS	
DRUG CLASS	**INTERACTION EFFECT**
Central nervous system depressants ■ Benzodiazepines ■ Phenothiazines ■ Barbiturates ■ Antihistamines ■ Alcohol ■ Anesthetics Muscle relaxants	Respiratory depression and sedation
Agonist–antagonist opioids (buprenorphine)	Precipitates withdrawal reaction
Anticholinergics ■ Tricyclic antidepressants ■ Antihistamines ■ Phenothiazines	Urinary retention Constipation
MAOIs	Hyperpyrexia Respiratory depression Confusion
Serotonergic agents	Increased risk for serotonin syndrome
Opioid-favorable drug reactions	
Antiemetics	Reduced symptoms of nausea and vomiting

MAO Is, monoamine oxidase inhibitors.
Source: Adapted from Burchum, J. R., & Rosenthal, L. D. (2016). *Lehne's pharmacology for nursing care* (9th ed.). Elsevier.

and safety information. Dosing should be individualized and should "start low and go slow" with gradual increases to manage pain.

Definition of Terms
- *Opioid naive:* Patients who do not receive opioid analgesics on a chronic, daily basis
- *Opioid tolerance:* Defined as a daily requirement of morphine 60 mg PO, or other opioid equivalent every day at least for a week: 60 mg PO morphine/d; 25 mcg transdermal fentanyl/hr;

TABLE 19.8 SCHEDULE II CONTROLLED SUBSTANCES

MORPHINE SULFATE			
15–30 mg	PO	q4h (immediate release)	
15–30 mg	PO	q8–12h (sustained release)	
10 mg	IM	q4h	
2–10 mg	IV	q2–4h	
10 mg	SC	q4h	
CODEINE			
15–60 mg	PO	q4h	
HYDROCODONE/ACETAMINOPHEN (NORCO)*			
5/325 mg	PO	One to two tablets q4–6h	Maximum 8 tablets/d
7.5/325 mg	PO	One tablet q4–6h	Maximum 6 tablets/d
HYDROCODONE/ACETAMINOPHEN (VICODIN)*			
5/300 mg	PO	One to two tablets q4–6h	Maximum 8 tablets/d
7.5/300 mg	PO	One tablet q4–6h	Maximum 6 tablets/d
10/300 mg	PO	One tablet q4–6h	Maximum 6 tablets/d
OXYCODONE/ACETAMINOPHEN (PERCOCET)*			
2.5/325 mg	PO	Two tablets q6h	Maximum 12 tablets/d
5/325 mg	PO	One tablet q6h	Maximum 12 tablets/d
7.5/325 mg	PO	One tablet q6h	Maximum 8 tablets/d
10/325 mg	PO	One tablet q6h	Maximum 6 tablets/d
HYDROMORPHONE (DILAUDID)			
2–4 mg	PO	q4–6h (immediate release)	
1–2 mg	IM or SC	q2–3h	
0.2–1 mg	IV	q2–3h	
METHADONE (DOLOPHINE)—FOR SEVERE PAIN			
2.5 mg	PO	q8–12h	
2.5–10 mg	IM/IV/SC	q8–12h	
MEPERIDINE (DEMEROL)			
50–100 mg	PO	q3–4h	
50–150 mg	IM or SC	q3–4h	Maximum dose 600 mg/d
OXYCODONE (OXYCONTIN)			
5–15 mg	PO	q4h	
FENTANYL TRANSDERMAL SYSTEM (DURAGESIC)—FOR PAIN MANAGEMENT IN OPIOID-TOLERANT PATIENTS ONLY			
Dosage is individualized based on patient's prior treatment experience. Dosage is calculated based on the dose conversion guidelines in the product package insert, other reliable reference. Dose titration: Iinitial titration after 3 days based on the daily dose of supplemental opioid analgesics required by the patient on the second or third day of the initial application. Further titration should occur after no less than two 3-day applications as it may take up to 6 days for fentanyl levels to reach equilibrium.			

*Maximum acetaminophen dose is 4,000 mg/d.
IM, intramuscular; IV, intravenous; SC, subcutaneous.

TABLE 19.9 SCHEDULE III CONTROLLED SUBSTANCES

CODEINE PHOSPHATE–ACETAMINOPHEN (TYLENOL WITH CODEINE)			
30/300 mg	PO	One to two tablets q4h	Maximum 360/400 mg in 24 hours
60/300 mg	PO	One tablet q4h	
BUPRENORPHINE HYDROCHLORIDE (BUPRENEX)			
Initial dose: 0.3 mg IM or slow IV (over 2 minutes); may repeat once after 30–60 minutes then 0.3 mg IV/IM q6h			

IM, intramuscular; IV, intravenous.

TABLE 19.10 SCHEDULE IV CONTROLLED SUBSTANCES

TRAMADOL (ULTRAM)			
Class	Nonopioid centrally acting analgesic		
Mechanism	Binds to mu-opioid receptors. Inhibits reuptake of serotonin and norepinephrine in the central nervous system.		
50–100 mg	PO	q4–6h	Maximum 400 mg/d

30 mg PO oxycodone/d; 8 mg PO hydromorphone/d; 25 mg PO oxymorphone/d; or an equianalgesic dose of any other opioid

- *Morphine milligram equivalents (MME/d)*: Refers to the amount of morphine an opioid dose is equal to when prescribed. Is often used to gauge the potential for abuse and overdose based on the amount of opioid being given.

Opioid Conversion

Effective pain control may require switching from one opioid to another or changing from one route to another to maximize pain control and minimize adverse medication effects. Opioid conversion tables from reputable sources may be used to make these dosage calculations (see Sample Opioid Conversion Table With Calculation Instructions). Once the conversion dose is calculated, the new opioid starting dose should then be reduced by 25% to 50% to avoid unintentional overdose due to incomplete cross-tolerance and individual variations in opioid pharmacokinetics. The new dose can then be gradually increased as needed.

To calculate the total daily dose, do the following:

- Determine the total daily doses of current opioid medications (consult patient history, electronic health record, and prescription drug monitoring program [PDMP] as necessary).
- Convert each dose into MMEs by multiplying the dose by the conversion factor.
- If more than one opioid medication is used, add together.
- Determine equivalent daily dose of new opioid by dividing the calculated MMEs of current opioid by new opioid's conversion factor. Reduce this amount by 25% to 50% and then divide into appropriate dosing intervals.

Sample Opioid Conversion Table With Calculation Instructions

https://www.aafp.org/dam/AAFP/documents/patient_care/pain_management/conversion-table.pdf

Opioid taper: Slow taper minimizes withdrawal symptoms. Decrease the dose by less than 10% per week for patients taking opioids for longer 10 years. Once the smallest available dose is reached, extend the interval between doses. Opioids may be stopped when taken at a frequency of less than once a day. Collaborate with mental health providers during this period. Access www.aafp.org/dam/AAFP/documents/patient_care/pain-management/conversion-table.pdf for more information.

It is possible that a rapid tapering process could be required for patient safety under certain circumstances.

OPIOID ANTAGONISTS

- (Naloxone, naltrexone)

See Chapter 5, "Substance Use and Addiction," for more information.

NONOPIOID (ADJUVANT) ANALGESICS

- NSAIDs (see Chapter 13, "Musculoskeletal System")
  - Ibuprofen (Motrin), naproxen (Aleve), meloxicam
- Salicylates (see Chapter 13, "Musculoskeletal System")
  - Acetylsalicylic acid (aspirin)
- Antidepressants (see Chapter 15, "Psychobehavioral Disorders")
  - SSRIs
    - Fluoxetine (Prozac), citalopram (Celexa)
  - Aminoketones
    - Bupropion (Wellbutrin)
- Anticonvulsants (see Chapter 14, "Nervous System")
  - Gamma-aminobutyric acid (GABA) structural analogs
    - Gabapentin (Neurontin)
  - GABA analogs
    - Pregabalin (Lyrica)

REVIEW QUESTIONS

1. What are the most appropriate interventions to minimize the risk for falling?
   - A. Ensure the patient doesn't get out of bed.
   - B. Behavioral and environmental modifications (improved lighting and removal of clutter) and physical therapy/strength training.
   - C. Use of a roll-belt and toileting before bed.
   - D. Hold medications that cause dizziness and keep lights on at night.

2. Frank is a 63-year-old man with parotid cancer who has had major surgery, including resection and reconstruction. He is undergoing chemotherapy and radiation. He has severe neck and mouth pain and is no longer able to swallow; so he receives all nutrition and medications crushed through his percutaneous endoscopic gastrostomy (PEG) tube. His current pain regimen consists of oxycodone tablets 15 to 30 mg q4h as needed for pain. He has to awaken at nighttime to receive his pain medication. He rates his pain 8/10. What regimen might serve him better?
   - A. Oxycodone extended release BID
   - B. Norco liquid PRN
   - C. Transdermal fentanyl with lower dose oxycodone PRN for breakthrough pain
   - D. Recommend Lidoderm patch

ANSWERS

1. **Correct answer: B. Rationale:** Behavioral and environmental modifications (improved lighting and removal of clutter) and physical therapy/strength training would be the most appropriate interventions. The cause of gait instability and risk for falling need to be identified first, and then proper intervention selection can be implemented alone or together to minimize the risk for falling. Other interventions include walking, appropriate/well-fitting shoes, and assistive devices (cane, walker). Keeping the patient in bed is not appropriate as this will contribute to muscle weakness and atrophy. Although toileting before bed is appropriate, use

of a roll-belt or any restraint is not indicated. Holding medications are not appropriate and keeping lights on at night can contribute to an increased risk of delirium.

2. **Correct answer: C. Rationale.** Patient's pain is severe and transdermal fentanyl can provide long-acting pain relief, and there is the option for additional medication

if needed. Extended-release medications must not be crushed.

REFERENCES

The complete reference and additional reading lists appear in the digital version of this chapter, at https://connect.springerpub.com/content/book/978-0-8261-7417-8/part/part02/chapter/ch19

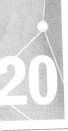

Maximizing Health for the Older Adult

Jennifer P. Colwell, Suzanne Purvis, Anita White, Donna Washburn, and Megan Siebert

PRUDENT HEART LIVING

OVERVIEW

Atherosclerotic cardiovascular disease (ASCVD), more commonly referred to as *heart disease* or *cardiovascular disease (CVD)*, is projected to continue to be a major cause of morbidity and mortality in the United States, despite improvement in care and outcomes (Benjamin et al., 2019). Experts from the American College of Cardiology (ACC) and the American Heart Association (AHA) have developed lifestyle guidelines geared at ASCVD prevention, to improve cardiovascular health (Lloyd-Jones et al., 2010).

KEY PRIMARY STRATEGIES FOR PRUDENT HEART HEALTH

- Encourage a healthy lifestyle over a lifetime as the first line of prevention against ASCVD, heart failure, and atrial fibrillation.
  - Promote a heart-healthy diet with a focus on vegetables, fruits, whole grains, nuts, lean protein, low-fat dairy, and fish. Replace saturated fat with mono and polyunsaturated fats in limited quantities. Minimize the intake of trans fats, processed meats, refined carbohydrates, and sweetened beverages.
  - Use counselling and calorie restriction for weight loss and management in obese and overweight adults.
  - Encourage recommended levels of activity to include 150 minutes of moderate intensity physical activity per week or 75 minutes of vigorous intensity activity per week.
  - Assess adults for tobacco use at every healthcare visit and assist as well as strongly advise users to stop.
  - Address stress reduction and sleep hygiene.
- Effective preventive strategies for clinicians to use in practice.
  - An individualized assessment of the social determinants of health should be done. To aid clinicians in screening patients and having discussions that are outside the norm of clinically focused conversations, tools, such as *the accountable health community screening tool* for nonmedical health-related social needs, are available (Billoux et al., 2017).
  - Routine 10-year ASCVD risk estimation must be done, using a pooled cohort equation for all adults 40 to 75 years of age. The risk estimation guides discussions of risk factors and management.
  - Testing, such as coronary artery calcium scanning, should be done for patients in certain categories who are reluctant to start or restart taking statins: patients who refuse

due to side effect concerns, older patients (men between 55 and 80 years and women between 60 and 80 years) with low risk, and middle-aged adults (40–55 years) with a 10-year ASCVD calculated borderline risk of 5% to <7.5% and with other individual risk enhancers of ASCVD.

- Other key strategies involve chronic disease management and decision points for starting pharmacotherapy.
  - Lifestyle changes for adults with type 2 diabetes mellitus (T2DM) include improving dietary eating habits and following physical activity recommendations.
  - Pharmacotherapy recommendations for T2DM, hyperlipidemia, and hypertension are outlined in Chapter 6 and Chapter 9.
  - Do not discontinue routine aspirin use for primary prevention without a careful risk–benefit consideration.

DISCUSSIONS OF CARDIOVASCULAR HEALTH AND RISK ASSESSMENT SCREENING DISCUSSIONS

According to the AHA, cardiovascular health is defined by the presence of both ideal health behaviors and ideal healthy factors (Table 20.1); together, these make up seven factors that AHA refers to as *Life's Simple 7* (Lloyd-Jones et al., 2010).

The pursuit of healthy behaviors and a healthy lifestyle is the crux of prudent heart health. Following a healthy lifestyle and changing familiar less healthy habits built over a lifetime can be complex. The ACC/AHA 2019 guidelines strongly stress the need for several approaches for optimal results, including increasing the regularity of these discussions at patient visits.

LIFESTYLE FACTORS

Lifestyle factors are heart-healthy behaviors that may lead to ASCVD risk reduction. Greater than 90% of adults older than 60 years of age do not meet most of the healthy lifestyle recommendations (Benjamin et al., 2109). The lifestyle factors that are emphasized for prudent heart health are

- Nutrition and diet,
- Exercise and physical activity, and
- Tobacco cessation (Arnett et al., 2019).

Nutrition and Diet

The current ACC/AHA 2019 guidelines outline that consuming a diet rich in vegetables, fruits, legumes, nuts, whole grains, and fish decrease the risk of ASCVD (Table 20.2). The recommended food choices are typical of Mediterranean diets (Arnett et al., 2019) and Dietary Approaches to Stop Hypertension [DASH] (Whelton et al., 2017).

TABLE 20.1 THE AMERICAN HEART ASSOCIATION'S FACTORS OF HEART HEALTH

IDEAL HEALTHY BEHAVIORS	
Nonsmoking status	**IDEAL HEALTHY FACTORS**
Maintain BMI <25 kg/m² with smart eating, watch calories and portions	Untreated total cholesterol <200 mg/dL
	Untreated BP systolic <120 mmHg/diastolic <80 mmHg
Heart-healthy eating with a focus on fruits, vegetables, lean protein; limiting salt, sugary foods/drinks and saturated or hydrogenated fats	Fasting blood glucose <100 mg/dL
Physical activity recommendations: at least 150 minutes of moderate intensity accumulated per week or 75 minutes of vigorous intensity per week	

BMI, body mass index; BP, blood pressure.

Source: Data from Lloyd-Jones, D. M., Hong, Y., Labarthe, D., Mozaffarian, D., Appel, L. J., Van Horn, L., Greenlund, K., Daniels, S., Nichol, G., Tomaselli, G. F., Arnett, D. K., Fonarow, G. C., Ho, P. M., Lauer, M. S., Masoudi, F. A., Robertson, R. M., Roger, V., Schwamm, L. H., Sorlie, P., ... American Heart Association Strategic Planning Task Force and Statistics Committee. (2010). Defining and setting national goals for cardiovascular health promotion and disease reduction: The American Heart Association's Strategic Impact Goal through 2020 and beyond. *Circulation, 121*, 586–613. http://doi.org/10.1161/CIRCULATIONAHA.109.192703

TABLE 20.2 AMERICAN COLLEGE OF CARDIOLOGY/AMERICAN HEART ASSOCIATION FOODS FOR HEART HEALTH

HEART-HEALTHY FOOD	SERVING SIZES DAILY/WEEKLY	UNHEALTHY FOOD CHOICES: USE SPARINGLY
Olive oil preferably rich in polyphenols	≥4 tbsp/d	Soda drinks <1 drink/d
Tree nuts and peanuts	≥3 servings/wk	Commercial bakery goods, sweets, and pastries <2 servings/wk
Fresh fruits	≥3 servings/d	Avoid trans fat <1 serving/d
Vegetables	≥2 servings/d	Red and processed meats <1 serving/d
Fish (such as salmon), seafood	≥3 servings/wk	Refined carbohydrates such as bread/pasta
Legumes	≥3 servings/wk	Limit alcohol consumption ≤1 glass for women and ≤2 glasses for men (12 oz beer; 4 oz wine)
Other recommendations: Eat whole grains Eat white meat and remove any visible fats Replace saturated fat with mono- and polyunsaturated fats Reduce dietary cholesterol and sodium intake (DASH)		

DASH, Dietary Approaches to Stop Hypertension.

Source: Data from Estruch R., Ros, E., Salas-Salvado, J., Covas, M., Corella, D., Aros, F., ...PREDIMED Study Investigators. (2018). Primary prevention of cardiovascular disease with a Mediterranean diet supplemented with extra-virgin olive oil or nuts. *New England Journal of Medicine, 378*, e34.

Along with healthy food choices, collaborating with dietitians and adding behavioral interventions for those patients who are overweight are suggested strategies (Bittner, 2019). Further recommendations are covered in Nutrition and Weight Management.

Exercise and Physical Activity

Actively discussing the benefits of physical activity and prescribing an activity regimen for patients with chronic diseases, such as diabetes and hypertension, in a primary care setting have been associated with short-term lifestyle changes (Babwah et al., 2018). Physical exercise has been linked to prudent heart health. Aerobic activity and resistance training exercises both provide benefits.

- Activity discussions are guided by current weight, body mass index (BMI), physical activity lifestyle behaviors, other CVD risk enhancers, and presence of chronic conditions.
- The ACC/AHA 2019 guidelines recommend assessment of BMI at least annually (Arnett et al., 2019), with consideration of waist circumference measurement, especially in women, to further aid in identification of those with cardio-metabolic risk.
- It is important to approach physical activity discussions with patients to reduce ASCVD risk, especially those with sedentary lifestyles (Arnett et al., 2019). Sedentary behavior is characterized by any waking behavior, such as sitting behaviors of watching television or playing video games, that result in very low energy expenditure (≤1.5 metabolic equivalents or METs) (Young et al., 2016).

- The recommended activity amounts have not changed since the last preventive guideline, namely, at least 150 minutes of moderate intensity accumulated per week or 75 minutes of vigorous intensity per week or some combination of both. Counselling for weight management should also include addressing psychosocial stressor mitigation and sleep hygiene (Grossman et al., 2017).
- Sleep hygiene is an important factor in cardiovascular health and includes duration plus quality of sleep and assessment of factors that impede sleep (Knutson, 2013).

Tobacco Use

The link between CVD and smoking is well known. The ACC/AHA 2019 guidelines reemphasize the need to screen for tobacco use routinely (Arnett et al., 2019). Clinicians should have active and ongoing discussions at every healthcare visit. The guideline outlines screening for tobacco use, strongly counselling patients to quit, and discussions of available treatment options.

Screening for tobacco use:

- Occurs at every healthcare visit.
- Includes not just smoking cigarettes but all forms of tobacco (Bittner, 2019), including electronic nicotine delivery systems or ENDS such as e-cigarettes.
- Identifies number of cigarettes smoked per day (CPD), which is important for determining pharmacologic treatment dosing.

Counselling for tobacco use:

- Advise to avoid secondhand smoke to reduce ASCVD risk in all adults regardless of tobacco use.
- Offer strong advice to patients who are using tobacco products to quit.
- Use of techniques, including motivational interviewing and shared decision-making, to tailor counselling (ACC/AHA, 2019).
- Identifying a support person or persons. Social support has a positive impact on chronic disease management and can improve prospects for smoking cessation success.
- Consideration of peer-to-peer coaching models for tobacco cessation (ACC/AHA, 2019).

Treatment options for tobacco use:

- Recommend using both pharmacologic and behavioral interventions to help with smoking cessation and improve quitting rates (Arnett et al., 2019).
- Pharmacologic options with Food and Drug Administration (FDA) approval, including nicotine replacement therapy (NRT), are available in various forms such as patches, gum, lozenges, nasal sprays, and oral inhalers; as well as bupropion and CHANTIX.
- ***NRT-specific management:*** NRT therapy is guided by CPD (1 CPD = 1–2 mg of nicotine). NRT is used with caution in patients who have had recent (<2 weeks) myocardial ischemia, infarct, angina, or serious arrhythmia and are pregnant, breastfeeding, or adolescent.
- Behavioral interventions are tailored for patient needs and may be offered in individual or group sessions.
- Tobacco cessation is not easy and most clinicians are ill prepared to guide and empower patients. The University of California San Francisco has an open source training program to train clinicians. Access at https://rxforchange.ucsf.edu/

CONCLUSIONS

The current primary preventive guidelines for CVD offer much more than pharmacotherapeutic management. These guidelines:

- Emphasize lifestyle changes early and throughout the trajectory of life and disease progression.
- Recognize the need for collaboration and team-based care.
- Include a 360° assessment of risk factors that is holistic.
- Focus on meeting the patient in settings where patient-centered care with shared decision-making may be provided.

APRNs have the skills and scientific background to provide holistic preventive care and are well suited to advance primary prevention of ASCVD and empower patients to lead healthier lives. Nursing associations, such as Preventive Cardiovascular Nurses Association, have useful tools to help clinicians promote prudent heart health; access at http://pcna.net/clinical-tools/tools-for-healthcare-providers/heart-healthy-toolbox.

SLEEP HYGIENE

OVERVIEW

Researchers agree that regularly obtaining a full night's sleep is essential to health and well-being (American Academy of Sleep Medicine, 2019; National Sleep Foundation, 2003). Common problems that interfere with getting enough sleep include difficulty falling asleep, frequently awakening with difficulty falling back asleep, snoring, and excessive daytime sleepiness (EDS; National Sleep Foundation, 2003). Education about the stages of the sleep–wake cycle and use of sleep hygiene measures has been shown to alleviate some sleep problems (American Academy of Sleep Medicine, 2019).

Lack of sleep has been linked to (Luyster et al., 2015; Neikrug & Ankoli-Israel, 2010):

- Inattention and poor executive functioning, leading to falls and accidents
- CVD
- Obesity
- Depression
- Cognitive decline and dementia

Risk factors for impaired sleep (Dean et al., 2016; Zdanys & Steffens, 2015):

- Anxiety and stress
- Environmental noise or temperature changes
- Psychiatric and neurologic disorders
- Polypharmacy
- Primary sleep disorders
- Chronic diseases and pain
- Use of alcohol, caffeine, or nicotine before bedtime
- Shift work
- Aging changes

Sleep Physiology

The normal sleep–wake cycle is controlled by the hypothalamus, which directs the body's circadian rhythms (Crowley, 2011). Circadian rhythms are those processes that occur on a regular basis and include changes in body temperature and sleep. Research has demonstrated two main phases of the circadian sleep–wake cycle: Non-REM sleep and REM sleep (Crowley, 2011). The sleep–wake cycle, including both non-REM and REM sleep, takes approximately 90 minutes. Table 20.3 outlines a complete sleep–wake cycle with aging changes that occur in each stage (Crowley, 2011; Neikrug & Ankoli-Israel, 2010).

PRIMARY SLEEP DISORDERS COMMON IN OLDER ADULTS

Primary sleep disorders, which can contribute to impaired sleep, need to be differentiated from aging changes in sleep architecture (Neikrug & Ankoli-Israel, 2010). These disorders include the following:

- Insomnia
- Sleep-disordered breathing (SDB)
- Restless leg syndrome (RLS)
- Periodic limb movement disorder (PLMD)
- REM sleep behavior disorder

Insomnia

Insomnia is a common sleep complaint that involves either difficulty falling asleep or staying asleep through all stages of the sleep cycle. Table 20.4 lists those factors that increase risk for development of insomnia, including some common medications that are associated with impaired sleep (Neikrug & Ankoli-Israel, 2010; Zdanys & Steffens, 2015).

Sleep Assessment

A sleep assessment involves obtaining a good medical history, including an objective sleep history. Self-report questionnaires

TABLE 20.3 STAGES OF THE NORMAL SLEEP CYCLE AND ASSOCIATED CHANGES WITH AGING

	DESCRIPTION OF SLEEP STAGE	SLEEP CHANGES WITH AGING
Non-REM sleep		
Stage 1	Lighter sleep	Time spent in lighter stages of sleep stays same or increases slightly.
Stage 2		
Stage 3	Slow-wave sleep	Less time spent in these deeper stages.
Stage 4	More difficult to awaken	
REM sleep		
Stage 5	Intense vivid dreams; no skeletal muscle movement	Less time spent in REM sleep.

Overview of sleep changes with aging:
- Less slow-wave sleep and less total sleep time
- Number of nocturnal arousals increases
- Longer duration of waking state after sleep onset
- Advanced sleep phase resulting in earlier bedtimes and early morning awakening

TABLE 20.4 FACTORS RELATED TO INSOMNIA

CHRONIC CONDITIONS OF AGING	ANTIHYPERTENSIVES
Anxiety and stress	Respiratory drugs
Lack of good sleep hygiene	Central nervous system stimulants
Shift work	Decongestants
Primary sleep disorders	Hormones
Polypharmacy	Psychotropics
Psychiatric disorders	

are often utilized to assist in the evaluation of sleep (Luyster et al., 2016):

- *Pittsburgh Sleep Quality Index:* Self-report questionnaire that assesses sleep quality at night.
- *Epworth Sleepiness Scale:* Self-report questionnaire that assesses for excessive sleepiness during the day by measuring the tendency to fall asleep while engaging in various activities.
- *Consensus Sleep Diary:* Gathers information on amount and quality of sleep.

A referral to a sleep expert may be needed to get more thorough objective testing, including actigraphy (measures movement during sleep) and polysomnography (overnight sleep study; Luyster et al., 2016).

Treatment of Insomnia

Nonpharmacologic management of insomnia should be tried before any medication due to risk of adverse reactions in older adults (Dean et al., 2016).

Nonpharmacologic Sleep Interventions

- Sleep hygiene measures include regular bedtime routines such as warm milk or bath, exposure to light early in the day, and regular bedtimes
- Exercise
- Relaxation, meditation, and imagery
- Limit daytime naps
- Monitoring environmental noise and temperature
- Avoiding alcohol, caffeine, nicotine at bedtime (Crowley, 2011; Dean et al., 2016; Zdanys & Steffens, 2015)

SLEEP-DISORDERED BREATHING

Sleep-disordered breathing (SDB) is more common in older adults. It can be mild and occur as simple snoring or appear in more severe manifestations all the way along a continuum of severity to obstructive sleep apnea (OSA; Neikrug & Ankoli-Israel, 2010). Risk factors for SDB include age, obesity, smoking, sedating medications, neurologic impairments, and alcohol use (Neikrug & Ankoli-Israel, 2010).

Etiology

Narrowing or relaxation of the pharyngeal airway while asleep occurs with either complete (apnea) or partial (hypopnea) closure and can result in desaturation, interrupted sleep, and EDS (Crowley, 2011). More severe cases, such as those seen with untreated OSA, have been linked in some studies to development of CVD and cognitive impairment (Crowley, 2011).

Assessment

- The severity of SDB is measured by the apnea–hypopnea index (AHI). An AHI of 5 to 10 is indicative of SDB (Neikrug & Ankoli-Israel, 2010).
- Evaluation should also include a complete history: assessing for presence of snoring as well as the frequency of daytime sleepiness.
- Screening tools for SDB can help to identify those with moderate to severe conditions. One commonly used tool for SDB used preoperatively is the STOP-BANG (Dean et al., 2016).
- For those who score positively, a history and physical together with laboratory sleep studies can help determine severity so treatment can be started if indicated.

Treatment

The gold standard for the treatment of SDB is continuous positive airway pressure (CPAP), which is known to reduce EDS by improving total sleep time and sleep quality (Neikrug & Ankoli-Israel, 2010). More research is needed on mouth devices currently sold on the market that hold the airway open during sleep to assure effectiveness and safe use. Evaluation by an expert before using them is recommended (American Academy of Sleep Medicine, 2019).

RESTLESS LEG SYNDROME

Symptoms of RLS occur in the legs when the patient lies down and the restlessness is only relieved with movement. Symptoms of RLS include the following (Crowley, 2011; Zdanys & Steffens, 2015):

- Tingling
- Leg cramps
- Unpleasant sensation in the legs

RLS is seen up to twice as often in women than in men, and age is an important risk factor. Other risk factors associated with RLS include low iron, Parkinson's disease, and end-stage renal disease (Crowley, 2011).

Treatment

Nonpharmacologic interventions that can help reduce symptoms of RLS include exercise, sleep hygiene practices, and reduction of caffeine (Crowley, 2011; Zdanys & Steffens, 2015). It is best to try nonpharmacologic interventions first, in order to avoid medications that can be potentially harmful in older adults. Some of the medications that can be used to treat RLS if indicated are dopamine agonists, anticonvulsants, and benzodiazepines (Neikrug & Ankoli-Israel, 2010).

PERIODIC LIMB MOVEMENT DISORDER

PLMD is characterized by repetitive leg movements during sleep that can cause arousal (Crowley, 2011). This results in complaints of sleep-onset difficulty and less restorative sleep. The risk for PLMD increases with age

Etiology

Age-related declines in dopamine receptors have been associated with PLMD, as well as comorbid venous insufficiency and iron deficiency anemia (Crowley, 2011).

Treatment

Nonpharmacologic sleep interventions as mentioned previously can be helpful and should be initiated first. In some cases, L-dopa has been shown to reduce the number of leg movements (Crowley, 2011).

REM SLEEP BEHAVIOR DISORDER

This sleep disorder involves muscle movements during REM sleep. Muscles are usually atonic during REM sleep. These muscle movements can include yelling or screaming, striking out, or even walking around while asleep (Neikrug & Ankoli-Israel, 2010). There have been reports of REM sleep behavior disorder where people have gotten out of bed and driven a car or ate a meal but not remembered it. This is more common in men and those with neurologic disorders (Neikrug & Ankoli-Israel, 2010).

PHARMACOLOGIC TREATMENT FOR SLEEP DISORDERS

The American Geriatric Society's 2019 Updated AGS Beers Criteria for Potentially Inappropriate Medication Use in Older Adults highly recommends against use of sleep medications as first-line treatment for SDB due to risk of daytime drowsiness and delirium (American Geriatric Society, 2019). Diphenhydramine (found in many over-the-counter sleep medications) and benzodiazepines are especially discouraged in older adults. Table 20.5 gives examples of commonly prescribed medications for sleep, different classes of medications, and a common herbal supplement that is also frequently used for sleep (Schroeck et al., 2016).

Prescribing and Management Guidelines

- Educate on need to sleep a full 7 or 8 hours when on prescribed sleep medications to avoid daytime drowsiness.
- Benzodiazepines are not recommended for older adults per the American Geriatrics Society's 2019 Updated AGS Beers Criteria for Potentially Inappropriate Medication Use in Older Adults (2019).
- Prescription sleep medications taken regularly should be tapered when discontinuing.
- Herbal supplements (e.g., Melatonin) must meet certain quality standards, but effectiveness is not guaranteed by the FDA.

TABLE 20.5 EXAMPLES OF COMMON PRESCRIPTION MEDICATIONS AND HERBAL SUPPLEMENT FOR SLEEP

MEDICATION	CLASS	MECHANISM OF ACTION	INDICATIONS AND CONTRA-INDICATIONS	DOSAGE	SIDE EFFECTS	SAFETY/ PATIENT EDUCATION
Temazepam	Benzodiazepine	Bind to GABA receptors	Increases total sleep time	7.5 mg at HS	Daytime drowsiness, falls, delirium, and dementia	Taper when discontinuing.
Zolpidem	Sedative or hypnotic	Binds to GABA receptors	Decreases sleep onset and improves total sleep time	5 mg, immediate release tablet and spray	Dizziness, drowsiness, delirium, falls, and night-time sleep behaviors	Report daytime drowsiness; abrupt withdrawal can cause rebound insomnia.
Trazodone	Atypical antidepressant	Alpha adrenergic and histamine blockade	Depression; prolongs slow-wave sleep and total sleep, interacts with warfarin	25–100 mg daily at HS	Mild dizziness, drowsiness, headache	Report daytime dizziness or sleepiness.
Melatonin	Dietary supplement and hormone	Naturally released; suppresses neuronal activity	Enhances the circadian rhythms	1–2 mg, immeiate release formula	Daytime sleepiness	Monitor for daytime drowsiness.

GABA, gamma-aminobutyric acid; HS, hours of sleep.
Note: GABA is the chief inhibitory neurotransmitter.

NUTRITION AND WEIGHT MANAGEMENT

OVERVIEW

Nutrition is defined as the process of how the body takes in and uses food to stay healthy (Cambridge, 2019).

- Only 12.2% of adults meet the daily requirement for fruit consumption and only 9.3% of adults meet the daily requirement for vegetable consumption (Centers for Disease Control and Prevention [CDC], 2018).
- Poor diet is linked to the most common chronic diseases for the United States: type 2 diabetes, some cancers, and obesity (CDC, 2018).
- Obesity affected approximately 93.3 million of U.S. adults in 2015 to 2016 (Hales et al., 2017).

Obesity-related conditions, such as heart disease, stroke, type 2 diabetes, and certain types of cancer, can lead to premature death; $147 billion was the estimated medical cost of obesity in 2008.

Physiology

The Five Process Stages of Nutrition

- **Ingestion:** Food enters mouth.
- **Digestion:** Large insoluble molecules are broken down into small soluble molecules.
- **Egestion:** Undigested particles are removed from the body.
- **Absorption:** Small molecules are absorbed into the blood.
- **Assimilation:** Absorbed food is utilized by the cells.

Primary Functions of Nutrition

- Provide energy.
- Maintain tissues.
- Regulate nutrients: Carbohydrates, fats, proteins, water, vitamins, and minerals.

Caloric balance is important to maintaining a healthy weight. The balance between physical activity and caloric consumption is important to health. Overweight individuals are at higher risk for premature mortality as well as increased incidence of CVD, hypertension, cancer, and more.

Nutrition is made up of macronutrients, providing bulk energy, and micronutrients, needed in small amounts, in addition to adequate water intake. Recommended daily consumption of the components of nutrients has been defined and broken down even further by the USDA (United States Department of Agriculture, 2005) into amounts recommended to match differing levels of caloric intake (Table 20.6).

Macronutrients

- **Carbohydrates**—45% to 65% of total caloric intake (whole grain, refined grain)
- **Protein**—10% to 35% total caloric intake (fish, lean meat, poultry, eggs, beans, peas, soy products, unsalted nuts, and seeds)
- **Fat**—20% to 35% total caloric intake (trans fats may contribute to heart disease; *n*-3 polyunsaturated fats are protective)
- **Fiber**—14 g/kcal (25–36 g/d if moderately active; replace refined grains, such as white rice and white bread, with whole grains such as brown rice and whole-wheat bread)

Micronutrients

- **Sodium**—<2,300 mg/d
- **Calcium and vitamin D**—calcium 1,200 mg for postmenopausal women and 1,000 mg for others. Vitamin D 500 International Units (IU) daily or 800 IU daily for individuals over 70 years
- **Folate**—0.4 mg daily for women in reproductive years
- Multivitamin

TABLE 20.6 RECOMMENDED DAILY CONSUMPTION

FOOD GROUP	DAILY AMOUNT BASED ON 2,000-CALORIE DIET/WEEK
Vegetables	**2.5 cups/day**
Dark-green vegetables	1.5 cups/week
Red and orange vegetables	5.5 cups/week
Legumes (beans and peas)	1.5 cups/week
Starchy vegetables	5 cups/week
Other vegetables	4 cups/week
Fruits	**2 cups/day**
Grains	**6 oz/day**
Whole grains	3 oz/day
Refined grains	3 oz/day
Dairy	**3 cups/day**
Protein foods	**5.5 oz/day**
Seafood	8 oz/week
Meats, poultry, eggs	26 oz/week
Nuts, seeds, soy products	5 oz/week
Oils	**27 g/day**
Calories for other uses	**270 Kcal/day**
Water	**1,500 mL for the first 20 kg of body weight plus 20 mL for every kilogram over 20 kg. Average fluid needs are 30–35 mL/kg or 1 mL//kcal of energy required.**

Source: Modified from U.S. Department of Agriculture. https://health.gov/sites/default/files/2019-09/2015-2020_Dietary_Guidelines.pdf

Energy Requirements—Estimated Energy Requirement

The balance between physical activity and caloric consumption is important to health. Calorie needs are calculated using the following equations:

- **Women:** $354.1 - (6.91 \times \text{age [y]}) + PAC \times (9.36 \times \text{weight [kg]} = 726 \times \text{height [m]})$
- **Men:** $661.8 - (9.53 \times \text{age [y]}) + PAC \times (15.91 \times \text{weight [kg]} + 539.6 \times \text{height [m]})$

Physical activity coefficient (PAC):

- Sedentary PAC = 1.0
- Low activity PAC = 1.12
- Active PAC = 1.27
- Very active PAC = 1.45

NUTRITION SCREENING AND ASSESSMENT

Nutritional screening is an initial step in the identification of those who are malnourished or at risk for becoming malnourished. Screening is also integral to the assessment for obesity. Being overweight does not equate to being nutritionally sound. The Joint Commission standards require nutritional screening within 24 hours of admission for inpatient hospitals and on initial visit for outpatient settings (2016).

Nutritional Screening

Several tools for nutritional screening are available with strength of reliability and validity (Table 20.7).

TABLE 20.7 SCREENING TOOLS

TOOL	STRENGTH	SETTING	USE
Nutrition Risk Screening (2002)	Sensitivity: 39%–70% Specificity: 83%–93%	Acute hospital, critically ill	Two components: (1) Screening assessment for under-nutrition, (2) estimate for disease severity
MST*	Sensitivity: 74%–100% Specificity: 76%–93%	Acute hospital, cancer patients	Ask two questions: "Have you been eating poorly because of a decreased appetite?" and "Have you lost weight recently without trying?"
MUST	Predictive validity in older adults, hospitalized patients, and mortality Sensitivity: 61% Specificity: 76%	Acute hospital, older adults	Incorporates BMI, weight loss (in 3–6 months), anorexia (for 5 days due to disease); commonly used in the United Kingdom; sensitive for protein energy undernutrition in hospitalized patients
NST	Sensitivity: 86% Specificity: 95%	Acute hospital	Dietitian screening tool
The SNAQ	Community: Sensitivity: 81.3% Specificity: 76.4% Long-term care: Sensitivity: 88.2% Specificity: 83.5%	Community-dwelling, long-term care residents	14-item screen for identification of older persons at risk for 5%–10% weight loss
SCREEN II	Sensitivity: 84% Specificity: 58% Test–retest reliability was adequate (ICC = 0.83). Inter-rater reliability was adequate (ICC = 0.83)	Seniors in community	17-item tool for nutritional risk by evaluating food intake, physiologic/social/functional barriers to eating, weight change (abbreviated eight-question version is also available)
MNA*	Widely validated and predictive of poor outcomes	All	Global assessment and subjective perception of health (health, diet, body measurements); MNA-SF uses six questions from the full MNA (substitutes calf circumference if no BMI available)

*The two screening tools with the highest sensitivity (>83%) and specificity (>90%) are the MNA-SF and the MST.

BMI, body mass index; ICC, intra-class correlation; MNA, Mini Nutritional Assessment; MNA-SF, Mini Nutritional Assessment—Short Form; MST, Malnutrition Screening Tool; MUST, Malnutrition Universal Screening Tool; NST, Nutrition Screening Tool; SCREEN, Seniors in the Community: Risk Evaluation for Eating and Nutrition; SNAQ, Simplified Nutrition Assessment Questionnaire.

A nutritional assessment follows the screening assessment consisting of integration of all findings:

- Review of body systems: medical, nutrition, and psycho-social histories (see Undernutrient Intake Conditions and Overnutrient Intake Conditions)
- Physical exam
- Anthropometric data: height, weight, BMI, and ratio of lean body tissue to body fat
- Functional outcomes
- Examination of energy intake and nutrients

Nutritional Assessment

- Functional assessment covering self-care abilities:
  - Eating preferences
  - Activities of daily living
  - Need of assistance with shopping, cooking
  - Nutritional status
  - Home environment
  - Activity

Weight Assessment

- Weight within normal range for height and body is measured by BMI. Several online calculators are available free for use.
- Body fat distribution needs to be equal.
  Serial measurements of body weight provide the best screening for nutritional sufficiency and early identification of change

of status with older adults. Weight loss in older adults is predictive of mortality (Gregg et al., 2003; Wallace et al., 1995; Wannamethee et al., 2005, Table 20.8).

Other laboratory studies may be utilized especially if utilizing parenteral nutrition (electrolytes, glucose, blood urea nitrogen, creatinine). If unexplained anemia is present, a further evaluation of iron levels and specific vitamin levels should be done. Serum calcium, magnesium, and phosphorous should also be assessed in the setting of poor oral intake or gastrointestinal loss.

Common Problems of the Nutrition System

Under-nutrient intake conditions
Over-nutrient intake conditions

UNDERNUTRIENT INTAKE CONDITIONS

Nutritional malnourishment is present in 38.7% of hospitalized patients (Kaiser et al., 2010). Many conditions are related to inadequate nutrient intake (Table 20.9). The normal aging process allows for physiologic factors affecting weight loss (Table 20.10).

- Older adults are less able to rebound from an episode of under-nutrition than younger adults.
- The impact of under-nutrition on outcomes inclusive of functional level, length of stay for hospitalized procedures, and complications is great with the highest risk associated with poor appetite, high BMI, and diagnosis of infection, delirium, or cancer (Mudge et al., 2011).

TABLE 20.8 LABORATORY ASSESSMENT OF PROTEIN STATUS

LAB VALUE	RANGE	HALF-LIFE	USE
Serum albumin	35–50 g/L (3.5–5.0 g/dL)	18–20 days	<2.2 g/dL Low serum album is a marker of a negative catabolic state and predictor of poor outcome.
Serum transferrin	204–360 mg/dL	8–9 days	Reflective of systemic inflammatory response, low iron status. Indicator of low protein status only in setting of normal serum iron.
Serum prealbumin (transthyretin)	15.7–29.6 mg/dL	2–3 days	Responds to catabolism or inflammation and rises when resolved.

Source: Seres, D. S. (2005). Surrogate nutrition markers, malnutrition, and adequacy of nutrition support. *Nutrition in Clinical Practice, 20*, 308. https://doi.org/10.1177/0115426505020003308

TABLE 20.9 CONDITIONS RELATED TO INADEQUATE NUTRIENT INTAKE

CONDITION	CAUSE	INTERVENTION
Social isolation at mealtime	One third of people over 65 years old live alone	Community groups, club activity enhancement; Family/significant other awareness
Social and/or financial limitations	Greater number of older adults live at poverty level	Community outreach programs; community assessment of poverty level and public health awareness
Medical malignancy	Decrease in taste and smell sensitivity or alteration in taste	Nutritional supplements; ensure meals meet individual tastes, lift dietary restrictions. modify diet
Psychiatric depression	Decreased desire for self-care inclusive of dietary needs	Nutritional awareness and assessment. Nutritional supplements; provide for small easy-to-carry food
Medical dysphagia related	Stroke, Parkinson's disease, amyotrophic lateral sclerosis, Zenker's diverticula, motility disorders	Assistance with feeding, medication intervention, consider enteral feeding
Medical	Endocrine (hyperthyroidism, new onset diabetes mellitus), End-organ disease (congestive heart failure, end-stage renal disease, COPD, liver failure) Gastrointestinal disorders (celiac, inflammatory bowel, peptic ulcer, gastroesophageal reflux)	Consider dietary requirements and ability to follow new restrictions; if unable to tolerate oral intake, assess enteral or parenteral need
Medical infections	Tuberculosis, rheumatologic disorders, neurologic (Parkinson's, chronic pain), Alzheimer's	Possible need for assistance with feeding due to disease progression
Drug or alcohol dependence		Vitamin supplements, enteral or parenteral nutrition
Medication side effects	Digoxin, opioids, serotonin reuptake inhibitors, diuretics	
Dental conditions	Dental caries, missing teeth	Connect to dental care

COPD, chronic obstructive pulmonary disease.

TABLE 20.10 PHYSIOLOGIC FACTORS FOR WEIGHT LOSS

FACTOR	RATIONALE
Age	Taste bud recognition of salt and other tastes decreases
Gastric emptying	Decrease in rate-prolonged antral distension causes reduced hunger and increased feeling of fullness
Central nervous system	Digestive hormones are less detected by brain with increased age (glucagon, GLP-1, cholecystokinin, leptin, ghrelin)
Impaired regulation of food intake	Decreased stimulatory effects of neurotransmitters in appetite, increased sensitivity to inhibitory effects of serotonin, cholecystokinin, and corticotropin-releasing factor

GLP-1; glucagon-like peptide-1.
Source: Adapted from Parker, B. A., & Chapman, I. M. (2004). Food intake and ageing—The role of the gut. *Mechanisms of Ageing and Development, 125*, 859. https://doi.org/10.1016/j.mad.2004.05.006

Three conditions resulting in loss of weight due to decreased appetite or muscle are defined in Table 20.11. Some patients may require appetite stimulants in order to increase nutrient intake (Table 20.12).

OVERNUTRIENT INTAKE CONDITIONS

Obesity is defined as BMI >30 (Table 20.13). Higher body weights are associated with a greater all-cause mortality.

- Obesity is associated with greater morbidity related to multiple disease conditions such as hypertension, coronary heart disease, stroke, gallbladder disease, dyslipidemia, type 2 diabetes, osteoarthritis, sleep apnea, respiratory problems, and various cancers.
- Worsening disability and function can be improved with weight reduction as well as some pain conditions affected by weight (Wee et al., 2011). Slow loss with regular exercise with

TABLE 20.11 ANOREXIA, CACHEXIA, SARCOPENIA

CONDITION	DEFINITION	CAUSE
Anorexia	Decreased in appetite	Physiologic changes, decreased energy requirements, reduced physical activity, loss of lean body mass; changes in taste and smell, illness, drugs, dementia and mood disorders, living in institutional settings, fewer teeth
Cachexia associated with increased morbidity	Loss of muscle with or without loss of fat mass	Anorexia, inflammation, insulin resistance, increased muscle protein breakdown; usually occurs with underlying illness: cancer, end-stage renal disease, COPD, heart failure, rheumatoid arthritis, AIDS
Sarcopenia: Can occur in overweight individuals	Loss of muscle mass, strength, and performance	Associated with increased rates of functional impairment, falls, disability, and mortality; disuse, endocrine function changes, chronic disease, inflammation, insulin resistance, nutritional deficiencies

COPD, chronic obstructive pulmonary disease.

TABLE 20.12 APPETITE STIMULANTS

MEDICATION	CLASS	MECHANISM OF ACTION	INDICATIONS AND CONTRAINDICATIONS	DOSAGE	SIDE EFFECTS	SAFETY/ PATIENT EDUCATION
Megestrol acetate	Progestational agent	Unknown	Beer's Criteria possibly inappropriate for 65 years and older. Only consider in older adults with cancer or AIDS.	800 mg daily	Edema, worsening heart failure, DVT, muscle weakness, impaired corticoadrenal axis function	Use as directed; report adverse reactions; if of childbearing age, utilize prophylactics, avoid pregnancy
Dronabinol	Cannabinoid	Complex effects on the central nervous system Metabolized by CYP2C9 and CYP3A4 enzymes	Useful for anorexia, nausea/vomiting with cancer or AIDS. Contraindicated in hypersensitivity to sesame oil. Avoid use in pregnancy.	2.5 mg BID 1 hour before lunch and dinner	Nervous system, seizures, tachycardia	Swallow whole, do not crush; may be habit forming; increased risk of falls
Mirtazapine	Antidepressant	Exact mechanism of action is unknown. Thought to enhance central noradrenergic and serotonergic activity Metabolized by cytochrome P450 enzymes, CYP1A2, CYP1D6, CYP3A4	For treatment of depression and weight loss. Do not take with tryptophan, MAOI.	15 mg once daily HS	Sleepiness, racing thoughts, blurred vision, sudden weakness, rash, strange dreams, dry mouth constipation, weight gain, mania	Increased suicide rates in children
Ghrelin mimetics	Growth hormone secretagogues	Stimulates appetite and increases fat-free mass	Weight gain to increase lean muscle mass, improve strength and function. Use in older adults with sarcopenia, cachexia, or weight loss. Prohibited in sports.	25 mg daily	Hyperglycemia, dizziness, nausea	Monitor blood glucose in diabetics

DVT, deep vein thrombosis; MAOI, monoamine oxidase inhibitor.

TABLE 20.13 OBESITY CLASSIFICATIONS AND BODY MASS INDEX

CLASSIFICATION	BMI	INTERVENTION BASED ON RISK AND BMI
Underweight	<18.5	
Normal	18.5–24.9	
Overweight	25–29.9	Diet, exercise, and behavior modification
Obese I	30–34.9	Diet, exercise, and behavior modification; consider drug therapy
Obese II	35–39.9	Diet, exercise, and behavior modification; consider drug therapy
Obese III	>40	Diet, exercise, and behavior modification; consider drug therapy and surgery

BMI, body mass index.

the addition of calcium and vitamin D supplements should be utilized. Loss of muscle mass loss and bone mineral density may be lessened with exercise.

- Lifestyle change is integral to sustained weight loss. Pharmacotherapy and bariatric surgery may be considered as adjuncts to comprehensive lifestyle change.

Use of motivational interviewing techniques and comprehensive lifestyle interventions, such as 12 contacts in 12 months, combined with dietary, physical activity, and behavioral strategies offer support to change.

Pharmacological therapy should be offered to those with BMI >30.

Prescribing and Management

- These medications listed in Table 20.14 have multiple drug interactions and risks; ensure patient education is complete.
- Phentermine or topiramate is to be avoided within 14 days following use of monoamine oxidase inhibitor (MAOI).
- Phentermine or topiramate is not recommended in patients with unstable cardiac or cerebrovascular disease.
- Orlistat requires more frequent monitoring of warfarin, levothyroxine, and anticonvulsant levels.

Nutritional issues in older adults consist of vitamin B_{12} deficiency. Some advocate for screening for B_{12} deficiency over the age of 65 years. Vitamin D deficiency is thought to be due to lack of sun exposure and impaired skin synthesis in older adults.

CANCER PREVENTION

OVERVIEW

Clinical nurse specialists (CNSs) have a unique opportunity to promote cancer prevention strategies and impact reduction of cancer morbidity and mortality in the older adult population. The older adult population, in comparison to other age groups, has the highest incidence of cancer and/or comorbid diseases that also impact cancer risk. Prevention may encompass a variety of strategies depending on individual risk factors, physical or functional ability, and psychosocial factors. Historically, older adults have been excluded from prevention efforts due to age bias.

Unavoidable Risk Factors and Preventive Measures

Advancing age is the single biggest risk factor for developing cancer (National Cancer Institute, 2015).

- Age-related changes in organs and damage in DNA structure allow abnormal cell mutation and reproduction:
  - Lifestyle choices that optimize health and mitigate the development of comorbid illness may help delay age-related changes in organs and DNA.

- Age-related general deconditioning of the immune system allows abnormal cell proliferation and metastasis. Infections can cause chronic inflammation, suppress the immune system, or directly cause abnormal cell proliferation (American Cancer Society, n.d.).
  - Healthy diet, exercise, and rest in combination with avoidance of tobacco smoke, limited alcohol intake, and avoiding infection are viable cancer prevention measures

Genetic Mutations

Older adults may also have a genetic mutation as not all people with genetic mutation develop the associated cancer;

- Genetically inherited cancers are related to specific mutations and only blood relatives are at risk for having a genetic mutation passed to them.

Breast and Ovarian Cancer

- Genetic mutations related to breast cancer (*BRCA1*, *BRCA2*) were among the first proven to be related to increased prevalence of cancer.
- Individuals with genetic risk for breast cancer may elect to have prophylactic mastectomy and/or begin treatment with a chemo-preventive, such as tamoxifen, in premenopausal women or an aromatase inhibitor for postmenopausal women (NCCN Clinical Practice Guidelines in Oncology, n.d.).
- Education is not gender specific for breast cancer preventive strategies due to increased risk for breast cancer in males, females, and transgender individuals with mutations. Males who develop breast cancer have a higher likelihood of genetic mutation in their blood relatives.
- Individuals should understand that prophylactic surgery alone reduces their risk but does not eliminate risk. Thus, more than one preventive strategy may be indicated.
- An oncologist referral is generally recommended to evaluate risk based on the type of mutation and to counsel the patient on current recommendations to make a shared decision regarding prevention strategies.
- Encourage the patient to ask about available clinical trials focused on prevention of genetic-related cancers prior to agreeing to surgery or other preventive treatments. Researchers are more likely to include older adults than in past years and clinical trials allow older individuals to be part of cutting-edge treatments.

Familial Cancer

Familial cancer refers to an increased prevalence of cancer in blood-related individuals but without an associated genetic mutation. The reasons behind increased prevalence of cancer in some families and not others is not always well understood.

TABLE 20.14 PHARMACOLOGIC INTERVENTIONS FOR OBESITY

MEDICATION	CLASS	MECHANISM OF ACTION	INDICATIONS AND CONTRAINDICATIONS	DOSAGE	SIDE EFFECTS	SAFETY/ PATIENT EDUCATION
Orlistat	Gastrointestinal lipase Inhibitor	Prevents absorption of fats. Inhibits gastric and pancreatic lipases, the enzymes that break down triglycerides in the intestine	Contraindication: Pregnancy, not recommended in breast-feeding mothers. May decrease cyclosporin concentrations. Monitor closely in patients taking warfarin and levothyroxine. Effect of anticonvulsant may be reduced.	120 mg TID	Increases GI motility when taken with diet high in fat.	Take with or within 1 hour of each meal containing fat. Must take daily multivitamin at least 2 hours prior to orlistat.
Lorcaserin	Anorexiant Serotonin 5-HT$_{2C}$ receptor agonist	Activates serotonin receptor in brain known to control appetite in the hypothalamus	Reduces appetite to reduce weight. Not recommended in severe renal impairment or end-stage renal disease. Contraindicated in pregnancy and breast-feeding mothers. Serotonin syndrome possible. Use with caution in patients with cardiovascular disease. Risk of hypoglycemia in diabetics.	10 mg BID with or without food. Consider stopping if no weight reduction after 12 weeks	Headache, dry mouth, nausea, back pain, low blood sugar, constipation	Do not crush.
Phentermine/ topiramate	Anorexiant, anticonvulsant, sympathomimetic	Phentermine: reduces appetite Topiramate: effects appetite suppression and satiety by multiple mechanisms, blocks sodium channels, enhances GABA(A) activity, antagonizes AMPA/kainite glutamate receptor, weakly inhibits carbonic anhydrase	Indications: Weight management in type 2 diabetes. Dose in renal impairment should not exceed 7.5 mg/46 mg once daily if creatinine clearance <50 mL/min. Dose in hepatic impairment should not exceed 7.5 mg/46 mg once daily. Contraindicated in pregnancy and breast-feeding mothers. Contraindications: MAOIsi-hyperthyroidism, glaucoma.	1 phentermine 3.75 mg/topiramate 23 mg extended-release capsule each morning for 14 days. Then 7.5 mg/46 mg each morning for 12 more weeks	Cardiovascular, glaucoma, hyperthermia, hypokalemia, hypotension, metabolic acidosis, suicidal ideations	Take in the morning. Most effective with low carbohydrate diet. Has multiple drug interactions. Parameters to monitor: weight, resting heart rate, blood pressure, serum bicarbonate, serum glucose, potassium, serum creatinine, suicidal and mood disorders.

AMPA, alpha-amino-3-hydroxy-5-methyl-4-isoxazole propionic acid; GABA, gamma-aminobutyric acid; GI, gastrointestinal; MAOIs, monoamine oxidase inhibitors.

- Familial cancer occurs primarily in older adult family members and may include similar cancers or a variety of unrelated cancers.
- Exposure to a common carcinogen, such as tobacco smoke, radon, or chemical pollutants, may explain some incidences of multiple cancer diagnoses in family members in a similar geographic location where there is no genetic mutation.
  - Public health education and surveillance of cancer-type clusters is important for prevention of cancers related to these exposures.

Avoidable Risk Factors and Recommended Preventive Measures

- Tobacco use is the greatest avoidable risk for cancer mortality worldwide (WHO, 2017):
  - Tobacco use in smoke or smokeless form is the primary cause of cancers of the lung, head, and neck. Exposure to secondhand smoke causes lung cancer in nonsmoking adults.
  - Tobacco use is also attributed to kidney, bladder, pancreas, stomach, and cervical cancers and acute myelogenous leukemia (PDQ Cancer Prevention Overview, 2019; WHO, 2017).
  - E-cigarette use, also known as vaping or Juuling, is still too new for assessing long-term risk. Contrary to popular belief, e-cigarettes are not nicotine free and may contain harmful chemicals. E-cigarettes are not approved by the FDA to aid in smoking cessation (Zborovskaya, 2017).
  - Lung cancer risk and other cancer risks decrease over time after smoking cessation.
  - Smoking cessation in adults aged 65 and older decreases risk for all-cause mortality compared to older adults who continue to smoke (Nash et al., 2017).
  - Preventative screening is important, especially with increasing age (Table 20.15).

Physical Inactivity, Dietary Factors, Alcohol Use, and Obesity

Decreased physical activity, poor diet, alcohol use, and obesity in adults aged 65 and older are strongly related to increased risk for cancer and other comorbid diseases. Obesity and other risk factors that promote and maintain inflammation in the body may be a causative factor. Increasing physical activity, eating a healthy diet, limiting alcohol intake, and maintaining a healthy weight can greatly improve health, decrease risk of cancer, and reduce risk of comorbid diseases.

- Older adults should follow the same physical activity guidelines as younger adults, including 150 minutes or more of physical activity a week and strength training in addition to balance training (ASH, 2019).
  - Adults aged 65 years and older are less likely to meet physical activity guidelines of 150 minutes of physical activity a week.
- Alcohol intake should be limited to one drink a day for women and two for men.

Infections

Infectious agents are estimated to cause 26% of cancers in developing nations and 8% in developed nations (National Cancer Institute, 2015).

- Individuals who undergo organ transplant are treated with immunosuppressants and are at increased risk for cancer.
- HIV increases risk of opportunistic cancers such as Kaposi's sarcoma.
- Infection with human papillomavirus (HPV) is correlated with cervical cancer as well as cancers of the penis, vagina, anus, and oropharynx (National Cancer Institute, 2015).
  - Vaccination for HPV is primarily given in the teens or early 20s. The vaccine is most effective when given prior to HPV exposure.
- Additional infections related to increased risk for cancer development include Helicobacter pylori (gastric ulcer disease and gastric cancer), hepatitis B and C (liver cancer), and Epstein-Barr virus (lymphoma).

Environmental and Occupational Exposure to Carcinogenic Chemicals

Pollution of air, water, and soil with chemicals contributes to development of cancer to differing degrees depending on geographical location (WHO, 2017):

- Clusters of cancers in families, neighborhoods, and industry have been linked to pollutants.
- Certain professions were more likely to develop occupation-related cancers prior to implementation of safety standards in the United States (CDC, n.d.).

TABLE 20.15 PREVENTIVE SCREENING

TYPE OF SCREENING	GOAL OF SCREENING	RECOMMENDED FREQUENCY
Colorectal	Colon cancer risk increases after age 50	Routine colonoscopy for patients ages 50–75 years old; findings may indicate need for more frequent exams
Prostate	Prostate cancer risk increases with age, especially after age 55	Annual PSA from age 55–69 years old; not recommended after age 70
Breast	Breast cancer risk	Annual mammogram for ages 45–54 years and every 2 years 55–69 years
Cervical	Cervical cancer	Women ages 21–65 years with cytology (**Pap smear**) every 3 years or for women ages 30–65 years who want to lengthen the **screening** interval; **screening** with a combination of cytology and **HPV testing** every 5 years
Glaucoma	Glaucoma risk increases after age 40 years	Baseline at age 40 years old, with annual eye exams
Osteoporosis	Older adults are more prone to osteoporosis; weakened bones place them at a greater risk for fractures, especially with falls	Postmenopausal women over age 65 DEXA scan no more frequently than every 2 years

DEXA, dual-energy x-ray absorptiometry; HPV, human papillomavirus; PSA, prostate-specific antigen.

- Exposure to asbestos found in older building materials is a well-known risk for development of mesothelioma.

Radiation

Radiation is energy in the form of high-speed particles or electromagnetic waves. Exposure to solar radiation is the primary cause of nonmelanoma skin cancers (PDQ Cancer Prevention Overview, 2019).

- Basal and squamous cell skin cancers are related to prolonged exposure to the sun and are common occurrences in older adults who work primarily out of doors (e.g., farming).
  - Prevention includes use of protective UV-rated clothing and sunblock as well as limiting exposure to UV rays.
- Major sources of population exposure to ionizing radiation are medical radiation (x-rays, CT, fluoroscopy, and nuclear medicine) and naturally occurring radon gas in home basements (PDQ Cancer Prevention Overview, 2019).
  - Testing homes for radon levels, sealing basements, and improving ventilation helps reduce radon-related cancer risk (WHO, 2017).

Cancer Prevention Education and Resources

- National Cancer Institute: www.cancer.gov/about-cancer
- Centers for Disease Control and Prevention: www.cdc.gov/cancer/dcpc/prevention/index.htm
- National Cancer Institute Division of Cancer Prevention: Clinical Trials Search: https://prevention.cancer.gov/clinical-trials/clinical-trials-search
- American Cancer Society Prevention and Early Detection Guidelines: www.cancer.org/health-care-professionals/american-cancer-society-prevention-early-detection-guidelines.html

FAMILY AND ROLE THEORIES

- Patient- and family-centered care is an approach to care that is mutually beneficial to healthcare providers, patients, and families. This approach includes planning, delivery, and evaluation of healthcare.
- Core concepts of patient- and family-centered care:
  - Dignity and respect
  - Information sharing
  - Participation
  - Collaboration
- The CNS considers patient- and family-centered care to assess and identify barriers and challenges for the active participation of the patient and family.
- The family is involved in decision-making.
- Examples of tools for assessing family assessment and functioning:
  - Family Inventory of Life Event and Changes (FILE): www.mccubbinresilience.org/measures.html
  - Family Inventory of Resources for Management (FIRM): www.mccubbinresilience.org/measures.html

FAMILY THEORY

- The concept of "who is the family" is subject to the influences of culture and society.
- The historical view of the "family" as a nuclear family has evolved to changing forms such as extended family, single-parent family, blended family, and alternative families.
- The structure and function of the "family" is important to consider for the health and well-being of the patient. An acute illness or chronic condition impacts the economic resources, emotional health, and resilience of the family.

- To provide patient-centered care, the CNS must consider the impact on the patient and "family."
- Family systems (Kerr, 2019):
  - Refers to the concept of looking at the family as a cohesive emotional unit.
  - Understand individuals by their relationships with the people in their family.
- Resiliency Model of Family Stress, Adjustment and Adaption (McCubbin & McCubbin, 1993):
  - Used to facilitate the role of the family in the care of the patient.
  - *Level 1:* Adjustment phase—"how the family views the illness"
  - *Level 2:* Family capacity to adjust to the challenge of the illness
  - *Level 3:* Looks at the impact of the illness on the family

CAREGIVER ROLE

- A caregiver provides help to an individual who requires assistance with daily living due to old age, disease, mental disorder, or disability. Often, the caregivers are providing unpaid healthcare to adults.
- Caregiver burnout or stress can be defined as a state of emotional, mental, and physical exhaustion related to the burden of caregiving.
- Approximately 34.2 million Americans have provided unpaid care to an adult aged 50 or older in the prior 12 months (The National Alliance for Caregiving and AARP Public Policy Institute, 2015).
- Caregiver strain and burden speak to the difficulties in assuming the role of the caregiver.
- Signs of caregiver strain and burden (Mayo Clinic, 2019):
  - Change in physical well-being (such as weight loss or gain, personal hygiene neglect, complaints of fatigue, headaches, or pain)
  - Change in health behaviors (such as increased smoking or drinking, eating less or more, difficulty sleeping, cutting back on personal leisure activities)
  - Changes in psychosocial behaviors (such as anger, irritability, anxiety)
  - Feelings of loss or inadequacy
- Strategies to manage caregiver strain and burden (Mayo Clinic, 2019):
  - Take steps to preserve your physical health.
  - Seek education and resources to support your role as a caregiver.
  - Ask for help from other family members or friends
  - Be realistic and flexible on what you can provide.
  - Respite care: short-term care provided for individuals to provide a break to their caregivers.
- Resources for caregivers:
  - Look for community resources such as Council on Aging and church-based programs
  - AARP: www.AARP.org
  - National Alliance for Caregiving: www.caregiving.org

ADULT IMMUNIZATIONS

- Vaccinations are a critical step to help adults with prevention against communicable diseases. Vaccinations are given throughout the life span, including in older adulthood (Table 20.16).

TABLE 20.16 ADULT VACCINATION SCHEDULE

VACCINE	POPULATION	ADMINISTRATION SCHEDULE	CONTRAINDICATONS	NOTES
Influenza	All adults	One dose annually	Hive-only egg allergy; if other egg allergy, administer in medical setting with preparations to manage reaction	
Td, Tdap (tetanus diphtheria, pertussis)	All adults	One dose Tdap, then Td booster every 10 years		One dose is recommended with each pregnancy, during weeks 27–36
MMR	All adults	One–two doses	Pregnancy, immunocompromised, HIV CD4+ count <200	
VAR	All adults	Twodoses	Pregnancy, immunocompromised, HIV CD4+ count <200	Administer to those without evidence of immunity to varicella Administer 4–8 weeks apart
RZV (preferred) or ZVL	>50 years >60 years	Two doses One dose	Pregnancy, immunocompromised, HIV CD4+ count <200	Administer 2–6 months apart
HPV	Up to age 26 years (female) Up to age 21 (male)	Two–three doses (depending on age at initiation of series)		
PCV13	≥65 years	One dose		1 dose PPSV23 at least 1 year after PCV13
PPSV23	≥65 years	One dose		Those <65 should get one–twodoses if other indications present
HepA	All adults if risk factors present	Two–three doses		For adults with specified risk factors
HepB	All adults if risk factors present	Three doses		For adults with specified risk factors Available three-dose HepB or combined HepA–HepB
Meningococcal (MenACWY)	All adults	One–two doses, then booster every 5 years		Dosing and frequency varies based on risk factors
MenB	All adults if risk factors present	Two–three doses		
Hib (*Haemophilus influenzae* type b vaccine)	All adults if risk factors present	One or three doses		Recommended for adults with sickle cell disease, hematopoietic stem cell transplant

Note: Adults are classified as age 19 years and older.

HPV, human papillomavirus vaccine; MMR, measles, mumps, rubella; PCV13, 13-valent pneumococcal conjugate vaccine; PPSV23, 23-valent pneumococcal polysaccharide vaccine; VAR, varicella; ZVL, zoster live-attenuated vaccine.

Source: Adapted from Centers for Disease Control and Prevention. (2019). *Recommended adult immunization schedule.* https://www.cdc.gov/vaccines/schedules/downloads/adult/adult-combined-schedule.pdf; Immunization Action Coalition. (2011). *Summary of recommendations for adult immunization.* http://www.immunize.org/catg.d/p2011.pdf

- Some vaccinations provide a near complete life-span immunity, whereas others require readministration periodically.
- The effects of vaccinations vary from protection against the disease to minimization of symptoms, if exposed.
- Vaccines are produced in oral, intranasal, and injection formats, of which most adult vaccinations are injections.

The most current vaccination schedules can be found on the Centers for Disease Control and Prevention (CDC) website.

REVIEW QUESTIONS

1. As a clinical nurse specialist you are assessing a newly admitted patient. The patient has been weak with nausea and vomiting as his chief complaint. His body mass index (BMI) is 38, and although weak, he is ambulating without difficulty. The patient states he has loss of appetite and has not eaten for the last 3 days. One of your primary concerns with this patient would be:
   A. Malnutrtion
   B. Risk of infection
   C. Immobility
   D. Fluid overload

2. Lack of sleep has been linked in studies to all of the following except:
   A. Depression
   B. Falls
   C. Weight loss
   D. Cardiovascular disease

ANSWERS

1. **Correct answer: A. Rationale:** Being overweight does not mean that the individual is nutritionally sound. Their intake could be made up of empty nutrients devoid of essential vitamins and minerals necessary for health. Because the patient has not eaten for 3 days, this is an even greater concern and can lead to many unnecessary complications. Risk of infection is always a concern, but there are no obvious sources or signs of infection at this time. Immobility is also a concern to address, but the patient is currently mobilizing appropriately. Fluid overload is not a concern; the patient is most likely dehydrated due to lack of intake.

2. **Correct answer: C. Rationale:** Lack of sleep is associated with obesity, not weight loss. Lack of sleep has been shown to increase the risk for depression, falls, and cardiovascular disease.

REFERENCES

The complete reference and additional reading lists appear in the digital version of this chapter, at https://connect.springerpub.com/content/book/978-0-8261-7417-8/part/part02/chapter/ch20

21 Advocating for Patients and Nurses

Melissa A. Wilson, Michelle J. Kidd, Lori Delaney, Jo. M. Tabler, Patricia Gilman, M. Jane Swartz, Theodore J. Walker, Jr., and Natalie Baird

CONSULTATION PRINCIPLES AND CONCEPTS

OVERVIEW

Definition of Consultation

A role or function used by clinical nurse specialists (CNSs) to offer their own clinical expertise to other colleagues or to seek additional information to enhance their own practice (Tracy & O'Grady, 2019). It refers to indirect provision of care through helping others implement change (Fulton et al., 2010):

- Case specific
- Individual
- Group specific to staff or patients or system
- Integrated into direct care roles
- Occurs in all specialties of advanced practice nursing
- Overview
- Consultation should be considered a core competency of all CNS roles

Purpose

The purpose is to improve outcomes, enhance healthcare delivery systems, extend the knowledge available to solve clinical problems, foster ongoing professional development of consultee, or a combination of these goals (Hamric 2019).

Conceptual Models of Consultation

- Benner's research on clinical expertise included *seven domains of practice* in which consultation is embedded:
  - Helping role
  - Administering and monitoring therapeutic interventions and regimens
  - Effective management of rapidly changing situations
  - Diagnostic and monitoring functions
  - Teaching–coaching function
  - Monitoring and ensuring the quality of healthcare practices
  - Organizational and work role competencies (Fulton et al., 2010)
- Barron and White—Degree of clinical responsibility
  - Consultation is distinguished by the degree to which the nurses assumes direct responsibility for clinical management.
  - Consultants are generally not responsible for direct management of the clinical dilemma for which they are consulting.
  - Consultee assumes responsibility for the clinical outcome and is free to use or not use the advice offered by the consultant.
- Caplan's four models of consultation—Center of focus
  - Client-centered case consultation (most common)
  - Consultee-centered case consultation
  - Program-centered administrative consultation
  - Consultee-centered administrative approach

Outcome Evaluation of Clinical Nurse Specialist Consultation

- The consultation role is often integrated into other work tasks and is sometimes difficult to quantify.
- It is essential to show quantifiable results/outcomes of CNS practice.
- The literature supports the efficacy of CNS consultants' promotion of cost savings and improved patient outcomes (Zuzelo, 2010).
  - Higher quality of care
  - Improved continuity of care
  - Augmented consistency in therapeutic interventions

Professional and Personal Attributes for the Clinical Nurse Specialist Consultation Role

- Manage conflict constructively and come to effective resolutions.
- Develop good interpersonal skills.
- Manage and value diversity (of patients, staff, organizations).
- Be culturally competent.
- Be autonomous, independent, and accountable.
- Develop self into a collaborative colleague.
- Work with and possibly disagree with other healthcare providers such as physicians, allied health therapists, and organizational administrators.
- Be comfortable with power
- Use power to create win–win situations

Through consulting, the CNS as a content expert provides an array of approaches to improve clinical outcomes. In addition to the many skills required in the CNS role, confidence, motivation, and negotiation skills are particularly important for consultation (Zuzelo, 2010).

Summary of the Statement on CNS Practice and Education

- Consultation concepts are the essential core content for CNS curricula.
- Content area focuses on consultation theory and research and the associated skills of serving as a clinical expert.

The complete reference and additional reading lists appear in the digital version of this chapter, accessible at https://connect.springerpub.com/content/book/978-0-8261-7417-8/part/part02/chapter/ch21

- Consultation skills are essential when working with patients/clients, nurses, or other healthcare providers.
- Consultation activities promote collaboration with other healthcare professionals, solving complex patient problems, developing best practice models, and improving systems of care (National Association of Clinical Nurse Specialists [NACNS], 2004).

INTERPROFESSIONAL COLLABORATION

Caring for the adult and aged population entails assisting clients with complex physical, emotional, social, cognitive, and financial issues associated with chronic diseases. When disciplines try solving problems from a singular perspective, the results are often fragmented and poorly coordinated. An interprofessional approach allows for integration of each discipline's strengths to coordinate a comprehensive plan of care for client problems.

Research has shown that more patients die when nurses and physicians fail to communicate. Collaboration is key for safe patient care and pivotal to the success of the CNS role. Positive patient outcomes are achieved through caring practices, clinical inquiry and judgment, facilitation of learning, responding to diversity, and serving as a change agent using systems thinking. Outcomes are best realized when the CNS uses expert knowledge and skills in collaboration with other professionals (Foster, 2007).

Definition of Terms

- **Collaboration:** A dynamic interpersonal process in which two or more individuals make a commitment to each other to interact authentically and constructively to clarify complex patient problems, find solutions to those problems, and provide services to achieve identified goals, purposes, or outcomes (Hanson & Spross, 2019).
- **Interprofessional team**: A group of healthcare (physicians, nurses, pharmacists, dieticians) and social care (behavioral specialists, social workers) professionals working together to provide patient-centered care (Szafran et al., 2018).
- **Patient-centered care:** Care provision that is respectful of, and responsive to, individual patient preferences, needs, and values and that ensures that patient values guide clinical decisions (Institute of Medicine [IOM], 2015).

Domains of collaboration—CNSs execute the collaboration competency in several domains (Hanson & Spross, 2019):

- **Individuals**—Forming partnerships with patients/families and individual clinicians
- **Teams/groups**—Facilitating teamwork to ensure delivery of effective, high-quality care
- **Organization**—Shaping advanced practice nursing and clinical care
- **Global arenas**—Working across countries to provide patient care and volunteer

Characteristics of collaboration: Characteristics overlap and interlink because many are mutually dependent on others for full collaboration (Summer, 2014).

- Clear goals that everyone on the team works toward
- Clarity about each team member's role and contributions
- Clear and open communication
- Effective decision-making
- Engagement of all members in the work of the team
- Appreciation of diversity in terms of generation, culture, and thinking
- Effective conflict management
- Trust among members

- Cooperative relationships
- Participative leadership
- Collaboration is *not* (Hanson & Spross, 2019)
  - Parallel communication,
  - Parallel functioning,
  - Information exchange,
  - Coordination,
  - Consultation,
  - Comanagement, or
  - Referral.

Types of Collaboration

- **Multidisciplinary**—Different disciplines but staying *within* their boundaries
- **Interdisciplinary**—*Between* disciplines, into a coordinated whole
- **Transdisciplinary**—*Across* disciplinary boundaries to provide integrated services to clients

Benefits of Collaboration

- For patients
  - Improved quality of care
  - Increased patient satisfaction
  - Lower mortality rate
  - Improved patient outcomes
  - Patients feel more secure, cared for, and closer to nurses
- For nurses
  - Improved clinical expertise
  - Crisis management
  - Managing life-sustaining functions in unstable patients
  - Decreased turnover
  - Monitoring quality and identifying gaps
  - Improved clinical leadership and mentoring
- For providers
  - Increased sharing of responsibility
  - Increased sharing of expertise
  - More mutually satisfying problem solving
  - Increased personal satisfaction
  - Increased quality of professional life
  - Enhanced mutual trust and respect
  - Improved management of chronic diseases
  - Avoidance of redundant care and ensures coverage

Consequences of Failure to Collaborate

- For organizations
  - Lack of or uncoordinated teamwork and "handoffs"
  - Disruption of continuity of care
  - Increase in disruptive behaviors
- For individual providers
  - Negative job satisfaction and attitudes
  - Increased turnover (Hanson & Spross, 2019)

Barriers to Collaboration

- Disciplines learning and working in silos
- Ineffective communication
- Team dysfunction–disruptive behavior
  - Absence of trust and respect
  - Fear of conflict
  - Lack of commitment
  - Avoidance of accountability
  - Inattention to results
- Lack of clearly defined roles
- Misalignment of patient goals
- Lack of team skills and input (Szafran et al., 2018)

Strategies for Successful Collaboration

- Individual strategies
  - Listen and encourage others
  - APRNs promote their exemplary nursing practices
  - Participate in interdisciplinary quality-improvement initiatives
  - Evaluation of evidence-based practice guidelines
  - APRNs role model their practice strategies
  - Work together on joint projects
  - Social opportunities at conferences
  - Collaboratively developed practice guidelines (Hanson & Spross, 2019)
- Team strategies
  - Team activities to build trust
  - Build a group of like-minded individuals; be a role model for those who are not engaged in collaboration
- Organizational strategies
  - Magnet requirements
  - Joint Commission requirements
  - Create tool kits to facilitate the adoption of evidence-based practice guidelines
  - Take action to eliminate disruptive behavior

ADVOCATING FOR NURSES AND THE CLINICAL NURSE SPECIALIST ROLE

TERMS

Public policy: Policy made at the legislative, executive, and judicial branches of federal, state, and local levels of government that affects individual behaviors under the respective government's jurisdiction. These policies include congressional legislation signed by the president, legislative amendments, and court's judicial decisions. Defense policy, domestic policy, and foreign policy are the three major sectors that are categorized by allocative or regulatory type.

Health policy: The development by government and other policy makers of present and future objectives pertaining to healthcare and the healthcare system and the articulation of arguments and decisions regarding these objectives in legislation, judicial opinions, regulations, guidelines, standards, and so forth that affect healthcare and public health (National Institutes of Health [NIH], n.d.). Health policy falls under domestic policy and includes programs within the Department of Health and Human Services.

Healthcare reform: The ongoing process of change involving those who receive care, why and how they receive care, and the payment structures around care delivery.

ADVOCATING FOR THE CNS ROLE

Although all four CNS groups are skilled in direct patient care, either as individual practitioners or as members of interprofessional teams, CNSs use their skills in systems and nursing practice spheres of influence in addition to patient care. CNSs are trained to view healthcare through a global systems perspective and to implement changes in processes with the intent to improve the health outcomes of individuals and populations. As a change agent, the CNS is adept at identifying inefficiencies in care processes, developing potential solutions, implementing change, testing, and evaluating processes to improve care

delivery and patient care outcomes efficiently and cost effectively. In addition, because of their education and skills, CNSs make ideal candidates for informing on public and health policy issues that relate to nursing practice, patient care, and system processes.

PUBLIC POLICY

For decades, nurses have been advocating for patients' rights, patient care, and for nurses' professional practice autonomy and recognition to use their education and knowledge within their specified scope of practice. Advocating for autonomy and recognition is reason enough to understand and participate in the policy-making process at any level. Part of the profession's moral and ethical code is to engage and advocate for public health and welfare (American Nurses Association [ANA], 2015). Furthermore, CNSs are mandated to promote initiatives that improve quality care and health outcomes (NACNS, 2004).

The need for nurses' voice at the public policy table has frequently been overlooked. At the national level, only five nurses have seats in the 116th Congress. At the community level, city council members may not be health professionals, limiting their understanding of the health needs of populations and individuals within a community. Including CNSs would provide valuable insight regarding population health, systems processes, and nursing practice when policy discussions are taking place at the local, state, and national levels. The contribution of the CNS as an expert clinician and public health advocate on community councils and boards provides awareness and advice on appropriate public services, programs, and healthcare. Moreover, CNSs can foresee the consequences of change in policy that otherwise might not be recognized and provide evidence-based guidance to stakeholders.

Involvement in policy requires networking and relationship building. It is helpful to get to know key individuals who work with legislators or stakeholders who might be able to provide information on upcoming initiatives and legislative activities. Keeping oneself informed of current legislative activity is important to timing the approach to stakeholders and lawmakers. State and the federal governments have websites describing the current agenda and legislation including the status of bills, amendments, laws, sponsors, and contact information. Professional nursing organizations often have political action committees that follow current policy agendas and activities to inform members of what is needed to push through an initiative. Getting involved and keeping abreast of the current policy climate through a professional nursing organization is one of the best ways to engage in policy work.

Public Policy Formation

Many factors influence policy making, including individuals; organizations; interest groups; social, environmental, and political preferences; bias; and the policy itself. The process is complex. Therefore, policies must be scrutinized, evaluated, and reevaluated for potential unintended consequences resulting from policy development or change. Longest (1998) described six phases of policy development, summarized as follows:

- **Problem identification and agenda setting:** The first step of policy making in which problems are ranked and compete for political support to be recognized on their merit to continue in the process. Also referred to as passing through the policy window (Kingdon, 1995).

- **Formulation and development:** The problem-solving phase where alternative policies are developed.
- **Adoption:** The acceptance of the policy alternative, including regulation and legislation; requires a legislative majority, agency directors' consensus, or court decision.
- **Implementation:** The compliance phase of policy formation, where administrations provide labor and fiscal resources to carry out adopted policy.
- **Assessment:** The evaluation phase to determine if the implemented policy follows statutory requirements and if the intended objective has been met.
- **Modification:** The decision whether to maintain, modify, or eliminate the policy.

The policy-making process is dynamic. Proposed policies can modulate between different phases at different times depending on the problem, the stakeholders involved, the level of importance, and timeliness of the process. Engagement with professional organizations is valuable because of their size and ability to monitor the political climate to take advantage of the appropriate time to introduce a problem and determine who would be the most suitable policy maker to approach for support. The National Association of Clinical Nurse Specialists (NACNS), in collaboration with other professional organizations, has set national policy recommendations for legislative and regulatory change related to the nursing workforce, health reform, and health information technology based on data that indicate a pressing need for change. Current advocacy includes targeting specific congressional committees to present legislative proposals that recognize the full scope of practice and prescriptive authority for APRNs in all healthcare settings across all states. Among the top initiatives supporting CNS practice and access to care are advocacy for changes in legislation and regulation that remove barriers and do not impose new barriers to CNS practice such as requiring supervision by medical doctors, osteopaths, or dentists. More information can be accessed on the NACNS website (https://nacns.org/advocacy-policy).

Healthcare Reform

Healthcare reform affects every aspect of the healthcare system. Federal and state government cutbacks on healthcare programs are large-scale factors that affect the ability of individuals to access care. CNSs are equipped to respond to the needs of healthcare systems, nursing practice, and patients and families across the healthcare continuum to facilitate optimal care delivery and outcomes.

Advanced practice professional organizations such as NACNS are advocating for healthcare reform to include CNSs in reimbursement for services across all settings, including home care. Other healthcare reform efforts in collaboration with nurse organizations include advocating for CNS recognition and validation as contributors in value-based purchasing, accountable care organizations, and primary care medical homes. CNSs are well educated as leaders of change and are essential contributors to the dialogue on healthcare reform.

Healthcare Technology

Advocating for innovative and appropriate use of technology to accommodate the needs of patients, staff, and systems is a significant role of CNSs. Additionally, as frontline leaders, CNSs are in the position to evaluate and inform national and state-level policy makers on the need for efficient practitioner-friendly software systems that contribute to appropriate and meaningful use of healthcare information technology to produce valuable data. Such data provide the bases for evidence-based practice, patient care, and research.

PROFESSIONAL PRACTICE

Accountability

Accountability is a required attribute of CNS practice to ensure appropriate and responsible use of patient, public, staff, and organization resources. CNSs should become familiar with system financial tools to develop an understanding of budgetary constraints that might affect the implementation of processes to improve patient care. Understanding resource allocation and prioritizing specific patient care and unit, staff, and system needs facilitate the ability to evaluate problems and provide appropriate solutions successfully (Tracy & Lindquist, 2007).

Certification

The federal government defines the CNS as a master's prepared nurse who has been educated in a clinical nurse specialist program with certification as an advanced practice nurse from an accredited credentialing organization and is the standard required to obtain Medicare provider status. State regulations are inconsistent, however, leading to confusion and inappropriate use of the CNS title. Some states require certification for licensure as a CNS and the privilege to use the CNS title. Other states do not recognize the CNS as an CNS and may not require certification or a master's degree for licensure.

Several certifying agencies offer CNS specialty certification examinations (see Chapter 1). Agencies acknowledge that there is a lack of certification exams for some specialties. A major contributing factor is the considerable cost associated with exam development.

Prescriptive Authority

CNSs are APRNs specializing in the care of complex conditions and vulnerable populations. The ability to provide safe, comprehensive care depends on the CNS's ability to use advanced skills in assessment, diagnosis, and interventions including pharmacologic and durable medical equipment therapies in an individualized plan of care. Advanced graduate-level course work in pharmacology, pathophysiology, and health assessment are required education for all certified APRNs, including CNSs who intend to practice at the advanced level. Each state has specific regulations regarding prescriptive authority. States regulate CNS prescriptive authority through their boards of nursing alone or in conjunction with boards of medicine and pharmacy (Federal Trade Commission, 2014). CNSs who intend to prescribe must be aware of the regulatory body and regulation within the state they practice (ANA, 2016).

Collaborative Practice

Collaboration is an essential standard of professional performance for the CNS (NACNS, 2004). The current state of healthcare necessitates collaboration in a quickly changing environment where optimal healthcare outcomes require input from multiple professional practitioners.

Legal Concerns

Legislative regulation of CNS practice includes both title protection and the scope of practice as specified in each state's regulation. State laws grant the CNS authority to practice and hold CNSs accountable for nursing practice at the advanced level. States that do not recognize the CNS title potentiate the misuse of the title by individuals who are not prepared and qualified to practice as APRNs. State regulation should recognize the CNS scope of practice with specificity and hold accountable those who practice as APRNs.

In 2008, the National Council of State Boards of Nursing APRN Advisory Committee and the APRN Consensus Work Group developed the APRN Consensus Model (2008). The Consensus Model is a framework to guide states in adopting uniform regulation and laws regarding CNS roles and practice. The objective is to have consistency from state to state for licensure, accreditation, certification, and education (LACE) for all APRNs. As of October 2018, 28 states and the District of Columbia have implemented recommendations set by the Consensus Model (Phillips, 2019). However, until all states establish consistent laws and regulations, APRNs, including CNSs, who practice in more than one state or live in one state and practice in another, must be aware of each state's requirements and differences and adjust their scope of practice accordingly.

ADVOCATING FOR PATIENTS, EQUITABLE HEALTHCARE, AND PATIENT RIGHTS AND PREFERENCES

OVERVIEW

Provision 3 of the American Nurses Association (ANA) *Code of Ethics* (2015) states, "The nurse promotes, advocates for, and protects the rights, health, and safety of the patient" (ANA, 2015, p. 9). The nurse must incorporate the following measures into practice to adhere to this provision:

- Protection of the rights of privacy and confidentiality
- Protection of human participants in research
- Performance standards and review mechanisms
- Professional responsibility in promoting a culture of safety
- Protection of patient health and safety by acting on questionable practice
- Patient protection and impaired practice

Equitable Healthcare

Advocating for patients includes working to ensure that healthcare is equitable for all people. Provision 8 of the ANA *Code of Ethics* (2015) states, "The nurse collaborates with other health professionals and the public to protect human rights, promote health diplomacy, and reduce health disparities" (ANA, 2015, p. 31). The nursing profession holds to the principle that health is a universal right; nurses commit to advancing the health, welfare, and safety of individuals and communities; nurses work with others to provide a robust response for creative solutions to reduce health disparities; and nurses are mindful of competing moral values and are working to bring attention to human rights violations.

Equitable healthcare is the access to resources needed to improve and maintain health by overcoming inequalities that infringe on fairness and human rights norms of individuals or groups, whether those groups are defined socially, economically, demographically, or geographically (World Health Organization [WHO], 2019). Removing health inequities is often a complex process that incorporates more than just delivering healthcare but also implementing interventions that redress the inequities such as law reform, economics, or social reform. In 2010, the passage of the Patient Protection and Affordable Care Act (ACA) required the U.S. healthcare system to accommodate an increase in demand for health services. It noted that nurses are in a unique position to lead these efforts for a better integrated healthcare system by providing patient-centered, accessible, and affordable care (IOM, 2011).

Patient Rights and Preferences

Patients have certain rights and preferences protected by federal and state law. For example, the Patient Bill of Rights, created by the Affordable Care Act (Medicare, 2011), gave patients protections related to insurance companies. There are other Patient Bill of Rights declarations that protect certain vulnerable populations such as Mental Health Bill of Rights, Hospice Bill of Rights, and Rights of People in Hospitals.

The CNS has the responsibility to incorporate patient and family values and preferences into care planning and delivery. The direct-care sphere of impact of CNS practice involves the patient/family; This practice includes reflecting the patient/family treatment preferences, weighed with available resources, into the treatment plan (NACNS, 2019).

Core Clinical Nurse Specialist Competencies for Advocating for Patients

A CNS has the responsibility to identify, articulate, and take action on ethical concerns at the patient, family, healthcare provider, community, and public policy levels.

At the system level, the CNS has the ethical responsibility to lead change, manage, and empower others to influence clinical practice and political processes both within and across systems. This includes fostering a healthy work environment (HWE), where nursing practice and system interventions can promote patient, family, and community health needs and safety.

Specific Adult-Gerontology CNS Competencies

- Advocates for the patient's preferences and rights.
- Analyzes the ethical impact of scientific advances, including cost and clinical effectiveness, on patient and family values and preferences.
- Advocates for equitable healthcare by participating in professional organizations and public policy activities.
- Advocates for ethical principles in protecting dignity, uniqueness, and safety of all.
- Advocates for equitable healthcare by participating in professional organizations and public policy activities.

ADVOCATING FOR ETHICAL PRINCIPLES

OVERVIEW

The overarching ethical framework for nurses is guided by the ANA *Code of Ethics* (2015). This is a nonnegotiable ethical standard of the ethical values, obligations, duties, and professional ideals of nurses individually and collectively (ANA, 2015). It expresses to society the ANA's commitment, beliefs, and values and provides a framework for ethical nursing practice.

One of the essential characteristics of CNS practice is ethical conduct (Fulton et al., 2014). To function optimally in the CNS role, the CNS must have an ethical foundation and be knowledgeable in ethical reasoning to make decisions. In the United States, a wide variety of ethical frameworks have shaped contemporary healthcare, such as utility-based ethics, duty-based ethics, virtue-based ethics, law-based ethics, rights-based ethics, and feminist ethics (Tong, 2007). Each of these ethical theories provides a certain viewpoint or framework to influence ethical practice and decision-making. According to the NACNS *Statement on Clinical Nurse Specialist Practice and Education* (2019), nursing's ethical framework and social mandate are fully described by the ANA *Code of Ethics* (2015). Adhering to this framework is a moral obligation of the CNS, and its concepts are directly connected to the provisions of ethical conduct for a nurse in the ANA *Code of Ethics* (2015; NACNS, 2019).

Advocating for ethical principles Includes the following:

- Fostering autonomy and truth telling
- Advocating for patients, families, and other nurses
- Assisting with patients and families to approach end-of-life issues with dignity
- Mentoring nurses and other professionals to deliver safe and equitable care
- Engaging in a formal self-evaluation process, seeking feedback regarding own practice from patients, peers, professional colleagues, and others
- Fostering professional accountability in self and others
- Facilitating resolution of ethical conflicts by
  - Identifying the ethical implications of complex care situations,
  - Considering the impact of scientific advances, costs, clinical effectiveness, patient and family values and preferences, and other external influences, and
  - Applying ethical principles to resolving concerns across the three spheres of influences.
- Promoting a practice environment conducive to providing ethical care
- Facilitating interdisciplinary teams to address ethical concerns, risks or considerations, benefits, and outcomes of patient care
- Facilitating patient and family understanding of the risks, benefits, and outcomes of proposed healthcare regimen to promote informed decision-making
- Advocating for equitable patient care by
  - Participating in organizational, local, state, national, or international level of policy-making activities for issues related to their expertise, and
  - Evaluating the impact of legislative and regulatory policies as they apply to nursing practice and patient or population outcomes.
- Promoting the role and scope of practice of the CNS to legislators, regulators, other healthcare providers and the public:
  - Communicating information that promotes nursing, the role of the CNS and outcomes of nursing and CNS practice through the use of the media, advanced technologies, and community networks
- Advocating for the CNS/APRN role and for positive legislative response to issues affecting nursing practice

ADVANCED COMMUNICATION CONCEPTS

OVERVIEW

A groundbreaking report was published by the National Academy of Medicine (NAM), formerly known as the *Institute of Medicine (IOM)*, entitled *To Err Is Human*, which called out communication as a major downfall of healthcare, resulting in massive errors and human demise (Kohn et al., 2000). A follow-on report entitled *The Future of Nursing: Leading Change, Advancing Health* (2011) identifies good communication skills as a key contributing factor to optimization of the healthcare

system and improving safety (IOM, 2011). The Joint Commission reports breakdown of communication is a major determinant of adverse health events (The Joint Commission, 2014). The CNS holds an integral role that requires use of advanced communication skills to navigate complex, unpredictable situations while caring for patients through the health continuum (NACNS, 2016). Throughout the CNS competencies, skilled communication techniques are required to optimize health outcomes. "To be a leader, the CNS must be a skilled communicator and educator who is capable of identifying patterns and using disciplined inquiry/research and ethical reasoning to make decisions, describe reality, and anticipate the future accurately" (NACNS, 2004, p. 18).

Critical Elements of Skilled Communication

The AACN Standards for Establishing and Sustaining Healthy Work Environments (American Association of Colleges of Nursing [AACN], 2016) identifies critical elements of skilled communication for healthcare organizations and practitioners.

Critical elements for organizations include the following:

- Support interprofessional education and coaching to develop critical communication skills.
- Zero-tolerance policies for abuse and other disrespectful behavior in the workplace.
- Ensure effective and respectful information sharing among patients, families, and the healthcare team.
- Formally evaluate the impact of communication on clinical and financial outcomes and the work environment.
- Require skilled communication as a criterion of performance appraisal and demonstration of skilled communication to qualify for professional advancement.

Critical elements for healthcare practitioners include the following:

- Focus on finding solutions and achieving desirable outcomes.
- Strive to protect and advance collaborative relationships among colleagues.
- Invite and hear all relevant perspectives.
- Call upon goodwill and mutual respect to build consensus and arrive at a common understanding.
- Demonstrate congruence between words and actions and hold others accountable for the same.
- Access and proficiently use appropriate communication technologies.
- Solicit input on communication style and strive to continually improve.
- Identify personal learning and professional growth needs related to communication skills (AACN, 2016).

Crucial Conversations

The newest *Statement on Clinical Nurse Specialist Practice and Education* (NACNS, 2019) specifically identifies "crucial conversations" as an important interpersonal communication skill of the CNS. Crucial conversations are discussions between two or more people where the stakes are high, opinions vary, and emotions run strong (Patterson et al., 2012). The ability to effectively communicate with patients/families, nurses, and nursing personnel and representatives from other disciplines at all levels of the system is essential for CNS practice (NACNS, 2019). Advanced communication skills within therapeutic relationships are utilized to improve care (AACN, 2010). The CNS must often build trust within a short period of time and utilize that trust to improve care. Building trust relies on effective communication and leadership skills (NACNS, 2019).

Conflict Management

The CNS utilizes skillful guidance and teaching to advance care. This will require the CNS to use leadership, team building, negotiation, and conflict resolution skills to build partnerships within and across systems, including communities (NACNS, 2016). Resolving conflict will often require the skills of an effective communicator, leader, and negotiator and may include situations that have ethical or moral contexts. Guiding ethical principles such as accountability, advocacy, autonomy, beneficence, fidelity, justice, nonmaleficence, and respect for persons should be utilized to lead amicable ethical conflict resolution.

Interviewing

Skilled interviewing techniques include the following (Bickley, 2017):

■ Building the relationship	■ Empathetic responses
■ Active listening	■ Validation
■ Guided questioning	■ Reassurance
■ Nonverbal communication	■ Partnering with the patient
■ Transitioning	■ Summarization
■ Empowering the patient	

Situations that require the CNS to adapt interviewing techniques are as follows:

■ The silent patient	■ The patient with a language barrier
■ The confusing patient	■ The patient with low literacy or low health literacy
■ The patient with altered cognition	■ The patient with hearing or vision impairment
■ The talkative patient	■ The patient with limited intelligence
■ The crying patient	■ The patient with personal problems
■ The angry or disruptive patient	■ The seductive patient

Topics requiring sensitive approaches are as follows:

■ Abuse of alcohol, prescription, or illicit drugs	■ Family interactions
■ Sexual practices	■ Domestic violence
■ Death and dying	■ Psychiatric illnesses
■ Financial concerns	■ Physical deformities
■ Racial and ethnic experiences	■ Bowel function

Source: Bickley, L. S. (2017). Bates' guide to physical examination and history taking (12th ed.). Lippincott, Williams & Wilkins.

MORAL AGENCY AND ADVOCATING FOR ETHICAL PRINCIPLES

OVERVIEW

Moral agency/advocacy is described as "Working on another's behalf and representing the concerns of the patient/family and nursing staff; serving as a moral agent in identifying and helping to resolve ethical and clinical concerns within and outside the clinical setting"(Reed et al., 2007, p. 6). Advocacy is defined as the "act or process of pleading for, supporting, or recommending a cause or course of action" (ANA, 2015, p. 41). Advocacy can apply to an individual, group, population, society or issue.

Upon being licensed, a nurse commits to a set of professional values guided by the ANA Code of Ethics (2015). According to this code, nurses are moral agents and charged with advocating for ethical principles. Barriers, either internal or external to the nurse, may prevent nurses from properly advocating for their patients. Moral distress is the loss of moral integrity within the nurse that results from the inability to advocate in a way that brings moral resolution.

Ethical challenges may arise in any of the three spheres of impact in CNS practice. Ethical questions that challenge the nurse's moral integrity can stem from patient, practice, and systems/organizational situations. The NACNS has established core and population-specific competencies related to ethics, advocacy, and moral agency (NACNS, 2019).

Moral Distress

There is an irrefutable link between HWEs, patient safety, and nurse recruitment and retention (AACN, 2001). Depending on the frequency or intensity of a moral distress situation, nurses can suffer, impacting the patient, nursing practice, and the system/organization. Nurses experiencing moral distress will distance themselves from patients and families, lose their capacity to care, fail to deliver good care, communicate poorly with coworkers, suffer emotional distress, and experience symptoms of burnout (AACN, 2008). Nurses who remain at an institution and suffer with unresolved distress can perpetuate increased costs and poor patient satisfaction (Cimiotti et al., 2012; Epstein & Hamric, 2009). This issue is so significant that the AACN issued a policy position stating that every nurse and every employer of nurses is responsible for implementing programs and mitigating the effects of moral distress (AACN, 2008). Assessment of moral distress and interventions to lessen its impact have been particularly challenging due to the subjective and personal nature of the experience.

Moral resilience has been proposed as a promising direction for mitigating moral distress and suffering. This concept entails an individual's ability to sustain or restore their moral integrity when encountering a moral distress situation (Rushton, 2016). It calls for individuals, nurse leaders, researchers, groups, and organizations to work together to transform the culture to create conditions where moral and ethical practices can prosper.

Implementing six essential evidence-based standards for creating a healthy work environment (HWE) has repeatedly demonstrated improvement in the overall health of the work environment, leading to better nurse staffing and retention, less moral distress, and lower rates of workplace violence (AACN, 2019). These essential standards include the following:

- Skilled communication
- True collaboration
- Effective decision-making
- Appropriate staffing
- Meaningful recognition
- Authentic leadership

SOCIAL DETERMINANTS OF HEALTH

OVERVIEW

Health is affected by individual characteristics, such as gender and genetics, and by behaviors, such as diet, exercise, social habits, immunizations, health screenings, and seeking care when ill or injured. However, health is also influenced by the social, economic, and physical conditions in which people are born, live, learn, work, and age. These conditions are known as the social *determinants of health* and can help explain why some people are healthier than others and why some are not as healthy as they could be (Centers for Disease Control and Prevention, 2018; Healthy People 2020, n.d.-a).

Key Domains of Social Determinants of Health

Economic stability

■ Poverty ■ Employment	■ Food security ■ Housing stability

Education

■ Early childhood education and development ■ High school graduation	■ Enrollment in higher education ■ Language and literacy

Social and community context

■ Workplace conditions ■ Civic participation	■ Discrimination ■ Community cohesion ■ Incarceration

Health and healthcare

■ Access to healthcare ■ Access to primary care	■ Health insurance coverage ■ Health literacy

Neighborhood and built environment

■ Quality of housing ■ Access to transportation ■ Availability of healthy foods	■ Quality of water and air ■ Neighborhood crime and violence

Examples of the Health Impact of Social Determinants

- Access to parks and safe sidewalks is associated with physical activity in adults.
- Education is associated with longer life expectancy and health-promoting behaviors, such as regular physical activity, not smoking, routine health exams, and recommended health screenings.
- Readily available supermarkets and grocery stores increase access to affordable, healthy foods.
- Discrimination, stigma, or unfair treatment in the workplace can increase blood pressure, heart rate, and stress and undermine self-esteem and self-efficacy.
- Bullying can result in depression, use of illegal drugs, and suicidal behavior.

Understanding the social determinants of health and working to establish policies and programs that positively influence social, economic, and physical conditions can substantially improve the health of individuals and populations (Healthy People 2020, n.d.-a).

HEALTHCARE DISPARITIES AND VULNERABLE POPULATIONS

OVERVIEW

Many health concerns such as heart disease, asthma, obesity, diabetes, HIV/AIDS, viral hepatitis B and C, infant mortality, and violence disproportionately affect certain populations. Healthcare disparities are differences in health outcomes that are closely linked with social, economic, and/or environmental disadvantages and occur in the context of broader inequality (Healthy People 2020, n.d.-c; U.S. Department of Health & Human Services, n.d.).

Healthcare disparities negatively affect groups of people who systematically experience greater obstacles to healthcare due to the following:

■ Racial or ethnic group ■ Religion ■ Socioeconomic status ■ Gender ■ Age	■ Mental health ■ Cognitive, sensory, or physical disability ■ Sexual orientation or gender identity ■ Geographic location ■ Other characteristics historically linked to discrimination or exclusion

Disparities in healthcare not only affect the groups dealing with the disparities but also limit overall gains in quality of care and health for the broader population and result in unnecessary costs. Efforts to reduce disparities focus on vulnerable populations, which are groups of people at higher risk for experiencing healthcare disparities (U.S. Department of Health & Human Services, n.d.).

Vulnerable populations include the following:

■ People of color ■ Low-income groups ■ Women ■ Children	■ Older adults ■ Individuals with special healthcare needs ■ Individuals living in rural and inner-city areas

Elimination of Healthcare Disparities

Healthcare systems and clinicians can
- Provide education to increase cultural and communication competence of healthcare providers, and
- Improve care coordination and quality of care.

Individuals and families can
- Participate in community-led prevention initiatives, and
- Utilize community resources to improve health literacy.

Government entities, community organizations, educational institutions, and businesses can also play a part in the reduction of healthcare disparities (U.S. Department of Health & Human Services, n.d.).

PREVENTING BIAS IN CARE

OVERVIEW

Healthcare inequity affects the LGBTQ population. Care requirements of the LGBTQ population have received significant attention as a result of the IOM and Healthy People 2020 emphasis on best practices when caring for the unique health issues of LGBTQ persons. Healthcare inequity is closely tied to sexual and social stigma. Sexual stigma can be defined as the negative regard, inferior status, and relative powerlessness that society collectively assigns to nonheterosexuality behavior, identity, relationship, or community (Herek, 2007). Since 2011, The Joint Commission has issued a standard that requires hospitals to prohibit discrimination based on sexual orientation and gender identity (www.jointcommission.org/lgbt). Also since 2011, the Conditions of Participation of the federal Centers for

Medicare & Medicaid Services (CMS) have required hospitals to permit patients to designate visitors of their choosing and to prohibit discrimination in visitation based on sexual orientation and gender identity. The American Association of Critical Care Nurses 2016 Webinar Series described barriers to healthcare in two distinct modes: (1) delays in seeking care—fear of discrimination, subjection to violence, and fear of breach of confidentiality and (2) difficulty accessing healthcare—lack of partner benefits, prejudicial policies and procedures, and lack of LBGT healthcare (AACN, 2016). Disparity exists in an overall higher incidence of chronic stress, depression, anxiety, suicide, and drug/tobacco/alcohol use. As our population ages, LGBT seniors have a higher rate of isolation due to lack of family or social support. Much of this stigma is a result of the 1973 American Psychiatric Association judgment that homosexuality was a mental health disorder (Levin, 2016). The Emergency Nurses Association (ENA) highlighted Espinoza et al.'s (2014) research on experiences and attitudes of the LGBTQ age group 45 to 75 years, noting that 3 million adults older than 55 years identify as LGBT and that number is expected to double over the next 20 years (ENA, 2017). Knowledge of the data, history, stigma, and bias of the LGBT communities leverages the CNS to positively influence the attitudes and beliefs of the patient, nurse, and system.

Definitions

Sexuality and gender are at the heart of human expression. The terms are complex, multidimensional, and nonbinary. Differentiating between gender and sexuality will help the CNS better advocate for and collaborate with patients, family, and staff. Understanding the terminology of identity, expression, and sexuality will assist the CNS to advocate for their patient's complex health needs. Gender is a biophysical conception that is actualized as a binary set of identities either male or female, man or woman, or masculine or feminine. Gender may be thought of as a medically assigned term. Gender is often confused for biological sex; however, gender is independent of anatomy. Sex, however, is a descriptor of the anatomical state medically as the two phenotypes of male versus female. Body parts and sexual anatomy are often looked to for the determination of sex, that is, does your patient have a penis or a vagina? Gender identity is with whom the patient identifies or the inner sense of being a man or a woman. Identity is an internalized concept regardless of external appearance. Gender expression is a set of behaviors that has been socially determined to be masculine or feminine or how we communicate our identity to the world. Sexual orientation is a set of attractions, behaviors, and romantic feelings for men, women, or both. Sexual orientation is also fluid and has a broad spectrum connotation but often minimalized to homosexual, heterosexual, and bisexual. *Lesbian* has been used to describe women who are primarily attracted to women. *Gay* is used to define both men and women who have same-sex attractions. *Bisexual* is used to delineate persons who are attracted to both men and women. *LGBTI* is the term with the addition of the intersex population. *Intersex* refers to differences of sexual development (DSD) for which there is a variation of sex phenotypes, chromosomal, hormonal, or anatomical, such that one's sex is not congruent with the society's male versus female anatomical binary status. *Intersex* is an older term that is transitioning to the preferred *DSD*. When Q is added, Q may represent *queer* or *questioning*. These terms are fluid. The CNS should seek to understand the person's perception of the letters they use to describe themselves (Eckstrand & Ehrenfeld, 2016). Multiple organizations refer to the *Genderbread person* to enhance understanding of the terminology (Figure 21.1).

Meaningful Use

In 2016, the U.S. Department of Health & Human Services took a momentous stance in addressing inequalities affecting LGBTQ people in healthcare by including sexual orientation and gender-identity data in the electronic health record (EHR) requirements certified under the **Meaningful Use** program. The CMS and the Office of the National Coordinator (ONC) for Health Information Technology final rules necessitate all EHR systems qualified under stage 3 of Meaningful Use to authorize users to record, change, and access structured data on sexual orientation and gender identity. This requisite is a portion of the 2015 edition's demographics certification measure and incorporates sexual orientation and gender identity data to the 2015 edition's base EHR definition. The advantage to Meaningful Use compliance allows the practitioners at a facility to engage in open, healthy discussions associated with the LGBTQ patient's unique health needs such as preventive screening, assessment of risky sexual behavior that can transmit infection and HIV, and behavioral concerns related to stigma, such as suicidality (HEI, 2018). Success in collecting sexual orientation and gender identity information relies on a robust training program for staff on how to maintain patient privacy and confidentiality while asking the questions and recording the answers in the EHR.

Demographics

Sexual and gender minorities span across all demographics. Regardless of the CNS's specialty or practice location, all healthcare providers care for sexual and gender minority patients. The 2014 CDC National Health Interview Survey on sexual orientation of more than 33,000 people between the ages of 18 and 64 found 96% identify as straight, 1.6% gay or lesbian, 0.7% bisexual, and 1% as something else. The transgender population has been more difficult to determine because of the historical "don't ask, don't tell" era that was repealed in 2011, which left the "t" often unaddressed. However, using alternative estimation and prevalence data from sexual reassignment surgery, the transgender population is approximately 0.2% (Eckstrand & Ehenfeld, 2018).

Research funded by the IOM and the National Institutes of Health (NIH) found that the LBGTIQ populations experience stigma associated with their sexual and gender minority status, disproportionate behavioral risks and psychosocial health problems, and higher chronic disease risk factors when compared to their heterosexual and cisgender counterparts. The largest focus of research to date is on increased risk and incidence of HIV/AIDS and sexually transmitted disease. Research on the sexual health of minority women and transgender population is limited. The CNS may work with the systems diversity office to conduct novel research that may assist in the care of the LGBTIQ population (Coulter et al., 2014).

Assessment of the Patient
Communication

- Healthcare assumptions of "male" or "female" appearance can negatively affect outcomes if pertinent assessments are not made. For example, a "male" enters your facility for abdominal pain. This person has been undergoing gender reassignment treatment with testosterone. The healthcare providers assume the patient to be a male and do not do a pregnancy test. The patient goes to x-ray for an abdominal

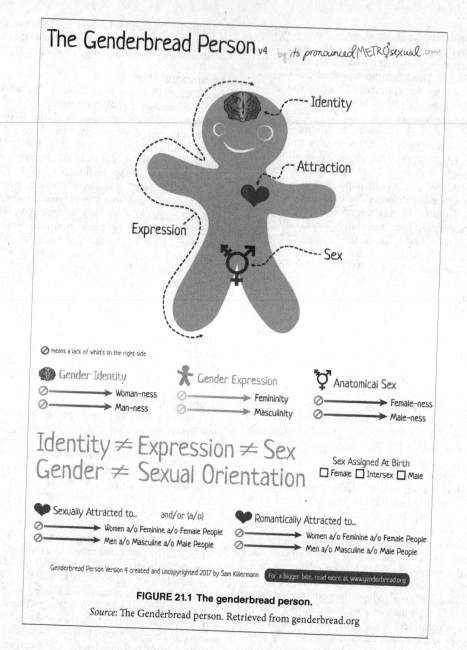

FIGURE 21.1 The genderbread person.

Source: The Genderbread person. Retrieved from genderbread.org

series. The x-ray technician sees fetal parts on the exam. Therefore, it is important to ask about sexual orientation and gender identity in your admission process and to relay only pertinent healthcare information to those needing information for healthcare-related interventions.

- Simply ask, "What is the patient's preferred name?" For instance, ask, "If I have to wake you from a deep sleep, what name would you prefer I shout? and "what pronoun do you use when you refer to yourself?"
- Identify the patient's support system. One approach is, "I see you have support here with you today. What are their names?"
- Using the patient language, identify the patient's partner by asking, "What do you call your partner, husband/wife, cousin?"
- Keep in line with Meaningful Use requirements. Your dialogue can start with, We ask this of all of our patients. "Do you think of yourself as straight or heterosexual, lesbian, gay or homosexual, bisexual, decline to answer, or not listed?" This is the sexual orientation descriptor in the electronic medical record (EMR) section.
- In addition, with Meaningful Use, ask, "What is your current gender identity?" Male, female, transgender male, transgender female, genderqueer neither exclusively male nor female, not listed, or decline to answer.
- Body language and a caring presence are needed to ensure your patient feels comfortable and welcome to answer the questions without fear of heterosexual bias.

Physical Assessment

- **Assess sexual organs only when necessary**: Assessment of sexual organs is only necessary when a complete history and physical is necessary or the chief complaints direct such assessment. For instance, if a person complains of abdominal pain, it is usual and customary to assess the abdomen and related sexual organs as part of the differential diagnosis. However, it is not usual and customary to assess the abdomen and related sexual organs for a simple sprained ankle.

- **Educate** the patient on the purpose of a **thorough healthcare exam** and the purpose of knowing what body parts exist and why they need to be examined. For instance, we need to rule out pelvic infections, we need to rule out testicular torsion, and so forth only as clinically relevant in the differential diagnosis.
- Discuss with the patient the importance of a **thorough medication review**. Reduce the incidence of medication-related interactions for those medications that may not be listed in an EMR or medication reconciliation list. Ensure any antiretroviral therapy (ART), nucleoside reverse transcriptase inhibitors (NRTIs), protease inhibitors, preexposure prophylaxis prevention (PrEP), or hormone therapy are listed.
- As appropriate, engage the partner in healthcare **multidisciplinary collaboration**. Older generations are less accepting of LGBTQ status because of strained relationships, bias, and stigma. Assist the patient to consider healthcare planning, power of attorney, medical power of attorney, and end-of-life decisions if the traditional family is not or has not been present for family support.

Prevention of Bias and Promotion of Equality

- Respect each patient for their uniqueness.
- All patients should feel safe when receiving care.
- Examine your own belief system and attitude.
- Ensure you are using facts not stereotypes.
- Learn about LGBTQ terminology.
- Refer to practice group position statements on the care and treatment of LGBTQ patients.
- Acknowledge real and perceived barriers.
- Establish a trusting relationship through open dialogue.
- Use appropriate interview techniques (open-ended questions) and ensure information is confidential.
- Identify and validate the patient's support system.
- Listen to the patient as they describe their partner or relationship.
- Use inclusive language.
- Promote zero tolerance for discrimination. Use crucial conversations in a private setting for colleagues, caregivers and patients who display bias.

Key Points

- If you use the wrong name or pronoun, apologize authentically and state you will not misstep next time.
- Avoid assumptions based on heterosexual norms.
- Avoid questions/examinations concerning transgender patients unless medically necessary. Do not use the transgender patient to educate the healthcare practitioner on care requirements.
- Explain the "why" behind standard safety checks. Medication administration may enforce using, "What is your name and date of birth?" These are the two unique identifiers for medication safety.
- Inquire about hormone therapy on the premise that medication interactions and adverse reactions can be reduced if the care team is knowledgeable of medication history: taking, recently, or abruptly stopped.
- Ensure and advocate for the post nondiscrimination policy at all points of entry.

- Collaborate with leadership, risk, and social services to ensure any policies are in alignment to assign patient rooms according to the patient's identified gender.
- Unisex bathrooms assist to alleviate stigma and bias. Moral distress for the transgender person is alleviated.
- Consider safe zones. Signage of the LGBT communities may be a visual clue to the inclusiveness of the organization.
- Collaborate with human resources and risk management to ensure that equal visitation policies are inclusive of all.
- Sensitivity training should include key audiences of leadership, nursing, registration, patient relations, human resources, legal, risk, and social work.
- Support groups allow for crucial conversations surrounding bias and stigma reduction to be discussed and solutions to be formulated by the diversity team.

Clinical Practice Resources

- ENA—Topic brief on care of the gender-expansive and transgender patient in the emergency care setting
- https://www.eeoc.gov/laws/guidance/what-you-should-know-eeoc-and-protections-lgbt-workers—Equal employment and opportunity related to the LGBTQ population
- Healthcare Equity Report—Provides purposeful focused interventions to guide healthcare systems provide friendly, welcoming environments
- *Standards of Care for the Health of Transsexual, Transgender, and Gender-Nonconforming People* by the World Professional Association for Transgender Health (WPATH; Coleman et al., 2012) offers clinical practice guidelines for hormone therapy dosing guidelines

CULTURAL COMPETENCE

OVERVIEW

Addressing the cultural beliefs of individuals in a multicultural society while providing high-quality healthcare presents a significant challenge for the CNS. In 2015, the ANA introduced the professional standard of Culturally Congruent Practice to meet the demands of the nursing profession's social contract with an increasingly diverse society:

- Standard 8: Culturally Congruent Practice—"The registered nurse practices in a manner that is congruent with cultural diversity and inclusion principles" (ANA, 2015a, p. 69).

Definition of Terms

- *Culturally congruent practice* is the "application of evidence-based nursing that is in agreement with the preferred cultural values, beliefs, worldview, and practices of the healthcare consumer and other stakeholders" (ANA, 2015a, p. 31).
- *Cultural competence* represents "the process by which nurses demonstrate culturally congruent practice. Nurses design and direct culturally congruent practice and services for diverse consumers to improve access, promote positive outcomes, and reduce disparities" (ANA, 2015a, p. 31).
- *Ethnicity* refers to a shared identity related to social and cultural heritage including values, language, geographical space, and racial characteristics.
- *Race* refers to common biologic attributes shared by a group.
- *Ethnocentrism* is the belief that one's own way of life is superior to all others' and can be the source of biases and prejudices.

Competencies for Culturally Congruent Practice (Standard 8)

- **For all nurses:** Demonstrate respect, equity, and empathy for all healthcare consumers; understand how nursing care of vulnerable cultural groups can be impacted by discrimination and oppression.
- **For graduate-level prepared nurses:** Ensure that healthcare organizations value diversity and inclusion and reflect respect and equity in their policies, services, and practices.
- **For APRNs:** Assume leadership roles in identifying cultural needs and promoting shared decision-making solutions for the consumer (ANA, 2015a, pp. 69–70).

Organizational Resources for Cultural Competence

Some public and governmental organizations provide standards and guidelines to help nurses and healthcare organizations meet patient cultural needs and achieve cultural competence. Healthcare providers and healthcare systems need to challenge themselves to gain competence in order to provide delineated care addressing the specific patient's, population's, or social system's need for cultural relevancy.

Transcultural Nursing Society

The Transcultural Nursing Society (TCNS) helps meet the changing global needs related to transcultural nursing and healthcare (Transcultural Nursing Society [TCNS], 2019). The organization's website (https://tcns.org/) contains key resources and information to enhance individual and organizational cultural competence. The TCNS endorses the following standards:

- Knowledge of cultures
- Education and training in culturally competent care
- Critical reflection
- Cross-cultural communication
- Culturally competent practice
- Cultural competence in healthcare systems and organizations
- Patient advocacy and empowerment
- Multicultural workforce
- Cross-cultural leadership
- Evidence-based practice and research

Culturally and Linguistically Appropriate Services

The National Standards for Culturally and Linguistically Appropriate Services (CLAS) were developed by the U.S. Department of Health and Human Services, Office of Minority Health, for the purpose of advancing health equity in a culturally diverse nation (Office of Minority Health, Health and Human Services,

2013). The CLAS standards (see Table 21.1) were designed as a guide for both healthcare providers and systems and offer a foundation for cultural competence.

Nursing Considerations for Key Cultural Groups

Table 21.2 illustrates major points related to differences and similarities between key cultural groups. Each group has additional specific items that cannot be mentioned within a single table format study tool. The references and websites listed in this chapter are excellent resources for current standards and additional cultural detail. Table 21.2 shows several commonalities across cultural groups that can form a foundation for successful patient interactions. Remember to exercise patience and approach individuals without preconceived ideas. Use an interpreter if indicated. Treat all patients, family, and extended family members with respect. Empathy is essential to provide quality healthcare interventions.

STAFF EDUCATION, COACHING, AND MENTORING

OVERVIEW

Staff Education

- A process to influence the behavior of the healthcare staff to impact their knowledge, skills, and attitudes.
- The learning outcomes can be in the cognitive, affective, and psychomotor domains.

Adult Teaching and Learning

- Learning is individualized
- Four types of learners: visual, auditory, reading/writing, and kinesthetic
- Knowles's adult learning principles (andragogy)
  - Adults need to be involved in the planning and evaluation of their instruction.
  - Life experiences (positive and negative) are the basis for the learning activities.
  - Adults are most interested in learning subjects that have immediate relevance and impact on their job or personal life.
  - Adult learning is problem centered.
- Teaching strategies for adults
  - Provide content relevant to their lives.
  - Connect the learning to past experiences.
  - Utilize extrinsic (outside the learner) motivators (such as acknowledgment of progress or praise).
  - Nurture intrinsic (within the learner) motivators (such as improvement in health, self-determination, personal value).

TABLE 21.1 CULTURALLY AND LINGUISTICALLY APPROPRIATE SERVICES STANDARDS

Principal standard 1	Provide effective, equitable, understandable, and respectful quality care and services that are responsive to diverse cultural health beliefs and practices, preferred languages, health literacy, and other communication needs.
Governance, leadership, and workforce	Standards 2 through 4: Organizations promote CLAS and health equity through culturally and linguistically appropriate policies and practices.
Communication and language assistance	Standards 5 through 8: Ensure free language assistance to individuals with limited English proficiency and/or other communication needs, to facilitate timely access to all healthcare and services; provide materials in languages commonly used in the service area.
Engagement, continuous improvement, and accountability	Standards 9 through 12: Organizations implement, evaluate, sustain CLAS to ensure services that respond to the cultural and linguistic diversity of populations.

CLAS, culturally and linguistically appropriate services.

Source: Adapted from National CLAS Standards https://minorityhealth.hhs.gov/omh/browse.aspx?lvl=2&lvlid=53

- Use problem solving to enhance learning.
- Facilitate learning rather than being the content expert.
■ Key learning principles
  - Active participation by the learner promotes learning.
  - Learning is influenced by the motivation and readiness of the learner.
  - Learning is influenced by the environment in which it occurs.
  - Positive and immediate feedback can facilitate the learning.
  - Learning is the shared responsibility of the learner and the teacher.

Designing Education Initiatives
The ASSURE Model (Rega)
■ The ASSURE Model is helpful to organize and implement an educational activity.
  - Analyze the learner.
  - State the objectives.
  - Select the instructional methods.
  - Use the instructional methods.
  - Require learner performance.
  - Evaluate the teaching plan and revise as necessary.

Planning
■ Determine the educational need. Conduct a gap analysis. What is desired state versus the current state?
■ Determine whether the gap is *do not know* (knowledge), *do not know how* (skill), or *unable to do in practice* (practice) or a combination.
  - **Example:** Knowledge gap—A novice nurse asks why a patient with an elevated blood glucose is receiving a fluid bolus.
  - **Example:** Skills gap—A new glucose-monitoring device is being implemented on a nursing unit.
  - **Example:** Practice gap—Following a chart audit, the CNS determines that 10% of the charts did not have documentation on the intervention for an elevated blood glucose.
■ Consider the value of interprofessional continuing education to promote interprofessional collaborative practice.
■ Select individuals to assist with the planning process.
■ Determine the target audience.
■ Sources for planning, implementing, and evaluation of continuing education activities:
  - **American Nurses Credentialing Center:** www.nursingworld.org
  - **Joint accreditation:** www.jointaccreditation.org

Design
■ Determining the gap will help drive the design.
■ Consider the characteristics of the target audience (e.g., profession, experience, licensed vs. unlicensed).
■ Identify the learning outcome. A learning outcome(s) is written as a statement that reflects what the learner will be able to do because of your learning activity. A learning outcome(s) is observable and measurable.

Development
■ Determine the content.
■ Consider the venue for the activity such as face to face, web-based learning, or simulation.
■ Judge the cost (return on investment) of the venue chosen.
■ Content is based on the most current evidence.

■ Content is balanced and unbiased. If providing contact hours, the content must be free of commercial interest.
■ Select the instruction method to meet the learning outcome and the needs of the target audience. Examples include the following:

- Lecture	- Demonstration and return demonstration
- Team-based learning	
- Seminar	- Simulation
- One-to-one instruction	- Role modeling
	- Independent study

Implementation
■ Incorporate active learner engagement strategies. Examples include the following:

- Case studies	- Self-assessments
- Group discussion questions/answer	- Gaming
	- Role-playing
- Problem-based learning	
- Reflection	

■ Retention of information increases based on the level of learner involvement.
■ Integrate strategies to support the learner to retain the content after the activity. Examples include handouts, key points, reminders, visuals, coaching, and checklists.
Evaluation
■ Learning outcome(s) may be assessed at the end of the learning activity or at a later date.
■ Examples of short-term evaluation options are as follows:

- Posttest	- Active participation
- Intent to change practice	- Case study analysis
- Return demonstration, role-play	

■ Examples of long-term evaluation options are as follows:
  - Self-reported change in practice
  - Change in a quality indicator
  - Return on investment
  - Direct observation of performance.

Coaching and Mentoring
■ Mentoring in nursing implies pairing an experienced nurse with a less experienced nurse. The mentor provides guidance and support to learn a new position or develop in a role.
■ Mentoring and preceptorship are sometimes intertwined. A preceptorship is usually a short-term relationship between a novice and an experienced person (e.g., an academic student to CNS), whereas mentoring usually involves an ongoing professional relationship.
■ The purpose of the mentor is as follows:

- Transfer knowledge and skills.	- Serve as a role model.
- Provide feedback.	- Encourage continuing professional development.
- Offer psychosocial support.	

■ Preceptors and mentors may use coaching in working with staff.
■ Coaching is a strategy to transfer skills and knowledge.

TABLE 21.2 NURSING CONSIDERATIONS FOR KEY CULTURAL GROUPINGS

NURSING CARE FOCUS	ASIAN	AFRICAN/AFRICAN AMERICAN	EUROPEAN	AMERICAN INDIAN	ALASKAN NATIVE	SOUTH AMERICAN
Patient advocacy	Religious beliefs must be considered especially for patients not highly Westernized. The role of the food may not agree with Western medicine. Provide an open supportive environment to call for religious rites, ceremonies, and food prescriptions to be part of the patient's care.	African and African American are two distinct cultural groupings, even if genetically similar. Dependence on spirituality and intense family involvement may be perceived as needing acute medical or mental health intervention related to responses around disease state or condition (O'Rourke, McDowell, 2018).	Very broad category almost impossible to isolate. Advocate for patient modesty and discomfort with nudity. Extended family is important. Many healthcare issues are the same for Western Europe and United States.	Family is extremely important. Traditional healing is passed down through generations by visions, dreams, and stories. Healing may include alternative medicine, including sweat lodges, talking circles, drumming, ceremonial smoking, potlatch ceremonies, herbalism, animal spirits and vision quests (International Association of Providers of AIDS Care [IAPAC], 2014). Allow the practice of Native religions and Native medicine (Metropolitan Chicago Healthcare Council [MCHC], 2004).	Multiple Alaskan Native peoples including different dialects within the indigenous population. The healthcare system can be too fast in speech. Alaskan Natives are direct and concise in conversation. Providers must allow time for communication to happen or all information that is needed may not be obtained (Stanford, 2019).	Learned cultural attributes of kindness, respect, politeness, conflict avoidance, and modesty can prevent them from getting complete healthcare in the United States. Providers must acknowledge these attributes but continue to question and support to allow for complete patient interaction (Juckett, 2013).
Cultural knowledge	Five main categories within the term *Asian*. Over 55 distinct cultures and nationalities. Ranging from Pakistan in the west to Japan in the east, China to the north and Singapore to the south (Lim, 2015).	Lack of trust with Western medicine and healthcare providers. May be a generalized fear that any cancer surgery may cause it to spread. Pain may be area of concern. Religion should not be underestimated. Religion may prevent organ donation. May attempt prayer, healers, and advice from extended family (O'Rourke, McDowell, 2018).	Healthcare access and expectations may be different related to national socialized healthcare than to free enterprise economic-based healthcare with primary insurance coverage.	Native American healing is recognized by the National Institutes of Health. Based on the practice of living in harmony with the earth and has a place side by side with western medicine (Koithan & Farrel, 2010). Elders are looked to for leadership in making healthcare decisions. Therapeutic relationship must include respectful acceptance of elders and if requested to do so by the patient.	Native Alaskans may still mistrust Western medicine related to the history of distant boarding schools and stories of the early treatment of TB. Story telling used to pass along herbals, traditional medicine, and the respect that is given to elders, the earth, plants, and animals. The use of alcohol to initially treat physical and mental feelings has led to many people developing alcohol-related disease processes (IAPAC, 2014).	*Latinx* refers to multiple nationalities of Latin/Spanish descent. Nationalities include Mexico, Central America, South America, Cuba, and Puerto Rico. Take the time to develop a therapeutic relationship, which will prepare for interactive patient teaching and decreasing the cultural gap (Juckett, 2013).

(continued)

Cultural competence	Health and disease are defined differently. The scientific method is highly valued though interventions may be starkly different. Rather than surgery or rehabilitation the patient may feel the need for restitution to another person, rituals of forgiveness, or ceremonies to appease spirits (Lim, 2015). Special attention should be applied to needs related to mental health or socioeconomic impacts (APA, 2006).	Treatment of pain differs for the African and African American. African Americans may perceive a direct relationship between treatment of pain and spirituality. Strong influence of spirituality in a Christian tradition combined with social existential factors changes the way the body and mind respond to pain (Booker). The eCALD website is an excellent resource for different cultural beliefs of African countries. eCALD allows selection of both overall region and specific African countries. https://www.ecald.com	Awareness is key. Ask if the patient sees a medicine man, uses hallucinogens or traditional medicine. If having surgery, does the patient use the sweat lodge? Recognize that problems with alcohol and diabetes have a higher prevalence in the Native American population (American Academy of Orthopedic Surgeons [AAOS], 2019).	Give patients time to explain the chief complaint. Access to specialized care may be quicker with Western healthcare. This may not allow sufficient time for objective patient decision-making. Drug names are different.	Culturally competent treatment includes 10 specific items: "1. Show respect to others, each person has a special gift. 2. Share what you have. Giving makes you richer. 3. Know who you are. You are a reflection on your family. 4. Accept what life brings. You cannot control many things. 5. Have patience. Somethings cannot be rushed. 6. Live carefully. What you do will come back to you. 7. Take care of others. You cannot live without them. 8. Honor your elders. They show you the way in life. 9. Pray for guidance. Many things are not known. 10. See connections. All things are related" (Stanford, 2019).	*Hispanic paradox:* term for role of diabetes, hypertension, and obesity in health of the Latinx population. Significant stress in those newly immigrated to the United States. Many immigrate without a fixed job and with family, spouse/significant other; with or without children. Illness may be caused or exacerbated by this stress. Mental health issues especially PTSD can be blamed on issues related to religion, such as "soul loss." Certain medical issues may have been treated with traditional herbalism (Juckett, 2013).
Communication across cultures	Begin with the eCALD website. Can also be used as a PDF or live on electronic media. https://www.ecald.com/assets/Resources/Chapter-2-Introduction-to-Asian-Cultures.pdf	Actively engage patient in care to reduce stress. Healthcare disparity issues may result in underutilization of services (O'Rourke & McDowell, 2018). When there is a lack of care the patient may experience progression of illness and be more difficult to treat and communicate the severity of the situation.	Use of an interpreter may be the only way to get solid informed consent for healthcare. Even spoken English from different countries may be hard to understand, so slow down, speak, and listen with intent.	The greeting is very important. Direct eye contact may be considered rude. Fleeting passes of eye contact is appropriate. Don't expect a handshake unless you have an existing relationship. Avoid large movements and hand gestures. Use an interpreter as needed. It is quite appropriate to use drawings and provide direct written communication and may increase respect (AAOS, 2019).	Most Alaskan Natives, except those of extremes in age, can speak English. However, there is a stoic nature especially with regard to pain. Nonverbal communication needs to be observed (Stanford University, 2019).	Language barriers remain an issue. Healthcare literacy even if written materials are in Spanish may be difficult for some to understand or read. Formal Spanish is different from deviations of the language with inclusion of other Native languages and may not allow for adequate informed consent (Juckett, 2013).

APA, American Psychological Association; PDF, portable document format; PTSD, post-traumatic stress disorder; TB, tuberculosis.

- Coaching is a strategy to partner with others to inspire them to reach their greatest potential.
- **CNS competency:** Refers to skillful guidance and teaching to advance the care of patients, families, and groups of patients and the profession of nursing.
- The CNS utilizes coaching with a knowledge of adult teaching/learning theory.
- In coaching interactions with staff, the CNS considers Benner's stages of clinical competence:
  - **Stage 1:** Novice
  - **Stage 2:** Advanced beginner
  - **Stage 3:** Competent
  - **Stage 4:** Proficient
  - **Stage 5:** Expert
- Outcomes of effective coaching
  - Deepen the understanding of a concept or skill.
  - Promote critical thinking to consider possible alternatives.
  - Improve individual performance.
  - Build confidence.
- Coaching strategies

• Demonstrate the behaviors you expect • Display mutual trust and respect • Be present to offer gestural support and verbal prompts • Role-play or simulation activities • Practice active listening • Ask open-ended questions to support problem solving • Reflect your observations to encourage the person to think about the situation and their response to the situation • Avoid giving the answers • Convey confidence and support to the person • Help individual focus on key points (three to four at the most in each encounter)	• Use Socratic questions to clarify concepts, identify implications, and validate their understanding • Identify barriers to the individual's learning • Storytelling, case study, and visual pictures can clarify complex situations • Link a new concept to prior knowledge • Participate in debriefing sessions after critical events • Aid the individual in identifying and setting concrete and sustainable goals • Provide timely and genuine feedback • Acknowledge successes to motivate the individual toward future learning and professional growth

REVIEW QUESTIONS

1. The interdisciplinary team approach to assisting clients with healthcare issues is preferable to an individual discipline approach because
   A. individual disciplines promote integrated problem solving.
   B. teams with interdisciplinary focus promote integrated problem solving.
   C. the individual discipline will focus on seamless planning.
   D. the interdisciplinary team will promote fragmented care.

2. The clinical nurse specialist (CNS) has been asked to colead a geriatric resource nurse program with one of the nurses from the hospital to provide education on geriatric-related issues. This is an example of which role of the CNS?
   A. Collaboration
   B. Consultation
   C. Research
   D. Direct care

3. The local community council in a rural area has been asked to establish a public health center for members of the community. Most individuals are of retirement age and older and are unable to travel long distances for healthcare that would be available only in larger cities. A smaller portion of the community is made up of low- and middle-income families with a mix of small children and teenagers. The council is made up of community leaders, none of whom are healthcare professionals. The clinical nurse specialist (CNS) works for a large multisystem healthcare organization and was asked by a council member to provide some guidance for this project as a paid consultant. What is the most appropriate action?
   A. Submit a proposal for a program that you would administer on a fee-for-service basis for all community members.
   B. Consent to attend the next council meeting to assess the council's activities related to researching and data gathering, the project's funding needs, goals, and consequences to the community and all community members, including any conflict of interest or bias.
   C. Decline to get involved because you have limited exposure to public policy or lack experience in managing a community health program, and it is outside of your scope of practice.
   D. Call some of the providers that you work with to expand their practice to include the local community.

ANSWERS

1. **Correct answer: B. Rationale:** Collaboration among the interprofessional team enables the knowledge and skills of all team members to synergistically influence the patient care being provided rather than having just one perspective. Individual disciplines working independently do not promote integrated problem solving or seamless planning with other disciplines. Interdisciplinary teams promote integrated care.

2. **Correct answer: B. Rationale:** CNS consultation is defined as offering knowledge, expertise, and experience in a specialty practice. The CNS is acting as the geriatric specialty consultant in this case. Collaboration is a dynamic interpersonal team process to clarify complex patient problems and find solutions to those problems. The CNS is not performing research, nor providing direct patient care in this situation.

3. **Correct answer: B. Rationale:** The CNS must first establish that the council has done due diligence in determining the need for such a program and that the program would benefit the whole community, not excluding those who might also need services. Second, the CNS should research the resources available for providing services to remote rural areas from county and state agencies and others about which the council

might not have knowledge (mobile clinics, telehealth, or mobile imaging, etc.). Identify any unintended consequences that might arise from the project such as providing services for some community members but not others, low-income individuals who may feel ashamed to access the program, how to address health problems that need to be managed outside of the community, and how individuals will access such services. Submitting a proposal for a program that you would administer on a fee-for-service basis for all community members is exploiting the council and community because it takes advantage of the situation without investigating other

options. Nurses are obligated to public service, so the CNS should not decline to get involved. Even if the CNS is not an expert, they can provide resource information that could facilitate the project. Calling providers that the CNS works with is incorrect because it uses their influence to promote friends' or colleagues' professional interest.

REFERENCES
The complete reference and additional reading lists appear in the digital version of this chapter, at https://connect.springerpub.com/content/book/978-0-8261-7417-8/part/part02/chapter/ch21

Section III
Organizations and Systems

Systems Leadership

Marianne Benjamin

OVERVIEW

Systems leadership is a core competency of clinical nurse specialist (CNS) practice. The CNS must not only be able to manage change but, more important, must demonstrate ability to lead and empower others to influence clinical practice and political processes both within and across systems. The CNS should possess knowledge of their own areas of influence and how they integrate into the system as a whole. This knowledge and self-awareness increase the likelihood of sustainability when working with and through change.

ORGANIZATIONAL PRINCIPLES

Systems Theory
- Systems are composed of interrelated parts.
- These parts when arranged or configured result in a unified whole.
- A system can be open or closed.
  - Closed systems occur only in physical science (e.g., circulatory system).
  - Open systems interact internally and externally with the environment.
- Organizations are open systems comprised of inputs, throughputs, and outputs.
  - Staff, patients, equipment, supplies, financial resources, and so forth are inputs.
  - Throughput is the process(es) performed to create a product.
  - Output is the product or outcome. In healthcare systems, the output might be reduction in hospital-acquired conditions.

Systems thinking focuses on how systems interrelate with each part, thereby affecting the entire system. In leading or facilitating teams, the CNS must help team members understand the interrelatedness of all members of the larger organization. A change in a subcomponent of the larger system can affect other subcomponents as well as the larger organization.

- **A complex system** is a highly connected network of entities from which higher-order behavior emerges. Complex systems are characterized by unpredictability and nonlinearity.
- **Complex adaptive systems** are complex systems that can learn and adapt to change over time. The structure of the system itself can be changed over time as a result (Clancy et al., 2008). Healthcare and healthcare organizations are considered complex adaptive systems.

HEALTHY WORK ENVIRONMENT

A *healthy work environment* (HWE) is defined as one in which members of the healthcare team have good working relationships, where nurses are involved in decision-making regarding their practice, and where the organization listens and responds to nurses when patient care issues of concern are identified (Johansen et al., 2019).

An HWE is deemed essential for the provision of safe, quality, competent, and compassionate nursing care. An unhealthy work environment can be a contributor to medical errors, ineffective delivery of care, and conflict and stress among the healthcare team (American Association of Critical-Care Nurses [AACN], 2016). Failure to foster a HWE for nurses can cause harm to patients and families (Heath et al., 2004). The AACN (2016) developed a framework that comprises six standards for establishing and sustaining HWE.

- **Skilled communication**—The competency of being able to communicate effectively is just as important to patient safety as clinical skills.
- **True collaboration**—Recognizing and valuing the unique knowledge and abilities of other healthcare team members and their contributions to quality patient care.
- **Effective decision-making**—Nurses must be involved in making decisions about their own practice and patient care.
- **Appropriate staffing**—Matching patient needs with nurse competencies must be a priority to improve patient outcomes and nurse satisfaction.
- **Meaningful recognition**—Mutual respect and recognition must be implemented to promote the value brought by each person to the organization.
- **Authentic leadership**—Nurse leaders must embody HWE standards and engage others to as well.

The CNS contributes to a HWE by forming trusting and respectful relationships with multiple stakeholders within their area of influence and by modeling examples of effective communication among and across individuals and teams. As a means to enhance collaboration, the CNS should encourage and model peer-to-peer recognition and cultivate in the RN an appreciation and understanding of the roles and contributions of physicians, members of the patient care team, staff, and employees. The CNS, being mindful of generational differences, directly provides and/or recommends meaningful recognition for nurses who deliver excellence in patient care (Scruth et al., 2018).

INFLUENCING CHANGE

The CNS leads interdisciplinary teams in applying synthesized evidence to initiate clinical decisions and practice changes to improve the health of individuals, groups, and populations (Melnyk & Fineout-Overholt, 2019). The role of the CNS as a leader of change cannot be understated. While there are many theories on managing change, two listed here are common in the nursing literature (Roussel, 2013).

- **Lewin's theory**—The theory involves three stages: unfreezing, moving, and refreezing. The unfreezing stage occurs when some disequilibrium happens in the system that creates a need for change. The problem causing the disequilibrium is identified, and the best solution to the problem is selected. The moving stage is characterized by gathering information and buy-in from knowledgeable, respected, or influential persons in an effort to help in solving the problem. During the refreezing stage, solutions for change are integrated and stabilized as a part of the value system of the group. Driving and restraining forces are at work to either facilitate or attempt to impede the change. The leader as change agent must identify and work with these opposing forces in order to firmly establish and sustain the change.
- **Rogers's theory**—The theory modified Lewin's work by adding two additional phases.
  - Phase 1: Awareness (corresponds to Lewin's unfreezing stage)
  - Phase 2: Interest
  - Phase 3: Evaluation
  - Phase 4: Trial (Lewin's moving stage)
  - Phase 5: Adoption (Lewin's refreezing stage). It is here that the change is accepted or rejected.

For change to be successful, Rogers's theory describes five factors.

1. The result of the change must have an advantage over the current state.
2. The change must be compatible with existing values.
3. The change must have complexity. The theory posits that while simple change can be implemented more easily, a complex change persists.
4. The change must have divisibility. Small tests of change are introduced first.
5. The change must be easy to communicate in order to spread.

Rogers provides a description of the adopters in any change process.

- **Innovators** are the risk-takers. They might jump all in when it comes to change. The innovator is not concerned with the opinion of others.
- **Early adopter** is a respected opinion leader who is effective in translating the innovator's message for the early majority.
- **Early majority** are deliberate and will adopt new ideas before the average persons in the group. They do not seek out information independently but will follow the early adopter.
- **Late majority** tend to be suspicious and skeptical. They are influenced by peer pressure and then change accordingly.
- **Resistors** are the last to adopt to a change, paying little attention to the opinion of others. The resistor can be valuable in a change effort, forcing the change agent to listen to possible/probable barriers and then to act accordingly.

The CNS works with individuals and teams in an increasingly complex environment of fast-paced change. It is important for the CNS to be able to recognize and understand how people respond to change in order to make the most impact. Persons who experience major organizational change are likely to exhibit one of four response patterns: entrenched, overwhelmed, poser, or learner (Bunker, 2014; Table 22.1).

LEADERSHIP

Theories on leadership are often described in four categories: trait, behavioral, contingency, and contemporary.

- **Trait theory**—Focuses on the personal characteristics of the leader. Leaders deemed successful tend to be described as driven, persistent, self-confident, and resilient. These leaders are creative problem solvers, take initiative, accept the consequences of one's actions, possess the ability to influence others, act with integrity and tact, and demonstrate emotional intelligence (EI). Leaders who demonstrate EI are more sensitive to their personal emotions and the subsequent impact their emotions have on others (Northouse, 2010).
- **Behavioral theory**—Focuses on what leaders do or how they behave. Common styles of behavioral leadership include the following:
  - **Autocratic**—The leader attempts to change the behavior of followers/subordinates through use of positional authority, coercion, power, and punishment.
  - **Democratic**—The leader appeals to followers/subordinates through engaging and involving them in participation, goal setting, and collaboration.
  - **Laissez-faire (permissive)**—Assumes that followers/subordinates are able to make their own decisions and conduct work without specific direction or facilitation from the leader.
  - **Bureaucratic**—The leader uses organizational rules and policies to influence or change follower/subordinate behaviors.
  - Autocratic and bureaucratic leaders believe followers/subordinates are predominantly motivated by external factors.
  - Laissez-faire and democratic leaders believe that change is a result of internal motivation of followers/subordinates.
- **Contingency theory**—Or situational leadership—employs different styles based on the situation. As an example, a leader might use democratic style to engage followers/subordinates during a team-building retreat but employ autocratic tactics during an emergency.
- **Contemporary**—Theories of leadership are just that: more modern and befitting of complex environments. To be effective, today's leaders must be flexible and adaptable to meet the demands of the workplace.

Types of Leadership

- **Transformational leadership** transforms an organization through contextual and cultural changes. Leaders engage and encourage staff in risk-taking to move beyond the current reality. Transformational leaders create an environment of supportive trust and self-actualization for all employees. The transformational leader is compassionate and enthusiastic with the ability and skill to provide a vision, to motivate, and to inspire others (Melnyk & Fineout-Overholt, 2019). The American Nurses Credentialing Center's Magnet Recognition Program is based on transformational leadership.
- **Servant leadership** places other people and their needs before the leader's own self-interests. These leaders are attentive to the concerns of their followers, demonstrating empathy, care, and nurturance. The servant leader has a social responsibility to be concerned with inequalities and injustices and works to remove them. The servant leader uses less institutional power and control while shifting authority to those being led (Northouse, 2010).

TABLE 22.1 RESPONSE PATTERNS

RESPONSE PATTERN	DESCRIPTION	CHARACTERISTICS	CNS ACTION
Entrenched	May appear to be in denial, feel anxious, angry, or frustrated, or blame the organization for changing something that to them was fine as is.	Hoping to ride out the change, they can continue to work hard relying on past learning strategies and practices. They may admit the need for change but can resist changing their own behavior.	The CNS should be clear in communicating what is actually going to change and why, help them to see what they must let go of, and convey understanding, providing help in dealing with stress and frustration; the CNS must teach new behaviors through carefully paced learning activities conducted in a safe environment—such as in a simulation lab; provide effective role models; and provide frequent, positive feedback along the way.
Overwhelmed group	Report feeling powerless and depressed. They might appear withdrawn from the group, display resistive and passive–aggressive behavior, blame and complain, and have difficulty learning what's needed in the new state.	The overwhelmed person can have a negative impact on others in learning a new change.	The CNS should clearly communicate the specifics of the change and will need to provide continuous assistance through all phases of the change. A phased transition with connections to the old way of doing things is best with the overwhelmed group. A phased, slower approach with recognition of small successes to boost confidence is likely needed. Providing effective role models is a key strategy.
The poser group	Will attest to a high level of confidence about how they can handle change, often boasting and self-promoting and overestimating their strengths.	The poser's actual competence, however, does not equal their own sense of self and ability. The poser doesn't learn well. Posers are anxious to get started and will become frustrated with others who are complaining.	The CNS should provide external checks and balances with posers, as they tend to get off track due to lack of self-awareness. Frequent, objective assessment of their skills and learning needs should be made. Avoid expanding the role of the poser in the change process, insisting on incremental steps.
Learners	See life as a continual learning experience. They will feel optimistic and challenged when extended but remain in control of their destinies. Learners are not afraid of making mistakes.	They are resilient and will seek out learning opportunities. Learners prefer to solve problems rather than blame others. Learners are often the "go-to" people. Caution needs to be taken, as the learner can become "burned out" when relied upon over and over without a break. The learner will need periodic relief.	The CNS should give learners high-impact roles in the change process, allowing them to teach and lead others through transition. They are effective role models. Learners should be recognized and rewarded for their support and contributions.

CNS, clinical nurse specialist.
Source: From Bunker, K. A. (2014). *Responses to change: Helping people manage transition*. American Nurses Association.

- **Authentic leadership** is morally grounded, transparent, and responsive to people's needs and values. An authentic leader is a role model, focusing on the ethical and right thing to do. This type of leader prioritizes the development of others and ensures that their communication is transparent and is comprehended as intended. Authentic leaders build trust and HWEs by exemplifying four behaviors: balanced processing, internalized moral perspective, relational transparency, and self-awareness (Melnyk & Fineout-Overholt, 2019).

The Five Practices of Exemplary Leadership

Kouzes and Posner (2017) describe characteristics that are essential in a leader. These authors state that the majority of people will follow a leader whom they believe to be honest, competent, inspiring, and forward looking. By engaging in "the five practices of exemplary leadership" (Kouzes & Posner, 2017), the CNS can exemplify excellence in leadership.

- **Model the way:** Begin by clarifying your own personal values and guiding principles. When leading others, ascertain and affirm the shared values of the group.

- **Inspire a shared vision:** Envision a future of exciting possibilities, enlisting others in a common vision by appealing to shared aspirations.
- **Challenge the process:** Look outward for improvement innovations. Listen more. Create and expect an environment for experimentation, risk-taking, challenging the status quo of the system, and recognizing and acting on good ideas.
- **Enable others to act:** Engage others by fostering collaborative, trusting relationships. Attend to serving others' needs rather than your own. Develop and strengthen others' competence.
- **Encourage the heart:** Recognize, show appreciation, and celebrate the contributions of others.

PRINCIPLES OF GROUPS AND TEAMS

Group Dynamics

Group dynamics refer to a system of behaviors and psychologic processes occurring within a social group or between social groups. Groups are described as moving through five phases with associated behaviors (Forsyth, 2019; Table 22.2). For teams (groups) to be most effective, strong leadership is required. As a leader, the CNS can make an impact at each phase of the group dynamic.

Team Building

There are six critical factors that are necessary for teams to be able to perform at their highest level (Grimes, 2011).

- A clearly defined team objective
  - The purpose of the team must be clearly understood.
  - If a team gets off track, the leader must revisit the purpose/objective.
  - Signs that the team lacks understanding of purpose include defensive responses to constructive criticism, focusing on the unimportant, questioning the worth of the team's contributions, and inability to describe team outcomes and successes.
- Individual goals and tasks aligned to team objective
  - Team members understand their role on the team and how it relates to work performed by other team members.
  - Individual team member alignment impacts engagement in the common goal by providing members confidence in how their contribution leads to success of the team.

- Creative, nimble leaders who challenge team members are caring and participative
  - Leaders must possess EI and situational awareness in order to adapt their style of leadership to the particular needs of the team.
  - Signs that can mean a team requires more of its leader include resistance and ongoing disagreement, conflict over who should be in charge or play what role, self-serving activities that are not in line with the team's purpose, and lack of communication.
- Communication that is multidirectional and encouraged
  - A lack of communication erodes trust.
  - In the absence of communication, important concerns, issues, or problems are not addressed. The result may be rumor spreading, hearsay, untruths, distrust.
  - Signs a team is negatively impacted by lack of/insufficient communication include unpreparedness and duplication of efforts during meetings, lack of delegation, bottlenecking of information (multiple meetings without forward progress), excessive email messages and email strings, and forming cliques or gossip circles.
- An environment of trust and team loyalty
  - Trust allows team members to be comfortable pushing themselves to the fullest potential.
  - When working in a trusting environment, team members will "give the benefit of the doubt," rather than judging another as having acted with meanness or poor intent.
  - Signs of lack of trust include posturing against team members, elevating or promoting self-interests over the team's, and decreased engagement.
- Accountability and recognition
  - Discretionary effort by the individual is directed at the onset by setting clear expectations on an individual's expected contributions.
  - Clarifying roles, deliverables, and metrics for success allows members to be more fully engaged and more confidently interact with other team members.
  - Clearly set boundaries will contribute to a healthier sense of accountability.
  - Recognition for good outcomes and a job well done helps members remain loyal to the team and engaged in the work.
  - Recognition must be meaningful to the individual (see standards for HWEs earlier in this chapter).

TABLE 22.2 GROUP DYNAMIC CHARACTERISTICS

Orientation phase (forming)	Exchange of personal information, uncertainty, tentative communication	Leader is relied upon to set the direction of the group.
Conflict phase (storming)	Dissatisfaction, disagreement, challenges to leader and procedures	Leader assists the group to work through conflict.
Structure phase (norming)	Cohesiveness, agreement on procedures, identifying improved communication	Leader focuses on building relationships.
Performance phase (performing)	Focus on the work of the group, task completion, decision-making, cooperation	Leader provides feedback on work of the group, redirects efforts as needed, and strengthens relationships.
Dissolution phase (adjourning)	Departures, withdrawal, decreased dependence, regret	Leader recognizes collective accomplishments and individual strengths/contributions.

Source: From Forsyth, D. R. (2019). *Group dynamics* (7th ed.). Cengage Learning Inc.

- Signs of lack of accountability and recognition include continually asking for guidance rather seeking out their own solutions, asking permission to make decisions that are within the scope of one's role, taking excessive liberties beyond their scope, inability to acknowledge accomplishments made by other members, not taking responsibility for personal errors, and complaining regularly about lack of time and resources.

REVIEW QUESTIONS

1. What best describes the transformational style of leadership?
   A. Rotating leaders to allow for different perspectives in the leadership role
   B. A pyramid leadership structure with one person leading and all the rest following
   C. Leadership raising the motivation and morality among those under them to empower them
   D. Multiple leaders who come to consensus regarding management decisions

2. While leading a team in the ICU to implement a new enteral nutrition protocol, the CNS identifies some team members who are acting out during discussions. Which of the following should the clinical nurse specialist (CNS) recognize?
   A. When a team member resists the change—continuing to practice according to their old ways—they likely would benefit from repeating the mandatory education.
   B. Team members who complain about too many fast-paced changes may act out by displaying passive–aggressive behaviors. In reality, they may feel powerless and overwhelmed.
   C. Team members who act overly confident and self-promote themselves as an expert are the best persons to include on the planning and implementation team.
   D. High-functioning team members who regularly embrace learning that comes about with change are self-motivated. These staff are best kept to themselves and would intimidate others if allowed a formal role in the change process.

ANSWERS

1. **Correct answer: C. Rationale:** The transformational leader motivates their followers to participate in making decisions, encouraging them to develop ideas and problem-solving skills. This style of leadership empowers others to take responsibility for problems and create productive solutions. Rotating leaders and pyramid leadership do not motivate individuals or empower them to act. Multiple leaders coming to consensus demonstrates collaboration but does not empower others to act.

2. **Correct answer: B. Rationale:** Team members who might be overwhelmed with frequent and/or fast-paced change can have a negative impact on others and easily derail the change process. The CNS should provide clear, ongoing communication and assistance and might consider a phased approach to implementation. A slower approach tactic coupled with positive recognition of successful small steps can benefit the overwhelmed. Only providing education is not effective in making change. High-functioning team members who are self-motivated should be encouraged to be involved in the change and not excluded.

REFERENCES

The complete reference list appears in the digital version of this chapter, at https://connect.springerpub.com/content/book/978-0-8261-7417-8/part/part03/chapter/ch22

23 Quality Improvement and Safety

Lynne Marie Kokoczka, Dianna Jo Copley, Joan Miller, JoAnne Phillips, Melissa Lowder, Adrianne Opp, and Jennifer Embree

NURSING QUALITY EVOLUTION

Nursing quality has evolved through the years, benefitted by work done by the American Nurses Association's (ANA's) adoption of the use of quality assurance methods and Donabedian's structure, process, and outcomes model (Donabedian, 1996). ANA evaluated linkages to nursing staffing and quality in the early 1990s and launched the Patient Safety and Quality Initiative. Through a series of pilot studies, 10 nurse-sensitive indicators were developed (Montalvo, 2007).

NURSE-SENSITIVE INDICATORS

Nurse-sensitive indicators refer to outcomes that improve through either nursing care quality or quantity. Nurse-sensitive indicators include patient satisfaction, falls, pressure injuries, ventilator-associated pneumonias (VAPs), central line associated bloodstream infections, and urinary catheter associated infections.

- The **National Database of Nursing Quality Indicators (NDNQI)** was established by the ANA as a means to collect and compare knowledge of nursing-sensitive indicators and the impact to nursing care. The NDNQI mission aids nursing in quality improvements and patient safety initiatives by providing unit-level comparison data of nursing outcomes among like patient care areas. Hospitals track a variety of nurse-sensitive quality indicators and use the nationally benchmarked data to provide Magnet® Recognition program–compliant data.
- **Press Ganey** is a market analysis company that provides patient experience benchmarking analytics (Press Ganey, 2015). NDNQI also provides survey data regarding nursing retention.
- **The Joint Commission (TJC)** provides oversight and accreditation for multiple venues for healthcare provision. TJC approval and accreditation is a requirement for any recipient of federal funding, such as Medicare (The Joint Commission, 2019).
- Other indicators of quality may be reflected in patient satisfaction or patient experience scores, as well as adherence to clinical practice guidelines and prevention guidelines.

Clinical nurse specialists (CNSs) should understand the quality goals and measures within the organization, in addition to awareness of the performance level targets, and the potential to have an impact in the development of strategies or evidence-based solutions.

Hospital-Acquired Conditions

With the release of the Institute of Medicine (IOM) report *To Err Is Human: Building a Safer Health System* (IOM, 2000), preventable errors were identified as causing harm and even death to thousands of patients.

In 2008, the Centers for Medicare & Medicaid Services (CMS) implemented a series of payment reforms as a response to Congress's Deficit Reduction Act of 2005. The inpatient prospective payment system (IPPS) denies additional payment to hospitals for hospital-acquired conditions (HAC) that were not present on admission (POA) by linking financial disincentives to harm event occurrence.

- Eight events were identified as high-cost and high-volume preventable events by the Department of Health and Human Services (Thirukumaran et al., 2017). The CMS's intent was for hospitals to develop evidence-based practice interventions to prevent harmful events and thereby avoid withheld payments.

Nonpayment for Hospital-Acquired Conditions: Inpatient Prospective Payment System

As of 2013, the following HACs are cause for denial of payment

- Foreign object retained after surgery
- Air embolism
- Blood incompatibility
- Falls and trauma: fractures, dislocations, intracranial injuries, crushing injuries, burns
- Stage III and IV pressure ulcers
- Catheter-associated urinary tract infection (CAUTI)
- Vascular catheter-associated infection
- Surgical site infection—mediastinitis after coronary artery bypass graft surgery (CABG)
- Manifestations of poor glycemic control
- Surgical site infection following bariatric surgery for obesity
- Surgical site infection following certain orthopedic procedures
- Surgical site infection following cardiac implantable electronic device
- Deep vein thrombosis (DVT) or pulmonary embolism (PE) following certain orthopedic procedures
- Iatrogenic pneumothorax with venous catheterization (CMS.gov, 2019)

Safety Initiatives

Patient safety became the focus in response to awareness of preventable harm occurring within hospitals in the United States in the late 1990s. With the lack of payment for harm events, the patient safety movement inspired the creation of national organizations:

- National Patient Safety Foundation (NPSF)
- Institute for Healthcare Improvement (IHI) and National Quality Forum
- TJC

Regulatory agencies developed requirements for monitoring and recording errors through incident reporting, as well as compliance with benchmarked standards of care (TJC, 2019).

Healthcare patient safety improvements initially focused on individual performance. Emphasis has shifted toward work environment, cultures, and complexity of the healthcare environment as key contributors to near-miss-and-harm events to sustain improvements (Table 23.1).

Development of evidence-based practice is fueled by the increasing public and professional demand for accountability in safety and quality improvement within healthcare.

The analysis of adverse events identifies the environmental and system factors that contribute to events, despite best intentions and efforts. CNSs provide leadership to utilize best practices from other highly reliable industries, whose emphasis for improvement stems around human factors and system knowledge, such as mindfulness and risk resilience (Ebright, 2014).

CNSs have the ability to influence safety in five ways:

- Role-modeling nonpunitive safety behaviors
- Facilitation of learning about complex adaptive systems
- Understanding healthcare worker resiliency

- Managing complexity through change management strategies
- Staying up to date with current evidence related to patient safety (Ebright, 2014)

Safety work involves investigation to determine the actual course of events and restructuring the staff's recall of an event. Quality management tools, such as Lean methodology, help to identify waste, defects, and inefficiencies that lead to errors (Table 23.2).

Organizational and Accreditation Standards

There are multiple accreditation agencies within healthcare that provide oversight and guidelines as well as standards for the provision of safe and evidence-based care. Table 23.3 provides a summary of the organization, mission/vision, purpose, and safety oversight or initiatives.

HOSPITAL-ACQUIRED CONDITIONS AND PREVENTIVE MEASURES

OVERVIEW

HACs are undesirable conditions or situations that can impact a patient's safety and health that arise during a hospital stay or that occur at a medical facility. HACs are conditions that are high cost, high volume, or both; they are typically associated with high-cost diagnostic-related groups (DRGs) and could be prevented with application of evidence-based guidelines. Fourteen categories have been in place since 2013; this is evaluated annually, and hospitals will not receive reimbursement for any of these conditions or the care of the patient as it relates to the HAC. Correct assessment and documentation are essential to coding conditions that are considered POA to avoid nonreimbursement.

While recent reports have demonstrated a downward trend, nearly three million HACs were reported in 2014, which greatly impacts morbidity, mortality, and overall healthcare costs. Healthcare organizations should have reporting structures in place to identify and improve prevention efforts related to HACs.

TABLE 23.1 SIX AIMS FOR FUNDAMENTAL CHANGE IN CARE

AIM	DESCRIPTION
Safe	Avoid injury from care.
Effective	Match care to science.
Patient centered	Honor and respect patient choice and preference.
Timely	Reduce waiting for patients and staff.
Efficient	Reduce waste.
Equitable	Close racial and ethical gaps in healthcare.

Source: From Ebright, P. (2014). *Foundations of clinical nurse specialist practice* (p. 184). Springer Publishing Company, LLC.

TABLE 23.2 TOOLS FOR ANALYZING FAILURE AND WORK COMPLEXITY WITH ADVERSE EVENTS

TOOLS	DEFINITION
Root cause analysis	Process for identifying basic or contributing underlying causal factors due to variations in performance associated with near-miss or adverse events (AORN, 2019; https://www.patientsafety.va.gov/professionals/publications/glossary.asp).
Event-flow diagram	Diagram used to show the nature and flow of events leading to a near-miss or adverse event.
Data mining	Analysis of large amounts of data to identify relationships that have not previously been discovered and increase understanding of work complexity.
Healthcare FMEA	A prospective assessment that identifies and improves steps in a process, thereby reasonably ensuring a safe and clinically desirable outcome. A systematic approach to identify and prevent product and process problems before they occur (www.va.gov/ncps/SafetyTopics/FHMEA/HFMEAIntro.pdf).
Workflow analysis: Process mapping	The analysis and representation of clinical work processes from the perspective of the staff.
Positive deviance	Data are viewed to identify extraordinarily successful groups or individuals and bring the isolated success strategies of those "positive deviants" into the mainstream (www.12manage.com/methods_pascale_positive_deviance.html).
Risk resilience	Assessment of organizational strength and weakness to adapt to variation and manage risk.

FMEA, failure mode and effects analysis.
Source: From Ebright, P. (2014). *Foundations of clinical nurse specialist practice* (p. 194). Springer Publishing Company, LLC.

TABLE 23.3 OVERVIEW OF KEY REGULATORY AND OVERSIGHT ORGANIZATIONS

ORGANIZATION	MISSION/VISION	PURPOSE	SAFETY INITIATIVES
CMS (within the U.S. Department of Health and Human Services), a federal agency	CMS seeks to strengthen and modernize the nation's healthcare system, to provide access to safe, high-quality, affordable care.	Provides oversight and administration of Medicare healthcare Medicaid healthcare administered with local state government CHIP Health insurance marketplace Enforcement and compliance of Health Insurance Portability and Accountability Act (HIPPA)	Implements quality initiatives for benefit to Medicare and Medicaid recipients. Data reported to CMS are accessible to the public. Data are reported from hospitals, outpatient clinics, and provider practices. Reimbursement is based upon quality outcomes, with the advent of the Deficit Reduction Act (2005) and IPPS (CMS.gov, 2019).
NICHE—For acute care and long-term care (NICHE Healthcare of the Elderly, 2019)	Improve care of hospitalized older adults through consultation and education for nursing and interprofessional teams.	Improve care through consultation and education by becoming a member of the organization, access to education toward specific geriatric nursing competency.	Education of nurses and LPN/LVN's in long-term care regarding best practices for care of adult adults. Leadership training program can help to defray costs of membership (NICHE Healthcare of the Elderly, 2019).
Magnet—ANCC, a subsidiary of the ANA, ANCC Magnet Recognition Program	Global nursing care delivery is guided by Magnet organizations with emphasis on knowledge, expertise, and grounding in core Magnet principles that revolve around the patient, family, and community and strive for excellence in discovery and innovation in practice. The five key aspects of the model are transformational leadership; structural empowerment; exemplary professional practice; new knowledge, innovations, and improvements; and empirical outcomes.	Recognizes healthcare organizations that provide the highest levels of excellence and professionalism in the nursing practice. Provides mechanism for sharing best practices and strategies for quality care in a nursing practice environment.	Requires tracking of nurse-sensitive indicators based upon Magnet reporting standards and benchmarks. Provides oversight of Magnet Designation, demonstrating that excellence in nursing outcomes are achieved and maintained over time (one component of the forces of magnetism; ANCC, 2019).
TJC/JCAHO—The Joint Commission, formerly known as *The Joint Commission on Accreditation of Healthcare Organizations*, provides accreditation to healthcare providers regarding the provision of service to patients	"To continuously improve health care for the public, in collaboration with other stakeholders, by evaluating health care organizations and inspiring them to excel in providing safe and effective care of the highest quality and value" (https://www.jointcommission.org/about-us/#:~:text=The%20mission%20of%20The%20Joint,the%20highest%20quality%20and%20value).	TJC accreditation is a condition of licensure and for receipt of Medicare and Medicaid reimbursement in the majority of states. TJC promotes safety through NPSGs. The NPSGs' quality solutions are evidence based and system focused and have become a way for TJC to enforce changes in quality and safety. TJC accreditation is received after a site visit and review of policies, procedures, and processes; patient tracing is used to understand patient experiences.	TJC ORYX initiative integrates performance measurement data into accreditation process. ORYX measurement requirements support TJC-accredited organizations in quality improvement efforts (The Joint Commission, 2019)

ANA, American Nurses Association; ANCC, American Nurses Credentialing Center; CMS, Centers for Medicare & Medicaid Services; HIPAA, Health Insurance Portability and Accountability Act; IPPS, inpatient prospective payment system; JCAHO, The Joint Commission on Accreditation of Healthcare Organizations; NICHE, Nurses Improving Care for Healthsystem Elders; NPSG, National Patient Safety Goals; TJC, The Joint Commission.

HOSPITAL-ACQUIRED CONDITIONS

Foreign Object Retained After Surgery

Foreign objects retained after surgery or procedures, also known as retained foreign bodies (RFBs), are unintentionally left inside a patient. These items include soft goods, sharps, surgical instruments, device fragments, and miscellaneous items, such as guidewires (Association of periOperative Nurses [AORN], 2019). RFBs can result in long-lasting physical and emotional distress and in severe cases even death (Hariharan & Lobo, 2013).

Etiology and Pathophysiology

The body can have a wide range of pathologic findings depending on the type of item that is retained and its location or migration in the body (Hariharan & Lobo, 2013; Umunna, 2012).

- **Aseptic fibrous response:** Cotton material is encapsulated aseptically into granulomas or adhesions; the material slowly decomposes over time; the patient may remain symptomatic (Umunna, 2012).
- **Exudative:** an inflammatory response that triggers infection from abscess formation (Umunna, 2012).

Risk Factors

Patient

- High body mass index (BMI; Hariharan & Lobo, 2013; Umunna, 2012)
- High blood loss (Umunna, 2012)
- Abdominal, pelvic or vaginal surgery

Environment

- Lengthy procedure (Hariharan & Lobo, 2013)
- No surgical count or incorrect surgical count (Hariharan & Lobo, 2013; Umunna, 2012)
- Emergent procedure (Hariharan & Lobo, 2013; Umunna, 2012)
- Unplanned change in the procedure (e.g., laparoscopic converted to open surgery; Hariharan & Lobo, 2013; Umunna, 2012)

Prevention

- Effective communication among team members must occur when an item is unaccounted for and all team members are responsible for locating the item (AORN, 2019).
- Team members must be encouraged to speak up when there is a count discrepancy or ensure there is an uninterrupted count.
- Adherence to counting procedures of soft goods, sharps, and miscellaneous items (AORN, 2019):
  - Disruptions should be minimized during all phases.
  - Counting should be both audible and visible.
  - Counts should take place during the different phases of the procedure by two personnel.
- Use soft goods with radiopaque markers for identification of RFBs on imaging studies (Hariharan & Lobo, 2013; Umunna, 2012).
- Exploration of the surgical wound/cavity prior to wound closure (AORN, 2019).
- Examine all surgical tools and instruments for integrity before and after use (AORN, 2019).
- Account for devices that are implanted and explanted during the same surgery, such as surgical clips, prior to wound closure (AORN, 2019).
- Use a surgical safety checklist (Anderson et al., 2014).
- Develop policies and procedures for counting soft goods, sharps, miscellaneous items, and device fragments and processes for incorrect counts (AORN, 2019).
- Consider new technology to enhance but not replace manual counting (Hariharan & Lobo, 2013):
  - Radiofrequency tags
  - Computer-assisted sponge count devices

Assessment and Treatment

If there is an incorrect count during a procedure (AORN, 2019), the following should be done:

- Attempts should be made to locate the item in the patient, on the sterile field and on nonsterile areas, such as kick buckets.
- If the item is not located, an intraoperative x-ray should be completed.
- If the item is located in the patient before final skin closure, attempts should be made to retrieve the item.
- A RFB found after final skin closure should be discussed with the patient and reported per the hospital/facility polices.
- Once a RFB is discovered after final skin closure, the surgeon must decide whether or not to retrieve the object depending on its effects on the patient and if surgically retrieving the item will cause more harm than leaving the object in the body (Hariharan & Lobo, 2013).
- The patient should be treated for any associated symptoms, such as pain and infection, per evidence-based guidelines.

Clinical Practice Guidelines

- Association of periOperative Nurses—*Guidelines for Perioperative Practice* (AORN, 2019)

Air Embolism

Air embolism following infusion, transfusion, and therapeutic injection is considered an HAC (Centers for Medicare & Medicaid Services [CMS], 2018).

Etiology and Pathophysiology

Air embolisms are either venous or arterial and occur when air enters the circulatory system. Air enters actively through accidental injection or passively such as during a central venous access device (CVAD) removal if the patient is in Fowler's position (Cook, 2013).

Risk Factors

Environment

- Poor technique or inexperienced practitioner
  Patient
- Patent foramen ovale (PFO) (Cook, 2013)
  - Severity of the air embolism will be increased.

Prevention

Air embolisms related to vascular access are rare and the primary focus should be on prevention (Gorski et al., 2016).
Insertion of Central Venous Access Device

- Patient placed in supine or Trendelenburg position, so the insertion site is at or below the level of the heart (Cook, 2013; Gorski et al., 2016).

Removal of Central Venous Access Device

- Have patient perform Valsalva maneuver (Cook, 2013; Gorski et al., 2016).
  - Valsalva increases intraabdominal and intrathoracic pressure and may be contraindicated.
  - If contraindicated, use Trendelenburg, left lateral decubitus position, or have the patient hold their breath.
- Hold pressure until hemostasis is achieved (Gorski et al., 2016).

- Apply sterile, petroleum-based ointment for at least 24 hours to the site (Cook, 2013; Gorski et al., 2016).
- Patient should remain flat or in a reclining position for 30 minutes (Gorski et al., 2016).

Maintenance

- Healthcare providers and those trained in management of intravenous (IV) access should maintain vascular access devices (VADs) (Gorski et al., 2016).
- Scissors, razors, or other sharp instruments should not be used near VADs (Gorski et al., 2016).
- Air should be expelled from all access devices prior to using (Cook, 2013; Gorski et al., 2016).
- Do not leave IV fluids connected to unprimed tubing at the bedside (Cook, 2013).
- Education of patients to avoid disconnection of VAD connections (Gorski et al., 2016).
- Use Luer-Lok devices (Gorski et al., 2016).
- Assess the VAD for any compromises including cracks in the catheter (Cook, 2013).

Assessment and Treatment

Air embolisms can produce cardiopulmonary and/or neurologic signs and symptoms including chest pain, acute dyspnea, tachypnea, cough, light-headedness, anxiety, tachycardia, and hypotension. If air embolism is suspected, patients should be immediately positioned onto their left side and placed in the Trendelenburg position unless the patient has known increased intracranial pressure (Cook, 2013; Gorski et al., 2016).

Clinical Practice Guidelines

- Infusion Nurses Society—2016; Infusion Therapy Standards of Practice

Blood Incompatibility

The CMS (2018) identifies blood incompatibility due to transfusion of blood/blood components not compatible with the patient, which may result in acute or delayed hemolytic transfusion reactions.

Etiology and Pathophysiology

Blood incompatibility occurs due to failure to correctly match recipient's blood group with that of the blood/blood components, causing an immune response.

Risk Factors

- Misidentification of the patient
- Mislabeled specimens resulting in "wrong blood in tube"
- Handling multiple patients' samples
- Testing or issuing errors by the blood bank
- Multiple blood products stored in one area
- Deviation from established facility procedures

Red Blood Cells

Red blood cells (RBCs) are typed for ABO and Rh(D) (AABB [formerly American Association of Blood Banks], 2018; Table 23.4).

- Recipients who are Rh(D) positive may receive Rh(D) positive or negative RBCs.
- Recipients who are Rh(D) negative generally receive Rh(D) negative units only.
- Plasma must be ABO identical or ABO compatible (AABB, 2018; Table 23.5).

Platelets

Platelets express ABO antigens, and it is recommended to provide group-specific products (AABB, 2018; Bachowski et al.,

TABLE 23.4 ABO MATCHING: RED BLOOD CELLS

RECIPIENT	BLOOD DONOR			
	O	A	B	AB
O	Compatible			
A	Compatible	Compatible		
B	Compatible		Compatible	
AB	Compatible	Compatible	Compatible	Compatible

Sources: From AABB. (2018). *Primer of blood administration.* American Association of Blood Banks; Bachowski, G., Borge, D., Brunker, P. A. R., Eder, A., Fialkow, L., Fridey, J. L., Goldberg, C., Hopkins, C. K., Lightfoot, T., Morgan, S. M., Stramer, S., Wagner, S. J., & Westphal, R. (2017). In J. L. Fridey (Ed.), *A compendium of transfusion practice guidelines* (3rd ed.). American Red Cross.

TABLE 23.5 ABO MATCHING: PLASMA

RECIPIENT	BLOOD DONOR			
	O	A	B	AB
O	Identical	Compatible	Compatible	Compatible
A		Identical		Compatible
B			Identical	Compatible
AB				Identical

Sources: From AABB. (2018). *Primer of blood administration.* American Association of Blood Banks; Bachowski, G., Borge, D., Brunker, P. A. R., Eder, A., Fialkow, L., Fridey, J. L., Goldberg, C., Hopkins, C. K., Lightfoot, T., Morgan, S. M., Stramer, S., Wagner, S. J., & Westphal, R. (2017). In J. L. Fridey (Ed.), *A compendium of transfusion practice guidelines* (3rd ed.). American Red Cross.

2017). In general, Rh(D) negative individuals should receive Rh(D) negative platelets, particularly women of childbearing age (Bachowski et al., 2017).

Prevention

Only transfuse blood/blood components when supported by practice guidelines (Bachowski et al., 2017; Gorski et al., 2016). If an ABO incompatibility exists, presentation usually occurs before the first 50 mL have infused, making the first 10 to 15 minutes of a transfusion the most critical (AABB, 2018). Focusing on correct identification is paramount to preventing incompatibility reactions.

- Label specimens and verify blood/blood components in the presence of the recipient prior to transfusion (Gorski et al., 2016).
- Perform baseline assessment of vital signs, respiratory assessment, and any risk for transfusion-related adverse reactions such as volume overload (AABB, 2018; Gorski et al., 2016).
- A competent practitioner performs recipient and blood/blood component verification to include the following:
  - At least two independent patient identifiers (AABB, 2018; Gorski et al., 2016)
  - ABO and Rh(D) type of recipient and blood/blood component (AABB, 2018; Gorski et al., 2016)
  - Expiration date and if applicable expiration time (AABB, 2018; Gorski et al., 2016)
- Monitor for reactions 5 to 15 minutes after transfusion start and for 4 to 6 hours after completion.

- Implement policies for specimen obtainment, cross-matching of blood/blood components, and transfusion administration (AABB, 2018; Bachowski et al., 2017).

Assessment and Treatment

In patients suspected of having a transfusion reaction related to incompatibility, the transfusion must be immediately stopped and the reaction reported to the patient's provider and the blood bank (AABB, 2018). Perform an immediate clerical check to ensure the patient received the correct unit (AABB, 2018). Signs/symptoms of incompatibility include fever, chills, chest or back pain, cardiopulmonary instability, or shock (AABB, 2018).

Clinical Practice Guidelines

- AABB—2018: *Primer of Blood Administration*
- American Red Cross—2017: *A Compendium of Transfusion Practice Guidelines*
- Infusion Nurses Society—2016: *Infusion Therapy Standards of Practice*

Pressure Injuries (Stages 3 and 4)

See Chapter 12, "Integumentary System"

Falls and Trauma

This HAC category is very broad and includes falls in the hospital setting (CMS, 2018). It also includes other trauma that may or may not be present with falls, such as fractures, dislocation, head injuries, burns, or other traumas including lacerations, hemorrhage, frostbite, corrosions, and asphyxiation (CMS, 2018). Falls, as defined by the NDNQI, are unplanned descents to the floor and may or may not be associated with an injury (Agency for Healthcare Research and Quality [AHRQ], 2013).

Etiology and Pathophysiology: Falls

Falls are classified as physiologic (patient related) and/or environmental (AHRQ, 2013).

Risk Factors

Environment

- Unfamiliar environment
- Clutter and/or medical equipment
- Improper use of assistive devices
- Lighting

Patient/Physiology

- Weakness, fatigue
- Gait and/or balance disorders
- Vision and/or hearing impairments
- History of falls
- Cognitive impairment
- Older age
- Dizziness, vertigo, and/or postural hypotension
- Polypharmacy
- Use of diuretics, sedatives, opiates, and/or cardiovascular medications (American Geriatrics Society & British Geriatrics Society [AGS & BGS], 2011; Degelau et al., 2012)

Prevention

While not all falls can be prevented, there is extensive literature on efforts that clinicians and healthcare organizations can utilize to reduce falls in the acute care setting (Degelau et al., 2012).

- Complete fall risk assessment on admission, each shift, with changes in the patient's condition or location including after a fall occurs.
  - Communicate this risk to other team members involved in the patient's care.

- Educate the patient on their unique fall risk factors.
- Establish a safe environment.
  - Remove excessive equipment.
  - Place assistive devices, personal care items, and call lights within reach.
- Perform rounding hourly and implement a targeted toileting schedule if indicated.
- Establish policies for risk assessment and fall prevention.
- Utilize standard fall risk assessment tool.

Etiology and Pathophysiology: Trauma

Risk Factors

Environment

- Poor technique, inexperienced practitioner, or non adherence to safety checklists
- Presence of an ignition source (e.g., electrocautery or Bovie)
- Use of flammable skin preparation (e.g., alcohol-based solutions)
- Open oxygen source (e.g., nasal cannula or face mask)

Patient

- Procedure performed above the xiphoid process

Prevention

Prevention will vary based on the clinical setting and trauma. Following are recommendations to prevent fires and subsequently burns in the intraoperative setting (AORN, 2019).

- Allow sufficient drying time for flammable skin preparation solutions.
- Avoid pooling of flammable skin preparation.
- Configure drapes to reduce the accumulation of oxidizers.
- Moisten sponges/gauze when used in proximity of ignition sources.
- Announce when an ignition source is activated: Team members should reduce the oxygen concentration as needed and stop the use of nitrous oxide.
- Use grounding pads with electrosurgical devices.
- Use a safety checklist that includes risk for fire.

Assessment and Treatment: Falls and Trauma

Initial response should include an assessment for injuries. Depending on the severity of the trauma, supportive therapy including cardiopulmonary resuscitation should be undertaken immediately. Patients should not be moved if an injury is suspected. Fall injuries are often classified using the NDNQI levels (Table 23.6; AHRQ, 2013). Treatment and additional assessments will vary on the type of injury:

- Fractures: See Chapter 16, "Multisystem Disorders"
- Dislocations
- Head injuries: See Chapter 14, "Nervous System"
- Burns (Chapter 12): The immediate intervention should be to stop the source of the burn

Clinical Practice Guidelines

- American Geriatrics Society/British Geriatrics Society—2010: *Clinical Practice Guideline—Prevention of Falls in Older Persons*
- Association of Peri-operative Registered Nurses—2013: *Recommended Practices for a Safe Environment of Care*
- Institute for Clinical Systems Improvement—2012: *Health Care Protocol Prevention of Falls (Acute Care)*

Manifestations of Poor Glycemic Control

See Chapter 8, "Endocrine System."

TABLE 23.6 NATIONAL DATABASE OF NURSING QUALITY INDICATORS: FALL LEVEL OF INJURY

None	No signs or symptoms of injury; if imaging performed, no findings of injury noted
Minor	Application of a dressing, ice, limb elevation, cleaning of a wound; bruising or an abrasion; potential medications including topical and for pain
Moderate	Closure of skin using steri-strips, suture, or glue; or a muscle/joint strain
Major	Surgery, casting, or traction needed; neurologic consult required; internal injuries such as a rib fracture; or requirement of blood products related to the fall
Death	Death from injuries sustained from the fall; does *not* include physiologic events that may have led to the fall in which the patient then died

Deep Vein Thrombosis/Pulmonary Embolism Following Total Knee Replacement and Hip Replacement

Definition

Major orthopedic surgery is one of the most common causes of venous thromboembolism (VTE). Postoperative VTE are considered HACs by CMS for VTE after total knee replacement (TKR) and total hip replacement (THR). VTE can occur in any patient population especially with prolonged immobility.

Etiology and Pathophysiology

There is increased risk of developing a VTE, independent of other risk factors, after TKR and THR. Refer to Chapter 9, "Hematopoietic System" for additional VTE risk factors.

Risk Factors

- Activation of the coagulation cascade from tissue and bone injury
- Reduced venous emptying due to the intraoperative use of tourniquets
- Immobilization (Cionac Florescu et al., 2013)

Prevention

- THR or TKA should have 10 to 14 days of postoperative antithrombotic prophylaxis.
  - Low-molecular-weight heparin is the preferred medication.
  - Alternative medications include fondaparinux, apixaban, dabigatran, rivaroxaban, low-dose unfractionated heparin, glucuronidation adjusted-dose vitamin K antagonist, and aspirin.
  - Intermittent pneumatic compression device (IPCD) for a minimum of 18 hours per day in conjunction with pharmacological prophylaxis.
- Consider antithrombotic prophylaxis for up to 35 days postoperatively (Falck-Yitter et al., 2012).
- Patients with an increased risk for bleeding should have mechanical prophylaxis with IPCD alone.

Healthcare Organizations

- Consider policies and procedures to ensure every patient with TKR and THR has mechanical and/or pharmacologic VTE prophylaxis in the perioperative period and upon discharge.

Assessment and Treatment

Refer to Chapter 7, "Respiratory System," and Chapter 9, "Hematopoietic System," for the assessment and treatment of DVT and PE.

Clinical Practice Guidelines

- American College of Chest Physicians—2012: *Prevention of VTE in Orthopedic Surgery Patients*
- Association of periOperative Nurses—2019: *Guidelines for Perioperative Practice*

Iatrogenic Pneumothorax With Venous Catheterization

CVADs are intravascular catheters that terminate close to the heart or in one of the great vessels. A serious but preventable complication of CVAD insertion is pneumothorax. Iatrogenic pneumothoraxes occur during CVAD insertion when the needle, dilator, or guidewire punctures the lung, causing air to enter into the pleural space (Troianos et al., 2011).

Etiology and Pathophysiology

A life-threatening tension pneumothorax may occur if the insertion causes a one-way valve to occur, trapping air inside the lungs. This causes high pressure in the lungs and shifting of intrathoracic structures, which causes a loss of venous return of blood to the heart.

Risk Factors

Patient

- High BMI
- Underlying comorbidities such as congestive obstructive pulmonary disease (COPD) or coagulopathy
- Mechanical ventilation
- Inability to follow commands
- Restlessness
- Congenital abnormalities, operations, trauma, or radiotherapy to the anatomic region of the insertion site (Troianos et al., 2011; Tsotsolis et al., 2015)

Environment

- Site of attempted access (subclavian or internal jugular)
- Poor technique or inexperienced practitioner
- Insertion without ultrasound guidance
- Insertion under emergent situation
- Multiple insertion attempts
- Large catheter diameter

Prevention

- Prevention of iatrogenic pneumothoraxes focuses on training and ultrasound use.
  - Use of ultrasound for CVAD placement with real-time needle guidance into the desired vessel (Troianos et al., 2011; Tsotsolis et al., 2015)
  - Risk versus benefit of site selection (internal jugular vein has less risk of pneumothorax during CVAD insertion but the subclavian vein has a lower infection risk; Tsotsolis et al., 2015)
  - Standardized insertion method (Troianos et al., 2011)
  - Post-procedure imaging to confirm absence of pneumothorax (Tsotsolis et al., 2015)
  - Use of a safety checklist (Anderson et al., 2014)
  - High-quality training programs for practitioners who insert CVAD that include didactic and simulation training along with supervision during insertion (Troianos et al., 2011)
  - Credentialing and privileging of practitioners for CVAD insertion procedures

Assessment and Treatment

A pneumothorax may or may not be evident after insertion of a CVAD. Tension pneumothorax are life threatening and typically has immediate signs and symptoms; patients may require cardiopulmonary resuscitation if not quickly treated (Tsotsolis et al., 2015). Please refer to Chapter 7, "Respiratory System," for the assessment and treatment of pneumothorax and tension pneumothorax.

Clinical Practice Guidelines

- The American Society of Echocardiography and the Society of Cardiovascular Anesthesiologists (2011): *Guidelines for Performing Ultrasound Guided Vascular Cannulation*

HEALTHCARE-ASSOCIATED INFECTION

Healthcare-associated infections (HAIs) fall under the broader category of HACs. HAI definitions and treatment guidelines are updated on an ongoing basis: practitioners should refer to the most specific guidelines for inclusion/exclusion criteria and current treatment recommendations.

Catheter-Associated Urinary Tract Infection

Urinary tract infections (UTIs) include symptomatic or asymptomatic infection of the urinary system including the urethra, bladder, ureters, and kidneys. If the UTI is related to a urinary catheter, it is considered a CAUTI.

Signs and symptoms are as follows (Centers for Disease Control and Prevention [CDC], 2019):

- Fever greater than 38 °C
- Suprapubic tenderness
- Costovertebral angle pain or tenderness
- Urinary urgency, urinary frequency, and/or dysuria

Etiology and Pathophysiology

CAUTIs occur when breakdown in insertion or maintenance technique allows bacteria to enter the urinary system. Indications for a urinary catheter include the following (Gould et al., 2019):

- Acute urinary retention or bladder outlet obstruction
- Need for accurate measurement of urinary output in critically ill patients
- Perioperative use in selected surgical procedures:
  - Urologic surgery or other surgery on contiguous structures of the genitourinary tract
  - Prolonged duration of surgery
  - Anticipated intraoperative use of large-volume infusions or diuretic
  - Need for intraoperative monitoring of urinary output
- To assist in healing of open sacral or perineal wounds in incontinent patients
- Patient requires prolonged immobilization (e.g., unstable thoracic or lumbar spine; multiple traumatic injuries)
- Comfort for end-of-life care if indicated

Risk Factors

Environment

- Poor technique or inexperienced practitioner
- Poor catheter maintenance including not maintaining a closed drainage system
- Incorrect positioning of drainage tubing and/or bag

Patient

- Severity of illness
- Older age
- Female gender
- Comorbidities including diabetes mellitus, renal dysfunction, and impaired immunity
- Fecal incontinence

Prevention

Indication for urinary catheter should be assessed daily, and the urinary catheter should be removed as soon as clinically indicated (Gould et al., 2019).

- Follow proper insertion practices including hand hygiene, aseptic technique, antiseptic or sterile solution for peri-urethral cleaning, and a single-use packet of lubricant for insertion.
- Secure the urinary catheter after insertion to prevent movement and urethral traction.
- Maintain a closed drainage system with unobstructed urinary flow.
- Perform daily metal surface cleaning.
- Promptly remove unnecessary urinary catheters and use daily audits to determine if the catheter is still indicated.
- Utilize alternatives to urinary catheters such as external urinary collection devices when clinically appropriate.
  - Consider programs that have demonstrated success, including nurse-directed urinary catheter and guidelines for perioperative catheter management.
  - Consider the use of bundles with all needed supplies.

Assessment and Treatment

CAUTIs may occur despite all preventative measures being in place. If CAUTI is suspected, the urinary catheter should be removed, replaced if clinically indicated, and a urine specimen should be obtained for culture. Antibiotics should be administered based on the sensitivity of organisms and patient condition. See Chapter 16, "Multisystem Disorders," for a list of anti-infective agents. See Chapter 11, "Renal System" for additional information on treatment of UTIs.

Clinical Practice Guidelines

- Centers for Disease Control—(2009): *Guidelines for Prevention of Catheter-Associated Urinary Tract Infections*

Vascular Catheter-Associated Infection

Bloodstream infections that are related to an intravascular device, when the device is a CVAD, are known as *central line associated bloodstream infections (CLABSIs)*.

Etiology and Pathophysiology

CLABSIs may occur due to breakdown in insertion or maintenance technique, contaminated fluids, and/or skin flora, which allows bacteria or viruses to enter the bloodstream.

- Indications for a CVAD include the following (Gorski et al., 2016):
  - Clinical instability of the patient and or/complex infusion regimen
  - Episodic chemotherapy, anticipated duration of longer than 3 months
  - Continuous infusion therapy including parenteral nutrition, blood, fluid, and/or electrolytes
  - Invasive hemodynamic monitoring
  - Long-term intermittent infusion therapy (e.g., antibiotics)

- Failed or difficult peripheral venous access (ultrasound previously attempted)
- Apheresis or dialysis

Risk Factors

Environment

- Emergent catheter insertion
- Poor technique or inexperienced practitioner
- Catheter type, lumen size, and duration
- Frequency of catheter access
- Care settings, such as the ICU, have higher rates of infection

Patient

- Severity of illness
- Compromised skin integrity
- Femoral insertion sites (highest risk of infection)

Prevention

Assessment of indications for CVADs should be ongoing, and the CVAD should be removed as soon as clinically indicated (Gorski et al., 2016; O'Grady et al., 2011).

- Follow proper insertion practices, including hand hygiene, aseptic technique, maximal sterile barrier, preparation of the insertion site with at least 0.5% chlorhexidine (CHG), placement of a sterile dressing over the insertion site, and use of a CHG-impregnated dressing (O'Grady et al., 2011).
- Handle and maintain central lines appropriately, including the following:
  - Bathe ICU patients with CHG daily (Talbot et al., 2017)
  - Aseptic access of the CVAD (Gorski et al., 2016; O'Grady et al., 2011)
  - Change dressings aseptically that are wet, soiled, or dislodged (Gorski et al., 2016; O'Grady et al., 2011)
- Use designated, competent personnel for insertion and maintenance of CVADs.
- Use safety checklists to ensure adherence to aseptic insertion practices.
- Consider the use of bundles with all needed supplies.

Assessment and Treatment

CLABSIs may occur despite all preventive measures being in place. If CLABSI is suspected, peripheral blood cultures should be promptly obtained and antibiotics administered based on the sensitivity of organisms and patient condition. The CVAD should be removed and if indicated replaced per the healthcare organizations protocols.

Clinical Practice Guidelines

- Centers for Disease Control (2011): *Guidelines for the Prevention of Intravascular Catheter-Related Infections*
- Centers for Disease Control (2017): *Updated Recommendations on the Use of Chlorhexidine Impregnated Dressings for Prevention of Intravascular Catheter Related Infections*
- Infusion Nurses Society (2016): *Infusion Therapy Standards of Practice*
- National Kidney Foundation (2006): *Clinical Practice Guidelines for Vascular Access*

PUBLIC RESOURCES FOR PROCESS IMPROVEMENT

As healthcare transitions from volume to value, clinicians must seek resources to examine current processes and practices and to critically evaluate their efficiency, effectiveness, and impact on outcomes.

- Process improvement is a proactive approach to improving processes and practices to influence outcomes (AABB, 2018), by addressing human performance across organizations (AGS & BGS, 2011).
- Numerous resources are available from organizations, such as the CMS, TJC, IHI, and AHRQ, to support the work of process improvement (Table 23.7). The IHI provides an Improvement Project Roadmap with step-by-step guidance on conducting an improvement project (Box 23.1).

EVALUATING PATIENT OUTCOMES

OVERVIEW

The only way to know whether an intervention or strategy you implemented made a difference is to measure outcomes.

- Determining what will be measured is part of the planning process.
- All outcome measures should be determined prior to any implementation of steps.
- Determining and validating the problem is essential before you can determine appropriate outcomes.
- The difference between an outcome measure and a process measure needs to be appreciated.
  - An outcome measure shows the impact to the organization, staff, or patients. It can also be referred to as a metric.
  - Process measures are often confused with outcome measures but really only tell us if the intervention or strategy was indeed applied.
  - Process measures are equally important because without them, we would not know if the outcome measure is a true reflection of whether our intervention or strategy made a difference.

For example, "central line dressings are not applied properly" is not a problem. The result of those actions is a problem.

The outcome measure of the previous example would be the CLABSI rate. The process measure would be how many dressings are applied correctly.

Measurement and Outcomes

Patient outcomes can be broken down into four subgroups (Doran et al., 2010):

- Clinical-symptom management and prevention of complications; morbidity/mortality
- Functionality, quality of life, ability to participate in activities of daily living
- Perception: patient satisfaction/experience
- Cost: use of resources

Outcome considerations for the CNS

- Are the outcomes short term or long term? Typically, there should be a mixture of both.
- Are the data already available or will they have to be collected? Again, the outcomes and the plan for obtaining data should all be outlined and agreed upon by the team prior to implementing any intervention or strategy. Some data may not be feasible or practical to obtain.
- How will I report outcome data and whom will I report it to? This comes back to stakeholders and keeping the staff engaged.
- Are there outcomes that are required? Some outcome metrics, such as infection rates, are publicly reported and organizations are required to collect and report the data in a particular way (Table 23.8).

TABLE 23.7 PUBLIC RESOURCES FOR PROCESS IMPROVEMENT

ORGANIZATION	RESOURCES/WEBSITE
AHRQ National Quality Strategy: Better care Health People/Healthy Communities Affordable care	AHRQ: The National Quality Strategy https://innovations.ahrq.gov/issues/2016/06/15/national-quality-strategy-guiding-efforts-improve-health-care-quality
AHRQ Talking Quality offers guidance on producing comparative information on healthcare quality that is understandable / useful to consumers.	AHRQ Talking Quality https://www.ahrq.gov/talkingquality/index.html
ANA: Overview of ANA's work on nursing quality and useful related resources. Includes links with resources: Quality organizations Research and measurement, including a research toolkit and resources on the link between nursing and quality Advocacy Education on quality, including links to NDNQI and QSEN	ANA Nursing Quality https://www.nursingworld.org/practice-policy/nursing-excellence/quality/
ASQ: International organization, not focused on healthcare. Provides case studies, webcasts, journal articles, and resources for certification in quality. The resources on the ASQ website provide a wide variety process improvement tools.	ASQ https://asq.org/quality-resources
CMS Hospital-Acquired Conditions (Present on Admission Indicator): CMS currently has identified 14 conditions that result in higher costs and could have reasonably been prevented. Hospitals that perform in the bottom quartile will have their payments ↓ by 1%.	CMS Hospital-Acquired Conditions https://www.cms.gov/Medicare/Medicare-Fee-for-Service-Payment/HospitalAcqCond/index.html
CMS HACRP: Health and Human Services adjusts payments to the lowest performing hospitals in two domains: patient safety indicators and hospital acquired infections.	CMS HACRP https://www.cms.gov/Medicare/Medicare-Fee-for-Service-Payment/AcuteInpatientPPS/HAC-Reduction-Program.html
CMS Quality Measures: Tools to help the government measure or quantify healthcare processes, outcomes, patient perceptions, and organizational structure and/or systems.	CMS Quality Measures https://www.cms.gov/Medicare/Quality-Initiatives-Patient-Assessment-Instruments/QualityMeasures/index.html
Hospital Compare: Sponsored by CMS, provides information on the quality of care at over 4,000 Medicare certified hospitals. This resource is used by patients and families to assess the quality of care of hospitals and healthcare organizations.	Hospital Compare https://www.medicare.gov/hospitalcompare/about/what-is-hos.html
IHI: Focus is on improving the quality of health care for all populations. Created the triple aim for healthcare: improving population health; improving the experience of care for that population; and decreasing the per capita cost of health care. Promotes the science of patient safety through the development of programs and processes that improve care and decrease cost. NPSF: Conducts education, research, and advocacy in support of patient and workforce safety. IHI and NPSF merged in 2017	IHI http://www.ihi.org//resources/Pages/default.aspx Free resources include: Model and measures for process improvement Change for Improvement Process improvement tools IHI White papers on performance improvement Audio and video resources National Patient Safety Foundation https://www.npsf.org/

(continued)

TABLE 23.7 PUBLIC RESOURCES FOR PROCESS IMPROVEMENT (*continued*)

ORGANIZATION	RESOURCES/WEBSITE
ISMP: Nonprofit organization whose work has resulted in changes in clinical practice, public policy, and drug labeling and packaging. Gold standard for medication safety standards.	ISMP https://www.ismp.org/resources?field_resource_type_target_id%5B33%5D=33#-resources--resources_list Key Guidelines: Medication safety High alert medications Infusion pump safety Automated dispensing cabinets Intravenous push medications Subcutaneous insulin use
TJC manual for National Hospital Inpatient Quality Measures: Collaboration between TJC and CMS to identify hospital performance measures.	TJC https://www.jointcommission.org/specifications_manual_for_national_hospital_inpatient_quality_measures.aspx
TJC National Patient Safety Goals: A program to help organizations identify and address specific patient safety issues. They are reviewed and updated annually, based on reported events and feedback from practitioners and providers.	TJC https://www.jointcommission.org/standards_information/npsgs.aspx
TJC Pioneers in Quality: A program to assist Joint Commission-accredited hospitals toward eCQM adoption and reporting. Includes the Proven Practices Collection.	TJC Pioneers in Quality https://www.jointcommission.org/facts_about_pioneers_in_quality/
NAHQ: Organization dedicated to the development of healthcare quality professionals.	NAHQ https://nahq.org/about/about-national-association-healthcare-quality
National Council for Medication Error Reporting and Prevention: The NCC is an independent body of 27 national organizations whose aim is to maximize the safe use of medications and increase awareness of medication errors through open communication, increased reporting, and promotion of medication error prevention strategies.	National Council for Medication Error Reporting and Prevention NCC http://www.ihi.org/resources/Pages/OtherWebsites/NCCMERP.aspx
NDNQI: Sponsored by Press-Ganey, examines the relationship between nursing care and patient outcomes. Essential data for hospitals who are ANCC Magnet credentialed.	NDNQI https://nursingandndnqi.weebly.com/ndnqi-indicators.html
National Quality Forum: Establishes the standard for measurement of healthcare quality. Sets priorities for performance measurement. Recommends measures used in payment and public reporting.	National Quality Forum http://www.qualityforum.org/about_nqf/work_in_quality_measurement/ https://www.qualityforum.org/what_we_do.aspx

AHRQ, Agency for Healthcare Research and Quality; ANA, American Nurses Association; ANCC, American Nurses Credentialing Center; ASQ, American Society for Quality; CMS, Centers for Medicare and Medicaid Services; eCQM, electronic clinical quality measure; HACRP, Hospital-Acquired Condition Reduction Program; IHI, Institute for Healthcare Improvement; ISMP, Institute for Safe Medication Practices; NAHQ: National Association of Healthcare Quality; NCC, National Coordinating Council; NDNQI, National Database of Nursing Quality Indicators; NPSF, National Patient Safety Foundation; QSEN, Quality and Safety Education for Nurses; TJC, The Joint Commission.

Sources: From Agency for Healthcare Research and Quality. (2013). *How do you measure fall rates and fall prevention practices?* https://www.ahrq.gov/professionals/systems/hospital/fallpxtoolkit/fallpxtk5.htm; Agency for Healthcare Research and Quality. (2017). *Estimating the additional hospital inpatient cost and mortality associated with select hospital-acquired conditions.* AHRQ Publication No. 18-0011-EF; Anderson, D. J., Podgorny, K., Berríos-Torres, S. I., Bratzler, D. W., Dellinger, E. P., Greene, L., Nyquist, A.-C., Saiman, L., Yokoe, D. S., Maragakis, L. L., & Kaye, K. S. (2014). Strategies to prevent surgical site infections in acute care hospitals: 2014 update. *Infection Control and Hospital Epidemiology, 35*(6), 605–627. https://doi.org/10.1086/676022; Association of periOperative Nurses. (2019). *Guidelines for perioperative practice.* Association of periOperative Nurses; Centers

(*continued*)

TABLE 23.7 PUBLIC RESOURCES FOR PROCESS IMPROVEMENT (continued)

for Disease Control and Prevention. (2019). *National Healthcare Safety Network (NHSN) patient safety component manual*. https://www.cdc.gov/nhsn/pdfs/pscmanual/pcsmanual_current.pdf; Centers for Medicare & Medicaid Services. (2018). Hospital acquired conditions. https://www.cms.gov/Medicare/Medicare-Fee-for-Service-Payment/HospitalAcqCond/Hospital-Acquired_Conditions.html; Cionac Florescu, S., Anastase, D. M., Munte-anu, A. M., Stoica, I. C., & Antonescu, D. (2013). Venous thromboembolism following major orthopaedic surgery. *Maedica, 8*(2), 189–194; Cook, L. S. (2013). Infusion-related air embolism. *Journal of Infusion Nursing, 36*(1), 26–36. https://doi.org/10.1097/NAN.0b013e318279a804; Degelau, J., Belz, M., Bungum, L., Flavin, P. L., Harper, C., Leys, K., Lundquist, L., & Webb, B. (2012). *Prevention of falls (acute care)*. Institute for Clinical Systems Improvement; Falck-Ytter, Y., Francis, C. W., Johanson, N. A., Curley, C., Dhal, I. E., Schulman, S., Ortel, T. L., Pauker, S. G., & Colwell, C. W. (2012). Prevention of VTE in orthopedic surgery patients. *Chest, 141*(2), e278S–e325S. https://doi.org/10.1378/chest.11-2404; Bachowski, G., Borge, D., Brunker, P. A. R., Eder, A., Fialkow, L., Fridey, J. L., Goldberg, C., Hopkins, C. K., Lightfoot, T., Morgan, S. M., Stramer, S., Wagner, S. J., & Westphal, R. (2017). In J. L. Fridey (Ed.), *A compendium of transfusion practice guidelines* (3rd ed.). American Red Cross; Gorski, L., Hadaway, L., Hagle, M. E., McGoldrick, M., Orr, M., & Doellman, D. (2016). Infusion therapy standards of practice. *Journal of Infusion Nursing, 39*(1S), S1–S159; Gould, C. V., Umscheid, C. A., Agarwal, R. K., Kuntz, G., Pegues, D. A. & the Healthcare Infection Control Practices Advisory Committee. (2009). *Guidelines for prevention of catheter-associated urinary tract infections 2009*. Centers for Disease Control. https://www.cdc.gov/infectioncontrol/pdf/guidelines/cauti-guidelines-H.pdf; Hariharan, D., & Lobo, D. N. (2013). Retained surgical sponges, needles and instruments. *Annals of the Royal College of Surgeons of England, 95*(5), 87–92. https://doi.org/10.1308/003588413X13511609957218; Mangram, A. J., Horan, T. C., Pearson, M. L., Silver, L. C., & Jarvis, W. R. (1999). Guideline for prevention of surgical site infection, 1999. *American Journal of Infection Control, 27*(2), 97–134. https://doi.org/10.1016/S0196-6553(99)70088-X; O'Grady, N. P., Alexander, M., Burns, L., Dellinger, E. P., Garland, J., Heard, S. O., Lipsett, P. A., Masur, H., Mermel, L. A., Pearson, M. L., Raad, I. I., Randolph, A., Rupp, M. E., Saint, S., & the Healthcare Infection Control Practices Advisory Committee. (2011). *Guidelines for the prevention of intravascular catheter-related infections, 2011*. Centers for Disease Control. https://www.cdc.gov/hai/pdfs/bsi-guidelines-2011.pdf; Talbot, T. R., Stone, E. C., Irwin, K., Overholt, A. D., Dasti, M., & Kallen, A. (2017). *2017 Updated recommendations on the use of chlorhexidine impregnated dressings for prevention of intravascular catheter related infections*. Centers for Disease Control. https://www.cdc.gov/infectioncontrol/pdf/guidelines/c-i-dressings-H.pdf; Troianos, C. A., Hartman, G. S., Glas, K. E., Skubas, N. J., Eberhardt, R. T. Walker, J. D., & Reeves, S. T. (2011). Guidelines for performing ultrasound guided vascular cannulation: Recommendations of the American Society of Echocardiography and the Society of Cardiovascular Anesthesiologists. *Journal of American Society of Echocardiography, 24*(12), 1291I–1318. https://doi.org/10.1016/j.echo.2011.09.021; Tsotsolis, N., Tsirgogianni, K., Kioumis, I., Pitsiou, G., Baka, S., Papaiwannou., A., Karavergou, A., Rapti, A., Trakada, G., Katsikogiannis, N., Tsakiridis, K., Karapantzos, I., Karapantzou, C., Barbetakis, N., Zissimopoulos, A., Kuhajda, I., Andjelkovic, D., Zarogoulidis, K., & Zarogoulidis, P. (2015). Pneumothorax as a complication of central venous catheter insertion. *Annals of Translational Medicine, 3*(3), 40. https://doi.org/10.3978/j.issn.2305-5839.2015.02.11

Box 23.1 Improvement Project Road Map

Set an aim: What are you trying to accomplish?
Develop an improvement strategy.
Develop and pilot a reliable standard process of care tasks
Implement the standard care process; monitor performance
Spread the new standard throughout the system

TABLE 23.8 EXAMPLES OF OUTCOMES

PATIENT	STAFF	ORGANIZATION
Decreased infections	Nursing engagement and satisfaction, job enjoyment	Cost (length of stay, reimbursement, use of resources, readmission rate, etc.)
Improved functional status	Nursing time	Use actual cost if known or documented averages
Increased satisfaction	Nursing knowledge	Reputation of the hospital: ratings, accreditations

CNSs and Nurse-Sensitive Outcomes

Nurse-sensitive outcomes are those things that "reflect nursing's unique contribution to patient care and are necessary for demonstrating the quality of nursing practice" (Duffy, 2002, p. 70). Nurses impact so many outcomes in the hospital, but these outcomes are those that can be empirically tied to the care provided by nursing.

Common Nurse-Sensitive Patient Outcomes

- CLABSI
- CAUTI

- VAP
- HAPI (hospital-acquired pressure injury)
- Patient falls
- Failure to rescue
- Patient perception of pain

Other common patient outcomes CNSs impact:

- Surgical site infections
- Glycemic control
- Medication errors
- Restraint usage

CNSs possess the competencies necessary to impact patient-related outcomes. CNSs frequently lead the multidisciplinary groups that manage these outcomes.

When leading the efforts in a nurse-sensitive outcome, CNSs should do the following:

- Understand the problem and current state; they must have some level of data-driven validation.
- **Lead a group in the effort:** CNSs are skilled in leading groups and facilitating meetings.
- **Communicate effectively:** Communication is key to the success of any outcome effort. Communicate with all stakeholders and those involved in impacting the outcome.
- **Be a change agent:** Have an understanding of change theories and apply them to the strategies.
- **Be a mentor:** Demonstrate the behaviors that are desired to produce desired outcomes.
- **Analyze and present data:** Know how to communicate outcomes so that the stakeholders can understand the outcomes and what is needed from them to either hardwire current state or work to improve to obtain the desired outcome.

Validity and Reliability Measures

Before thinking about the validity and reliability of an instrument, first consider that there are two different types of instruments.

- Instruments that are used to collect information by a researcher or an investigator
  - Examples of these include observation forms, checklists, and rating scales
- Instruments that are completed by subjects
  - Examples of these include questionnaires, surveys, and tests

Validity and reliability are important any time you are using a data collection instrument. These measures help determine the quality of the data collected.

Validity

The validity measurement indicates to what degree the instrument is measuring what it was intended to measure. There are many different types of validity but the most common are the following:

- **Content**—Do items in the instrument adequately measure or represent what you are trying to measure?
- **Construct**—Does the instrument accurately measure a construct (something that cannot be measured directly, such as a belief)?
- **Criterion**—Does the score of the instrument correlate with an outcome?

How to Test Validity

- **Content**—Have the instrument reviewed by a subject matter expert.
- **Construct**
  - **Convergent validation**—When the instrument has a high correlation with another test that measures the same thing
  - **Divergent validation**—When the instrument has a low correlation with another test that measures something different
  - **Factor analysis**—Formal statistical test
- **Criterion**—Compares instrument scores to an outcome measure

Reliability

The reliability of an instrument is its ability to produce consistent results.

For example, a scale is valid if it yields the correct weight. It is reliable if it yields the same weight each time it is used. A scale that is off by 5 lbs would not be valid but could be reliable if it was **always** off by 5 lbs.

How to Test for Reliability

- **Test for internal consistency**—Most common is Cronbach's alpha (higher the better, greater than .70 or .80 acceptable)
- **Test–retest measures**—Administering the instrument multiple times (with *no* intervention between testing) to the same sample and comparing scores to ensure consistency
- **Inter-rater reliability**—Comparing scores between individuals in a sample. This is particularly helpful when multiple individuals are using a tool or protocol to collect information. Inter-rater reliability helps ensure consistency among individuals.

INFORMATION TECHNOLOGY

OVERVIEW

Information technology (IT) may be used as an umbrella term to conceptually describe any number of things that utilize electronic processes to receive and/or deliver information.

Health information technology (HIT) is the use of IT for the receipt, delivery, and utilization of health information in electronic systems (Office for Civil Rights, 2019). HIT is the division of IT that pertains more specifically to IT in the many and various health sectors, for example, devices, the electronic health record (EHR), Health Information Exchange (HIE) networks, and telecommunications.

- The Office of the National Coordinator (ONC) was established in 2009 to carry out the requirements to ensure the meaningful use of interoperable EHR throughout the United States as a critical national goal to improve the quality, safety, and efficiency of healthcare (American Recovery and Reinvestment Act [ARRA], 2009).
- **Interoperability** is the "ability of different information systems, devices or applications to connect, in a coordinated manner, within and across organizational boundaries to access, exchange and cooperatively use data amongst stakeholders, with the goal of optimizing the health of individuals and populations" (Healthcare Information and Management Systems Society [HIMSS], 2019).

HIT is growing as a necessity of the care delivery system to deliver the highest quality of care at the lowest cost. HIT is needed to derive positive patient outcomes, patient experiences, and the most efficient care processes; it is imperative that the CNS be knowledgeable of HIT and its relationship with CNS practice.

OVERVIEW OF INFORMATICS

The American Medical Informatics Association (AMIA) describes health informatics as an interdisciplinary applied research and practice domain within a larger context: informaticsis, a driver of innovative IT solutions for knowledge and information management based upon data generated by people in all sectors related to health (American Medical Informatics Association [AMIA], 2019).

NURSING INFORMATICS

The ANA defines *nursing informatics (NI)* as "the specialty that integrates nursing science with multiple information and analytical sciences to identify, define, manage and communicate data, information, knowledge and wisdom in nursing practice" (2015, p. 8).

The specialty of NI has grown in all areas, with the most prevalent impacts on clinical application utilization from development to optimization in EMR and computerized physician order entry (CPOE; HIMSS, 2017).

There are key attributes of NI that perhaps sum the role up best (Sensmeier, 2012):

- Experienced users of the nursing process
- Experts at using their analytical, critical thinking skills
- Excellent project managers using technology and information systems
- NI is a partner to nurses and nursing departments in the analysis and evaluation of technologic design and function to meet process needs and aid nurses in the efficient capture of documentation, while ensuring policies are upheld and regulatory required elements of nursing best practices are designed efficiently.
- NI is also the role by which innovative and transformative solutions have been demonstrated (Nelson & Parker, 2019).
- NI may assist nurses' understanding of HIT functionalities and provides an avenue by which IT knowledge, system functionality, and workflow design are understood.

EHRs and their data are expected to drive efficiencies in care processes while protecting patients' health information and ensuring the best patient safety, quality of care, and outcomes.

Definitions

Electronic medical records—A digital version of the paper charts in the clinician's office. An electronic medical record (EMR) contains the medical and treatment history of the patients in one practice (Garrett & Seidman, 2011).

Electronic health record—Focuses on the total health of the patient: going beyond standard clinical data collected in the provider's office and inclusive of a broader view on a patient's care (Garrett & Seidman, 2011).

Two key methodologies of HIT are targeted to facilitate improvements in the improved access to healthcare services, namely, a person's experience of care and consumer expectations related to these barriers: telehealth and patient portals.

TELEHEALTH

Telehealth offers the opportunity to meet consumers' increasing desire and demand for more convenient and affordable care. Telehealth and telemedicine services are reshaping the scope of learning for clinicians, who must remain competent in all realms of care delivery processes to ensure the safe, best, and most efficient patient care that meets the expectations of increasingly better-informed consumers.

Definitions

Telehealth—Refers to "the use of electronic information and telecommunications technologies to support and promote long-distance clinical health care, patient and professional health-related education, public health and health administration" (Office of the National Coordinator [ONC], 2019a, p. 15).

Telemedicine—Remote clinical services (ONC, 2019b).

There are several types of devices that may be used for telehealth, including the following:

- Smartphones and their apps
- Wearables such as activity trackers
- Telephone or computer-based automated reminders
- Continuous blood glucose monitors
- Important to ensure that clinicians have ample opportunity for training and educational opportunities to ensure their understanding of functionalities, security implications, employer expectations, and legislative controls
- Healthcare systems utilize telemedicine technologies to extend into underserved areas whose residents may not have access to the same levels of care more urbanized areas experience (HIMSS, 2019) and to populations who need or expect access in a much more convenient form of delivery (HIMSS, 2019)
- Telehealth services use technology for improved patient access to services, do not require in-person visits, and may allow for assessment and monitoring via a virtual platform such as e-ICUs, remote telemetry monitoring, and follow-up video visits
- Barriers to telehealth (Baggot et al., 2019):
  - Lacking consistency in the definition of telehealth
  - Services considered to be telehealth
  - Reimbursement of services delivered via telehealth platforms
- Consumer adoption

Consumerism and better, faster care demand the use of HIT and telehealth services. There will always be a necessity for clinical expertise in the design of HIT for best clinical outcomes. With HIT in the hands of patients, the CNS must be a knowledge expert at the patient, nurse, and system levels to ensure evidence-based standards of care are incorporated within the systems used.

PATIENT PORTALS

Definition

The HIE allows healthcare professionals and patients to securely access and share patients' medical information electronically (ONC, 2017).

- An integral component of HIE is the uptake and integration of patients' data.
- Patient portals, a secure, online avenue by which patients engage with and may enter their own protected health information (PHI) through a patient-accessed portal of the EHR, are growing as an expected option for consumers to know about their PHI and engage with it as a core member of the care team (ONC, 2017).
- Direct-to-consumer applications and devices are readily available and enable many health and wellness features, diet and physical activity tracking, and symptom analysis. While there has traditionally been a clear segregation between a personal device and EHRs, there is an increase in the demand for connectedness between the traditionally siloed sectors all related to a person's health (Sharp, 2019).

The CMS intends to put patients at the center of their healthcare, enabling patient engagement opportunities and interoperability of systems, including the following:

- Increasing efficiencies for patient's use of portals by ensuring timely sharing of healthcare information
- Improve data sharing between payers for timely coordination of benefits
- Increased access to prices and costs of healthcare services for informed decision-making
- Utilizing application programming interfaces (API) to connect third party software with EMRs for seamless and more timely interfacing between systems

The Medicare Incentives program Incentives for Adoption and Meaningful User of Certified EHR Technology is described as using technology to improve patient self-management, communication, and access. Meaningful Use has incentivized the HIT infrastructure to achieve greater than 450,000 eligible professionals and hospitals' use of EHRs (Desalvo, n.d.); there are now new functionalities to improve patient engagement functionalities to improve health outcomes (ONC, 2016).

The ONC has identified seven key steps outlined in an easy-to-use *Patient Engagement Playbook,* collecting best practices and clinical feedback regarding patients' engagement with portals (Box 23.2; ONC, 2019).

There are several HIT tactics to improve usability and interoperability with patient portals:

- Patient's understanding and utilization as well as clinicians' in the various and many healthcare fields where portals can be used.

Box 23.2 Seven Key Steps for Patient Portal Engagement

1. Facilitate easy enrollment.
2. Activate portal features that meet patient needs.
3. Ensure all patients can access and understand information.
4. Allow portal access for caregivers.
5. Integrate patient-generated health data and EHRs.
6. Leverage APIs and other health IT.
7. Improve appointments with health IT.

API, application programming interfaces; EHR, electronic health record; IT, information technology.

Source: Office of the National Coordinator. (2019). *Patient engagement playbook.* https://www.healthit.gov/playbook/pe

- Patient awareness of portals while advocating for their best and highest level of functionality available.
- Using technologic efficiencies while improving patient engagement and consumer satisfaction is imperative to our nursing field.
- Advocating for our nursing discipline, ensuring technologies are used to shift nursing to practice at the top of license and improving patient engagement and satisfaction are paramount endeavors.

The CNS, a leader in nursing, must understand the applicability of IT and HIT in their domains of practice:

- At the system level, the CNS must know the healthcare landscape, including strategic legislative direction with financial, privacy-, and consumer-related policies, advocating for HIT solutions that deliver high-quality care and positive patient outcomes
- At the nurse level, the CNS will understand how to integrate top of license nurse work in a meaningful way with more efficient and technologic processes that are evidence based to drive positive outcomes
- At the patient level, the CNS will, in their daily lives as a consumer of IT, know IT functionalities that are applicable to a person's needs while managing their health; the CNS will seek HIT solutions that ensure the best patient privacy, safety, and care that allow for the patient to function as an engaged member of their care team.

FINANCIAL STEWARDSHIP, COST–BENEFIT ANALYSIS, AND HEALTHCARE FINANCING

OVERVIEW

Financial stewardship is defined as wise management of resources (Bosner, 2019) and stewardship itself is defined as "careful and responsible management" (Merriam Webster, 2019). CNSs possess the skills and competencies to meet the needs of the public based on allotted healthcare financing while improving quality, safety, and care and maintenance of those with chronic illnesses and wellness and also reducing care costs (National Association of Clinical Nurse Specialists [NACNS], 2019).

CNS Effectiveness

Unique advanced-level CNS competencies in developing quality improvement projects and programs result in cost reduction across the care continuum. Whether developing programs, evaluating current programs, or analyzing ways to reduce expenses, CNSs always are respectful stewards of resources.
CNSs demonstrate cost effectiveness through the following:

- Educating and mentoring nurses and nursing students, leading to enhanced nurse retention and recruitment and cost savings for an organization
- Increasing access to community-based care through Nurse Managed Health Care Centers, providing expert clinical care in private offices and community clinics, and demonstrating program effectiveness in slowing down disease progression and decreasing healthcare costs
- Coaching those with chronic illness, promoting self-care, reducing illness costs, and improving access to wellness and prevention services, thus reducing hospital readmissions (NACNS, 2019)

Cost–Benefit Analysis

- Cost–benefit analyses (CBAs) financially operationalize how evidence-based programs can decrease cost and expenses over current programs in practice.
- The ability to develop CBAs is part of the CNS's responsibility as a financial steward for organizations. Performing a CBA helps CNSs identify all direct and indirect costs of developing an intervention, which will result in a positive outcomes, and focus on costs associated with intervention implementation and return on investment.
- CBA is an applied economic mechanism that assesses outcomes in terms of using money to improve societal welfare, such as through CNS-developed programs.
- CBAs provide full program cost, identify benefits and expenses against the program's monetary cost, and evaluate the success of potential goals of a proposed change.

There are many challenges of quantitatively capturing all benefits and costs; the CBA can proactively guide program business decisions (Carroll & Shabana, 2010; Swenty et al., 2011).

- A CBA uncovers pertinent issues impacting the program's potential success or failure and proactively guides decision-making (Newcomer et al., 2015).
- The CBA helps translate health outcomes into financial values (i.e., willingness to pay).
- The CBA tells CNSs the difference rather than a ratio, and tells them about dollars spent on an intervention minus dollars saved in benefits (Finkler et al., 2007).
- Potential benefits from the CBA are related to the decision about commencing a new project or implementing a change related to the costs of a program decision.
- In a CBA, the decision makes sense if the benefits related to the decision will exceed the costs (Newcomer et al., 2015) or if the intervention has a positive benefit–cost ratio and adds value to the organization.

To determine both a positive benefit and a cost–benefit ratio, monetary values must be assigned to both costs and benefits. Assigning monetary values to healthcare outcomes is difficult. Measuring life's value and health outcomes that are tied to immediate risk of life and death is also difficult.

The project benefit–specific dollar value of advantages must be estimated, including incremental values that will result from the project, such as more patients who could be provided for or increased revenue. The CBA can also identify if the number of patients and revenue outweigh the expenses when adding additional costs to support the increased volume and revenue (Schmidek & Weeks, 2005).

Steps, key elements, and considerations when conducting a CBA are identified in Boxes 23.3 to 23.6 (Gupta, 2011).

- The CBA steps can be a challenge since assigning a dollar value to many items may be difficult.
- Subtracting the benefit created from an action or a program by the cost of the program reflects the program's net benefit.
- If the benefits of the program divided by the costs are greater than 1, then the program has a positive benefit–cost ratio, suggesting it can add value and merits further program

Box 23.3 Steps of a Cost–Benefit Analysis

- Determining monetary program benefits
- Calculating the total program costs
- Weighing benefits versus costs
- Completing the decision analysis

Box 23.4 Key Elements for a Cost–Benefit Analysis

- Identifying the need for program change
- Collecting information and data regarding the mission
- Human resources
- Necessary data for the program
- Stakeholder analysis to assure important voices are at the table for insight
- Identifying the key assumptions of the CBA for consideration, approval, indirect and direct costs, salaries, and benefits
- Discussion around what might be unknown savings

CBA, cost–benefit analysis.

Box 23.5 Considerations for a Cost–Benefit Analysis

- Timely and structured literature review
- Market analysis
- Advertising, internal and external marketing
- Human resources, orientation and training, effects on productivity
- Data collection costs
- Meeting costs to determine program goals and objectives and consideration of the anticipated outcome
- Program and participant benefit estimations
- Effects of actions: cost versus benefit
- Measuring and valuing identified effects, process, and outcome
- Discounting future costs and benefits relative to the flow/present

Box 23.6 Cost–Benefit Analysis

- Compares benefits related to decision about a new program or the change to the costs of that decision
  - Decision makes sense if benefits related to decision will exceed the costs.

$$\frac{\text{Benefits}}{\text{Costs}} > 1$$

investigation. If less than 1 there is a negative benefit–cost ratio and the program should be reconsidered.

- The CNS should compare alternatives and choose the program with the greatest cost–benefit ratio (Finkler et al., 2007). The decision analysis should be completed based upon the cost–benefit analysis.
- Operating costs must be identified for ongoing running and maintenance of intervention: hiring new personnel, maintaining equipment and space, and monitoring performance (Schmidek & Weeks, 2005).
- Identifying opportunity cost is looking at the cost of the best alternative that is foregone because a particular course of action is pursued (Schmidek & Weeks, 2005).
- Identifying incremental direct costs or costs incurred solely for intervention implementation may include personnel training and purchase of new machinery or software; there is anticipated decreased productivity during the start-up phase (Schmidek & Weeks, 2005).
- Direct costs are those costs incurred while employed and are easily identified and relate directly to recruitment, temporary replacement, and hiring (O'Brien-Pallas et al., 2006).
- Indirect costs are incurred for the overall organizational benefit with additional focus of leadership on the program (Schmidek & Weeks, 2005).
- Determine the estimated total cost of the intervention.
- Calculate the anticipated annual return on the investment (Schmidek & Weeks, 2005).

The National Association of Clinical Nurse Specialists has a Cost Analysis Toolkit available on their website (https://nacns.org/professional-resources/toolkits-and-reports/cost-analysis-toolkit).

REVIEW QUESTIONS

1. What is the best statement about the National Database for Nursing Quality Indicators (NDNQI) nurse-sensitive quality indicators and hospital-acquired conditions (HAC)?
   A. Both NDNQI nurse-sensitive indicators and HAC describe quality-improvement initiatives.
   B. Measures are tracked and compared at the unit-level for comparison of quality outcomes.
   C. Payment may be withheld if conditions are not present on admission or preexisting to a hospital stay.
   D. NDNQI and HAC only affect nurses and should not include other disciplines in prevention.

2. The nurse manager of a hospital-based department asks the clinical nurse specialist (CNS) to lead an effort to decrease the number of medication errors taking place in her department. What is the first thing the CNS should do?
   A. Pull together a multidisciplinary group and begin drafting a charter.
   B. Begin outlining possible strategies and interventions to decrease medication errors.
   C. Have the nurse manager thoroughly explain her perception of the problem and validate the problem with data.
   D. Decide on desired outcomes related to medication errors.

ANSWERS

1. **Correct answer: C. Rationale:** NDNQI describes nursing-sensitive indicators, as does HAC, which are potential harm events; HACs have spurred the development of

prevention and quality improvement initiatives but are not in and of themselves quality improvement initiatives. Only NDNQI measures are tracked and compared at unit level for comparison, like hospitals and units. Payment may be withheld for HAC and nursing-sensitive indicators, since they overlap, as in CAUTI, CLABSI, VAP, and pressure injuries. NDNQI and HAC are best addressed using an interprofessional process-improvement process.

2. **Correct answer: C. Rationale:** Understanding and clarifying the perception of the problem and then validating the problem with data should be the first thing the CNS does. Pulling together a multidisciplinary group, drafting a charter, outlining possible strategies, and deciding on desired outcomes are all important steps that follow the clarification and validation of the problem. A CNS must first understand the problem before planning on how to address it.

REFERENCES

The complete reference and additional reading lists appear in the digital version of this chapter, at https://connect.springerpub.com/content/book/978-0-8261-7417-8/part/part03/chapter/ch23

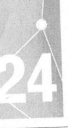

Evidence-Based Practice and Research

Julie Cahn and Karen S. March

EVIDENCE-BASED PRACTICE

OVERVIEW

Evidenced-based practice (EBP) is an approach integrating the best research available, clinical expertise, and patient preferences and values in order to change practice (Association of periOperative Registered Nurses [AORN], 2012; Melnyk & Fineout-Overholt, 2015).

Primary Functions

- Decrease uncertainty by providing evidence for interventions (Melnyk & Fineout-Overholt, 2015).
- Increase the likelihood of a patient achieving a desired outcome (Melnyk & Fineout-Overholt, 2015).
- Provides a systematic problem-solving approach to answering clinical questions (Melnyk & Fineout-Overholt, 2015).

Components

- Evidence from different levels of research, clinical guidelines, and expert opinions (AORN, 2012; Melnyk & Fineout-Overholt, 2015)
- Evidence from the patient assessment data (e.g., history and physical, lab reports, radiological findings; Melnyk & Fineout-Overholt, 2015)
- Knowledge from the practitioner's clinical expertise (AORN, 2012; Melnyk & Fineout-Overholt, 2015)
- Patient's preferences and values (Melnyk & Fineout-Overholt, 2015)

EBP Models

There are many different models of EBP; a few are listed in the following (AORN, 2012).

- Stetler Model of Research Utilization to Facilitate EBP
  - Includes five phases
    - Preparation
    - Validation
    - Comparative evaluation or decision-making
    - Translation and application
    - Evaluation
- Iowa Model of EBP to Promote Quality of Care
  - Includes problem-focused and knowledge-focused triggers
- Johns Hopkins Nursing EBP Model
  - Includes three phases
    - Practice question
    - Evidence
    - Translation
- ACE Star Model of EBP
  - Five-point star
    - Discovery
    - Summary
    - Translation
    - Integration
    - Evaluation

Overview of Steps in EBP

1. Identify a need for change in practice.
2. Create a specific PICO(T) question.
3. Search the evidence using key words from the PICO question.
4. Collect the most relevant and best evidence (AORN, 2012).
5. Critically appraise the evidence (AORN, 2012).
6. Review the results of the evidence from the appraisal process (AORN, 2012).
7. Design a practice change based on the best available evidence and clinical expertise (AORN, 2012).
8. Implement the practice change using each patient's values and preferences.
9. Evaluate the practice change and associated patient outcomes, including unintended consequences.
10. Change the practice again if needed or integrate and continue to monitor.
11. Disseminate the outcome (Melnyk & Fineout-Overholt, 2015).

PICO(T)

There are several different formats a PICO(T) question may be written in depending on what knowledge is being sought (American Association of Critical-Care Nurses [AACN]). Careful formulation of a PICO(T) question leads to key words that can be used for a systematic evidence search.

Each part of PICO(T) stands for a different part of the question being asked (AACN).

- P—Patient population (e.g., pediatrics, oncology patients)
- I—Intervention (independent variable)
- C—Comparison (compared to the intervention)
- O—Outcome
- T—Time frame (not always needed)

Levels of Evidence

Once a clinical question has been developed into a PICO(T) question, key words can be generated from the PICO(T) question to use during the search of the medical literature databases (AORN, 2012; Melnyk & Fineout-Overholt, 2015). There are many databases, including PubMed, Cumulative Index to

The complete reference and additional reading lists appear in the digital version of this chapter, at https://connect.springerpub.com/content/book/978-0-8261-7417-8/part/part03/chapter/ch24

Nursing and Allied Health Literature (CINHAL), Joanna Briggs, Cochrane Clinical Trials Register, and Scopus (AORN, 2012; Melnyk & Fineout-Overholt, 2015). Once the studies are obtained, the literature is critically appraised (AORN, 2012; Melnyk & Fineout-Overholt, 2015). It is important to note that a systematic review of any type of study (randomized controlled trials [RCTs], quasi-experimental, or nonexperimental) is always a stronger form of evidence than a single study from that same category (e.g., experimental, quasi-experimental, nonexperimental; AORN, 2012). See Box 24.1.

Other types of evidence that are not research based may also be found in medical database searches (AORN, 2012):

1. Clinical practice guidelines
2. Consensus or position statements
3. Literature reviews
4. Case reports
5. Expert opinion articles
6. Organization experience (i.e., quality improvement articles)

Next Steps

- Review the evidence and determine the highest and best quality evidence available (AORN, 2012; Melnyk & Fineout-Overholt, 2015).
- If there is sufficient evidence, design a practice change based on that evidence, clinical expertise, and patient values (Melnyk & Fineout-Overholt, 2015). Incorporate the practice change into standard practice and then evaluate the results (e.g., outcomes, unintended consequences; Melnyk & Fineout-Overholt, 2015).
- Adjust the practice as needed and then disseminate (e.g., publish) your findings (AORN, 2020; Melnyk & Fineout-Overholt, 2015; Parkosewich, 2013).
- If there is not sufficient evidence to change the practice, the clinical nurse specialist (CNS) may need to develop their own innovative solution and/or conduct research to determine if there is a better solution to the problem identified.

BOX 24.1 Strength of Evidence—Strongest to Weakest

Systematic Review of Randomized Control Trials With Meta-analysis
Systematic review of randomized control trials without meta-analysis
Randomized control trial (experimental study with randomization)
Systematic review from quasi-experimental studies with or without meta-analysis
Quasi-experimental studies (experimental study without randomization)
Systematic review from correlational studies with or without meta-analysis
Correlational studies (nonexperimental)
Qualitative studies
Descriptive surveys

ANOVA, analysis of variance.
Source: Association of periOperative Registered Nurses. (2012). *Evidence rating*. https://www.aorn.org/guidelines/about-aorn-guidelines/evidence-rating

RESEARCH

OVERVIEW OF THE RESEARCH METHODOLOGY

Both the *Future of Nursing* (Institute of Medicine [IOM], 2010) report and the Magnet® Recognition Program of the American Nurses' Credentialing Center (ANCC) have provided a focus on and impetus for nurse participation in research. *Research* is a process by which one may investigate phenomena, describe or quantify certain aspects of the phenomena, or answer specific questions related to the phenomena of interest. To that end, *research methods* provide structure and guidance for researchers to plan a study and then gather and analyze data in order to answer specific research questions (Polit & Beck, 2017). The steps of the research process may include the following:

- Search for and read relevant literature.
- Develop a research idea based on what is reflected in the literature.
- Generate a research hypothesis.
- Determine an appropriate design for the study.
- Conduct the study.
- Analyze data obtained during the study.
- Decide whether the hypothesis was supported.
- Disseminate results.

The *scientific method* guides progress through a research study via a rigorous approach to provide order and discipline in the pursuit of knowledge acquisition. Two major paradigms (or lenses) for nursing research include *quantitative* research and *qualitative* research.

- *Quantitative* research is concerned with evidence that is objective and grounded in reality. Usually, quantitative evidence is comprised of numeric information that can be analyzed using statistical procedures.
- *Qualitative* research focuses on understanding the dynamic nature of human experience.
- Quantitative and qualitative research have common features (Polit & Beck, 2017):
  - Goals of both involve gaining a more thorough understanding of phenomena.
  - Researchers of both methods collect and analyze evidence empirically.
  - Both methods rely on human participation and cooperation.
  - Practitioners of both forms of research may be concerned with ethical dilemmas.

The selection of a specific research method to be employed often depends both on the personal philosophy of the researcher and on the research question.

New knowledge is generated through research. Nurses who are involved in research and EBP must develop a degree of familiarity with statistical principles in order to fully consider outcomes.

Types of Research Designs

- **Experimental design:** Includes random assignment, manipulation of an independent variable(s), and a control group
- **Quasi-experimental design:** Controlled trials but lack randomization or a control group
- **Nonexperimental design**—Researchers collect data but do not intervene for example observational studies (Polit & Beck, 2017)

Variables in research studies are identified as independent or dependent (Polit & Beck, 2017):

- **Independent variable**—Variable being manipulated or presumed to be the cause
- **Dependent variable**—Presumed effect or outcome of interest

OVERVIEW OF STATISTICAL PRINCIPLES

APRNs must understand, measure, and interpret findings from research studies or EBP projects in the context of the likely influence of chance on outcomes. It is only through an understanding of statistical principles that the APRN can determine whether an effect occurred by chance or whether it occurred because of some other reason (such as an intervention). In the case of evidence-based projects in healthcare, it is important to know whether observed outcomes occurred due to the effects of an intervention or the influence of chance (Dancey et al., 2012).

CNSs may serve as principal investigators in healthcare research projects or they may serve as a resource for nurses involved in EBP projects. In either case, the CNS needs to have at least a basic working understanding of statistics.

Descriptive or Inferential Statistics

- *Descriptive* statistics are used to describe data (Conner & Johnson, 2017; Giuliano & Polanowicz, 2008; Hedges & Williams, 2014; Main & Ogaz, 2016).
- *Inferential* statistics are used in an attempt to generalize findings from a sample to a population (Allua & Thompson, 2009; Giuliano & Polanowicz, 2008; Hedges & Williams, 2014; Main & Ogaz, 2016).

Decisions about appropriate statistical testing depend upon levels of measurement of variables that are utilized within a study or project (Allua & Thompson, 2009; Polit & Beck, 2017).

Levels of Measurement

In research studies or EBP projects, data may be grouped for analysis. Although there may be rationale for such a decision, it is important to note that such grouping may result in movement from a higher level of measurement to a lower level of measurement (Table 24.1).

- Researchers should be aware that this results in information loss and fewer options for statistical testing (Polit & Beck, 2017).
- Data with a higher level of measurement can always be converted to a lower level of measurement, but the reverse is not true.
- It is always best to use the highest level of measurement to achieve the most powerful and precise analysis.

Given a set of data, one method for initially examining the data may include running a frequency distribution, which is discussed in the following.

Frequency distribution—An arrangement of values from lowest to highest within a group; consists of observed values plus the number of cases at each value (Polit & Beck, 2017). Frequency data can be displayed in graphs—histograms and frequency polygons—and are often presented as the "bell-shaped" curve. A look at the frequency distribution on a graph allows the researcher to further assess attributes of the data set. For example, examination of the shape of the frequency distribution reveals whether or not the variable occurs along a normal distribution—is the frequency distribution symmetrical? In other words, are both sides mirror images of each another? If so, the researcher understands that the data are normally distributed (Polit & Beck, 2017). This information is very useful in determinations about the type of statistical testing that can be accomplished.

Key features distinguish the *normal curve*:

- Most scores or data points cluster around the middle of the curve.
- The curve is symmetrical; both halves are mirror images of each another.
- The mean, median, and mode fall at exactly the same point.
- The relationship with the standard deviation is symmetrical on both sides of the curve.

If the shape of the distribution is *skewed* to one side, this means that the peak of the distribution falls to one side and the tail is longer on the opposite side. When this occurs, the CNS cannot assume that the data are normally distributed. This, too, impacts decisions about statistical testing that may be considered for use (Polit & Beck, 2017).

Central tendency—Term used to describe averages. In research, there are three measures of central tendency: the *mean*, the *median*, and the *mode* (Giuliano & Polanowicz, 2008; Polit & Beck, 2017).

Mean—The most stable measure of central tendency (Conner & Johnson, 2017; Giuliano & Polanowicz, 2008; Hedges & Williams, 2014; Polit & Beck, 2017); derived by adding all of the values in a frequency distribution and dividing by the total number of values; if the distribution is *skewed*, the mean gets pulled toward the long tail.

Example: 1, 2, 3, 4, 5, 6, 7, 8, 9

$$Mean = \frac{1+2+3+4+5+6+7+8+9}{9} = 5$$

Median—The place within a frequency distribution that is situated so that precisely 50% of values fall above it and 50% of values fall below it (Conner & Johnson, 2017; Giuliano & Polanowicz, 2008; Hedges & Williams, 2014; Polit & Beck, 2017); by representing an average position within a series of numbers, the median is not sensitive to extremes; median is *the preferred measure of central tendency for a skewed distribution.*

Example: 1, 2, 3, 4, 5, ⑥, 7, 8, 9

Median = 5

Mode—The most frequently occurring value within a frequency distribution (Conner & Johnson, 2017; Giuliano & Polanowicz, 2008; Hedges & Williams, 2014; Polit & Beck, 2017); less stable than mean or median.

Example: 1, 2, 3, 4, 4, 4, 5, 6, 6, 9

Mode = 4

Variability—The degree to which values within a data set are spread (Giuliano & Polanowicz, 2008).

- *Heterogenous* variability suggests that data points are highly varied and the curve is broad on the baseline, while *homogenous* variability suggests that data points are very similar and the curve is narrower along its baseline (Polit & Beck, 2017).

TABLE 24.1 LEVELS OF MEASUREMENT

LEVEL	CONSIDERATIONS	DESCRIPTION	EXAMPLES	USEFUL STATISTICAL TESTS
Nominal	Numbers are assigned to organize characteristics into categories; are symbolic representations of equivalence or non-equivalence only. Numbers assigned to categories represent no quantitative value (i.e., 0 = male; 1 = female)—therefore, these numbers cannot be treated mathematically (i.e., cannot calculate average gender). Instead, it is best to describe data by percentages within each category. Numbers have no intrinsic meaning—data cannot be used to determine measures of central tendency (mean, median or mode)	Categorical—distinct and nonoverlapping; exhaustive categories	Gender, yes/no, seasons, marital status	*Frequencies, percentages; modes* **Nonparametric–Chi-square (χ^2)** can be used to compare *two or more* groups; **Fisher's exact test** is used to compare *two* groups (Pett, 2016)
Ordinal	Attributes are sorted according to *order or relative rank*; categories are mutually exclusive; while certain ranks are notably higher or better than others, there is *no way to quantify how much higher or better one is over another*—offers relative ranking of the attribute only (i.e., moving up by one level is better than baseline, but there is no way to quantify by how much)	Mutually exclusive categories or groupings are rank ordered and exhaustive; for example, level of distress noted in a patient prior to undergoing a medical procedure—from 1—*not at all distressed* to 5—*extremely distressed*	Ranges of family income across a group; any attribute rated along a Likert scale	*Non-parametric—Mann-Whitney test* for two independent groups; *Kruskal–Wallis test* for three or more independent groups; *Spearman's rho* for correlation (Pett, 2016) *Use of parametric tests (means, standard deviations) with ordinal-level data is viewed as controversial
Interval	Attributes are rank ordered; values are equidistant from one another; since there is no absolute zero, distances between values do not uniformly carry the same meaning—consider that a change in body temperature from 97 °C–100 °C is not meaningful in the same way as a change in body temperature from 100 °C–103 °C; there is no ability to describe the absolute magnitude of a relationship (50 °F is not twice as hot as 25 °F); referred to as a *continuous* variable. Averages can be used to describe data. Options for mathematical analysis are increased—parametric tests can be used effectively	Mutually exclusive, exhaustive groups with rank ordering at equidistant intervals; therefore, can quantify the amount of difference between a certain score and another.	Temperature measured in degrees Fahrenheit; self-efficacy scores; coping scores; pain scores	*All measures of central tendency and variance; Parametric statistics*—t test; ANOVA; Pearson product–moment correlation coefficient;
Ratio	Highest level of measurement; also referred to as a *continuous* variable All mathematical analysis is acceptable and effective.	Mutually exclusive, exhaustive groups with rank ordering at equidistant intervals; Has a meaningful and absolute zero point (absence of the specific attribute)	Weight; blood pressure; other physical measures; central venous pressure; pulmonary artery pressure	*Parametric statistics*

*Important considerations include sample size and shape of distribution of dependent variable.

ANOVA, analysis of variance.

Sources: From Allua, S., & Thompson, C. B. (2009). Inferential statistics. *Air Medical Journal, 28*(4), 168–171. https://doi.org/10.1016/j.amj.2009.04.013; Giuliano, K. K., & Polanowicz, M. (2008). Interpretation and use of statistics in nursing research. *AACN Advanced Critical Care, 19*(2), 211–222; Hedges, C., & Williams, B. (2014). Anatomy of research for nurses. Sigma Theta Tau International; Main, M. E., & Ogaz, V. L. (2016). Common statistical tests and interpretation in nursing research. *International Journal of Faith Community Nursing, 2*(3), article 2. http://digitalcommons.wku.edu/ijfcn/vol2/iss3/2; Pett, M. A. (2016). *Nonparametric statistics for health care research: Statistics for small samples and unusual distributions* (2nd ed.). Sage; Polit, D. F., & Beck, C. T. (2017). *Nursing research: Generating and assessing evidence for nursing practice* (10th ed.). Wolters Kluwer.

- The *range* is a measure of variability determined by subtracting the lowest value from the highest value within a frequency distribution (Conner & Johnson, 2017; Hedges & Williams, 2014).
- *Standard deviation* is a frequently used measure of variability that describes the spread of data points away from the mean (Conner & Johnson, 2017; Giuliano & Polanowicz, 2008; Hedges & Williams, 2014; Polit & Beck, 2017); in calculation of standard deviation, every score is used.

Correlation—Can be used to determine whether a relationship exists between two variables (ordinal, interval, or ratio measures)

- Correlations between two variables can be described using scatter plots on a horizontal and vertical axis; the direction of the scatter plot slope reveals the direction of the correlation (Hedges & Williams, 2014; Polit & Beck, 2017).
- **Pearson's r** product–moment correlation coefficient is the most frequently used correlation statistic; it requires interval or ratio measures of variables (Allua & Thompson, 2009; Polit & Beck, 2017).
- **Spearman's rho (ρ)**—Used to determine correlation when assumptions for parametric tests are not met or when data are ordinal level; values range from −1.00 to +1.00 (Allua & Thompson, 2009; Pett, 2016; Polit & Beck, 2017). This correlation index is useful when data are ordinal level (Allua & Thompson, 2009).

Confidence intervals—Indicate both a probability (%) of correctness and a range of values within which a parameter exists; that is, "CI 95% = ($23.4 \leq \mu \leq 29.54$)" would be written in a research report as "95% CI (23.4, 29.54)" and it would be interpreted as "the confidence is 95% that the population mean is between 23.4 and 29.54" (Giuliano & Polanowicz, 2008; Polit & Beck, 2017).

Level of significance—These represent the probability of incorrectly rejecting a null hypothesis (Giuliano & Polanowicz, 2008; Polit & Beck, 2017); referred to as *alpha* (α); an α of 0.05 indicates that if 100 samples are drawn from a population, chance dictates that a true null hypothesis would be rejected 5 times, whereas an α of 0.01 similarly indicates that, based on the same 100 samples drawn from a population, chance suggests that a true null hypothesis would be rejected just once (Hayat, 2010; Kalinowski & Fidler, 2010). Setting the level of significance reduces the chance of committing a type I error, rejecting a true null hypothesis. However, by setting a stricter level of significance, a researcher increases the chance of committing a type II error—accepting a false null hypothesis (Giuliano & Polanowicz, 2008; Polit & Beck, 2017). For a given study, p = the probability of observing the data if the null hypothesis is true. When $p < \alpha$, the value is considered *statistically significant* (Giuliano & Polanowicz, 2008; Hedges & Williams, 2014; Kalinowski & Fidler, 2010; Mellis, 2018; Polit & Beck, 2017). Based on the first example here, this means that the data have even fewer than 5 chances in 100 of being consistent with the null hypothesis.

Statistical significance—Based on p value less than a stated α; implies that results are not likely due to chance at the specified level of probability (Giuliano & Polanowicz, 2008; Hedges & Williams, 2014; Kalinowski & Fidler, 2010; Mellis, 2018; Polit & Beck, 2017); the researcher should be careful, however, to include information about the magnitude of the effect—that is, *confidence interval*—which provides an interval within which the population parameter is believed to be contained (Giuliano & Polanowicz, 2008; Hayat, 2010; Kalinowski & Fidler, 2010; Mellis, 2018; Polit & Beck, 2017).

Parametric tests—Estimate a parameter; require level of measurement on interval or ratio scale; assume that variables demonstrate a normal distribution; more powerful than nonparametric tests; more preferred (e.g., t test; ANOVA; Pearson's r; Allua & Thompson, 2009; Polit & Beck, 2017).

t test—Tests for differences in group means (of two independent groups) on a continuous dependent variable (Allua & Thompson, 2009; Hedges & Williams, 2014; Main & Ogaz, 2016).

Analysis of variance (ANOVA)—Tests differences between means in three or more groups (Allua & Thompson, 2009; Giuliano & Polanowicz, 2008; Hedges & Williams, 2014; Main & Ogaz, 2016).

Pearson's r—Test for correlation when both the independent and the dependent variables are interval or ratio levels of measure (Allua & Thompson, 2009; Main & Ogaz, 2016).

Nonparametric tests—Do not estimate a parameter; no requirement for variable to demonstrate normal distribution—less restrictive; useful in situations with nominal or ordinal level data or with smaller sample size (e.g., Mann-Whitney U test; Fisher's exact test; Kruskal-Wallis test; Friedman's test; Spearman's rho; Giuliano & Polanowicz, 2008; Pett, 2016; Polit & Beck, 2017)

Mann-Whitney U test—Tests for differences in group means (of two independent groups) on a dependent variable on an ordinal scale; this is the nonparametric equivalent of the independent group t test (Pett, 2016; Polit & Beck, 2017).

Kruskal-Wallis test—Tests for differences in group means in more than two groups (Pett, 2016; Polit & Beck, 2017).

Chi-square—Tests for differences in proportions between groups when the dependent variable is on a nominal scale and samples are small; calculated by comparing observed frequencies and expected frequencies (if no relationship exists between the variables; Hedges & Williams, 2014; Main & Ogaz, 2016; Pett, 2016; Polit & Beck, 2017)

Fisher's exact test—Tests for differences in proportions between groups when the dependent variable is on the nominal scale; used instead of chi square if sample size is small (<30; Pett, 2016; Polit & Beck, 2017)

Power analysis—Used to help estimate sample size needed and to avoid type II errors (null hypothesis is wrongly accepted; Polit & Beck, 2017).

OVERVIEW OF PROTECTION OF HUMAN SUBJECTS

Human subjects' protection refers to certain government regulations that serve to protect participants in research studies (Polit & Beck, 2017). Initially, a code of ethics was developed and adopted by the National Commission for the Protection of Human Subjects of Biomedical and Behavioral Research in 1978. The same Commission issued the *Belmont Report*, which serves as the guide to regulations affecting government-sponsored research in the United States. The report may be read online on the Health and Human Services website (www.hhs.gov/ohrp/regulations-and-policy/belmont-report/index.html) and is available in printable pdf version. For those who prefer another option, a video on this report is also available on the site.

Belmont Report—A statement of a set of principles on which standards of ethical conduct in research in the United States are based: *beneficence, respect for human dignity*, and *justice* (U.S. Department of Health and Human Services, 2016; Polit & Beck, 2017).

- *Beneficence* implies that the researcher must minimize harm and maximize benefits to the patient (Polit & Beck, 2017). This principle states that the researcher has an obligation to avoid, prevent, or minimize harm (nonmaleficence) to participants in a research study.
- *Respect for human dignity* provides for two specific rights to participants of research—the right to self-determination and the right to full disclosure (Polit & Beck, 2017).
  - *Right to self-determination* means that participants have the right to choose to partake in a study and that those same participants have the right to choose not to provide any information and to withdraw from a study when and if they see fit.
  - *Right to full disclosure* requires the researcher to fully describe the study, the person's right to refuse participation, the responsibilities of the researcher, and possible risks or benefits that have been foreseen.
- *Justice* provides for participants' rights to fair treatment and right to privacy (Polit & Beck, 2017). Specifically, this principle requires the researcher to protect the interests of vulnerable individuals and to avoid exploitation of the individual. Further, researchers are required to minimize intrusiveness and assure that individual privacy is protected.

Resources for Human Subjects Protection

Additional resources on the protection of human subjects may be found on government websites.

- The Health Resources and Services Administration (HRSA) website, contains links to a free online training module sponsored by the National Institutes of Health (NIH) as well as a link to webinars offered by the Office of Human Research Protections (OHRP).
- The Department of Health and Human Services (DHHS) specifically highlights requirements for protection of human subjects.
- The Association of Clinical Research Professionals (ACRP) also offers free training on human subjects' protection and ethics for research.
- Some healthcare organizations obtain professional level training for staff from paid sites such as the Collaborative Institute Training Initiative (CITI) program.

Procedures for Protecting Study Participants

- Conduct a risk–benefit assessment.
- Individuals who are considering participation must be provided a summary of risks and benefits (*minimal risk* is defined as not greater than one would encounter ordinarily in life or in routine care settings).
- Obtain informed consent from the participants—participants have adequate information about the study, they understand the information, and therefore they can consent or decline participation voluntarily.
- Maintain confidentiality.
- Consider the need for debriefing.
- Protect the rights of vulnerable individuals such as
  - Children,
  - Mentally or emotionally disabled,
  - Severely ill or physically disabled,

- Terminally ill,
- Institutionalized individuals, and
- Pregnant women.
- Submit for review to the institutional review board (IRB; Polit & Beck, 2017).

Requirements for Informed Consent—Implies that participants have sufficient information about the study, have ability to comprehend the information provided, and have the ability to offer or refuse consent voluntarily (Polit & Beck, 2017).

Information That Must Be Shared With Participants

- Healthcare activities that are routine and those activities that are treatments for the study
- The goals of the research project
- The type of data to be collected during the study
- Expectations for data collection and any other procedures that will occur
- Expected time commitment for each contact and the total number of expected contacts
- Who is sponsoring/funding the study; if the study is part of an academic requirement, participants should be made aware
- Any foreseeable risks (physical, psychologic, social, or economic) or discomforts as well as any efforts undertaken to minimize risks or discomfort
- Potential benefits to themselves or others
- Alternative treatments that might be of benefit to them, if available
- Stipends or reimbursements that will be provided
- The fact that participants' privacy will be protected at all times
- The fact that participation is voluntary and that failure to volunteer will not result in penalty
- The fact that they have the right to withdraw from or withhold information from the study at any time after consent
- Whom they may contact with questions, comments, or concerns throughout the study (Polit & Beck, 2017)

Skills for Dissemination of CNS Work

It is critically important to share the outcomes of CNS work (Melnyk & Fineout-Overholt, 2015; Parkosewich, 2013). The main reason for dissemination is to share results with individuals who may be looking for answers to the same question. Additionally, dissemination may allow the findings to positively impact a wider patient population than one healthcare facility or system. Other reasons for dissemination include promotion of the CNS role, recognition, and resume building.

There are many ways to disseminate work (Parkosewich, 2013):

1. Poster presentations at the facility and the health system at the local, regional, national, or international levels (AORN, 2020)
2. Podium presentations at the facility and the health system at the local, regional, national, or international levels
3. Publication of articles or studies in peer-reviewed journals

Poster Presentations

Poster presentations are one of the easiest ways to start dissemination of CNS work. Poster presentations are also a good place to start for people who may have difficulty speaking in front of groups. Many healthcare systems and local, regional, national, and international conferences accept abstracts for poster presentations (AORN, 2020). If the conference accepts poster presentations, be sure to read the conference guidelines about how to set up a poster presentation. Poster presentations are typically set up with headers similar to what is in a research paper (Table 24.2). Ensure that the poster is a visually appealing and has a balance between the "white space" and text. Consider the poster to be more like a bulleted PowerPoint presentation than a paper. People new to creating posters should seek out a mentor who has had success as a poster presenter. Poster authors also are typically expected to attend the conference, hang the poster, and represent the poster during specific times (AORN, 2020).

Podium/Oral Presentations

Podium presentations are an important tool for the CNS. Podium presentations provide opportunities to engage audience members in the outcomes of CNS work (Parkosewich, 2013). Many healthcare systems and local, regional, national, and international conferences accept abstracts for podium presentations. Review the conference requirements for podium presentations and inquire about the audience who will be participating. Another good place to start is at local professional association chapter meetings. Local meetings of professional associations often put out calls for speakers as part of a continuing education program. Specific community groups may also have an interest in certain topics (e.g., churches, diabetes prevention groups, weight loss groups).

When setting up a podium presentation, consider the following questions (Melnyk & Fineout-Overholt, 2015; Parkosewich, 2013):

- What does the audience want to know and what do they already know?
- What is the audience education level?
- How would audience members use the information in their work?
- How will you be able to engage the audience (e.g., small group discussions, role-play activities, polling questions)?
- Will you be expected to provide handouts and what would be most meaningful?

Panel Presentations

Panel presentations are another type of venue to convey different experiences or perspectives on a topic. Panel presentations may use one type of professional (e.g., CNS) from many different facilities or an interdisciplinary panel. Panel presentations are typically moderated by a specific person outside the group of panelists who will prompt discussions or ask targeted questions. Panels may also take questions from the audience.

Publishing

Publishing an article, study, chapter, or book at first may seem like a lengthy process. However, publishing is not something that must be done alone. Finding a mentor who has had success in publishing the type of document you want to work on is a good way to start (Melnyk & Fineout-Overholt, 2015; Parkosewich, 2013). Also, starting small can help with faster completion and help keep up motivation. For instance, organizational experience articles describe EBP projects and are often found published in professional journals. Publishing also offers an opportunity to strengthen writing skills, build expertise on a subject, and show growth on a résumé.

Consider the following key points prior to publication (Melnyk & Fineout-Overholt, 2015; Parkosewich, 2013):

- Subject matter of your article.
- Existing evidence on the subject.
- Review the structure, content, and writing style of articles like yours.
- Determine which peer-reviewed journals would be most interested in this subject.
- Consider the amount and type of readers and the impact factor (how much the journal is cited) for each journal.
- Look for "calls for abstracts" and special issues from the journals you are interested in.
- Review the journal guidelines for the type of article you are considering.
- Matching your content to what the journal is looking for will increase the chance of your work being accepted.
- Don't be afraid of rejection or lots of editing; both are normal in journal publication. The key is to keep trying.

REVIEW QUESTIONS

1. What are three key factors of evidence-based practice (EBP)?
   A. Clinical expertise, patient values, and provider resources
   B. Provider knowledge, patient values, and research evidence
   C. Best available research, clinical expertise, and patient preferences
   D. Patient assessment data, clinical resources, and best available research

2. An arrangement of values from lowest to highest within a group plus the number of cases at each value defines which of the following?
   A. Mean
   B. Standard deviation
   C. Frequency distribution
   D. Confidence interval

ANSWERS

1. **Correct answer: C. Rationale:** EBP takes into consideration the best evidence available as well as clinical expertise and patient preferences. Although patient values and

TABLE 24.2 POSTER HEADER EXAMPLES

EBP POSTER	RESEARCH POSTER
Clinical problem/significance	Problem/purpose
Background	Literature review
Clinical question	Research question/hypothesis
Description of evidenced-based protocol	Conceptual framework
Implementation of evidence-based protocol	Methodology
Results	Data analysis
Conclusion/discussion	Results
Nursing implications	Conclusions/discussion
References	Nursing implications
N/A	References

EBP, evidenced-based practice.
Source: Association of periOperative Registered Nurses (AORN). (2020). Poster criteria by type. https://www.aorn.org/surgicalexpo/perioperative-nurse-education/posters

research evidence are integral for EBP, provider resources and knowledge are not key elements to be included.

2. **Correct answer: C. Rationale:** A frequency distribution is an arrangement of values from lowest to highest within a group plus the number of cases at each value. Mean is the mathematical average of a group of numbers. Standard deviation is a statement of variability. Confidence interval is a range of values within which a parameter exists and a statement of probability.

REFERENCES

The complete reference and additional reading lists appear in the digital version of this chapter, at https://connect.springerpub.com/content/book/978-0-8261-7417-8/part/part03/chapter/ch24

Section IV
Practice Exam

Practice Exam

Jaime A. Hannans and Tiffany Losekamp

1. A female patient with Guillain-Barré syndrome (GBS) has paralysis affecting the respiratory muscles, requiring mechanical ventilation. When the patient asks the nurse about the paralysis, how should the nurse respond?
   A. It must be hard to accept the permanency of your paralysis.
   B. You may have difficulty believing this, but the paralysis caused by this disease is temporary.
   C. You'll have to accept the fact that you're permanently paralyzed. However, you won't have a sensory loss.
   D. You'll first regain use of your legs and then your arms.

2. A 78-year-old female is admitted with a 10-day history of gastrointestinal (GI) virus and acute oliguric renal failure. The clinical nurse specialist (CNS) knows that this clinical scenario is associated with electrolyte imbalances and it is important to observe for:
   A. EKG changes with peaked T waves
   B. EKG changes with flattened or inverted T waves
   C. Central nervous system changes
   D. Muscle fatigue

3. The clinical nurse specialist (CNS) receives a pain management consult for a patient post laparoscopic cholecystectomy experiencing right shoulder pain. The patient is currently taking 10 mg of oxycodone q4h PO. What intervention would you consider first for this patient?
   A. Contact the provider for an increase in oxycodone dose.
   B. Encourage mobility and apply heat to the shoulder.
   C. Contact the provider for an x-ray of the shoulder.
   D. Contact the provider for an order for physical therapy.

4. A patient is admitted for elective scheduled surgery and reports a history of myasthenia. What is an important teaching point the patient should be made aware of for any procedure or surgery?
   A. The patient will experience more fatigue than usual.
   B. Physical therapy will be required for every patient.
   C. Certain types of anesthesia may exacerbate the crisis for a patient.
   D. The patient may require a specific type of intubation.

5. Which are a constellation of symptoms indicating a pericardial tamponade?
   A. Muffled heart tones, jugular venous distention, diminished breath sounds in the left chest
   B. Narrowed pulse pressure, hemoptysis, and absent breath sounds in the left chest
   C. Muffled heart tones, jugular venous distention, and pulseless electrical activity
   D. Hemoptysis, chest pain, and flat neck veins

6. The clinical nurse specialist (CNS) will follow all the following principles when caring for a patient with subcutaneous Remodulin infusion **except**:
   A. Change the subcutaneous site when red.
   B. Prescribe H1 and H2 blockers daily to keep the inflammation down.
   C. Expect infusion site pain in the first week of therapy.
   D. Prescribe topical anesthetic agents and/or vasoconstrictive agents PRN to relieve site pain.

7. A 43-year-old female with acute asthma is admitted to the ICU in acute distress. On assessment, she has decreased breath sounds bilaterally and is using accessory muscles; heart rate (HR), 110; SpO$_2$, 85% on a nonrebreather. Multiple nebulizers have been used with no effect; she is fatigued and unable to speak in full sentences. What are suggested mechanical ventilation settings?
   A. Volume-controlled ventilation (A/C, CMV)
   B. Pressure-controlled ventilation (PCV)
   C. Continuous positive airway pressure (CPAP)
   D. Mandatory minute (MMV), auto mode

8. A 52-year-old male is diagnosed with a viral hepatitis infection that was contracted from injection drug use. Treatment includes antiviral therapy and ongoing supportive care. What type of hepatitis is this patient likely experiencing?
   A. Hepatitis A
   B. Hepatitis B
   C. Hepatitis D
   D. Hepatitis E

9. A 76-year-old woman has symptoms of middle stages of Alzheimer's disease. What medication should be given to aid in processing memory and learning?
   A. Ketalar (ketamine)
   B. Requip (ropinirole)
   C. Aricept (donepezil)
   D. Dextromethorphan (DM)

10. What are the most consistently seen geriatric syndromes throughout literature?
    A. Delirium, dementia, gait instability/falls
    B. Delirium, skin breakdown/pressure injury, urinary incontinence
    C. Dementia, frailty, urinary incontinence
    D. Gait instability/falls, skin breakdown/pressure injury, sleep problems

11. How does nursing informatics (NI) blend the wisdom of clinical expertise and information technology (IT)?
    A. Nurse informaticists are experienced users of the nursing process; experts at using their analytical, critical

thinking skills; and excellent project managers using technology and information systems.

B. NI requires 10 years of clinical experience combined with at least 5 years of informatics experience.

C. NI informs nursing managers of the best care processes using HIT solutions.

D. Nurse informaticists have worked in a variety of clinical settings with people from all backgrounds who use IT in their daily lives.

12. The *Belmont Report* espouses which of the following principles on which standards of ethical conduct in research are based?
A. Nonmaleficence
B. Justice
C. Anonymity
D. Patient confidentiality

13. Frank is a 63-year-old man with parotid cancer who has had major surgery including resection and reconstruction. He is undergoing chemotherapy and radiation. He has severe neck and mouth pain and is no longer able to swallow, so receives all nutrition and medications crushed through his percutaneous endoscopic gastrostomy (PEG) tube. His current pain regimen consists of Oxycodone tablets 15 to 30 mg q4h as needed for pain. He has to awaken at nighttime to receive his pain medication. He rates his pain 8/10. What regimen might serve him better?
A. Oxycodone extended release BID
B. Norco liquid PRN
C. Transdermal fentanyl with lower dose oxycodone PRN for breakthrough pain
D. Recommend Lidoderm patch

14. After administration of oral vancomycin, an adult patient develops severe bronchospasm with stridor and diffuse erythema. The patient is alert and oriented to person, place, and time. Vital signs are as follows: heart rate (HR) 119 in sinus tachycardia, blood pressure (BP) 140/85 mmHg, mean arterial pressure 70 mmHg, respirations 30/min, oxygen saturation 92% via a nonrebreather mask. What medication order would be the first priority for this patient? What dose of epinephrine should be administered?
A. Epinephrine 3 mg of 1:10,000 dilution IV
B. Benadryl 25 mg IM
C. Epinephrine 0.3 mg of 1:1,000 dilution IM
D. Benadryl 50 mg PO

15. Which of the following can definitively diagnosis myocarditis?
A. EKG
B. Echocardiography
C. Cardiac magnetic resonance imaging
D. Endomyocardial biopsy (EMB)

16. A 74-year-old patient with end stage metastatic breast cancer reports feeling short of breath. Which of the following statements best describes the clinical nurse specialist's rationale for using oxygen to treat dyspnea symptoms in this case?
A. Correction of hypoxia correlates with the degree of symptomatic benefit the patient experiences with oxygen therapy.
B. A pulse oximetry measurement is required prior to initiating oxygen therapy.

C. Patients and families benefit psychologically when oxygen therapy is utilized.
D. Improved oxygen saturation affects the respiratory center, decreasing the sensation of breathlessness.

17. Which of the following actions is indicated by the nurse caring for a patient receiving Infliximab?
A. Order an videonystagmography (VNG) prior to first dose of the drug.
B. Recommend patient take all doses at the same time each day.
C. Teach the patient to sit before standing to avoid the effects of orthostatic hypotension.
D. Teach the patient signs and symptoms of infection.

18. What is the single biggest risk factor for developing cancer?
A. Aging
B. *BRCA 1* mutation
C. Exposure to chemotherapy
D. Working in a job that uses chemical agents for cleaning

19. A patient has had MS for 15 years. What change in health history would need to be a priority to address by the provider?
A. Poor appetite
B. Numbness and tingling to upper extremities
C. Injection site reaction
D. Shingles diagnosis

20. A patient is seen in a pain clinic with complaints of pain specific to his right upper back. What nonopioid intervention can the clinical nurse specialist (CNS) recommend?
A. Caudal injection
B. Fascia iliaca block
C. Facet joint injection
D. Trigger point injection

21. When is financial stewardship a foundational expectation of clinical nurse specialist (CNS) practice?
A. Only when developing new programs
B. When determining clinical outcomes only at the system level
C. In the practice of mentoring others
D. In all CNS practice

22. A 45-year-old male patient presents with blood pressure (BP) of 145/95 mmHg. He is mildly overweight and a non-smoker. Which of the following interventions should be recommended?
A. Smoking cessation.
B. Work with patient to create a meal plan based on low sodium, lean meats, and 4 to 5 servings of fruits and vegetables.
C. Walk 30 minutes 1 to 2 times per week.
D. Drink no more than 3 alcoholic beverages per day.

23. A 86-year-old male with a history of angina pectoris and early onset cognitive impairment was admitted for dehydration and urinary tract infection (UTI). He complains of chest pain. After assessing him, what is an appropriate dosage of nitroglycerin to administer?
A. 0.1 to 0.2 mg SL q5m, up to 2 times
B. 0.3 to 0.6 mg SL q5min up to 3 times
C. 0.8 to 1.0 mg SL q5min up to 3 times
D. 0.3 to 0.6 mg PO q5min up to 3 times

24. An 86-year-old patient with a history of nonalcoholic steato-hepatitis (NASH) cirrhosis and grade 1 ascites presents to the ED with worsening shortness of breath. The patient's son informs the clinical nurse specialist (CNS) of a 2-week history of progressive shortness of breath. Recent illness includes a viral respiratory infection that responded to over-the-counter medication 3 months ago. No other acute illness was reported. The patient is compliant with NASH treatment. While in the ED, the patient is unresponsive to noninvasive positive pressure airway measures and undergoes endotracheal intubation and mechanical ventilation support due to hypoxic respiratory failure. The patient is sedated and without ventilator asynchrony; however, O_2 saturation remains in the low 80s. A chest x-ray confirms the presence of fluid in the right lower lung. Bedside ultrasound identifies a large pocket of fluid in the right middle lung. Based on patient's history and clinical picture of this patient, the adult-gerontology clinical nurse specialist (AG-CNS) suspects that hypoxia is due to
    A. Undiagnosed COPD
    B. Incomplete resolution of viral infection
    C. Pancreatitis
    D. Hepatic hydrothorax

25. What is the purpose of the patient needing to use chlorhexidine to wash prior to surgery?
    A. To help with prevention of surgical site infections
    B. To make sure your patient takes a bath tonight
    C. To prevent catheter-associated urinary tract infections (UTIs)
    D. To ensure the patient does not have an allergic reaction to skin anesthetic

26. An 82-year-old patient was admitted to the hospital 3 days ago for a urinary infection and dehydration. She recently started having periods of disorientation, hallucinations, and pulling at her intravenous (IV) line. She has not been sleeping well at night and has been found up out of bed several times the past 2 nights. The nurse has consulted the clinical nurse specialist (CNS) to help manage the patient. What is the first step for managing the patient appropriately?
    A. Assure patient is restrained so she does not get up at night and fall.
    B. Prescribe Haldol 5 mg PRN.
    C. Determine etiology of delirium; make sure patient has lights on during the day and lights off at night.
    D. Prescribe Ambien 5 mg QHS for sleep.

27. Identify the intervention in the following PICO(T) question: *In a pediatric surgical patient, what is the effect of the presence of the parent at induction on anxiety rates compared with not having the parent present?*
    A. Pediatric surgical patient
    B. Anxiety rates
    C. Presence of the parents
    D. Not having the parents available

28. An example of a patient care scenario involving a health inequity would be:
    A. A community in Ohio does want immunizations because of their religious beliefs.
    B. A student entering college is required to get a physical assessment before acceptance.
    C. An older adult is unable to drive anymore and therefore unable to get to the clinic for their yearly flu shot.
    D. A flu pandemic has affected 25% of the local population, exhausting local resources.

29. A patient presents with ongoing nonmenstrual abdominal pain that she has had for 7 months. What interventional procedure can be performed to manage the pain?
    A. Antiemetic medication
    B. Celiac plexus block
    C. Paravertebral nerve blocks
    D. Steroid injection

30. A post–ischemic stroke patient is being discharged on an oral anticoagulant (Coumadin). You are teaching the patient and family about drug food interactions, specifically to avoid which food?
    A. Tomatoes
    B. Lima beans
    C. Sweet potatoes
    D. Spinach

31. A patient with cancer is experiencing acute diarrhea. The clinical nurse specialist (CNS) recognizes this as osmotic diarrhea. The CNS recommends that the patient:
    A. Increases fiber
    B. Take multivitamins
    C. Avoid foods containing sugar
    D. Take loperamide

32. Which of the following is contraindicated when prescribing diuretics for older adults?
    A. Slowly taper medication doses.
    B. Monitor BUN and creatinine.
    C. Recommend decreasing fluid intake to limit urine frequency.
    D. Monitor for orthostatic hypertension.

33. Which of the following is **not** a possible treatment for hyperthyroidism?
    A. Methimazole
    B. Propranolol
    C. Levothyroxine
    D. Radioactive iodine therapy

34. A patient with a long history of alcoholic liver cirrhosis is being admitted for excessive blood loss due an upper gastrointestinal (GI) bleed. The clinical nurse specialist (CNS) is assisting the nurse in anticipating interventions that will be necessary for the patient. In addition to replacing volume blood losses, which initial measure will be critical for this patient?
    A. Immediate placement of balloon tamponade device
    B. Administration of vitamin K
    C. Airway protection via endotracheal intubation
    D. Placement of an arterial line to continuously monitor blood pressure

35. Which vessel contributes to a characteristic clinical picture found in patients with stroke?
    A. Left internal carotid artery
    B. Right vertebral artery
    C. Right middle cerebral artery
    D. Left anterior cerebral artery

36. A 68-year-old patient presents with symptoms of dizziness, orthopnea, and edema. The focused assessment of this patient begins with the:
    A. Cardiovascular system
    B. Respiratory system
    C. Neurologic system
    D. Reproductive system

37. A patient has been scheduled for a synchronized cardioversion. What cardiac rhythm would the patient likely have to be scheduled for this procedure?
    A. Asystole
    B. Wide complex ventricular tachycardia
    C. Third-degree heart block
    D. Atrial fibrillation

38. A 78-year-old female with a history of chronic obstructive pulmonary disease (COPD) and type II diabetes is admitted to the ICU for urosepsis, dehydration, hypotension, and mental status change. She is currently on supplemental oxygen, IV fluids, and IV piperacillin/tazobactam. Which of the following ICU-acquired weakness (ICU-AW) early-prevention strategies is **not** appropriate at this time?
    A. Glycemic control (110–180 mg/dL)
    B. Fluid and electrolyte balance
    C. Prevention of organ failure
    D. Seizure precautions

39. A 75-year-old male with a history of arthritis presents with altered mental status and complains of "ringing in the ear," with stable vital signs with the exception of an increased respiratory rate (RR). His daughter reports the patient accidentally took his two types of his arthritis medicine BID with his daily dose of Pepto Bismol about 4 hours ago. She found him confused and breathing quickly. Which of the following arterial blood gasses do you expect of find?
    A. pH 7.55, PCO_2 50 HCO_3^- 24
    B. pH 7.46, PCO_2 22 HCO_3 16
    C. pH 7.25, PCO_2 65 HCO_3 38
    D. pH 7.35, PCO_2 32 HCO_3^- 20

40. The body adapts to potentially stressful challenges by activating response mechanisms in the autonomic nervous system. The stress response begins in which area of the brain?
    A. Amygdala
    B. Hypothalamus
    C. Thalamus
    D. Cerebral cortex

41. Which of the following is the appropriate initial treatment of tension pneumothorax?
    A. Chest tube insertion
    B. Needle decompression
    C. Needle aspiration
    D. Emergency video-assisted thorascopic surgery (VATS) procedure

42. A 47-year-old female is admitted to the medical unit with acute pancreatitis and hypertension. The clinical nurse specialist (CNS) performs an initial assessment and notes flexion of the thumb and hyperextension of fingers with inflation of the blood pressure cuff. The CNS suspects which potential complication of acute pancreatitis?
    A. Hypoglycemia
    B. Hypomagnesemia
    C. Hyperkalemia
    D. Hypocalcemia

43. A clinical nurse specialist (CNS) on the cardiac unit can identify a heart failure patient by which key findings?
    A. Clear lung sounds and fluid volume deficit
    B. Not tolerating ambulating and has fluid retention and dyspnea

C. Normal sinus rhythm and requiring oxygen 2 L via nasal cannula
D. Atrial fibrillation and dyspnea

44. The clinical nurse specialist (CNS) is caring for a patient who is taking both warfarin and bile acid sequestrants. What teaching does the CNS need to ensure is completed for the patient?
    A. Take other oral medications 1 hour before or 4 to 6 hours after bile acid sequestrants.
    B. All oral medications should be taken together
    C. Do not drink grape juice while taking the medications.
    D. Limit the intake of vitamins A, D, and E in food while on bile acid sequestrants.

45. A patient presents with complaints of fatigue, anxiety, and palpitations. His lab work reveals a thyroid-stimulating hormone (TSH) of <0.1 mIU/L (normal range 0.4–4.0 mIU/L), free T4 of 2.1 ng/dL (normal range 0.89–1.76 ng/dL), and free T3 of 5.7 pg/mL (normal range 2.3–4.2 pg/mL). Physical exam is notable for diaphoresis, tachycardia, tremors, slight, and symmetrical enlargement of the thyroid gland without nodules and protrusion of the eyes. What is the mostly likely diagnosis?
    A. Primary hypothyroidism
    B. Toxic multinodular goiter (MNG)
    C. Myxedema coma
    D. Hyperthyroidism

46. Which of the following is the nonparametric equivalent of the t test?
    A. Kruskal-Wallis test
    B. Spearman's rho
    C. Mann-Whitney's U
    D. Fisher's exact test

47. In Native American cultures, there are many interactions that may not be appropriate but quite common to use with other cultures. It is important to recognize issues that could become barriers to the therapeutic relationship. Which of the following items are specifically found to be possible pitfalls when developing a nursing therapeutic relationship?
    A. Modesty is key; ask how they want to be addressed, herbs and alternative treatments are very important, and the practitioner may need to work with a traditional healer.
    B. They prefer to be addressed as Native or Native American; modesty is only important with females, traditional medicine may be used, and a traditional healer may also be used.
    C. The traditional healer may recommend against surgery; modesty is directed toward the older adult only, the practitioner may speak too fast or attempt too much eye contact to develop trust with the patient, and travel may be difficult from a traditional reservation or isolated rural area.
    D. Travel is easy and always arranged by the tribal council or health corporation, alcoholism is always an issue, diabetes will occur in all Native Americans at some point, traditional rituals have removed any need for modesty in the population.

48. A patient with a history of nonadherence to the prescribed medical plan is admitted to the hospital for reoccurring infection of a nonhealing diabetic foot ulcer. The clinical nurse

specialist (CNS) specializing in care of patients with diabetes is consulted to see this patient. When assessing the patient, the CNS learns that the patient has little assistance at home, limited financial and social resources, and a low literacy level. In order to impact adherence to the plan after discharge, the CNS should:

A. Have the patient verbalize understanding of the plan of care.

B. Give the patient written instructions for dressing changes.

C. Determine whether the patient is eligible for home care assistance for wound dressing changes.

D. Provide web-based diabetes self-management resources prior to discharge.

49. Opioid-induced sedation can be detected by

A. End tidal CO_2 monitoring and the Pasero Opioid Sedation Scale (POSS) tool

B. O_2 saturation monitoring

C. Monitoring respiratory rate (RR)

D. Asking a family member if the patient is snoring

50. A 66-year-old female is admitted to the hospital following a fall. She has a history of Alzheimer's disease. Her husband is a primary caregiver. He tells the clinical nurse specialist (CNS) he left her alone to go to the grocery store. What is the best intervention for the CNS to provide?

A. Recommend admission to a long-term care facility specializing in care for patients with Alzheimer's disease

B. Consult with hospice for end-of-life care

C. Contact the Alzheimer's Association for resources or adult day care services

D. Do an assessment for elder abuse

51. When developing interventions to decrease healthcare disparities, the CNS working in a prenatal clinic located in a neighborhood with many Burmese individuals will include:

A. Staff education about Burmese health beliefs

B. Obtaining low-cost medications

C. Improving public transportation

D. Updating equipment and supplies for the clinic

52. The clinical nurse specialist (CNS) is leading a hospital-wide change to implement a new evidence-based care bundle for patients with sepsis and intends to use Lewin's change theory in planning the phases of the project. To best sustain the change in practice, the CNS should plan to:

A. Encourage subgroup opposition to the change so many viewpoints can be considered.

B. Help staff come to a total consensus regarding the change.

C. Include naysayers on the planning team.

D. Be available to support those affected by the change until refreezing occurs.

53. The clinical nurse specialist (CNS) is seeing a patient who has a history of bipolar depression. The patient is currently experiencing symptoms of diarrhea, vomiting, increased thirst, and hand tremors. The CNS suspects side effects from which of the following?

A. Lithium

B. Depakote

C. Sertraline

D. Carbamazepine

54. All patients should receive a malnutrition screening assessment to aid in the identification of those patients at nutrition risk. Select the tool that would be appropriate to aid in your assessment.

A. Braden Scale

B. BMI

C. Malnutrition Universal Screening Tool (MUST)

D. Confusion Assessment Method (CAM)

55. How would a clinical nurse specialist (CNS) describe the options of a hypercapnic patient who has an advanced directive for do not resuscitate (DNR)/do not intubate (DNI) with trial noninvasive ventilation?

A. The patient can have an endotracheal tube placed at the bedside.

B. The patient can have temporary bilevel positive airway pressure (BiPAP) or continuous positive airway pressure (CPAP) via a mask.

C. The patient can only have oxygen via nasal cannula.

D. There are no options to assist this patient.

56. A patient who had a myocardial infarction is going to cardiac rehabilitation where progressive exercise is monitored by healthcare professionals. When would this patient be most vulnerable to injury and complications?

A. Between 5 and 9 days

B. Between 10 and 14 days

C. Between 15 and 20 days

D. Between 20 and 30 days

57. Which test definitively diagnoses pulmonary arterial hypertension (PAH)?

A. Transthoracic echocardiogram (TTE)

B. Sleep study

C. Cardiac MRI

D. Right heart catheterization (RHC)

58. A young adult has been prescribed Depakote (divalproex sodium) for new onset of seizures. Which of the following side effects would be most concerning needing additional reevaluation?

A. Headache

B. Dyspepsia

C. Nosebleed

D. Low blood sugars

59. A patient's ABG results are as follows: pH 7.33, PCO_2 39 HCO_3 15. These results:

A. are common in patients with vomiting or nasogastric suctioning.

B. are characterized by renal bicarbonate retention.

C. can be caused by diuretic therapy.

D. can be caused by renal failure.

60. A 78-year-old male has just been admitted to your unit from a nursing home after emergent laparotomy. As you assess the patient, you note which of the following age-related changes as your most concerning finding?

A. Decreased gastrointestinal motility

B. Loss of epidermal elasticity

C. Improved cognitive function

D. Loss of lean muscle mass

61. Which government organization sets the recommendations for adult vaccination schedules?

A. American Medical Association (AMA)

B. Centers for Disease Control and Prevention (CDC)

C. Centers for Medicare & Medicaid Services (CMS)

D. National Institutes of Health (NIH)

62. The clinical nurse specialist (CNS) who manages acute stroke at a hospital knows that providing care for a person who has experienced a stroke may at times include strong moral viewpoints from the staff. The CNS knows that it will be important to implement which of the following interventions for a healthy work environment on the stroke unit?

A. A firm, authoritarian style of leadership

B. Clear steps and processes for everyone to implement the same care for everyone

C. A workshop to learn effective team communication skills

D. Review of the current policy and procedure manual

63. What does *PICO(T)* stand for?

A. Population, Intervention, Comparison, Outcome, Time Frame

B. Procedure, Intervention, Contrast, Outcome Rates, Time

C. Patients, Intention, Contrast, Outcome, Time Frame

D. Population, Intersession, Comparison, Time Frame

64. Hyponatremia in cirrhosis leads is caused by:

A. Reduced water secretion and reduced serum osmolality

B. Increased water absorption and increased serum osmolality

C. Increased sodium reabsorption, free water retention, and reduced serum osmolality

D. Decreased sodium reabsorption and increased serum osmolality

65. A patient has decompensated liver disease and is declining in the ICU due to sepsis. Which is a symptom that would indicate the patient has a complication of decompensated liver disease?

A. Ascites

B. Spontaneous bacterial peritonitis (SBP)

C. Decreased bowel sounds

D. Interstitial hypovolemia

66. A patient with Parkinson's disease takes levodopa, vitamin C, Lisinopril, and baby aspirin. What food type should the patient avoid in high amounts?

A. Carbohydrates

B. Fiber

C. Fats

D. Protein

67. Second generation antipsychotics require monitoring of which of the following?

A. Blood pressure and electrolytes

B. Lipids and blood glucose

C. Potassium and sodium only

D. White blood cell count

68. A 53-year-old female with no past medical history presents to the urgent care clinic complaining of general malaise and hot flashes and painful urination. Her vitals are as follows: temperature is 36.7° C heart rate (HR) is 96 bpm, respiratory rate (RR) is 28 breaths/min, blood pressure (BP) is 101/56 mmHg, mean arterial pressure (MAP) is 71 mmHg, SpO$_2$ 96% on room air. The provider is concerned and draws a lactate; the result is 2.3. What assessment finding is most

concerning for this patient and will determine the next priority intervention?

A. Temperature, BP, and RR

B. Genitourinary assessment, HR and RR

C. Lactate, HR and RR

D. RR, temperature, HR

69. Roy's adaptation model places emphasis on the person's own coping abilities to achieve health in an environment with what three types of stimuli?

A. Focal, facial, and emotional

B. Focal, contextual, and residual

C. Contextual, chemoreceptor, and sensory

D. Contextual, sensory, and residual

70. A 65-year-old female with a history of poorly controlled type 2 diabetes and neuropathy presents with a sprained ankle, after slipping on ice on the way to her mailbox early this morning. Select the priority intervention for her initial care.

A. Elevate affected limb.

B. Encourage her to rest her ankle over the next few days.

C. Apply ice to the ankle for 15 minutes qh.

D. Refer to occupational therapy for evaluation and assistance with mobility needs.

71. The clinical nurse specialist (CNS) is seeing a client who presents with a history of drug abuse and is complaining of muscle cramps, loss of balance, constipation, muscle stiffness, impulsiveness, and low energy. The CNS suspects which of the following?

A. Decreased production of dopamine

B. Hypoglycemia

C. Hyponatremia

D. Hypothyroidism

72. A 76-year-old female has hypertension and presents with shortness of breath, crackles, and bilateral lower edema. Which class of antihypertensives should be strictly avoided for this patient?

A. Beta blockers

B. Dihydropyridine calcium channel blockers

C. Ace inhibitors

D. Nondihydropyridine calcium channel blockers

73. A patient has a blood glucose of 38 mg/dL but is asymptomatic. What is the best course of action?

A. The patient is asymptomatic, so no intervention is necessary.

B. Give the patient a snack with carbohydrates, protein, and fat.

C. Administer 25 mL of D50 intravenously.

D. Give 20 g of carbohydrates as juice.

74. A patient presents to the burn unit with full thickness wounds that are circumferential around one arm. While monitoring circulatory status diligently, there may also be a need for:

A. Fasciotomy

B. Surgical debridement

C. Physical therapy consult

D. Escharotomy

75. Due to the extreme fatigue caused by interferon-based medications, what is a strategy to optimize activity levels?
    A. Time injection administration to allow for patient/family activities.
    B. Prescribe Provigil to allow for increased energy levels.
    C. Decrease the interferon medication dosage.
    D. Teach the patient that previous activities cannot be accomplished now that they are diagnosed with multiple sclerosis (MS).

76. A patient with a past medical history of asthma and possible allergic reaction to IV contrast needs a routine CT of the head with IV contrast. What is an appropriate premedication regimen prior to the CT scan?
    A. Prednisone 50 mg PO 13 hours, 7 hours, and 1 hour prior to the CT and diphenhydramine 50 mg PO 1 hour prior to the CT
    B. Methylprednisolone sodium succinate 40 mg IV and diphenhydramine 50 mg IV qh prior to the CT
    C. Dexamethasone sodium sulfate 7.5 mg IV immediately, and then q4h until the CT and diphenhydramine 50 mg IV 1 hour prior to the CT
    D. Diphenhydramine 50 minutes IV 7 hours and 1 hour prior to the CT

77. What is the acronym used to help remember the sequence used during cardiopulmonary resuscitation (CPR)?
    A. **A**irway **B**reathing **C**irculation
    B. **C**irculation **A**irway **B**reathing
    C. **A**irway **C**irculation **B**reathing
    D. **B**reathing **A**irway **C**irculation

78. What is an evidence-based approach, included in the gastrointestinal (GI) enhanced recovery after surgery (ERAS) recommendations, to prevent postoperative ileus?
    A. Insertion of a nasogastric tube post surgery
    B. Keeping the patient NPO (nothing by mouth) for 3 days post surgery
    C. Gum chewing
    D. Manage pain with IV dilaudid or morphine

79. When necrotizing fasciitis is diagnosed, which is the recommended approach to antibiotic therapy?
    A. Antibiotics only after identifying the bacteria with a blood culture
    B. A narrow-spectrum antibiotic aimed at the most likely bacteria
    C. Early administration of broad-spectrum antibiotics
    D. No antibiotics until after surgical debridement

80. Which antidepressants may prolong QT interval?
    A. Sertraline and Fluoxetine
    B. Citalopram and Escitalopram
    C. Sertraline and Citalopram
    D. Fluoxetine and Paroxetine

81. When considering the most recent laboratory evaluation of nutritional status, which lab value will provide the best results?
    A. Serum albumin
    B. Serum transferrin
    C. Serum prealbumin
    D. Serum Hgb

82. A hospital has a higher-than-expected rate of hospital-acquired infections (HAIs). The clinical nurse specialist (CNS) has been tasked with reducing the HAIs. What should the CNS's *first* task be?
    A. Review hospital policies for inclusion of most recent guidelines
    B. Identify stakeholders and call an interdisciplinary meeting
    C. Provide just-in-time education at the bedside
    D. Analyze HAI trends for the past 2 years

83. A cost–benefit analysis should identify:
    A. How government funding impacts patient outcomes
    B. Whether an intervention would be financially beneficial over the current practice
    C. How societal welfare was previously impacted
    D. The expenses of the current practice

84. The potential pathophysiologic consequences of pulmonary embolism (PE) includes:
    A. Right ventricular stress/cor pulmonale
    B. Low V/Q (ventilation/perfusion) ratio
    C. Pulmonary arterial hypotension
    D. Left ventricular hypertrophy

85. When caring for a patient with chemotherapy-induced mucositis, which intervention would be most appropriate?
    A. Ensure that the patient is NPO until the lesions heal.
    B. Encourage frequent alcohol-based mouth rinses.
    C. Administer a monoclonal antibody.
    D. Provide frequent oral care using a disposable mouth swab.

86. Which of the following is **not** a characteristic of osteoarthritis (OA):
    A. Pain
    B. Progressive loss of cartilage
    C. Swollen, hot joints
    D. Joint deformity

87. A patient presents with a history of abdominal trauma, left upper quadrant pain, tenderness upon palpation, and left shoulder pain. What lab work would be your first priority to evaluate?
    A. CBC
    B. LFTs
    C. PT/partial thromboplastin time (PTT)
    D. Chem 7

88. Adults who are immunocompromised, or have an HIV with CD4 count <200, should **not** receive which of the following vaccinations?
    A. Meningococcal, MMR, HiB
    B. MMR, human papillomavirus (HPV), ZVL
    C. MMR, HPV, influenza
    D. Tdap, MMR, HPV

89. Your 81-year-old patient states that she is a lifelong runner and still jogs around her neighborhood 6 miles a day, 5 days a week. What is appropriate advice to help her mitigate cancer risk?
    A. None. She is obviously a very healthy person and has low risk for developing cancer.
    B. Utilize protective UV blocking clothing and sunblock to reduce risk of skin cancers from prolonged sun exposure.

C. Advise her to cut back on this intense exercise. It is dangerous at her age to jog such a long distance and 150 minutes per week is recommended as a sufficient amount of exercise.

D. Advise her that short distance runs would be best to avoid fall risk.

90. Which of the following studies has the highest strength of evidence?

A. Quasi-experimental study (experimental study without randomization)

B. Experimental study (randomized control trial)

C. Clinical practice guideline

D. Systematic review of randomized control trial studies without meta-analysis

91. Which of the following is **not** a requirement for provision of informed consent?

A. Participants should be assured that privacy will be protected at all times.

B. Participants must be informed about the potential benefits to themselves or others.

C. Participants must be informed about the volume of data that will be collected.

D. Participants must be informed which healthcare activities are routine and which are treatments for the study.

92. The clinical nurse specialist (CNS) is assessing a client with a history of alcohol abuse. The client presents with a taut, distended abdomen. When assessing the abdomen, the CNS would anticipate:

A. Flatness over the liver region

B. Dullness over the region of the spleen

C. Bladder fullness

D. Fluid wave and shifting dullness

93. A medical-surgical unit nurse approaches the clinical nurse specialist (CNS) to discuss a patient status change. The patient, who has been hospitalized for 3 days, is now complaining of bone and muscle pain, chills, and restless legs. After reviewing the patient's medical record, the adult-gerontology clinical nurse specialist (AGCNS) suspects the patient is withdrawing from which of the following class of drugs?

A. Benzodiazepines

B. Opioids

C. Sedatives

D. Depressants

94. The clinical nurse specialist (CNS) assesses a patient with pulmonary arterial hypertensin (PAH) for objective signs that goals of treatment are reached. The CNS knows the patient is therapeutic on intravenous Veletri (prostacyclin) when

A. the patient has less syncope and reports improved exercise tolerance.

B. a 6-minute walk test distance is greater than 440 meters and BNP level is 100 pg/mL.

C. right atrial pressure (RAP) is 20 mmHg and mean pulmonary artery pressure (PAP) is 35 mmHg.

D. the patient has not had any bloodstream infections from her Hickman catheter.

95. A patient will need to be premedicated prior to a blood transfusion. The clinical nurse specialist knows that the premedications should be given:

A. 15 minutes before the transfusion

B. Immediately before starting the transfusion

C. 5 minutes after beginning the transfusion

D. 30 minutes before staring the transfusion

96. A patient hospitalized for the past week is noted to have blanchable redness to the sacrum. What would be the most appropriately treatment?

A. Massage the area vigorously

B. Place a hydrogel dressing on the wound

C. Relieve pressure over the area

D. Debride the wound

97. Which lab test is most important in early determination of the degree of traumatic shock?

A. Hemoglobin

B. Lactic acid

C. Partial prothrombin time

D. Anion gap

98. Benzodiazepines are not recommended as a sleep aid for older adults per the Beers List of Potentially Inappropriate Medications for the Elderly because they have increased potential to cause:

A. High blood pressure

B. Insomnia

C. Diabetes

D. Delirium

99. Which vaccinations are recommended for all adults?

A. HepA, HepB, Tdap, MMR, meningococcal

B. Influenza, Tdap, VAR, HepA

C. Influenza, Tdap, MMR, HPV

D. Influenza, Tdap, MMR, VAR, meningococcal

100. How is telemedicine related to telehealth?

A. Telemedicine is the use of remote services for HIT, and telehealth is the use of remote services for IT.

B. Telehealth describes all remote health-related services including nonclinical and administrative functions and telemedicine is one focus of it that pertains to remote clinical services.

C. Telehealth is the delivery of all clinical services, and telemedicine is a branch of that delivering medication-related healthcare services.

D. Telemedicine is the delivery of health-related services by physicians, and telehealth is the delivery of health-related services by all clinicians.

101. A patient still has dysphagia post ischemic stroke. The patient has a gastrostomy (G) tube for feedings and medications. Which medication ordered would you question?

A. Niacin (vitamin B_3)

B. ASA (aspirin)

C. Atorvastatin (Lipitor)

D. Coumadin (warfarin)

102. A patient with recurrent bouts of acute pancreatitis complaints is readmitted to your unit with complaints of abdominal pain and foul-smelling diarrhea. The results of the fecal elastase is 120 Cg/g. This result is:

A. Normal

B. Low and indicative of chronic pancreatitis

C. High and indicative of pancreatitis

D. Low and indicative of acute hepatitis

103. The clinical nurse specialist's patient's fasting blood glucose this a.m. was 207 mg/dL. Lunch, dinner, and evening blood glucoses yesterday were 178, 152, and 183 mg/dL. The patient received 4 units of correctional insulin. The

patient is currently on 25 units of insulin glargine daily, 8 units of insulin lispro with meals, and an insulin lispro medium dose correctional scale. Which of the following insulins needs adjustment?
A. Insulin glargine
B. Prandial insulin lispro
C. Correctional scale insulin lispro
D. No adjustment is necessary

104. Research has elucidated many of the risk factors associated with coronary heart disease. As a result of decades of epidemiologic work, which of the following was **not** determined to be a risk factor?
A. Hypotension
B. Male aged 50 years or more
C. Smoking
D. Sedentary lifestyle

105. A patient presents to the ED with dyspnea on exertion, dizziness, and fatigue over the past week or so. No complaints for chest pain. Vital signs: heart rate (HR) 125 bpm, blood pressure (BP) 80/40 mmHg, respiratory rate (RR) 26. Patient has an oxygen saturation of 87% on room air. Crackles are heard on the lower base of both lungs, jugular distention present, and heart sounds are distant. Which of the following is the best initial management of this patient?
A. Pericardiocentesis
B. Angiogram
C. Intravenous (IV) fluids
D. Beta blocker

106. The clinical nurse specialist (CNS) is caring for a patient with a blood glucose level of 42; the patient is currently asymptomatic. After looking at the medications, the CNS suspects which one could be causing symptoms?
A. Rosuvastatin
B. Pantoprazole
C. Furosemide
D. Metoprolol

107. The clinical nurse specialist (CNS) is caring for a postrenal transplant patient who recently started taking cyclosporine. The CNS knows the discharge teaching plan should include which of the following:
A. Monitor for low pulse rate (bradycardia).
B. Alert physician for weight gain or loss of 10% or more so the dose can be adjusted.
C. Notify the care team if any headaches, tremors, or seizures are noticed.
D. Take acetaminophen for any flu-like symptoms.

108. A 32-year-old female is diagnosed with acute hepatitis after an episode of acetaminophen (Tylenol) poisoning. Which of the following treatment interventions would you initiate?
A. Valproic acid (Depakene)
B. Prednisone
C. Acetylcysteine (Mucomyst)
D. Lorazepam (Ativan)

109. A patient in the ICU has continuous intracranial pressure (ICP) monitoring post operative day 1 after a craniotomy secondary to a head injury. The priority assessment for this patient is
A. Repeated neurologic assessment hourly
B. Neurologic assessment per shift

C. Monitoring lab values and trends
D. Musculoskeletal assessment with early mobility

110. Your patient has been prescribed Topamax (topiramate) for seizures. What adverse effect would warrant an immediate action?
A. A change in blood glucose reading
B. Blurred vision or visual disturbances
C. Tinnitus
D. Frequent stools and abdominal pain

111. A 23-year-old male is brought to the ED by his friends after running a marathon on an 80° day. His friends tell the clinical nurse specialist (CNS) that they can't believe he beat all of them because he barely trained. The patient is reporting "really sharp" bilateral lower extremity muscle cramps and has a temperature of 101 °F. What is the priority intervention?
A. Aggressive fluid rehydration to maintain urine output of 2 to 3 mL/kg/hr
B. Pain medication for the muscle cramping
C. Cooling blankets for his temperature
D. Oral rehydration with electrolyte-containing solutions

112. Objective data obtained in a patient encounter are usually recorded:
A. By body systems
B. In the problem list
C. In the health history
D. Before the health history

113. How could the clinical nurse specialist (CNS) describe pronation therapy to a family member of a patient in the ICU?
A. Proning a patient allows for better circulation to the lung in a patient with acute respiratory distress syndrome (ARDS).
B. Pronation is the only treatment for ARDS.
C. Pronation is a therapy to treat asthma.
D. Mechanical ventilation is a contraindicated when proning a patient.

114. A patient with grade 2 ascites returns to the ED with hepatic encephalopathy and fever after being discharged to an extended care facility 3 days ago. Cultures on ascites fluid and blood and urine are sent. The result of a diagnostic paracentesis reveals a polymorphonuclear (PMN) cell count greater than 250 cell/mm³. Which course of treatment is best for this patient?
A. Delay treatment until culture results are returned.
B. Treat fever with antipyretics.
C. Treat with IV cephalosporin agent (cefoxitin) or alternative therapy for 30 days.
D. Treat with IV cephalosporin agent (cefoxitin) or alternative agent for 7 to 10 days.

115. A 67-year-old male presents to the clinic with acute pain involving the right great toe. The patient states he has experienced this type of pain in the past. He reports having just returned from an out-of-town reunion of fellow retirees, where he admits to overeating and consuming more alcohol than usual. Physical exam reveals a swollen, red, right metatarsophalangeal joint. Based upon subjective and objective findings, the clinical nurse specialist (CNS) knows that interventions may include:
A. Allopurinol, high-protein diet
B. Oxycodone, low-purine diet

C. Allopurinol, low-purine diet

D. Oxycodone, warm compresses

116. You are caring for a patient who has been admitted to the hospital while receiving home hospice care but has revoked hospice in order to have a broken hip repaired. You understand that the patient has a general prognosis of which of the following?
    A. 3 months or less to live
    B. 6 months or less to live
    C. 12 months or less to live
    D. Weeks or less to live

117. Which nutritional screening tool offers the best validity?
    A. MNF
    B. MUST
    C. MNA
    D. SCREEN II

118. One of the nurses on the unit is concerned about her patient's heart rate (HR) of 40 beats per minute (bpm) and a BP of 90/65 mmHg. The patient is here for a scheduled cholecystectomy in the morning. The nurse is seeking assistance from the cliinical nurse specialist (CNS). What should the first intervention be from the CNS?
    A. Call the rapid response team.
    B. Ask the nurse to retake the patient's vitals.
    C. Order digoxin and ask for a transfer to the ICU.
    D. Go assess the patient.

119. The clinical nurse specialist (CNS) is caring for a patient with a history of an arrhythmia who has come in with dizziness and hypotension. What does the CNS suspect is the issue?
    A. Side effects from antiarrhythmic medication
    B. Decreased dopamine levels
    C. Complications from liver disease
    D. Stevens–Johnson's syndrome

120. Thyroid-stimulating hormone (TSH) is produced by the following gland:
    A. Hypothalamus
    B. Pituitary
    C. Thyroid
    D. Adrenal gland

121. A 78-year-old female is admitted to the unit for possible sepsis. Her daughter is the primary caregiver for her mother and concerned about her care. The daughter tells the clincal nurse specialist (CNS), "I really miss going to church on Sunday." What priority action should the CNS take?
    A. Assess for caregiver strain.
    B. Ask if the daughter has loss faith in her church.
    C. Inform her when the next church service is scheduled at the hospital.
    D. Enter a consult with case management for possible home services.

122. The local community council in a rural area has been asked to establish a public health center for members of the community. The clinical nurse specialist (CNS) has been asked to provide guidance to the council as a paid consultant. The CNS recognizes from the council member's request that the county and state that they live in has a need to support rural healthcare and they want to participate in the public policy solution. The most appropriate action is:
    A. Report the issue to the attorney general and ask for an investigation.
    B. Research the U.S. Health and Human Services Agency (HHS) databases for information on public health programs that would be available in the community.
    C. Contact the community council and recommend that they raise taxes to fund the community health clinic.
    D. Find out more information by researching appropriate databases. Research available funding programs. Develop a strategy to propose a solution. Continue to monitor the legislative process and report changes to the council.

123. What is the difference between health information technology (HIT) and information technology (IT)?
    A. IT is related to all technology and HIT is related to health.
    B. HIT more globally describes how IT should be used.
    C. HIT is the use of IT for the receipt, delivery, and utilization of health information in electronic systems.
    D. HIT is used by government entities to describe IT in healthcare.

124. A patient presents to the hospital in a depressive state; she reports a history of bipolar disorder and that she has not taken her medications for the past week. The appropriate treatment would include:
    A. Zolpidem (Ambien) 5 mg q12h
    B. Bupropion HCl (Wellbutrin) 100 mg q8h
    C. Naltrexone/Bupropion HCl (Contrave) 2 tablets PO q12h
    D. Quetiapine (Seroquel XR) 200 mg PO q12h

125. Cancer can cause changes in what component of Virchow's triad?
    A. Blood coagulability
    B. Blood viscosity
    C. Capillary leak
    D. Blood flow

126. When would a life vest be an appropriate intervention for a patient?
    A. Recently placed in hospice care
    B. At risk for sudden cardiac arrest and awaiting long-term trajectory
    C. Prior to having orthopedic surgery
    D. After having an implantable cardiac defibrillator placed

127. An 85-year-old male has multiple admissions to the unit for chronic obstructive pulmonary disease (COPD) exacerbation. His current diagnosis is failure to thrive. The clinical nurse specialist (CNS) reviewed the patient's plan of care with the care team. Which of the following should be done first?
    A. Pulmonary rehabilitation
    B. Case management consultation for an extended care placement
    C. Placing a do-not-resuscitate order
    D. Consulting palliative care for management

128. A 76-year-old woman weighs 43 kg. She has poor appetite and low albumin level. Which characteristic would be aligned to the concern related to nutrition for this patient?
    A. Weight gain
    B. Pressure Injuries

C. Loss of muscle mass

D. Pedal edema

129. A patient presents to the ED with severe headache and right-sided weakness. Further testing reveals the patient has suffered an intracranial hemorrhage (ICH). Upon questioning the family, it is discovered that the patient has been taking Coumadin (warfarin). The INR is 5.3. What is the next step in treating this patient?

A. More intensive imaging to further determine the cause of bleeding

B. An antiepileptic drug for seizure prophylaxis

C. Therapy to replace vitamin K–dependent factors

D. A bedside swallow exam to determine aspiration risk

130. A 52-year-old female presents to the clinic with a complaint of bilateral pain in wrists and distal interphalangeal (DIP) joints. The patient reports that her pain has come on gradually over a period of months along with generalized body aches. Pain and stiffness are worse in the early morning, lasting for at least 1 hour. Physical exam shows swollen DIP joints. Based on subjective and objective findings, the clinical nurse specialist (CNS) knows that interventions may include:

A. Tylenol, exercise

B. Ibuprofen, Methotrexate

C. Tylenol, ultrasound treatment

D. Ibuprofen, glucosamine supplement

131. All of the following diagnoses have potential for acid–base imbalances based upon abnormal ABG results and symptomatic presentation. Identify which of the following has a different acid–base imbalance than the other three options?

A. Asthma

B. Neuromuscular disorders

C. Severe obesity

D. Hyperventilation

132. The clinical nurse specialist (CNS) is interviewing a patient regarding their medication history to provide patient education. Which of the following statements by the patient indicates that the CNS should inquire further to obtain more information?

A. I take acetaminophen for my headache and nonsteroidal anti-inflammatory drugs (NSAIDs) for my arthritis.

B. I keep my pills in a pill box to make sure I take the correct medication and dose daily.

C. I take multiple herbal medicines because I know they have safe side effects.

D. I know that I have to watch my acetaminophen intake when taking my Darvocet.

133. The clinical nurse specialist (CNS) is rounding on an 80-year-old female, who was admitted yesterday with fevers and malaise for possible urinary tract infection (UTI). The patient's family stated they had not heard from her in 2 days and were concerned because she lives alone. They were exploring options for support at home because she has been very unsteady. The patient adds that while she remembers falling, she does not know how long she was on the ground before the firefighters came to help. What laboratory test should you consider as a priority concern that may further explain the patient's symptoms?

A. Urine culture

B. Creatinine kinase

C. Troponin

D. Hemoglobin and Hematocrit

134. One of the common age-related changes to the sleep–wake cycle is:

A. Less time in deeper, slow-wave sleep

B. More time in stages 1 and 2

C. Vivid dreaming stage is longer

D. Increased total sleep time

135. What is the best statement about the National Database for Nursing Quality Indicators (NDNQI), nurse-sensitive indicators and hospital-acquired conditions (HAC)?

A. Both NDNQI, nursing-sensitive indicators, and HAC describe quality-improvement initiatives.

B. Measures are tracked and compared at the unit level for comparison for quality outcomes.

C. Payment may be withheld if conditions are not present on admission or preexisting to a hospital stay.

D. NDNQI, nursing-sensitive indicators, and HAC are only monitored annually.

136. The clinical nurse specialist (CNS) is counseling a 71-year-old male regarding cancer risk reduction. Which recommendation is appropriate?

A. Avoid aging, exercise 150 minutes a week, avoid alcohol intake, and maintain a healthy body weight.

B. Avoid marrying into a family with genetic risk and take measures to reduce chance of radon exposure.

C. Limit exposure to the UV rays of the sun and make an appointment for genetic counseling following a recent diagnoses of breast cancer.

D. Question any tests ordered that involve radiation exposure and make an appointment for an HPV vaccination.

137. A 49-year-old woman has inoperable pancreatic cancer. Before the diagnosis, she enjoyed cooking and eating. Her husband is quite distraught about her lack of appetite and weight loss. The patient is resentful and feels pressured. Supplements are not to her liking. Which interventions are most appropriate?

A. Encourage the family to coerce the patient to drink protein shakes.

B. Insert a nasogastric tube to prepare for delivery of artificial nutrition.

C. Request an order for lorazepam for anxiety.

D. Discuss the option of Megestrol 200 mg BID to stimulate appetite.

138. The clinical nurse specialist (CNS) is working with a novice nurse on the care of a patient recently admitted with diabetic ketoacidosis. The CNS focuses the conversation with the novice nurse on the priorities of nursing care and asks the novice nurse to recall the interventions provided to past patients with diabetes. What is the rationale for the CNS actions?

A. Applying adult learning theory

B. Conducting a gap analysis

C. Employing Socratic questioning

D. Advocating for the patient

139. Which of the following is a role of the clinical nurse specialist (CNS) in managing nurse-sensitive indicators?

A. Lead a group of clinical nurses in determining how to implement strategies to decrease the risk of falls in an inpatient hospital unit.

B. Counsel nurses who are repeatedly not compliant with performing oral care on mechanically ventilated patients.

C. Communicate outcomes to select stakeholders in relation to glycemic control in the post–open heart surgery population.

D. Apply change theory concepts to further engagement and adherence to interventions and strategies that address employee adherence to job descriptions or policy.

140. A 35-year-old patient is admitted to the ICU with acute necrotizing pancreatitis and sepsis. On assessment, a large area of ecchymosis is noted in the umbilical region. This hallmark sign is called
A. Murphy's sign
B. Ranson's sign
C. Cullen's sign
D. Grey-Turner's sign

141. The clinical nurse specialist suspects that a patient may be anemic. Which of the following diagnostic tests should be ordered?
A. Prothrombin time and international normalized ratio (PT/INR)
B. Complete blood count (CBC)
C. D-dimer
D. Thrombin time (TT)

142. A clinical nurse Specialist has developed a tool to assist the nurses in the cardiac unit to identify patients who present with right-sided heart failure. Which statement would indicate that the tool is helping nurses understand the pathophysiology of right-sided heart failure? CNSs more frequently identify.
A. Patients who present with a respiratory rate (RR) of 32 and PaO_2 of 48 mmHg
B. Patients who present with rales auscultated from the lungs bilaterally
C. Patients presenting with mental changes with cool and pale skin
D. Patients presenting with increased central venous pressure and jugular vein distension

143. The clinical nurse specialist (CNS) has a client who has a history of blood clot. The client presents with bleeding from the gums when brushing the teeth, brown urine, and increased bruising. The CNS orders which test?
A. Prothrombin time (PT)
B. Digoxin level
C. Vitamin K level
D. Thyroid stimulating hormone (TSH)

144. A patient presents with complaints of fatigue, depression, and weight gain. Her lab work reveals a blood glucose of 101 mg/dL, TSH of 7.65, T4 of 9.2, and Na^+ of 136 mEq/L. The most likely cause of her symptoms is a new diagnosis of:
A. Diabetes mellitus
B. Adrenal insufficiency
C. Primary hypothyroidism
D. Subclinical hypothyroidism

145. A 58-year-old female is admitted to the ICU for gastro-intestinal (GI) bleed. She is emergently intubated for respiratory distress, given fluid boluses, and started on vasopressors for blood pressure management. She has a history of chronic kidney disease (CKD) with a baseline serum Cr 1.5 mg/dL and estimated glomerular filtration rate (eGFR) of 58. Other laboratory values show a hemoglobin of 6.0 g/dL, blood urea nitrigen (BUN) 65 mg/dL and serum creatinine (serum Cr) of 3.0 mg/dL, blood glucose of 155 mg/dL, potassium 4.0 meq/L, sodium 138 meq/L, and chloride 100 meq/L. She is currently taking a combined ipratropium/albuterol inhaler, metoprolol, and metformin.

According to the patient's BUN and serum Cr levels, which of the following is the most likely cause of the acute kidney injury (AKI)?
A. Prerenal: AKI due to medication
B. Postrenal: AKI due to CKD
C. Intrarenal: AKI due to diabetes
D. Prerenal: AKI due to GI bleed

146. A patient has arrived to the ED; the patient was found unresponsive with empty medication bottles around them. You order an arterial blood gas (ABG) and serum chemistry to evaluate the cause of the patient's unresponsiveness, suspecting a possible ingestion and acid–base imbalance. You receive the following values:
pH: 7.34
$PaCO_2$: 36
HCO_3^-: 18
Na: 137
Cl: 96
K: 4.0
Based on these values and patient history, which acid–base imbalance do you suspect?
A. Nonanion gap metabolic acidosis
B. High-anion gap metabolic acidosis
C. Metabolic alkalosis
D. Respiratory acidosis

147. When the clinical nurse specialist (CNS) is educating nursing staff on cognitive assessment for the older adult, it is important to make sure the nurse understands
A. Geriatric patients should be assessed for cognitive impairment
B. All geriatric patients are confused
C. Geriatric patients have incontinence issues
D. All geriatric patients are at risk for falls

148. A clinical nurse specialist (CNS) is seeking feedback from others to complete a self-evaluation of their own clinical practice to ensure they are effectively practicing ethical care. The CNS should seek feedback from all of the following people **except**:
A. A fellow CNS who serves on many of the same committees together
B. The family of a patient that the CNS was involved in the treatment for the patient when they refused care at the end of life
C. The security officer who works at the hospital that greets the CNS qam and can attest to the CNS showing up early for work with a smile on their face each day
D. A research coordinator working with the CNS for the past year on a project to evaluate the outcome of a new admissions process for patients with dementia

149. What is a patient portal?
  A. A patient's ability to access a hospital network via a virtual private network password
  B. Patient portals allow electronic health records (EHRs) users to access all their patients' medical records whenever they need to
  C. Portals allow patients to browse the internet for health tips during appointments or hospitalizations
  D. A patient portal is a secure, online avenue by which patients engage with and may enter their own PHI through a patient-accessed portal of the EHR

150. A 92-year-old patient with advanced dementia has had three episodes of aspiration pneumonia in 5 months. The patient has no written advance directives. A speech therapist recommends feeding tube placement. One of the patient's adult sons would like a feeding tube placed, while the other is unsure, and the patient's spouse states the patient would never want a feeding tube. The clinical nurse specialist's first action is to:
  A. Bring the case to the attention of the ethics committee.
  B. Emphasize to the son that a feeding tube will decrease recurrent pneumonia.
  C. Obtain a surgical consult to schedule a feeding tube placement.
  D. Organize a family and staff meeting to discuss the risks and benefits and consider the patient's wishes.

151. The clinical nurse specialist (CNS) is assessing a 35-year-old female patient who experienced multiple major stressful events in her childhood. The CNS knows early childhood stressors can impact adult health and ensures that the patient assessment includes:
  A. Lung cancer screening
  B. Blood glucose monitoring and BMI
  C. Ulcerative colitis screening
  D. Liver function tests

152. A new physician group was hired at a medical facility. They are requesting that the hospital purchase new equipment for the post-op unit. The chief executive officer (CEO) of the hospital asked the clinical nurse specialist (CNS) to look into the adoption of the new equipment. Based on this request, the CNS knows the best way to proceed would be with the following action:
  A. Refuse to "look into it" and tell the CEO that the current equipment is sufficient.
  B. Talk to the nurses on the unit and determine their preferences for the equipment.
  C. Speak to the physician group personally to get the background on their preferences for the equipment.
  D. Assemble an interprofessional team to perform a literature and market review of current equipment for recommendation to the hospital CEO.

153. The clinical nurse specialist (CNS) is rounding on a patient who mentions that he has had a sharp pain developing in his left forearm over the last "little while." He appears in significant pain and he had an IV removed from the left forearm yesterday after an extravasation. He reports decreased sensation in his hand, weakness in his arm, and the forearm feels rigid. What is the priority intervention?
  A. Warm compresses for 20 minutes qh to alleviate the swelling
  B. Increased physical therapy to assist with the weakness the patient is experiencing

C. Continue to monitor as the symptoms should resolve over the next 24 hours
  D. Obtain an emergent surgical consult for possible fasciotomy

154. Some immunosuppression therapy agents increase the risk of heart disease. For this reason, the clinical nurse specialist knows that they need to:
  A. Administer all doses with antacids.
  B. Recommend diet changes to avoid such things as grape juice.
  C. Dose according to body weight and make dose adjustments frequently.
  D. Start patients slow and on the lowest dose possible.

155. A patient returns from surgery with an open surgical incision that is pink and moist, and there is no necrotic tissue present. The order states daily wet-to-dry dressing changes. What is the most appropriate action?
  A. Follow the order as instructed.
  B. Change the order because you know there is a better dressing option.
  C. Contact the surgeon to inquire if this should be a wet-to-moist dressing to promote wound healing.
  D. Contact the operating room charge nurse to inquire about the incision being without a dressing.

156. A 75-year-old female patient from a nursing home has arrived with reports of confusion, cough, and fever. Her initial vital signs are as follows: heart rate (HR) is 111 bpm, blood pressure (BP) is 89/45 mmHg, temperature is 101.2°F, and respiratory rate (RR) is 22 breath/min. When selecting intravenous (IV) fluids, adequate crystalloid fluid resuscitation is required for this patient because of the:
  A. Loss of intravascular tone related to vasodilation
  B. Need to circulate antibiotics
  C. Risk of microthrombi formation
  D. Priority to reduce lactate

157. During a history intake, a patient tells the clinical nurse specialist (CNS) that she has a history of cervical dystonia. What type of injection should the CNS recommend?
  A. Local anesthetic
  B. Botulinum
  C. Morphine
  D. Steroid

158. What is the most important intervention to minimize the development of delirium?
  A. Keep the patient sedated.
  B. Implement preventive measures.
  C. Do not allow visitors.
  D. Complete vital signs at least q4h 24 hours a day.

159. A 63-year-old Hispanic male is being readmitted to the unit for poorly controlled diabetes mellitus. The primary nurse assigned to the patient tells the clinical nurse specialist (CNS) this is the third time this patient has required hospitalization due to his non-adherence with his prescribed diet and medication regimen. The CNS might ask the patient all of the following questions to determine the underlying cause for his readmission **except**:
  A. Do you need help paying for medications?
  B. Do you have access to transportation to the grocery store?

C. Do you have trouble understanding the English language?

D. When did you last check your fasting blood sugar level?

160. The clinical nurse specialist (CNS) contributes to a healthy work environment by:

A. Including the clinical pharmacist on the nursing team writing evidence-based discharge instructions for patients with atrial fibrillation

B. Working independent of the nursing unit staff council to roll out a new blood-sparing lab draw product

C. Including only the CNS's name on a presentation describing a committee project

D. Not getting involved when a charge nurse assigns a complex patient to a novice nurse recently off orientation

161. Which of the following would indicate that the measurement tool/instrument the clinical nurse specialist (CNS) wants to use is reliable?

A. A Cronbach alpha test result of .80

B. Having a content expert review the tool

C. The instrument has a high correlation with another test that measures the same thing

D. The instrument has a low correlation with another test that measures something different

162. What is information technology (IT)?

A. IT is a department in a hospital that installs printers.

B. IT describes any number of things that utilize electronic processes to receive and/or deliver information.

C. IT is the concept that pertains to computerized physician order entry.

D. IT is a field within the informatics program.

163. Which assessment tool is most appropriate when assessing an older adult with Alzheimer's disease?

A. Faces—Revised

B. Pain Assessment in Advanced Dementia (PAINAD)

C. Numeric Rating Scale

D. Checklist of Nonverbal Pain Indicators (CNPI)

164. On a medical-surgical unit, many patients are transferred to another unit for short-term rehabilitation services prior to discharge to home. Over the past 2 months, several problems and conflicts have arisen surrounding this transition of care. The unit manager calls upon the clinical nurse specialist (CNS) to do education to correct the problem. What is the first action taken by the CNS?

A. Call a meeting of all interested persons to plan the education.

B. Consider whether the content can be best delivered in person or web based.

C. Write the learning outcome and means to evaluate.

D. Conduct a gap analysis.

165. You are performing an interprofessional round on a patient who returned from surgery 2 hours ago for a bilateral knee replacement. The patient is difficult to arouse and only breathing 6 breaths per minute. What is the priority intervention for this patient?

A. Verify last medication administration for pain.

B. Administer oxygen via nasal cannula.

C. Stimulate the patient by sternal rub.

D. Encourage use of incentive spirometry (IS) q2h.

166. A 74-year-old male with a history of disease (chronic obstructive pulmonary COPD), diabetes, and congestive heart failure (CHF) comes to the ED for complaints of increasing shortness of breath, fatigue, and malaise over the past week. Chest x-ray shows right lower lobe infiltrate. Lab values include the following: Na^+ 149 mEq/L, K^+ 3.6 mEq/L, Cl^- 105 mEq/L, glucose 112 mg/dL, blood urea nitrogen (BUN) 29 mg/dL, creatinine 1.2 mg/dL, pH 7.34, $PaCO_2$ 55 mmHg, HCO_3^- 28 mEq/L, PaO_2 88 mmHg. The clinical nurse specialist (CNS) expects initial treatments to include IV antibiotics, supplemental oxygen, and:

A. Diuretic

B. Potassium supplement

C. IV fluid

D. Sodium bicarbonate

167. The clinical nurse specialist (CNS) would anticipate which plan of care for a patient with syncopal episodes, increased exercise intolerance, and signs of right heart failure?

A. Right heart catheterization and initiation of advanced pharmacotherapy

B. Cardiology consult and echocardiogram

C. Permanent pacemaker (PPM) insertion and diuresis

D. Cardiac rehabilitation for NYHA FC IV

168. First-dose syncope occurs in which of the following class of medications?

A. Calcium channel blockers

B. Beta blockers

C. Antiplatelets

D. Alpha adrenergic blockers

169. Hyperparathyroidism is associated with which electrolyte disturbances?

A. Hyperkalemia and hypomagnesemia

B. Hypernatremia and hypocalcemia

C. Hyperphosphatemia and hypocalcemia

D. Hypophosphatemia and hypercalcemia

170. Which of the following is an example of an outcome measure?

A. Adherence to required documentation of restraint assessment

B. Completion of a fall assessment for every patient in a given department

C. Number of rapid response team consultations

D. Number of patients with an intraoperatively acquired pressure injury

171. A 35-year-old female is referred for symptoms consistent with complicated grief. She tells the clinical nurse specialist (CNS) that a few months ago, her old college roommate passed away. On further exploration, she revealed that she and her roommate had an intimate sexual relationship. The patient has never been able to discuss this with her current spouse or family. They are unaware of her previous sexual orientation. This pattern of grief is most consistent with:

A. Chronic grief

B. Delayed grief

C. Exaggerated grief

D. Disenfranchised grief

172. A novice nurse asks the clinical nurse specialist (CNS) what steps are needed before procedures to ensure safety. What is the *best* response?

A. Safety checklists lead to lower rates of complications.

B. Safety checklists are used to improve compliance with hand hygiene before procedures.

C. Audits are completed to evaluate the procedural technique of the provider.

D. Two people verbally verify the safety checks including equipment and setup.

173. Which of the following protocols does **not** help reduce hospital-acquired pneumonia (HAP) cases?
     A. A robust oral care plan
     B. An interprofessional mobility program
     C. Pharmacy involvement in reduction of antibiotics
     D. Deep vein thrombosis (DVT) order sets

174. A 65-year-old Caucasian male has not seen a healthcare provider for several years. His blood pressure (BP_ is 160/90 mmHg with a repeat of 154/88 mmHg. Currently, he is not on any medications. He currently has no symptoms of chest pain, dizziness, light-headedness, or vision changes. Lab results reveal an estimated glomerular filtration rate (eGFR) of >90, $K^+ = 4.0$, and $Na^+ = 142$. His body mass index (BMI) is 29.6. Which medication listed here would be the most appropriate initial therapy to manage this patient's blood pressure?
     A. Atenolol
     B. Propranolol
     C. Spironolactone
     D. Hydrochlorothiazide

175. A patient is diagnosed with a tension pneumothorax. What is the immediate life-saving intervention?
     A. Large bore chest tube insertion
     B. Intubation with mechanical ventilation
     C. Emergency thoracotomy
     D. Pleural needle decompression

Answers and Rationales

1. **Correct answer: B.** You may have difficulty believing this, but "the paralysis caused by this disease is temporary" is a correct statement. Paralysis related to GBS is not permanent, and typically when mobility does return, arms will have function prior to legs.

2. **Correct answer: A.** Acute oliguric renal failure is commonly caused by dehydration due to fluid loss, which is consistent with this patient scenario. Hyperkalemia is an electrolyte disturbance consistent with acute oliguric renal failure and manifests as peaked T waves on EKG. Flattened or inverted T waves are consistent with hypokalemia. Central nervous system changes are a manifestation of hyponatremia, which can occur with fluid volume excess. Muscle fatigue is a common manifestation of hypophosphatemia and not applicable to this patient.

3. **Correct answer: B.** Right shoulder pain is most likely related to gas insufflation during laparoscopic surgery, which can be common postoperatively. Nonpharmacologic techniques such as mobility and heat application should be attempted first before medication dose adjustments are requested. Orders for physical therapy (PT) and x-ray would only be indicated when there is concern for a musculoskeletal injury.

4. **Correct answer: C.** The use of nondepolarizing agents for anesthesia may induce a myasthenic crisis, so anesthesia should be alerted to the patient's medications and history. Fatigue will be common but is not life threatening; physical therapy is contingent on the patient and while respiratory status is important, there should be no specific intubation modalities used other than usual endotracheal intubation unless the patient's anatomy denotes otherwise.

5. **Correct answer: C.** Muffled heart tones, jugular venous distention, and pulseless electrical activity are indicative of a pericardial tamponade. Muffled heart tones, jugular venous distention, and diminished breath sounds in the left chest are more likely indicative of a left-sided pneumothorax. Narrowed pulse pressure, hemoptysis, and absent breath sounds in the left chest are more likely indicative of a left-sided massive hemothorax. Hemoptysis, chest pain, and flat neck veins are more likely indicative of pulmonary contusion or hemothorax.

6. **Correct answer: A.** All of the answers are standards with Remodulin infusions except changing the infusion site due to redness. Redness of the subcutaneous infusion site is normal due to the vasodilatory effects of subcutaneous Remodulin. Sites should only be changed after weeks of successful therapy or signs of infection such as purulent drainage, fever, or increased white blood cell (WBC) count. Site pain needs to be controlled using various methods to increase adherence to therapy.

7. **Correct answer: A.** A volume-controlled ventilation mode is usually necessary as the initial mode of mechanical ventilation. High airway pressure is necessary to overcome the airway resistance of acute asthma. High peak airway pressures may be necessary but the plateau pressure can be maintained <28 cm H_2O (peak and plateau pressures can be directly monitored in this mode). Pressure-controlled ventilation can be used as asthma severity improves. Continuous positive airway pressure (CPAP) is a weaning mode. Mandatory minute ventilation (MMV) is appropriate for the operating room or postanesthesia settings.

8. **Correct answer: B.** Hepatitis B can be spread by injection drug use, which is a common way the virus is spread in the United States. Virus spreads via contact of an infected person's blood, semen, or other bodily fluids. Hepatitis B is usually left untreated until chronic condition at which time antiviral therapy may be initiated to reduce or minimize liver damage and other associated complications. Hepatitis A and E are transmitted through oral-fecal routes. Hepatitis D is only contracted when already infected with Hepatitis B.

9. **Correct answer: C.** Acetylcholine is a neurotransmitter that is essential for processing memory and learning. Thus medications such as Aricept are given to patients to increase acetylcholine levels within the body. Ketalar affects glutamate; Requip affects dopamine. Dextromethorphan affects N-methyl-d-aspartate (NMDA).

10. **Correct answer: A.** Throughout the literature, delirium, dementia, and gait instability/falls are listed consistently. Skin breakdown/pressure injury, urinary incontinence, frailty, and sleep problems are considered geriatric syndromes but vary among sources.

11. **Correct answer: A.** Nurse informaticists (NI) are experienced users of the nursing process, experts at using their analytical, critical thinking skills, and excellent project managers using technology and information systems. There is not a standard time period of clinical and/or informatics expertise required but rather a necessity for the skill set needed in the practice of NI. Nursing managers may be informed of ideal care processes using health information technology (HIT) solutions; however, the field of NI has a broader scope of expertise. NI experiences may include working with people who use information technology (IT) but should include more.

12. **Correct answer: B.** Justice is expounded upon within the *Belmont Report*; nonmaleficence, anonymity, and patient confidentiality are not central themes.

13. **Correct answer: C.** Patient's pain is severe and transdermal fentanyl can provide long-acting pain relief and there is the option for additional medication if needed. Extended release medications must not be crushed. Norco liquid is too short acting to work through the night. The Lidoderm patch is likely going to provide less relief than narcotics based on his current medication regime.

14. **Correct answer: C.** Intramuscular (IM) injection of epinephrine 0.2 to 0.5 mg 1:1,000 concentration is an appropriate dose for an awake, nonhypotensive patient. The dose concentration for IM epinephrine is 1:1,000 and for intravenous (IV) epinephrine is 1:10,000. Benadryl is an appropriate dose 25 to 50 mg IV but would not be a priority choice over administration of epinephrine first. Ensuring the correct concentration given in the correct route is vital when administering epinephrine for anaphylaxis.

15. **Correct answer: D.** Endomyocardial biopsy is the only way to definitively diagnose myocarditis. It provides the means to identify specific histotype of the myocarditis and assess the immunologic and virologic status of the myocardium and allows for individual tailored therapy The EKG will not provide direct information about myocarditis, but will note rhythm and electrical conduction irregularities. The echocardiogram provides information about structure and flow of the heart and valves. Cardiac MRI could provide insight about size and structure, perhaps indicating inflammation, but not definitively determine myocarditis

16. **Correct answer: C.** Oxygen therapy provides psychologic benefit to patients and their families as it can be associated with a form of treatment/medication, thus aiding the family in comfort. Correction of hypoxia has not been found to correlate with degree of symptomatic benefit; it does not improve oxygen saturation that affects the respiratory center, and pulse oximetry is not required to initiate.

17. **Correct answer: D.** Infliximab is an immunosuppressive drug. Regardless of their individual classes and mechanism of action, all drugs used for immunosuppression therapy target T-lymphocyte activity; therefore, all patients on immunosuppressive therapy are at increased risk of infection. The other choices are not associated with Infliximab.

18. **Correct answer: A.** Aging is the single biggest risk factor for developing cancer, according to the National Cancer Institute. Genetic mutations and exposure to chemotherapy are risks that are less common.

19. **Correct answer: D.** Many medications ordered for multiple sclerosis will alter immune reactions; thus a new onset of shingles (herpes) can be life threatening to a patient. Appetite alteration and injection site reactions are expected side effects of medication. Numbness and tingling can be a symptom of multiple sclerosis.

20. **Correct answer: D.** Trigger point injections involve the use of a local anesthetic to reduce pain at specific pinpointed locations. The fascia iliaca block, facet joint injection, and caudal injection would not alleviate pain specific to the right upper back.

21. **Correct answer: D.** Whether developing programs, evaluating current programs, or analyzing ways to reduce expenses, CNSs always are respectful stewards of resources.

22. **Correct answer: B.** The Dietary Approaches to Stop Hypertension (DASH) diet is a healthy way of eating and helps to decrease blood pressure (BP) through limiting salt intake and focusing on intake of fruits and vegetables. Walking for 30 minutes 3 to 5 times per week is recommended rather than 1 to 2 times per week; increasing physical activity both increases cardiac health and may have the added benefit of weight reduction. It is recommended that alcohol consumption be limited to 1 to 2 drinks per day as it may increase BP. The patient does not smoke.

23. **Correct answer: B.** The dosage of 0.3 to 0.6 mg sublingual is the standard dose and proper route of administration for symptoms of angina pectoris. The remaining doses and PO route of administration are not appropriate for this chest pain scenario.

24. **Correct answer: D.** The patient has a history of nonalocoholic steatohepatitis (NASH) cirrhosis and ascites. Hepatic hydrothorax symptoms are similar to those of acute respiratory distress. Undiagnosed chronic obstructive pulmonary disease (COPD) and pancreatitis are not supported by the information provided in this scenario. Viral respiratory infection occurred 3 months prior to the onset of these symptoms. Symptoms are not typical of pancreatitis

25. **Correct answer: A.** To help with prevention of surgical site infections. Chlorhexidine gluconate (CHG) is routinely used for skin preparation prior to surgery and specifically for open heart surgery and joint surgeries, to reduce potential skin infections at the surgical site post operatively. While hygiene and prevention of UTIs are also important, the CHG bath presurgery is specific to cleansing the skin overall.

26. **Correct answer: C.** The hallmark of delirium is a rapidly fluctuating level of consciousness (LOC), mood, and behavior; it tends to fluctuate in severity throughout the day and can be precipitated by dehydration and metabolic and electrolyte disturbances. Treatment should focus on identifying and managing causes. Determine etiology for delirium and treat accordingly. Pharmacologic treatment (especially in older adults) should only be considered after nonpharmacologic measures have failed or if the patient is a threat to their own safety or the safety of others.

27. **Correct answer: C.** The presence of the parents is the intervention in this PICO(T) scenario. Parents are not part of the PICO(T). Anxiety rates are the outcome. Not having the parents available is the comparison.

28. **Correct answer: C.** Health inequities can be determined by accessibility to healthcare. Vulnerable populations, such as older people, encounter difficulties that may prevent them from seeking healthcare. The other options are not indicative of health inequity. Refusing healthcare for religious reasons is not a health inequity; rather, it is a patient right. The clinical nurse specialist (CNS) can educate the community on the pros and cons of immunizations, but ultimately it is their right to refuse. The college student accepts the requirements of the college when they decide to apply to the college; therefore, it is not a health inequity. A flu pandemic is affecting the world population; there is no indication the local population is outside of what is being seen elsewhere.

29. **Correct answer: B.** Celiac plexus block. A celiac plexus block uses a local anesthetic to block pain signals in the abdomen from traveling to the brain. Paravertebral nerve blocks and steroid injections would not address the abdominal pain described. Antiemetics are used to treat nausea and vomiting rather than pain.

30. **Correct answer: D.** Patient is to avoid foods that are high in vitamin K (green leafy vegetables, that is, broccoli, kale, lettuce, spinach, etc.) as the high amounts of vitamin K can decrease Coumadin effects. Tomatoes, lima beans, and sweet potatoes are not high in vitamin K.

31. **Correct answer: D.** Osmotic diarrhea is usually self-limiting, lasting only a few days and generally responds well to loperamide. Increasing fiber, taking multivitamins, and avoiding foods with sugar are not supportive of osmotic diarrhea.

32. **Correct answer: C.** Decreasing fluid intake causes concentrated urine and places the patient at higher risk for infection and constipation. Slowly tapering medication doses, monitoring the blood urea nitrogen (BUN)/creatinine and kidney function, and monitoring for orthostatic hypertension due to dehydration are all appropriate.

33. **Correct answer: C.** Levothyroxine is synthetic T4 and is used to treat hypothyroidism. T4 lowers thyroid-stimulating hormone (TSH) levels by normalizing T4, thereby controlling the feedback loop and reducing secretion of thyroid-releasing hormone (TRH) and TSH. Methimazole is an anti-thyroid medication commonly used to treat hyperthyroidism. Propanolol is a beta blocker. Beta blockers are commonly prescribed to reduce signs of adrenergic stimulation such as tachycardia and tremors. Radioactive iodine therapy is used as a treatment for hyperthyroidism by causing thyroid cell destruction.

34. **Correct answer: C.** The most common reason for upper GI bleeding in patients with alcoholic liver cirrhosis is due to acute and active bleeding from esophageal varices that can be life threatening. Acute variceal rupture placed the patient at risk for aspiration. Endotracheal intubation will protect the airway. Monitoring BP and administering vitamin K will not protect the airway. Balloon tamponade device is utilized when bleeding cannot be controlled. Use of balloon tamponade requires the patient to have endotracheal tube. Balloon tamponade would be indicated if bleeding cannot be controlled by other measures or as a bridge to interventional measures such as esophagogastroduodenoscopy (EGD) or transjugular intrahepatic portosystemic shunt (TIPS). INR values are unknown. Vitamin K may be required if the INR is elevated. Arterial line placement may be needed if there is concern about BP accuracy via noninvasive measures, but this is not a critical initial measure

35. **Correct answer: C.** Right-middle cerebral artery is the correct answer as right hemispheric syndrome has a characteristic presentation. The other locations do not contribute to a characteristic clinical picture but present with symptoms specific to the location of the stroke or the vessel involved.

36. **Correct answer: A.** Key symptoms associated with cardiovascular system disorders include dizziness, syncope, orthopnea, angina, edema, and claudication. Dizziness accompanied by symptoms of orthopnea and edema in this patient scenario points to dizziness associated with a cardiovascular system problem. The focused assessment should therefore *begin* with the cardiovascular system. Subsequent assessment focus would include the respiratory system and neurologic system. The reproductive system is not pertinent to this patient scenario.

37. **Correct answer: D.** Atrial flutter and supraventricular tachycardia are also common rhythms that synchronized cardioversion could be utilized with the goal of returning the patient's rhythm back to their normal rhythm. Treatment for third degree heart block is a pacemaker placement. Asystole is a nonshockable rhythm. Treatment for wide complex ventricular tachycardia would be determined based upon patient assessment in addition to the rhythm and may include medications, electrolyte replacement, and supportive measures.

38. **Correct answer: D.** The patient's history of diabetes and dehydrated state support interventions for glycemic control and fluid–electrolyte balance. Hypotension is a risk factor for organ failure calling for close monitoring and prevention measures. Seizure precautions are not appropriate for this patient.

39. **Correct answer: B.** pH, 7.46; PCO_2, 22; HCO_3, 16. The leading diagnosis would be aspirin overdose, and most likely ASA chronic toxicity due to his history of arthritis and chronic ASA use as well as additional salicylates with Pepto-Bismol. He is symptomatic and although we did not state all of his lab findings, one can assume he shows respiratory alkalosis with his increased respiratory rate leading to a low pCO_2 and a metabolic acidosis with decreased bicarbonate. The pH is alkalotic, indicating respiratory compensation for a metabolic acidosis. If there was respiratory compensation, the pH would be low, as in option **D** this blood gas shows a primary metabolic acidosis with respiratory alkalosis as seen in diabetic ketoacidosis (DKA) or sepsis. Primary respiratory acidosis with bicarbonate retention is a sign that there is renal compensation; this is normally seen with patients with COPD and would have a blood gas as seen in option **C.**

40. **Correct answer: A.** The stress response begins in the amygdala, an area of the brain that contributes to emotional processing. The amygdala interprets sounds and images; when danger is perceived a distress signal is sent to the hypothalamus. The hypothalamus communicates the stress to the rest of the body through the autonomic nervous system. The fight-or-flight response is triggered and the body responds with a burst of energy to prepare to respond to the danger. The thalamus translates and relays neural impulses to the cerebral cortex.

41. **Correct answer: B.** Needle decompression is the appropriate initial treatment for tension pneumothorax followed by chest tube insertion. Needle aspiration is the treatment for symptomatic primary spontaneous pneumothorax. VATS is the treatment for recurrent pneumothorax.

42. **Correct answer: D.** Hypocalcemia occurs in up to 30% of cases when calcium binds to areas of fat necrosis around the pancreas. Positive Trousseau's sign (flexion of the wrist, hyperextension of the fingers, and flexion of the thumb after

inflating a BP cuff above the systolic BP) is a symptom of hypocalcemia. The remaining blood glucose and electrolyte imbalances are not associated with pancreatitis or the symptoms described in this case.

43. **Correct answer: B.** Signs and symptoms of heart failure include fatigue, weakness, and dyspnea. Patients with left sided-heart failure have poor ventricular function produces pulmonary congestion; patients will present with dyspnea due to the fluid backing up into the pulmonary system. Fluid volume deficit is not a clinical finding of congestive heart failure (CHF). Dyspnea or need for oxygen is not a key finding without other evidence of fluid overload, weight gain, fatigue, or activity intolerance.

44. **Correct answer: A.** Bile acid sequestrants can bind and decrease absorption of other drugs including warfarin. Due to this absorption, bile acid sequestrants should be taken 1 hour before or 4 to 6 hours after other medications. Grape juice does not interact with bile acid sequestrants or warfarin. Bile acid sequestrants reduce the absorption of vitamins A, D, and E. Limiting the intake of these vitamins would be contraindicated.

45. **Correct answer: D.** The low TSH and elevated T3 and T4 levels are consistent with hyperthyroidism. The protrusion of the eyes or exophthalmos is a hallmark sign of Grave's disease. The TSH level is low and not elevated, as seen with primary hypothyroidism. In addition, the T3 and T4 levels are elevated and would be low with primary hypothyroidism. The physical exam states a slight enlarged thyroid without nodules. With multinodular goiter (MNG), the thyroid is generally grossly enlarged with palpable nodules. The physical exam also lists exophthalmos, which is generally seen with Grave's disease. Myxedema coma is due to hypothyroidism. The labs demonstrate hyperthyroidism.

46. **Correct answer: C.** The Mann-Whitney *U* test is the nonparametric equivalent to the *t* test. Each of the other named tests are nonparametric tests, but none are correlates to the *t* test.

47. **Correct answer: A.** The Native American population is a large conglomeration of many different peoples, cultures, and ethnicities. That have become accustomed in many ways to being grouped together; however, they prefer to have their identity maintained. Modesty is typically very important to consider in all situations. Travel is often an issue that prevents access to specialized high-quality healthcare. Diabetes and alcoholism both have higher prevalence rates and should be considered but very few ethnic groups will all develop say diabetes; for example, the Pima Tribe may all develop some form of diabetes in their lifetime. Traditional healers, medicine men, shaman are all utilized still; however, the use may be mixed and combined in ways that are not traditional to one specific native ethnicity.

48. **Correct answer: C.** Obtaining additional support through home care visits will meet the patient's immediate need for assistance to perform dressing changes. Regular home visits allow for ongoing reinforcement of the care plan and improved adherence. A patient with a history of nonadherence, low-literacy, and a lack of resources may verbalize understanding of the plan of care but their actions are not demonstrating adherence; therefore, giving written instructions or having them verbalize a plan is not likely to produce changes.

49. **Correct answer: A.** End tidal CO_2 monitoring measures breath-to-breath ventilation and provides an accurate respiratory rate. The POSS tool can detect drowsiness that is present with opioid-induced sedation. Oxygen saturation and respiratory rate monitoring are important but end tidal CO_2 and POSS are more appropriate. Asking a family member is not appropriate in this case.

50. **Correct answer: C.** The husband could benefit from home services. Elder abuse and a need for hospice or long-term care are not indicated.

51. **Correct answer: A.** Healthcare disparities occur in the context of inequality and are linked to discrimination. Improving the cultural and communication competence of the staff can decrease healthcare disparities. While obtaining low-cost medications, improving public transportation, and updating supplies and equipment are important interventions for improving health outcomes, they do not address healthcare disparities.

52. **Correct answer: D.** Without support until the change is hardwired, it is likely that backsliding to the former state will occur. The successful CNS change agent recognizes the need to support and help staff stick with the new practice until the desired change has replaced the old way of doing things. Encouraging opposition, asking to come to a complete consensus, and including naysayers create issues with facilitating change or acting as a change agent.

53. **Correct answer: A.** Hand tremors, increased thirst and urination, diarrhea, vomiting, poor concentration, and drowsiness are all side effects of lithium. Lithium is used frequently to treat bipolar depression and is sensitive to hydration status. The symptoms listed are not associated with Depakote, Sertraline, and Carbamazepine.

54. **Correct answer: C.** The Malnutrition Screening Tool (MST) and Malnutrition Universal Screening Tool (MUST) are screening tools that are valid and reliable. Screening tools are suggested for all hospitalized patients to help further identify those at risk since it is not feasible for nutrition providers to do a thorough nutrition assessment on every patient. The Braden Scale is a skin assessment tool. The body mass index (BMI) is an indicator of body fat in children and adults but does not directly measure body fat. It is more often used to track patients who are overweight or at risk, over time. The Confusion Assessment Method (CAM) is used to evaluate confusion or altered mental status, often with patients on sedation or intubated.

55. **Correct answer: B.** Noninvasive positive airway pressure ventilation (NIPPV) can be an option for a hypercapnic DNI status patient to remove the excessive CO_2. The conversation with patient and family can be difficult and complex due to the multiple modalities available. A clear and concise decision is the goal in addressing advanced directive and clinical need to remove the excess CO_2. An endotracheal tube would be invasive. A nasal cannula would not support the needs of a hypercapnic patient. And there are options to support the patient.

56. **Correct answer: B.** After a myocardial infarction, healing takes place in a graduated fashion. Within 10 to 14 days, a collagen matrix is deposited as the beginning of a scar that is initially weak, mushy, and vulnerable to reinjury. It is during this time period, as the patient feels better and increases activity, that the scar is most susceptible to injury from

increasing stress. Therefore, any of the other time frame options are not correct.

57. **Correct answer: D.** Right heart catheterization (RHC) is the gold standard for pulmonary arterial hypertension (PAH) definitive diagnosis. Hemodynamic values mPAP >25, pulmonary vascular resistance (PVR) >3 Wood Units, and a pulmonary artery wedge pressure less than 15 mmHg confirm the diagnosis of PAH. Echocardiogram, pulmonary function test, CT, MRI, and sleep study are used to screen for PAH causes and structural abnormalities.

58. **Correct answer: C.** Patients on Depakote (Divalproex) may experience thrombocytopenia, mild in the sense of nose bleeds to severe coagulopathy. Depakote (Divalproex) is often prescribed for headache treatment; dyspepsia is not life altering, and the medication does not alter blood glucose.

59. **Correct answer: D.** During renal failure, the kidneys can fail to waste enough acid from the body, leading to metabolic acidosis. The other options occur in metabolic alkalosis rather than metabolic acidosis.

60. **Correct answer: D.** Decreased muscle mass is the most concerning as this will put the patient at a greater risk of falls and can lead to severe injuries. Decreased gastrointestinal (GI) motility is an age-related finding, but can be easily treated. Loss of epidermal elasticity is also an age-related change, but not as concerning. Age-related changes include a decrease in cognitive functioning, not improved.

61. **Correct answer: B.** The Centers for Disease Control and Prevention (CDC) sets the recommendations for vaccination schedules for adults, as well as for children and adolescence.

62. **Correct answer: C.** Learning team communication skills can improve the opportunity to resolve moral and ethical issues as they arise. Authentic leadership, which includes transparency, encouraging participation in key decision-making, engaging in mentorship, being enthusiastic, and adhering to standards, encourages a healthy work environment and generally lacks authoritarian-style leadership characteristics. Creating clear steps and processes so that the same care is implemented for each patient does not allow for effective decision-making or personalized, individualized patient care. Review of the policy and procedure manual is important for quality nursing care but does not address the moral complexities of caring for patients with acute stroke.

63. **Correct answer: A.** PICO(T) questions include population, intervention, comparison, and outcome along with time frame, if applicable.

64. **Correct answer: C.** High levels of aldosterone from the compensating renal angiotensin aldosterone system increases sodium reabsorption. Increased sodium reabsorption causes free water retention from reduced serum osmolality. This results in hyper or hypotonic hyponatremia.

65. **Correct answer: B.** Spontaeous bacterial peritonitis (SBP) is the result of translocated gut bacteria. In SPB, translocation is into the peritoneal cavity through the mesenteric lymph system. Ascites is fluid accumulation occurring from a cirrhotic liver. Not all individuals with ascites develop infection. Infected ascites fluid that leaks into the pleural space causes hepatic hydrothorax. Hepatic hydrothorax occurs individuals with portal hypertension. Sepsis, narcotics, and anesthesia, as well GI issues may impact bowel motility.

66. **Correct answer: D.** High amounts of protein can block levodopa absorption, in the gut as well as in the blood–brain barrier.

67. **Correct answer: B.** Second-generation antipsychotics have a risk of weight gain, increased BMI, and abnormal lipids. The other values do not require monitoring.

68. **Correct answer: C. Lactate, heart rate, and respiratory rate.** While she does meet 2/4 systemic inflammatory response system (SIRS) criteria based upon her increased heart rate (HR) and respiratory rate (RR), the potential infection (urinary tract infection [UTI]) and elevated lactate put her in the sepsis bucket. She is maintaining her BP and does not have further signs of organ failure, so she is not in shock or multiple organ dysfunction syndrome (MODS) yet.

69. **Correct answer: B.** The Roy Adaptation Model sees the person in continuous interaction with a changing environment. The environment includes focal, contextual, and residual stimuli. Facial, chemoreceptor, sensory, and emotional are not environmental stimuli described in Roy's adaptation model.

70. **Correct answer: A.** Elevating her leg will help reduce swelling and pain, as well as allow for examination. Resting her ankle the next few days and occupational therapy may be appropriate longer-term interventions. Ice is contraindicated for individuals who have decreased sensation.

71. **Correct answer: A.** The pleasure and reward center in the brain is stimulated in early drug use. Continued long-term use of drugs reduces the number of dopamine receptors in the brain called anhedonia. Regular drug use actually causes the brain to produce, absorb, and transmit less dopamine, resulting in a chemical imbalance. The signs and symptoms (s/s) of dopamine deficiency include muscle cramps, muscle stiffness, impulsiveness, and low energy. Hypoglycemia s/s are visual disturbances, confusion, shakiness, and sweating, Hyponatremia s/s are muscle weakness, headache, and nausea and vomiting. Hypothyroidism s/s include constipation, weight gain, fatigue, and increased sensitivity to cold.

72. **Correct answer: D.** Nondihydropyridine calcium channel blockers have the potential to slow the heart rate too much and should be avoided for patients with congestive heart failure. Based on the patient's age and symptoms, she presents with left congestive heart failure. Beta blockers, ace inhibitors, and dihydropyridine calcium channel blockers may be used to treat hypertension.

73. **Correct answer: C.** For severe hypoglycemia, IV treatment is the preferred option, even though the patient is asymptomatic (recall that beta blockers can mask the adrenergic symptoms of hypoglycemia). Administering a balanced snack may actually extend the time that the patient is severely hypoglycemic, as the protein and fat will delay absorption of carbohydrates through the GI tract.

74. **Correct answer: D.** Escharotomy is often necessary with circumferential burns to relieve pressure and avoid compartment syndrome from the response of the injured cells. Although fasciotomy also can relieve pressure to avoid compartment syndrome, it is often done related to damage to muscle or other tissue from a crush injury, where the escharotomy is specific to treat burns. The term *eschar* means

the leathery tissue after a full thickness burn. Surgical debridement and physical therapy will likely be future treatments to decrease scarring and increase mobility of the area.

75. **Correct answer: A.** Patients can still maintain activity levels while diagnosed and while taking medications. So the timing of medication administration can allow for patient's usual activity. Adding another medication is not optimal when med administration timing can work and decreasing interferon dosages will not be optimal for patients.

76. **Correct answer: A.** One correct premedication regimen for a planned, nonemergent procedure requiring radiographic contrast media (RCM) is Prednisone 50 mg PO 13 hours, 7 hours, and 1 hour prior to the CT and diphenhydramine 50 mg PO 1 hour prior to the CT. Both methylprednisolone sodium succinate/diphenhydramine and dexamethasone sodium sulfate/diphenhydramine are accelerated premedication regimens that are typically used for emergent, nonroutine procedures. Diphenhydramine without a steroid in addition would not be appropriate.

77. **Correct answer: B.** Recent guidelines recommend starting with circulation.

78. **Correct answer: C.** Gum chewing stimulates gut motility. Nasogastric (NG) insertion, NPO status, and administration of narcotics can decrease gut stimulation.

79. **Correct answer: C.** Early antimicrobial therapy is a critical consideration because necrotizing soft tissue infections (NSTI) are rapidly progressing and frequently caused by poly-microbial organisms including gram-positive, gram-negative, and anaerobic bacteria. Initiation of early, empiric, broad-spectrum antibiotics should not be delayed for organism identification or debridement.

80. **Correct answer: B.** Both Citalopram and Escitalopram have a risk for a prolonged QT. Sertraline, Fluoxetine, and Paroxetine do not have this as side effect.

81. **Correct answer: C.** Serum prealbumin responds to catabolism or inflammation and rises when resolved. Half-life is the shortest 2 to 3 days. Serum albumin has longer-term evaluation of protein intake. Serum transferrin and Hgb relate to hematology rather than protein or nutritional intake.

82. **Correct answer: D.** To address the system concern, the CNS must first understand the current state to identify opportunities and gaps in practice. Once data trends are analyzed, meeting with stakeholders and standardizing practice through policy utilizing current guidelines would address systematic concerns. Just-in-time education may be provided for any need and would not address the system issue.

83. **Correct answer: B.** Performing a cost–benefit analysis (CBA) helps CNSs identify all direct and indirect costs of developing an intervention that will result in a positive outcome and focus on costs associated with intervention implementation and return on investment rather than broader "government funding." Cost–benefit analysis is an applied economic mechanism that assesses outcomes in terms of using money to improve societal welfare, such as through CNS-developed programs.

84. **Correct answer: A.** Pulmonary capillary bed obstruction can cause increased RV afterload, dilation of the RV, and cor pulmonale. The left ventricle is not affected. PE is associated with pulmonary hypertension. High V/Q ratio is associated with PE.

85. **Correct answer: D.** Frequent gentle oral care with a soft, disposable mouth swab is appropriate. Ensuring NPO, alcohol-based mouth rinses, and monoclonal antibody are not supportive of mucositis.

86. **Correct answer: C.** Swollen, hot joints suggest septic arthritis, gout, or pseudogout, not OA. Pain is a characteristic of OA. On x-ray there is evidence of loss of cartilage in the joint. Joint deformity can be seen on physical exam as well as on x-ray.

87. **Correct answer: A.** Complete blood count (CBC) is correct. The left shoulder pain associated with abdominal trauma (Kehr's sign) along with left upper quadrant pain and tenderness is hallmark of splenic injury. To evaluate for a splenic injury, there would be associated decreased Hgb and Hct. LFTs would only be affected with liver injury or dysfunction. Liver injury would also have symptoms of pain and tenderness to right upper quadrant and right shoulder pain. Pancreatic injury would present with epigastric pain radiating to the back. Small bowel injury would have diffuse abdominal pain and possibly referred shoulder pain. Coagulation times would not be affected from splenic injury unless the patient injury was progressive leading to disseminated intravascular coagulation (DIC). Chemistry panel would be included in basic evaluation but meant to identify altered electrolytes, but not specific to recent splenic injury.

88. **Correct answer: B.** These vaccinations are not recommended for immunocompromised patients or pregnant patients. MMR and ZVL are live vaccines.

89. **Correct answer: B.** Utilize protective UV blocking clothing and sunblock to reduce risk of skin cancers from prolonged sun exposure. Prolonged exposure increases risk of skin cancer. It is ill advised to discourage someone from exercising or to advise they reduce exercise if they are clearly able to do so. Fall risk does not relate to cancer risk.

90. **Correct answer: D.** A systematic review of randomized controlled trials (RCTs) is stronger than any individual study alone; a guideline is not research evidence.

91. **Correct answer: C.** There is no requirement to disclose to participants details about the volume of data to be collected, but they should be informed about the types of data to be collected. Participants should be assured that privacy will be protected at all times. They must be informed about potential benefits to themselves or others. Prospective participants must also be informed about which healthcare activities are routine versus which are treatments specifically for the study.

92. **Correct answer: D.** The patient with history of alcohol abuse presenting with tautly distended abdomen is consistent with the clinical picture of alcoholic cirrhosis and ascites. Abdominal assessment findings consistent with cirrhotic ascites include fluid wave and shifting dullness. Liver percussion elicits a dull rather than flat sound. Bladder and spleen assessment is not pertinent to this scenario.

93. **Correct answer: B.** Restlessness, muscle/bone pain, insomnia, diarrhea, vomiting, cold flashes/goose bumps, and leg movements are consistent with signs of opioid withdrawal.

These are not the symptoms of benzodiazepine, sedative, or depressant withdrawl.

94. **Correct answer: B.** Objective signs that goals of treatment are reached include the following: patient obtaining FC I or II, 6-minute walk distance (6MWD) of greater than 380 to 440 meters, cardiopulmonary exercise test measured peak oxygen consumption greater than 15 mL/min/kg; ventilatory equivalent for carbon dioxide less than 45 L/min/L/min, BNP level toward normal, transthoracic echocardiogram (TTE) and/or cardiac magnetic imaging (MRI) demonstrating normal/near normal right ventricular (RV) size and function, hemodynamics showing normalization of RV function with right atrial (RA) pressure less than 8 mmHg, and cardiac index greater than 2.5 to 3 L/min/m². Syncope and reported exercise tolerance are subjective findings. Right atrial pressure (RAP) 20 mmHg and mean pulmonary artery pressure (PAP) 35 are high and reflect poor response to treatment. Prevention of central line-associated bloodstream infection (CLABSI) is a goal of perfect care not assessment of the effects of Veletri.

95. **Correct answer: D.** Thirty minutes before the transfusion for maximum impact and to allow the medication to work prior to transfusion. The other times frames don't allow for enough time.

96. **Correct answer: C.** Stage 1 wounds have intact skin; the goal is to prevent further progression. Relieving pressure is the best strategy for this goal. The other options will cause the area to worsen and impede healing.

97. **Correct answer: B.** Lactic acid demonstrates a degree of anaerobic metabolism and therefore is important in assessing degree of traumatic shock. Hemoglobin may indicate blood loss, but it does not immediately show acute hemorrhage and will not identify the patient in traumatic shock states. Partial prothrombin time does not determine degree of shock. Although anion gap can be useful in determining metabolic acidosis, it is not an early indicator of traumatic shock states.

98. **Correct answer: D.** One of the common side effects of benzodiazepines in older adults is delirium. High BP, insomnia, and diabetes are not side effects of benzodiazepines.

99. **Correct answer: D.** These vaccinations are recommended for all adults. HepA and HepB are only recommended for adults with risk factors. Human papillomavirus (HPV) vaccination is recommended as early as age 11 into adulthood but is minimally effective over age 26 and is not recommended over age 45.

100. **Correct answer: B.** Telehealth describes all remote health-related services, including nonclinical and administrative services. Telehealth and telemedicine both utilize HIT, health-related IT. All clinicians may utilize telemedicine as an HIT delivery method.

101. **Correct answer: A.** Niacin cannot be crushed, chewed, or broken due to the symptom of extreme flushing so it should not be given via G tube. Acetylsalicylic acid (ASA), Lipitor, and warfarin can be crushed and given via gtube.

102. **Correct answer: B.** Low and indicative of chronic pancreatitis. Normal fecal elastase level is above 200; high fecal elastase is above 500. Fecal elastase is not used to determine hepatitis.

103. **Correct answer: A.** First, assess basal insulin (insulin glargine) effectiveness. In this case, the patient has an elevated fasting blood glucose as well as high-normal to elevated post-prandial glucoses. This would suggest the patient does not have enough basal insulin. Adjusting prandial insulin will not have any effect on the fasting blood glucose. Correctional scale insulin would only be adjusted if the patient had a change in insulin sensitivity.

104. **Correct answer: A.** Hypotension is not a risk factor; hypertension is. Male aged 50 years or more, smoking, and sedentary lifestyle are all listed as risk factors associated with coronary heart disease in the Framingham Heart Study. Other risk factors determined by the study include age greater than 60 for women; obesity, family history of premature congenital heart disease (CHD); diabetes; and abnormal lipid levels.

105. **Correct answer: C.** Intravenous fluids. The patient is suffering from cardiac tamponade. Cardiac tamponade is a compression of the heart because of fluid accumulation in the pericardial sac. This fluid in the pericardia sac can cause enough pressure to prevent the atria and ventricles from filling completely during diastole. This results in decrease cardiac output (CO), stroke volume (SV), and hypotension. The body compensates with tachycardia. Eventually, the compensatory mechanisms fail, and hemodynamic instability ensues. Overall management of cardiac tamponade focuses on relieving pressure on the heart and improving CO. Treat as follows:
- Maintain airway
- Volume resuscitation to increase preload
- *Avoid* medication that decreases systemic vascular resistance (SVR) or preload (vasodilators)
- Severe hemodynamic compromise will require decompression with pericardiocentesis, but it is not the first or initial priority intervention

An angiogram evaluates blood flow throughout the cardiac vessels but is not indicated as a treatment for fluid accumulation in the pericardial sac. Beta blockers are intended to reduce BP, so this would not be an appropriate treatment when the patient is likely hypotensive.

106. **Correct answer: D.** Initially s/s of hypoglycemia are mediated by epinephrine and norepinephrine release. Beta adrenergic antagonists block the release of these and thus blunt early s/s of hypoglycemia. Metoprolol is the only beta adrenergic antagonist in this list.

107. **Correct answer: C.** Cyclosporin is an effective immunosuppressive agent used for renal transplants. The neurotoxic effects of calcineurin inhibitor drugs (CNIs), the drug class that includes cyclosporine, include symptoms ranging from headache to seizure with a reported incidence as high as 28%. Lowering the dose may decrease or reverse these symptoms. Bradycardia and weight gain are not side effects of cyclosporine. There is no interaction noted with acetaminophen and cyclosporine. However, due to the immunosuppressive effects of cyclosporine any flu-like symptoms should be reported to the provider.

108. **Correct answer: C.** Acetylcysteine (Mucomyst) is the standard of care treatment intervention for Tylenol poisoning, with dosage dependent on presentation and timeline of patient symptoms. The other medications listed are not related to treatment of Tylenol poisoning.

109. **Correct answer: A.** Ongoing neurologic assessments do include frequent neurologic assessments (more often than once per shift) as well as management of the intracranial pressure (ICP) equipment. Patients requiring ICP monitoring are at great risk for neurologic decline, and as this monitoring is invasive, infection is a great risk. The monitoring system has many moveable parts and can provide erroneous readings if there is not an intact system. If the patient is not positioned correctly when readings are taken, then the data will be elevated or less than accurate. Monitoring lab values, trends, and musculoskeletal assessment may be included, but these are not priority areas for assessment. The patient will be on bed rest with ICP monitoring.

110. **Correct answer: B.** Topiramate can cause visual changes such as myopia and secondary angle glaucoma warranting immediate physician care and discontinuation of medication. Tinnitus, blood glucose reading change, and frequent stools and abdominal pain are not side effects of topiramate.

111. **Correct answer: A.** The patient likely has rhabdomyolysis due to increased exertion and lack of training. The priority is aggressive fluid rehydration to prevent acute kidney injury (AKI). Oral rehydration could help but would provide an sufficient volume over time. The fluids will also reduce the patient's temperature, whereas cooling measures could help but will not address fluid loss. Pain medication may not be needed.

112. **Correct answer: A.** Objective data are collected during the examiner's physical assessment based on findings from inspection, palpation, percussion, and auscultation of each body system. These findings are then recorded by body system. The problem list is derived in part from the objective data findings in the physical examination. Physical assessment objective findings are a separate from the health history.

113. **Correct answer: A.** Pronation decompresses the weight of the abdomen thereby reducing the strain the lungs have to overcome to ventilate. Pronation is an appropriate treatment for a patient with ARDS but not the only option. Pronation is not appropriate for a patient with asthma. It is highly suggested to have an advanced airway secured before proning a patient.

114. **Correct answer: D.** Patient *symptomatic* with an elevated polymorphonuclear (PMN) count greater than 250 cell/mm^3 is indicative of spontaneous bacterial peritonitis (SBP). Symptoms include hepatic encephalopathy and fever. Additional contributing factors for SBP include nosocomial settings: recent hospitalization and discharge with 3 days stay in an extended care facility. A 7- to 10-day course of IV Cefoxitin is the treatment of choice; however, alternative therapy with Ciprofloxacin (2 days IV followed by 5 days oral) or 7 to 10 days of Piperacillin-Tazo in antibiotic-resistant individuals is also done. Do not delay treatment in symptomatic patients once cultures are obtained. Treatment delay is indicated only in asymptomatic individuals. Antipyretics such as nonsteroidal anti-inflammatory drugs (NSAIDs) should be used cautiously as these can cause further liver injury. Treatment course is 7 to 10 days, not 30 days.

115. **Correct answer: C.** The patient presentation is typical of gout. Allopurinol is a xanthine oxidase inhibitor that works by reducing the production of uric acid in the body. A low purine diet limits foods high in purine (meats, beer, grain liquors, seafood, fructose), which break down into uric acid when consumed. Oxycodone is not effective for gout pain. High-protein diet foods may exacerbate the gout flare. Topical ice packs may provide relief of gout discomfort.

116. **Correct answer: B.** A physician must certify that the patient has 6 months or less to live in order to qualify for hospice.

117. **Correct answer: C.** The two screening tools with the highest sensitivity (>83%) and specificity (>90%) were the Mini Nutritional Assessment (short form; MNA [SF]) and the Malnutrition Screening Tool (MST) as compared to the MNF, MUST, and SCREEN II tools.

118. **Correct answer: D.** It is important to remember that the patient's hemodynamic values are only a portion of the information needed to provide quality care. Assess the patient. Reassess. For a healthy athletic patient, it is possible this is the patient's normal trends at rest. Digoxin would potentially slow the heart rate. While the vital signs should be reassessed, the nurse is asking for the evaluation of the CNS. The rapid response team should only be contacted if the patient is in distress, so it is important to assess the patient first.

119. **Correct answer: A.** Hypotension is a side effect that is caused by most medications in the antiarrhythmic class. The other choices do not fit the listed symptoms.

120. **Correct answer: B.** The pituitary gland releases TSH. The hypothalamus secretes TRH. The thyroid gland releases T3 and T4. The adrenal gland releases mineralocorticoids, glucocorticoids, and adrenal androgens.

121. **Correct answer: A.** One of the signs of caregiver burden or stress is denying oneself pleasures. While the daughter reports missing church, it may not be therapeutic to question her faith as she may have only been physically unable to go to church due to feeling the demands to support her mother on Sundays. While offering church services that may be available at the hospital or support from the case manager are possible approaches for assistance, it is important to assess for caregiver role strain first, identifying what the daughter perceives she needs for support.

122. **Correct answer: D.** Legislators are busy people and they prioritize according to need and their constituents' priorities. Therefore, getting data, knowing stakeholders, and having a solid strategy and proposal are important and will provide the policy maker with the best background data to make a case. Follow-up and recommendations are important for program success and sustainability. Reporting the issue to the attorney general and asking for an investigation is incorrect because no strategy is in place and the attorney general would not be the appropriate resource. Although the U.S. Department of Health and Human Services (HHS) will have some information on programs and funding, it would be more appropriate to look at state and county data and programs to get information more relevant to the community. Although funding through raising taxes may help to support this project, it would not be the first action taken.

123. **Correct answer: C.** HIT is the use of IT for the receipt, delivery, and utilization of health information in electronic systems. HIT is related to the use of technology in health-related aspects and while HIT may describe the use

of IT in healthcare, IT more globally describes those functionalities available for HIT. HIT may be used by any entity, in any industry, for the delivery of health information using IT solutions.

124. **Correct answer: D.** Mood stabilizers or atypical antipsychotics plus antidepressants are commonly prescribed for patients with this disorder. There is no additional benefit from antipsychotic medications to decrease the effects of bipolar disorder, except for quetiapine (Seroquel). Bupropion, gabapentin, and nefazodone have been found ineffective in treating bipolar disorder. Ambien is not indicated. Cognitive-behavioral therapy and group therapy have also been found to be helpful for cooccurring bipolar disorder.

125. **Correct answer: A.** There is a clear connection between cancer and DVT. Many chemotherapy drugs can increase clotting factors and some of the genetic mutations that cause cancer increase clotting factors. The other choices are not affected by cancer.

126. **Correct answer: B.** Patients who are at risk for having arrhythmias that could lead to sudden cardiac arrest and awaiting a physician to decide long-term goals, such as an implantable cardiac defibrillator, would benefit from the life vest. Patients on hospice care would not use a life vest as the code status would be do not resuscitate (DNR). A patient would be monitored during orthopedic surgery, so a life vest would not be appropriate. A life vest is not needed if an automatic internal cardiac defibrillator is already in place.

127. **Correct answer: D.** The CNS is an advocate for the patient to reduce the symptoms associated with COPD. As the COPD patient's disease progresses and is end-stage, the CNS may be the palliative care advanced provider or may advocate for symptom reduction. The CNS can use motivational interviewing skills to understand the patient's wishes. Pulmonary rehabilitation, looking at extended care placement, and placing a do-not-resuscitate (DNR) order may be done after consulting palliative care.

128. **Correct answer: C.** Weight loss, loss of muscle mass, localized or generalized fluid accumulation, and diminished physical function. Malnutrition may be diagnosed when any two of the six defined characteristics (insufficient energy intake; weight loss; loss of muscle mass; loss of subcutaneous fat; localized or generalized fluid accumulation that may sometimes mask weight loss; and diminished functional status as measured by hand grip strength) are assessed and identified.

129. **Correct answer: C.** The reversal of the medication is the foremost factor in decreasing hematoma size. More imaging is not warranted at this time to determine source of bleed. The patient should not receive an antiepileptic drug as the patient has not had a clinical seizure and this follows the latest intracranial hemorrhage (ICH) guideline. A swallow exam is important when the patient will be taking oral medications; the patient may be NPO presently in the case of possible surgery after the INR normalizes.

130. **Correct answer: B.** The presentation of symmetrical joint pain, gradual onset over months, generalized aches, longer-lasting morning pain (>1 hour) in a female of middle age points toward rheumatoid arthritis (RA). Ibuprofen and methotrexate are treatments for RA. The remaining treatments are for OA. Morning joint pain in OA is of shorter duration and typically involves only one side of the body.

131. **Correct answer: D.** Respiratory acidosis can be caused by asthma, neuromuscular disorders, and severe obesity. Hyperventilation occurs in respiratory alkalosis.

132. **Correct answer: C.** "I take multiple herbal medicines because I know they have safe side effects." This statement by the patient indicates that the CNS needs to provide education. There is also concern for polypharmacy and a lack of informed understanding of prescribed and supplemental medications this patient may be taking. The CNS should advise the patient that there are many herbal medications that have interactions with over-the-counter and prescription medications. The CNS should also emphasize that the patient should report all meds including herbal meds with their provider before starting or continuing any of their herbal medication. Also, the CNS should state that many herbal medications have adverse side effects. Responses A, B, and D indicate the patient has knowledge about management of medications and/or interactions when taking multiple different medications.

133. **Correct answer: B.** Creatinine kinase. The patient may have developed rhabdomyolysis if she was laying on the ground for a prolonged period. Rhabdomyolysis is most commonly diagnosed by an elevated creatinine kinase. The urine culture can take up to 3 days for results and provides information about what bacteria may cause the UTI; however, it is not a priority. The Hgb and Hct could determine if the patient is anemic but that does not address her symptoms or provide information about length of time on the floor. The troponin may give you feedback about heart function is but not related to her current symptoms and story.

134. **Correct answer: A.** It is more common with aging to spend less time in the deeper stages of sleep. More time is spent in REM sleep stages or awake leading to increased issues with insomnia for geriatric patients. Light, nondreaming states are longer rather than vivid states, and total sleep times are less.

135. **Correct answer: C.** Payment may be withheld for hospital-acquired conditions and nursing sensitive indicators, since they overlap as in catheter associated urinary tract infection (CAUTI), CLABSI, VAP, and pressure injuries. An NDNQI describes nurse-sensitive indicators, as do hospital-acquired conditions, which are potential harm events, and have spurred the development of prevention and quality improvement initiatives but are not in and of themselves quality improvement initiatives. Only NDNQI measures are tracked and compared at the unit level for comparison to like units and hospitals. The monitoring occurs more frequently than annually, even daily for some indicators.

136. **Correct answer: C.** Limit exposure to the UV rays of the sun and make appointment for genetic counseling following a recent diagnoses of breast cancer. Reducing UV radiation may help prevent skin cancer, and males with breast cancer have a higher risk of genetic mutation and may benefit from prophylactic mastectomy and/or other preventive measures. There is no way to avoid aging. One may not know the genetic risk of whom they are marrying but at age 71, this is insignificant. Precautions for x-rays or other imaging that may have minor radiation exposure follows guidelines to protect patients. HPV vaccination does not have a related cancer risk.

137. **Correct answer: D.** Support by the whole team is necessary as the patient's condition continues its natural progression and negative effects on appetite. A trial course of an appetite stimulant is appropriate if the patient wishes to try. A NG tube is too invasive at this point, and lorazepam could increase sedation, thus reducing appetite further. Protein shakes may not be liked by the patient, and having the family coerce the patient to take in calories adds additional pressures, rather than providing education and support to the family about patients with cancer commonly having a decreased appetite.

138. **Correct answer: A.** The CNS is applying adult learning theory to focus on the priority problems and tie the new learning with prior experiences. Conducting a gap analysis is a process to identify an educational need and does not fit the scenario. Advocating for the patient does not fit here because the focus of the question is on the novice nurse not on the patient. Employing Socratic questioning is often used in simulation to help explore situations and concepts; this is not what is being described in the question.

139. **Correct answer: A.** CNSs should collaborate with formal leaders such as clinical or operational managers to address the performance of clinical staff. Speaking to staff who are not adhering to strategy and intervention expectations regarding barriers that may exist would be appropriate for a CNS. Counseling nurses who are still not implementing evidence-based strategies and interventions is not. All stakeholders should be included in communication of outcomes and the CNS may evaluate desired patient care outcomes with change theory rather than responsibilities aligned to human resources.

140. **Correct answer: C.** Cullen's sign is a large area of ecchymosis in the umbilical region. Murphy's sign is identified by performing an abdominal maneuver to assess for cholecystitis. The patient experiences pain on inhalation while the examiner's hand is firmly placed at the costal margin in the right upper abdominal quadrant. Ranson's criteria, not Ranson's sign, is used to determine the severity of pancreatitis on admission and 48 hours presentation. Grey-Turner's sign is flank ecchymosis that may be present in pancreatitis.

141. **Correct answer: B.** A CBC measures red blood cell (RBC), white blood cell (WBC), differential, hemoglobin (Hgb), hematocrit (Hct), platelet count, and mean corpuscular volume (MCV). Prothrombin time (PT)/international normalized ratio (INR), D-dimer, and thrombin time (TT) are associated with bleeding times.

142. **Correct answer: D.** Patients with right-sided heart failure present with increased central venous pressure and jugular vein distension; as the right ventricle decreases in function, fluid backs up into the supra and inferior vena cava causing venous congestion. Left-sided heart failure has respiratory impact that may lead to dyspnea, hypoxia, tachypnea, and rales. Mental changes may not be present unless the patient is significantly hypoxic, which also aligns to symptoms of left-sided heart failure.

143. **Correct answer: A.** With a history of blood clots, the client is most likely on an anticoagulant like warfarin. The s/s described, bleeding gums, brown urine, and increased bruising, are all indicative of a prolonged PT and bleeding issue. There is no indication the client is on digoxin. Vitamin K is the antidote to a warfarin overdose and the symptoms described are not associated with vitamin K. TSH is not appropriate to order with the symptoms described.

144. **Correct answer: D.** Lab results are consistent with subclinical hypothyroid because T4 level is normal. Blood glucose level is in the prediabetes range, not the diabetes range. Adrenal Insufficiency is not likely, given normal sodium levels. TSH is elevated but T4 is normal, so not consistent with primary hypothyroidism.

145. **Correct answer: D.** This patient has an acute event of GI bleed with supporting lab value of 6.0 g/dL indicating potential hypoxemia and hypovolemia. An increase in BUN levels suggests an impairment in kidney function due to multiple factors such as but not limited to CHF, acute and/or chronic kidney disease, dehydration, hypovolemia, shock, or excessive breakdown of protein in the blood (i.e., GI bleed or increased protein in the diet). The elevated serum Cr level indicates that the kidneys are not filtering effectively to remove the appropriate amount of creatinine from the body. Causes are similar to those for elevated BUN mentioned previously. Prerenal: AKI due to medication is incorrect because in this scenario, GI bleed is the primary, hypovolemic/low flow insult leading to AKI, not medications. Postrenal: AKI due to CKD is incorrect because the cause is due to the prerenal (not postrenal) acute insult from the GI bleed in this scenario. Intrarenal: AKI due to diabetes is incorrect because the cause is due to the prerenal (not intrarenal) acute insult from the GI bleed in this scenario.

146. **Correct answer: B.** The pH is below normal, indicating an acidemia. Bicarbonate is below normal, indicating this is a metabolic disorder. Anion gap is 27 [(137 + 4) − (96 + 18)]. Anion gap is elevated, indicating a high anion gap metabolic acidosis.

147. **Correct answer: A.** Dementia increases with age especially in those over 85 years old. There are many tools to evaluate cognitive function and if these tools raise suspicion for any cognitive impairment, additional evaluation is needed, such as neuropsychologic testing, bloodwork, or imaging. Not all geriatric patients are confused or have fall risk. Cognitive impairment and fall risk should be assessed individually. Incontinence issues are not normal for geriatrics and do not occur for all geriatric patients.

148. **Correct answer: C.** To ensure ethical clinical practice, the CNS will seek formal feedback from various professional colleagues as well as from patients and families that had the opportunity to see the CNS practice. While it may be nice to hear that the security officer has some good things to say about the CNS, it does not really attest to the CNS's ethical practice to show up to work early with a smile on their face.

149. **Correct answer: D.** A patient portal is a secure, online avenue by which patients engage with and may enter their own PHI through a patient-accessed portal of the electronic health record (EHR). Patients do not acquire network access through patient portals, and it is the device they're using that allows for browsing the internet for health tips. EHR users may also be consumers and as such have a patient portal for their own personal use; it is the

EHR itself that is used to access patient medical records for clinical decision-making.

150. **Correct answer: D.** The CNS has been asked to consult on a complex patient. The CNS is providing consultation recommendations to the family as a group so they understand risks and benefits of the feeding tube placement. This allows the family to be involved in the decision-making process based upon the wishes of the patient. Proceeding to surgical consult would depend upon the outcome of the family meeting. Referral to the ethics committee is only necessary if there is an unresolved ethical concern following the family meeting.

151. **Correct answer: B.** Children who experience chronic stressors have an increased risk for chronic low-grade inflammation, which in turn can contribute to obesity, insulin resistance, and other predisease states. Lung cancer, ulcerative colitis, and liver disease are not associated with chronic stressors in children.

152. **Correct answer: D.** Selecting the best equipment based on research is the optimal choice for patient care. An interdisciplinary team can consider best evidence, costs, equipment adoption, training, and so forth for potential implementation into a unit. While talking to the nurses and physician group for preferences is a good place to start the process, the best answer would be to consider the evidence from the literature, costs, safety, and risks–benefits. Refusing to address the issue will not promote the best outcome for the patient, employees, and system.

153. **Correct answer: D.** Obtain an emergent surgical consult for possible fasciotomy. Do not wait 24 hours. The patient appears to have developed compartment syndrome at the site of his IV extravasation. An emergent surgical consultation to determine the need for fasciotomy is the priority to preserve function of the extremity. Warm compresses and physical therapy do not address the immediate risk for compartment syndrome.

154. **Correct answer: D.** Several drugs used to treat rejection and diseases arising from autoimmune and inflammatory processes increase cardiovascular risk. This is due in part to increasing the risk of the following:

■ Hyperlipidemia
■ Hyperglycemia
■ Hypertension

Monitor patients at risk for these side effects and treat accordingly. Encourage healthy lifestyle changes. It is helpful to note that cyclosporin may increase statin concentration and toxicity such as myopathy. For this reason, start patients slow and on the lowest dose possible while monitoring for toxicity. Administering doses with antacids does not support cardiac health. Grape juice has no effect on cyclosporin. Dosage is decided on body weight but limit the frequency of dosage changes.

155. **Correct answer: C.** Contact the surgeon to inquire about the dressing change order should be the first step to clarify the purpose of the wet-to-dry dressing order. The order for a wet-to-dry dressing does not align to the described incision; therefore, following the order could have risks to the patient without clarification. Changing the order without discussion with the surgeon who wrote the order is not appropriate. The operating room (OR) charge nurse may or

may not have recall of the details about the patient, since the patient's OR record is likely on the unit, and the patient has been to the recovery room prior to return to the floor. In addition, the OR charge nurse cannot change the order written by the surgeon.

156. **Correct answer: A.** While the need to circulate antibiotics and the risk of microthrombi formation are true potentials, fluid administration does not augment these functions. This patient's vital signs indicate sepsis, which includes the need to provide adequate fluid resuscitation to respond to the infection and inflammatory response. Reduction of lactate will take time, so the next lactate will likely be re-evaluated in 2 hours and is not an immediate priority. With sepsis, there is vasodilation due to loss of vascular tone, so early fluid resuscitation supports management/stabilization of BP and HR.

157. **Correct answer: B.** Botulinum is Food and Drug Administration (FDA) approved to relax muscles to reduce pain of cervical dystonia. A local anesthetic, morphine, or a steroid, may or may not provide very short-term relief of pain rather than relaxation of the muscles involved.

158. **Correct answer: B.** Prevention is the best intervention to minimizing the development of delirium. The acute setting can be very disorienting to the older adult, coupled with an infection or illness, and they are at high risk for developing delirium.

159. **Correct answer: D.** Knowing when the patient last checked his fasting blood sugar will not help the CNS to determine the underlying cause for his readmission. The blood glucose is important information, but it does not provide an overall picture of the current situation. Questions about needing help paying for medication, access to transportation, and understanding English are focused on the social determinants of health and may help the CNS learn why the patient is unable to adhere to his prescribed treatment and why he has been readmitted. These questions offer a full view of the social determinants and health status.

160. **Correct answer: A.** The CNS contributes to a healthy work environment by forming trusting and respectful relationships with multiple stakeholders within their area of influence and by modeling examples of effective communication among and across individuals and teams. To enhance collaboration, the CNS should encourage and model peer-to-peer recognition and cultivate in the RN an appreciation and understanding of the roles and contributions of physicians, members of the patient care team, staff, and employees. Approaches that are independent of working groups, providing credit to one person, or poor delegation leads to potential conflicts and a sense of lacking value or support, which does not contribute to a healthy work environment.

161. **Correct answer: A.** A Cronbach alpha tests reliability. The other three options test validity.

162. **Correct answer: B.** IT describes any number of things that utilize electronic processes to receive and/or deliver information. IT may often be used as a term to describe a department within a healthcare setting but globally is not constrained to the function of installing printers. Computerized physician order entry may be understood as an IT

functionality but is not the only functionality of IT. Informatics are experts in technologic processes and use many and various IT methodologies; IT is not a field only within the Informatics specialty.

163. **Correct answer: B.** PAINAD is an observational data tool used to assess pain in noncommunicative patients and patients with advanced dementia. If the diagnosis of dementia is known and documented, it has more specificity than the Checklist for Non-Verbal Pain Indicators (CNPI). The Faces and Numeric Rating Scale tools require the patient's ability to interpret the measurements and provide a response.

164. **Correct answer: D.** Assess what is needed first. A gap analysis is a method to identify the difference between current knowledge, skill, and/or practice and desired best practice. Calling a meeting, considering content delivery, and writing learning outcomes are part of the process but are not the first action needed.

165. **Correct answer: C.** Patients who have received anesthesia and/or opioids are at risk for a decreased respiratory drive, one of the causes of respiratory acidosis. Priority treatment for respiratory acidosis for this patient is to increase the patient's respiratory rate and blow off CO_2. Sternal rub may temporarily awaken the patient; however, increased responsiveness will immediately increase respiratory rate, improving issues related to respiratory acidosis. Oxygen administration would be indicated if the patient is hypoxic; however, if the patient continues to have decreased respirations due to sedation, the patient may need further respiratory support to improve respiratory drive and/or reversal of anesthesia. While it may be helpful to evaluate the medications that have been given and the time frame of administration, that intervention will not improve the patient's current respiratory rate. The patient is not awake enough to adequately follow instruction for use of I.S.

166. **Correct answer: C.** The BUN–creatinine ratio is 24.2, which is consistent with dehydration and a 1-week history of malaise in older adults, which often involves inadequate PO intake. The potassium is normal and the sodium bicarbonate is slightly elevated, neither of which require intervention. Although the patient has a history of CHF, his current lab results indicate dehydration and a diuretic would be contraindicated.

167. **Correct answer: A.** Patients with syncopal episodes, increased exercise intolerance, and signs of right-heart failure need to be evaluated in a center of excellence for PAH specialty care. Right-heart catheterization and advanced therapy such as intravenous (IV) Veletri for patients with FC III and IV should be anticipated in patients that qualify for therapy. Cardiology consult may help a practitioner in the diagnosis of PAH but may also cause a delay in starting therapy. PPM is not the appropriate treatment for syncope related to PAH. Diuresis will help patients with fluid overload. Cardiac rehabilitation will help strengthen a patient after they are placed on appropriate therapy.

168. **Correct answer: D.** Some alpha blockers have a "first-dose effect." When a client begins taking the medication there can be pronounced hypotension and dizziness, which can have a syncopal effect. The other medications, calcium channel blockers, beta blockers, and antiplatelets, do not have this side effect.

169. **Correct answer: D.** Hyperparathyroidism is associated with hypophosphatemia and hypercalcemia. Hyperparathyroidism is characterized by hypersecretion of parathyroid hormone (PTH) leading to hypercalcemia and relative hypophosphatemia. The other imbalances are not consistent with hyperparathyroidism.

170. **Correct answer: D.** Adherence to required documentation of restraint assessment, completion of fall assessment, and number of renal replacement therapy (RRT) consultations are all process measures. They may be important metrics to your plan but only indicate how successful an intervention or strategy is implemented rather than providing an indication of an outcome.

171. **Correct answer: D.** Disenfranchised grief is characterized by the griever being deprived of validation and recognition of a loss because of social constraints in openly acknowledging the loss. Chronic grief is defined as grief that is excessive in duration. Delayed grief occurs when the griever does not deal with a loss at the time it happened. Exaggerated grief occurs when an intensification of normal grief occurs and the feelings are overwhelmed, resulting in emotional distress.

172. **Correct answer: A.** Safety checklists, such as the World Health Organization surgical safety checklist, have been shown to reduce compliance rates. Patient safety should be paramount during any procedure that can lead to patient harm. The checklists are not used to improve hand washing compliance or audit; however, part of quality assurance may review parts of charts such as the checklist to ensure that safety practices are being followed and maintained.

173. **Correct answer: D.** A deep vein thrombosis (DVT) order set is important but does not support a reduction in hospital-acquired pneumonia (HAP) cases. The CNS may collaborate with the interdisciplinary team to ensure the facility has care bundles and the bedside clinicians understand that bundling care may improve outcomes. HAP, whether nonventilator-associated hospital-acquired pneumonia (NVHAP) or ventilator-associated pneumonia (VAP), will benefit from a robust oral care program, mobility, and antibiotic stewardship initiatives and with elevating the head of bed.

174. **Correct answer: D.** Hydrochlorothiazide (HCTZ) is a thiazide diuretic. Thiazide diuretics, angiotensin-converting enzyme (ACE) inhibitors, angiotensin Ii receptor blockers (ARBs), and calcium channel blockers are considered first-line therapy for hypertension. Beta blockers, diuretics, alpha-1 blockers, direct vasodilators, and direct renin inhibitors are all second-line treatment medications. Based upon the American Heart Association (2017) treatment guidelines for managing hypertension, the patient falls under stage 2 hypertension with BP greater than or equal to 140/90.

175. **Correct answer: D.** Pleural needle decompression is the immediate life-saving intervention to relieve obstructive shock caused by tension pneumothorax. Although a chest tube may be inserted, this is not the immediate, life-saving intervention. Intubation is not an immediate, life-saving intervention for a tension pneumothorax. A thoracotomy is not indicated for a tension pneumothorax.

Index

Printed in the United States
by Baker & Taylor Publisher Services